COMPLICATIONS OF VITREO-RETINAL SURGERY

NOEMI LOIS, MD, PhD, FRCS(Ed), FRCOphth

Professor of Clinical Ophthalmology
Centre for Vision and Vascular Science
Queens University
Belfast, Northern Ireland,
United Kingdom

DAVID WONG, MB, ChB

Albert Young Bing Ching Chair Professor in
Ophthalmology
Head of the Department of Ophthalmology
LKS Faculty of Medicine
University of Hong Kong

. Wolters Kluwer | Lippincott Williams & Wilkins
Health

Philadelphia • Baltimore • New York • London
Buenos Aires • Hong Kong • Sydney • Tokyo

Acquisition Editor: Ryan Shaw
Product Manager: Kate Marshall
Production Project Manager: David Saltzberg
Senior Manufacturing Coordinator: Beth Welsh
Marketing Manager: Alexander Burns
Design Coordinator: Holly McLaughlin
Production Service: Aptara, Inc

Two Commerce Square
2001 Market Street
Philadelphia, PA 19103 USA
LWW.com

Printed in China

Library of Congress Cataloging-in-Publication Data

Complications of vitreo-retinal surgery / [edited by] Noemi Lois, David Wong.
p. ; cm.
Includes bibliographical references and index.
ISBN 978-1-4511-1938-1 (alk. paper)
I. Lois, Noemi, editor of compilation.   II. Wong, D. (David), 1952- editor of compilation.
[DNLM: 1. Vitreoretinal Surgery.   2. Intraoperative Complications.   3. Postoperative Complications.   4. Retinal Diseases—surgery.   5. Vitreous Body—surgery. WW 270]
RE551
617.7′35059–dc23

2013004404

Care has been taken to confirm the accuracy of the information presented and to describe generally accepted practices. However, the authors, editors, and publisher are not responsible for errors or omissions or for any consequences from application of the information in this book and make no warranty, expressed or implied, with respect to the currency, completeness, or accuracy of the contents of the publication. Application of the information in a particular situation remains the professional responsibility of the practitioner.

The authors, editors, and publisher have exerted every effort to ensure that drug selection and dosage set forth in this text are in accordance with current recommendations and practice at the time of publication. However, in view of ongoing research, changes in government regulations, and the constant flow of information relating to drug therapy and drug reactions, the reader is urged to check the package insert for each drug for any change in indications and dosage and for added warnings and precautions. This is particularly important when the recommended agent is a new or infrequently employed drug.

Some drugs and medical devices presented in the publication have Food and Drug Administration (FDA) clearance for limited use in restricted research settings. It is the responsibility of the health care provider to ascertain the FDA status of each drug or device planned for use in their clinical practice.

To purchase additional copies of this book, call our customer service department at (800) 638-3030 or fax orders to (301) 223-2320. International customers should call (301) 223-2300.

Visit Lippincott Williams & Wilkins on the Internet: at LWW.com. Lippincott Williams & Wilkins customer service representatives are available from 8:30 am to 6 pm, EST.

10 9 8 7 6 5 4 3 2 1

RRS1302

Contributors

Ehab Abdelkader, FRCS, FRCOphth
Lecturer of Ophthalmology
Department of Ophthalmology
Medical School
Menoufia University
Shibin El Kom, Egypt

Associate Specialist Ophthalmologist
Department of Ophthalmology
Aberdeen Royal Infirmary
Aberdeen, UK

Nur Acar, MD, FEBO
Associate Professor
Department of Vitreoretinal Disease
World Eye Hospital
Etiler, Istanbul, Turkey

Richard M. Ahuja, MD
Clinical Associate Professor
Department of Ophthalmology
Chicago Medical School
North Chicago, IL

Residency Director
Director of Vitreoretinal Services
Department of Ophthalmology
Stroger Cook County Hospital
Chicago, IL

Sofia Androudi, MD
Lecturer
Department of Ophthalmology
University of Thessaly
Larissa, Greece

J. Fernando Arevalo, MD, FACS
Professor
Wilmer Eye Institute
The John Hopkins University
Baltimore, MD

Chief
Vitreoretinal Division
The King Khaled Eye Specialist Hospital
Riyadh, Kingdom of Saudi Arabia

Alberto Arteaga, MD
Retina Fellowship
Retina and Vitreous Department
Instituto de Microcirugia Ocular
Barcelona, Spain

Ophthalmologist, Retina Specialist
Department of Ophthalmology
Clinica Oftalmologica
Madero, Tamaulipas, Mexico

Jose Garcia Arumi, MD
Professor
Department of Ophthalmology
Autonomous University of Barcelona
Barcelona, Spain

Chairman
Department of Ophthalmology
Hospital de la Vall d'Hebron
Barcelona, Spain

George William Aylward, FRCS, FRCOphth, MD
Consultant Vitreoretinal Surgeon
Moorfields Eye Hospital
London, UK

Augusto Azuara-Blanco, MD, PhD, FRCS(Ed), FRCOphth
Professor of Clinical Ophthalmology
Centre for Vision and Vascular Science
Queen's University Belfast

Honorary Consultant Ophthalmologist
Department of Ophthalmology
Belfast Health and Social Care Trust
Belfast, UK

Philip J. Banerjee, BMedSCi, FRCOphth
Vitreoretinal Research Fellow
Vitreoretinal Unit
Moorfields Eye Hospital
London, UK

Susanne Binder, MD
Professor
Department of Ophthalmology
Ludwig Boltzmann Institute for Retinology
  and Biomicroscopic Lasersurgery
Vienna, Austria

Chair, Director
Rudolf Foundation Clinic
Vienna, Austria

Silvia Bopp, PhD, DM
Senior Consultant, Assistant Professor
Augenklinik Universitaetsallee
MVZ GmbH
Bremen, Germany

Periklis Brazitikos, MD
Associate Professor
Ophthalmology
University of Thessaly
Larissa, Greece

Juan Diego Carpio, MD
Retina Fellowship
Retina and Vitreous Department
Instituto de Microcirugia Ocular
Barcelona, Spain

Ophthalmologist, Retina Specialist
Ophthalmology
Clínica Oftalmológica Oftalmolaser
Barcelona, Spain

Steve Charles, MD
Ophthalmology
Heritage Institute
University of Tennessee
Memphis, TN

David G. Charteris, MD, FRCS, FRCOphth
Consultant Vitreoretinal Surgeon
Vitreoretinal Unit
Moorfields Eye Hospital
London, UK

Ulrik Correll Christensen, MD, PhD
Fellow
Department of Ophthalmology
University of Copenhagen
Copenhagen, Denmark

Fellow
Department of Ophthalmology
Glostrup Hospital
Glostrup, Denmark

John B. Christoforidis, MD
Assistant Professor
Physician and Surgeon
Department of Ophthalmology
The Ohio State University College of Medicine
Columbus, OH

Lucienne Collet, MD
Retina Fellowship
Retina and Vitreous Department
Instituto de Microcirugia Ocular
Barcelona, Spain

Ophthalmologist, Retina Specialist
Department of Ophthalmology
Admira Vision
Barcelona, Spain

Inés Contreras, MD, PhD
Retina Specialist
Department of Ophthalmology
Hospital Universitario Ramón Y Cajal
Madrid, Spain

Borja Corcostegui, MD
Professor of Ophthalmology
European School of Advance Studies in
  Ophthalmology
Campus Lugano
Lugano, Switzerland

Medical Director
Instituto de Microcirugia Ocular
Barcelona, Spain

Sven Crafoord, MD, PhD
Associate Professor
Department of Ophthalmology
Orebro University Hospital
Orebro, Sweden

Lyndon da Cruz, MBBS, MA, FRCOphth, PhD, FRACO
Honorary Reader
UCL Institute of Ophthalmology
University College London
London, UK

Consultant Ophthalmic Surgeon
Vitreo-retinal and Medical Retina Department
Moorfields Eye Hospital NHS Foundation Trust
London, UK

Kunal K. Dansingani, MB, BS, MA, FRCOphth
Locum Consultant Ophthalmic Surgeon
Retina Department
Moorfields Eye Hospital
London, UK

Marc D. de Smet, MDCM, PhD, FRCSC, FRCOphth, FMH
Professor
Department of Ophthalmology
University of Amsterdam
Amsterdam, The Netherlands

Director
Retina and Inflammation
MIOS
Lausanne, Switzerland

Milton Nunes de Moraes-Filho, MD
Retina and Vitreous Fellowship
Department of Ophthalmology
Sao Paulo Hospital, Unifesp/EPM
Sao Paulo, SP, Brazil

Federica Genovesi Ebert, MD, PhD
Assistant
Ophthalmic Surgery Clinic
New Santa Chiara Hospital, Cisanello, Pisa
Pisa, Italy

Mostafa A. Elgohary, MBChB, MS, MD, FRCSI, FRCSEd, FRCOphth
Fellow
Department of Vitreoretinal Surgery
Moorfields Eye Hospital
London, UK

Marta S. Figueroa, MD, PhD
Retina Specialist
Department of Ophthalmology
Hospital Universitario Ramón Y Cajal
Madrid, Spain

Rhona Flin, PhD
Professor of Applied Psychology
Industrial Psychology Research Centre
University of Aberdeen
Aberdeen, Scotland, UK

John V. Forrester, MD, ChB
Emeritus Professor
Section Immunology and Infection, DAM
School of Medicine and Dentistry
University of Aberdeen
Aberdeen, Scotland, UK

Valentina Franco-Cardenas, MD
Association for Preventing Blindness in Mexico
Ophthalmology, Retina Department
Mexico City, Mexico

Arnd Gandorfer
Professor of Ophthalmology
Department of Ophthalmology
Ludwig Maximilians University
Munich, Germany

Medical Director
MVZ Memmingen Augen-MKG
Memmingen, Germany

Justin Gottlieb, MD
Associate Professor
Department of Ophthalmology and Visual Sciences
University of Wisconsin-Madison
Madison, WI

Zdenek J. Gregor, FRCS(Eng), FRCOphth
Consultant Vitreoretinal Surgeon
Moorfields Eye Hospital
London, UK

Eoin Guerin, FRCOphth, MD
Vitreoretinal Fellow
Department of Ophthalmology
Manchester Royal Eye Hospital
Manchester, UK

David Guyton, MD
The Zanvyl Krieger Professor of
    Ophthalmology
Department of Ophthalmology
The Krieger Children's Eye Center at The
    Wilmer Institute
The John Hopkins University School of
    Medicine
Baltimore, MD

Active Staff
Department of Ophthalmology
The John Hopkins Hospital
Baltimore, MD

Christos Haritoglou, MD
Professor
Department of Ophthalmology
Ludwig Maximilians University
Munich, Germany

**Richard Haynes, MB, BCh,
FRCOphth, DM**
Honorary Senior Lecturer
Academic Department of Ophthalmology
University of Bristol
Bristol, UK

Consultant Ophthalmic Surgeon
Retinal Department
Bristol Eye Hospital
Bristol, UK

Heinrich Heimann, MD
Honorary Senior Lecturer
Department of Eye and Vision Science
University of Liverpool
Liverpool, UK

Consultant Ophthalmic Surgeon
St Paul´s Eye Unit
Royal Liverpool University Hospital
Liverpool, UK

Andrew M. Hendrick, MD
Vitreoretinal Fellow
Clinical Instructor
Department of Ophthalmology
University of Wisconsin-Madison
Madison, WI

Kuhl Huh, MD, PhD
Professor
Department of Ophthalmology
Korea University
Guro Hospital
Seoul, Korea

Kazuaki Kadonosono, MD, PhD
Professor
Department of Ophthalmology
Yokohama City University
Yokohama-shi, Kanagawa, Japan

Chair
Ophthalmology
Yokohama City University Medical Center
Yokohama-shi, Kanagawa, Japan

**Anthony J. King, MD, MMedSci,
FRCOphth**
Honorary Associate Professor of Clinical
    Ophthalmology
Department of Ophthalmology
University of Nottingham
Nottingham, UK

Consultant Ophthalmologist
Department of Ophthalmology
Nottingham University Hospital
Nottingham, UK

Lazaros Konstantinidis, MD
Vitreo-Retinal Department
Royal Liverpool University Hospital
Liverpool, UK

Thomas C. Kreutzer, MD
Consultant
University Eye Hospital
Ludwig Maximilians University
Munich, Germany

Consultant
Department of Ophthalmology
Allgemeines Krankenhaus Linz
Linz, Austria

Lucia Kuffová, MD, PhD, FRCOphth
Senior Lecturer
Section Immunology and Infection, DAM
School of Medicine and Dentistry
University of Aberdeen
Aberdeen, Scotland, UK

Consultant
Department of Ophthalmology
Aberdeen Royal Infirmary
Aberdeen, Scotland, UK

**Morten la Cour, MD, FEBO,
Dr Med Scia**
Professor
Eye Department
University of Copenhagen
Copenhagen, Denmark

Consultant
Eye Department
Glostrup Hospital
Glostrup, Denmark

**Alistair Laidlaw, MD, FRCOphth,
FRCS(Glas)**
Consultant Vitreoretinal Surgeon
Department of Ophthalmology
St. Thomas' Hospital
London, UK

Wensheng Li, MD, PhD
Professor
Cataract and Retina
Eye Hospital
Wenzhou Medical College
Wenzhou, Zhejiang, China

**Noemi Lois, MD, PhD, FRCS(Ed),
FRCOphth**
Professor of Clinical Ophthalmology
Centre for Vision and Vascular Science
Queens University
Belfast, Northern Ireland, United Kingdom

Honorary Consultant Vitreoretinal Surgeon
Department of Ophthalmology
Belfast Health and Social Care Trust
Belfast, Northern Ireland, UK

Jose Lorenzo, MD, PhD
Vitreoretinal Consultant
Ophthalmology
Hospital POVISA
Vigo, Spain

Srilakshmi Maguluri, MD
Clinical Assistant Professor
Department of Surgery
University of Illinois
College of Medicine
Peoria, IL

Ophthalmologist
Department of Surgery
Thorek Memorial Hospital
Chicago, IL

Mauricio Maia, MD, PhD
Assistant Professor
Ophthalmology, Vitreoretinal Surgery Unit
Federal University of Sao Paulo
Sao Paulo, SP, Brazil

Director of Vitreoretinal Surgery
Department of Ophthalmology
Brazilian Institute of Fighting Against Blindness
Assis, SP, Brazil

Andre Maia, MD
Chief of Retina and Vitreous Department
Ophthalmology, Vitreoretinal Surgery Unit
Federal University of Sao Paulo
Sao Paulo, SP, Brazil

Director of Vitreoretinal Surgery
Department of Ophthalmology
Clinica Oftalmologica São Lucas
São Paulo, SP, Brazil

Pei Jian Miao, MD
Associate Chief Doctor
Xuzhou First People's Hospital
Glaucoma Department
Institute of Eye Disease Prevention and Control
Xuzhou, Jiangsu, China

Timothy G. Murray, MD, MBA, FACS
Founding Director, Professor
Murray Ocular Oncology and Retina
Jackson Memorial Hospital
Miami, FL

Yusuke Oshima, MD, PhD
Associate Professor
Department of Ophthalmology
Osaka University Graduate School of Medicine
Suita, Osaka, Japan

Ian Pearce, FRCOphth
Consultant Vitreo-Retinal Surgeon
St. Paul's Eye Unit
Royal Liverpool University Hospital
Liverpool, UK

Siegfried G. Priglinger, MD, FEBO
Professor of Ophthalmology
Department of Ophthalmology
Ludwig Maximilians University
Munich, Germany

Chairman
Department of Ophthalmology
General Hospital Linz, AKH
Linz, Austria

Adriana Ramirez, MD
Retina Fellow
Department of Ophthalmology
University of California, Los Angeles
David Geffen School of Medicine
Jules Stein Eye Institute
Los Angeles, CA

Stanislao Rizzo, MD
Chief
Ophthalmic Surgery Clinic
New Santa Chiara Hospital, Cisanello, Pisa
Pisa, Italy

Mario R. Romano, MD, PhD
Head of Vitreo-Retinal Service
Department of Ophthalmology
Istituto Clinico e Ricerca Humanitas
Milan, Italy

Steven D. Schwartz, MD
Ahmanson Professor of Ophthalmology
Jules Stein Eye Institute, Retina Division
University of California
Los Angeles, CA

Guy Shanks, MD, MA
Consultant Ophthalmologist
Department of Ophthalmology
Örebro University
Örebro, Sweden

Consultant Ophthalmic Surgeon
Department of Ophthalmology
Örebro University Hospital
Örebro, Sweden

Manoharan Shunmugam, FRCOphth
Vitreoretinal Fellow
Department of Ophthalmology
St. Thomas' Hospital
Westminster Bridge Road
London, UK

William E. Smiddy, MD
Professor of Ophthalmology
Ophthalmology
Bascom Palmer Eye Institute
University of Miami Miller School of
    Medicine
Miami, FL

Martin S. Spitzer, MD, PhD
Assistant Professor
Department of Ophthalmology
University Eye Hospital Tübingen
Tübingen, Germany

Theodor Stappler, MD
Honorary Clinical Lecturer
Eye and Vision Science
University of Liverpool
Liverpool, UK

Consultant Vitreoretinal Surgeon
St. Paul's Eye Unit
Royal Liverpool University Hospital
Liverpool, UK

David Steel, MBBS, FRCOphth
Honorary Senior Lecturer
Institute of Genetic Medicine
University of Newcastle Upon Tyne
Tyne and Wear, UK

Consultant Ophthalmologist
Sunderland Eye Infirmary
Sunderland, UK

Kevin K. Suk, MD
Instructor
Bascom Palmer Eye Institute
University of Miami
Department of Ophthalmology
Anne Bates Leach Eye Hospital
Miami, FL

Paul Sullivan, MBBS, MD, FRCOphth
Director of Education
Consultant Vitreoretinal Surgeon
Vitreoretinal Surgery
Moorfields Eye Hospital
London, UK

Chrysanthos Symeonidis, MD
Research Associate
2nd Department of Ophthalmology
Aristotle University of Thessaloniki
Thessaloniki, Macedonia, Greece

Associate Specialist
2nd Department of Ophthalmology
Papageorgiou General Hospital
Thessaloniki, Macedonia, Greece

Peter Szurman, MD, PhD
Head of Department
Department of Ophthalmology
Knappschaft's Eye Hospital
Sulzbach/Saar, Germany

Paul E. Tornambe, MD
Director
Retina Research Foundation of San Diego
Poway, CA

Jose Luis Vallejo-Garcia, MD
Consultant
Medical Retina and Vitreoretinal Department
Istituto Clinico Humanitas
Rozzano, Milan, Italy

Jan Van Meurs, MD, PhD
Professor of Ophthalmology
Department of Ophthalmology
Erasmus University Rotterdam
Erasmus Medical Center
Rotterdam, The Netherlands

VR Surgeon
Vitreoretinal Surgery
The Rotterdam Eye Hospital
Rotterdam, The Netherlands

Rachel Williams, PhD
Reader
Department of Eye and Vision Science
University of Liverpool
Liverpool, UK

Tom Williamson, MBChB, FRCS(Glas), FRCOphth, MD
Consultant
Department of Ophthalmology
St. Thomas' Hospital
London, UK

David Wong, MB, ChB
Chief of Service
Department of Ophthalmology
Queen Mary Hospital
Pok Fu Lam, Hong Kong

Ian Y. Wong, FCOphthHK, FHKAM
Clinical Assistant Professor
Eye Institute
The University of Hong Kong
Pok Fu Lam, Hong Kong

Honorary Associate Consultant
Queen Mary Hospital
Pok Fu Lam, Hong Kong

Roger Wong, MBBS, BA, FRCOphth
Vitreoretinal Consultant
Department of Ophthalmology
St. Thomas' Hospital
London, UK

Howard Ying, MD, PhD
Assistant Professor
Retina
Wilmer Eye Institute
Baltimore, MD

Assistant Professor
Department of Ophthalmology
John Hopkins Hospital
Baltimore, MD

Miguel Angel Zapata, MD
Associated Professor
Department of Ophthalmology
Autonomous University of Barcelona
Barcelona, Spain

Consultant
Department of Ophthalmology
Hospital de la Vall d'Hebron
Barcelona, Spain

Qinxiang Zheng, MD, PhD
Associate Professor, Associate Chief Doctor
Cataract Department
Eye Hospital
Wenzhou Medical College
Wenzhou, Zhejiang, China

Foreword

"Unfortunately, there were some complications." The phrase conjures the image of the surgeon, mask hanging down but still tied around the neck, speaking postoperatively to the patient's now-distressed loved ones. Yes, complications are certainly unwelcome and frequently eventful, even disastrous, in a given surgical situation, but to view them only negatively would be to miss the extraordinary value they have in guiding and improving our surgery. To attain this other vantage point requires that we study our complications carefully, try our best to understand every aspect, and most importantly, share our experiences and outcomes with one another. Seen in this positive light, complications are essential and informative features inherent in our surgical landscape like the crevasses that shape safe passage across a glacier. Indeed, the deep respect we feel when we are in the company of a distinguished surgeon is, in great measure, a respect for their lifelong experience, painful and triumphal, with every imaginable complication.

Vitreoretinal surgeons will welcome this marvelous book "Complications of Vitreo-Retinal Surgery" skillfully edited by Drs. Noemi Lois and David Wong and crafted with the help of a highly experienced group of distinguished surgeons. Each chapter has a simplified and uniform structure that includes concise introductory information followed by Pathogenesis/Risk Factors. Then, in the heart of each chapter, there are "Pearls on how to avoid it" followed by "Pearls on how to solve it." Each chapter concludes with a brief section on "Expected outcomes: what is the worst possible scenario?"; it was quite interesting to read these and see where the authors drew their line, although I, regrettably, could frequently envision something worse!

The information contained in this book is practical and useful in the extreme, and the enjoyment I found in reading it was most akin to discussing challenging surgical issues with a trusted colleague in an informal and congenial setting. Tables and illustrations are well done and thoughtfully used, and the overall impression of the book is one of remarkable clarity, innovation, and insight. Although many of the complications will always be with us and have been the subject of prior scholarly offerings, others have been most worthily assembled for the first time. To offer just a few examples, "Retinal Slippage" explains this often-mystifying subject in a way that every vitreoretinal fellow will welcome. "Poor View of the Fundus" is an excellent analysis of the most important part of every actual surgery, i.e., visualization of the tissues. "Refractive Changes Associated with Vitreoretinal Surgery" is an avant-garde treatment of a subject of growing importance due to the ever-increasing demand for improved visual outcomes in modern ophthalmic surgery. "Preventing Surgical Complications by the Use of Non-technical Skills" a thorough discussion of the complex and often underappreciated environment in which the surgery—and the surgeon—are embedded will be required reading on my service, as will the indispensable (though necessarily frightening) chapter on "Intraocular Bleeding."

I express my gratitude to Drs. Lois and Wong and the authors for this magnificent sharing of vitreoretinal complications in such an engaging and approachable format. I am certain that this volume will be read by the wide audience that it deserves, and that our surgeries, and our field, will move forward.

Donald J. D'Amico, MD
New York, NY

Preface

Vitreoretinal surgery is a fascinating, challenging and ever-changing field. Such a demanding subspecialty requires manual dexterity, surgical training, extensive knowledge, and sound reasoning. Many ordinary surgeons can perform vitreoretinal surgery well. The one attribute that distinguishes a great surgeon is perhaps the ability to avoid and to manage complications.

This book was conceived with the goal of compiling the best advice, given in a most succinct manner by leading vitreoretinal surgeons throughout the world, on what to do to prevent and treat surgical complications encountered in daily practice. It encompasses specific complications related to scleral buckling, pneumatic retinopexy, and 20-, 23-, and 25-gauge vitrectomy. It also covers general complications that can occur with any of these different surgical techniques. In each chapter, the complication is defined, its pathogenesis reviewed, and the risk factors for its occurrence are listed. Importantly, pearls on how to prevent and treat these complications are given in a clear, "bullet point" format.

This book has been written for vitreoretinal surgeons. Experienced surgeons may find it helpful as it contains approaches to prevent and treat complications that may be different or better than those they currently use. For newly trained vitreoretinal surgeons and fellows in training, this book may provide them with a useful guide to avoid complications and may add to their surgical armamentarium for handling complications when they do occur. Knowledge of these complications and tips to prevent them and solve them will help build confidence and achieve better surgical outcomes. We believe this book would be a great companion in the operating room. Outstanding scrub nurses may also enjoy reading this book; it will certainly increase their awareness of potential problems that can occur intraoperatively and help them anticipate the remedial actions surgeons may need to take when these complications occur. This book will provide useful background information for general ophthalmologists, residents, and optometrists who are involved in looking after patients before and after vitreoretinal procedures.

It is our hope that this book will help vitreoretinal surgeons to reduce the occurrence of complications associated with their procedures and to help them managing these complications in a more skillful and efficient manner, with the ultimate goal of improving patient's care.

Noemi Lois and David Wong

Acknowledgments

We are extremely grateful to all authors who have generously giving up their time to contribute with chapters for this book. We thank them for sharing their expertise on the subjects discussed and for providing us with their best "tips" to prevent and solve complications we may all encounter at some point during our daily practice of vitreoretinal surgery.

We would like to thank Ms Emilie Moyer and Ms Franny Murphy for their expert technical assistance on the elaboration of this book and to Ms Giovanna Santoni for her masterly performed drawings which illustrate this publication.

We would wish to thank Mr Jonathan Pine, Executive Editor, Lippincott Williams & Wilkins, for his support during the early stages of preparation of this book, and to Mr Ryan Shaw, Acquisitions Editor, Lippincott Williams & Wilkins for his expert technical assistance and advice throughout the publication process of this book.

Contents

SECTION II

PREVENTING SURGICAL COMPLICATIONS BY THE USE OF NON-TECHNICAL SURGICAL SKILLS 491

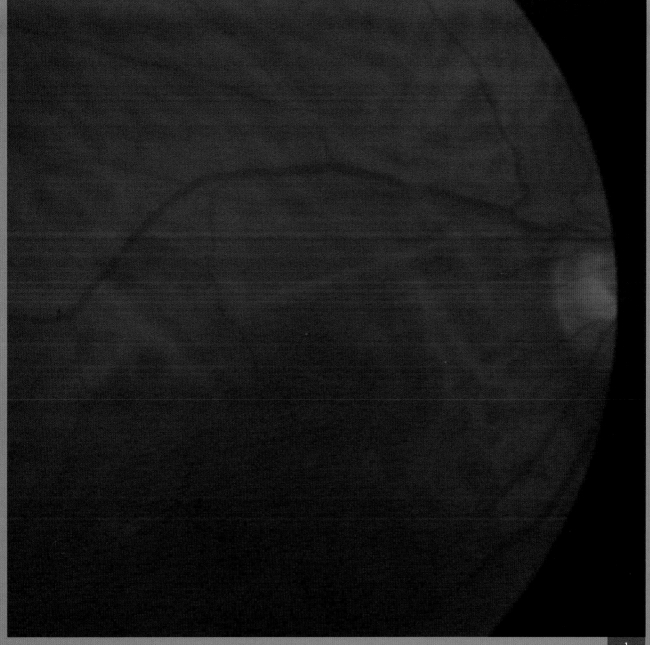

SECTION

I

COMPLICATIONS DURING OR FOLLOWING THE SURGICAL PROCEDURE

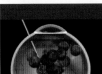

1

COMPLICATIONS ASSOCIATED with SUTURING the SCLERAL BUCKLE

LUCIENNE COLLET, ALBERTO ARTEAGA, JUAN DIEGO CARPIO, AND BORJA CORCOSTEGUI

◈ The Complication: Definition

Scleral buckling is considered an effective procedure for the management of rhegmatogenous retinal detachment. The most important factor related to the success of scleral buckling is the detection and treatment of all retinal breaks. Consequently, the accurate placement of the buckle on the scleral surface is critical.

The placement of the buckle may be either circumferential or radial. A circumferential peritomy is preferably performed 3 mm posterior to the limbus. Then, traction sutures with silk 3-0 are placed beneath the insertion of the rectus muscles to position the eye.

The sclera should be examined for thin areas in the four quadrants when an encirclement is being placed, or in the quadrant where a segmental buckle is planned. Scleral thinning and ectasia are considered important risk factors for globe perforation during scleral buckling procedures, especially while placing the sutures. Care must be taken to identify these areas; once found, if severe, the decision may be to abort the scleral buckling procedure and to convert into pars plana vitrectomy. However, if thinning is not considered to be severe, the surgeon may decide to continue with scleral buckling.

Globe penetration with the needle is an intraoperative complication of retinal detachment surgery; vitreous, choroidal, subretinal, and retinal hemorrhages, as well as vitreoretinal incarceration may be subsequently observed. Globe penetration has been estimated to occur during the placement of scleral sutures in 5% of cases and is often associated with thin sclera (see also Chapter 5).[1,2]

When operating in eyes with thin sclera, scleral cutout and scleral perforation can also occur which may lead to vitreoretinal incarceration, vitreous hemorrhage, suprachoroidal hemorrhage, subretinal hemorrhage, postoperative vision ≤20/200, proliferative vitreoretinopathy, and persistent or recurrent retinal detachment.[3]

◈ Vitreoretinal Incarceration

Vitreoretinal incarceration may occur during drainage of subretinal fluid (see Chapter 2) or, as stated above, by inadvertent penetration of the eye globe while placing the sutures for the scleral buckle or when raising the buckle in the eyes with thin sclera if suture cutout occurs. It has been reported as a rare intraoperative complication; however, in a recent study, it was observed with a frequency of 2%.[4] Clinically, it can be identified macroscopically by the presence of choroid–retina–vitreous coming out through the site of the needle penetration/suture cutout. Ophthalmoscopically, it can be seen as a characteristic dimple appearance of the retina at the site of the incarceration.

Pearls on How to Prevent It

- Case selection: Consider converting to pars plana vitrectomy in eyes with very thin and ectatic sclera.

- Avoid maneuvers that may increase intraocular pressure in the eye, such as pressing on the eye, while placing the scleral sutures.

- Make sure to see the tip of the needle while placing the suture through the sclera. Although full thickness and very deep scleral bites with the needle should be avoided, very shallow ones are neither recommended as these would have a higher chance to cutout through the sclera when raising the buckle. Follow the advice given below (see Sections "Scleral Cutout and Scleral Rupture" and "Pearls on How to Prevent It") with regard to placing the sutures in the sclera.

- In eyes with scleral thinning, avoid tightening the sutures too much and raising the buckles too high; these maneuvers may lead to scleral cutout and vitreoretinal incarceration.

Pearls on How to Treat It

- In cases where vitreoretinal incarceration is located anteriorly, it would be appropriate to support the area of vitreoretinal incarceration with the scleral buckle; if this is possible, other procedures may not be necessary.

- In cases where marked vitreoretinal incarceration has occurred, an encircling scleral buckle would reduce tractional forces and likely reduce the risk of retinal detachment secondary to vitreoretinal incarceration.

- In those cases where incarceration is located posteriorly, a vitrectomy with retinotomy may be necessary to prevent redetachment and proliferative vitreoretinopathy.

Choroidal Detachment and Suprachoroidal Hemorrhage

Choroidal detachment is defined as a separation of the uvea from the sclera and should be differentiated from suprachoroidal hemorrhage (see also Chapters 26C and 30). Suprachoroidal hemorrhage can happen during intraocular surgery or in the postoperative period, but it is still considered a rare event.[5] Systemic and ocular factors have been implicated for the development of suprachoroidal hemorrhage. In relation to systemic findings, sclerosis and fragility of choroidal vessels related to advanced age, systemic hypertension, and arteriosclerosis are considered predisposing factors.[6-8] The ocular conditions that may be associated with suprachoroidal hemorrhage are glaucoma, myopia, elevated intraocular pressure (IOP), aphakia, and inflammation.[9-11] These conditions can weaken the integrity of the long posterior ciliary arteries secondary to vascular necrosis. The incidence of suprachoroidal hemorrhage during or after scleral buckle procedures is difficult to determine. Delayed suprachoroidal hemorrhage is 10-fold greater than that of an intraoperative expulsive hemorrhage, and may vary from limited hematomas to massive hemorrhages that can be sufficiently large to produce central retinal apposition. The incidence of suprachoroidal hemorrhage in vitreoretinal surgery varies widely among different studies from 0.17% to 1.9%.[7,12–14]

For further details on risk factors, pathogenesis, and pearls on how to prevent and treat serous and hemorrhagic choroidal detachment, see Chapters 26C and 30.

⬥ Scleral Cutout and Scleral Rupture

Scleral cutout occurs most often in eyes with thin sclera. In these cases the suture can cut through the sclera usually at the time of raising the scleral buckle. When the sutures are tightened a partial or full thickness scleral defect may occur and can lead to other associated complications. Scleral rupture may also happen during dissection to expose the sclera in previously operated eyes, when exposing a previously placed scleral buckle or during scleral depression at the time of peripheral retinal examination, cryotherapy, or laser photocoagulation, most often in eyes with thin sclera, eyes that had previously failed retinal detachment surgery, or eyes with scleral pathology (see also Chapter 5).[15]

⬥ Risk Factors

Tabandeh et al.[3] found the main risk factors for scleral rupture during retinal detachment surgery to be reoperations after a failed retinal detachment surgery in 71% of cases and pre-existing scleral pathology in 29%. In this study, the site of the rupture was found to occur in the bed of the previously placed scleral buckle in all patients that had undergone a previous buckling procedure. Other studies have suggested that additional factors associated with scleral thinning, including inflammation and necrosis from previous cryotherapy and glaucoma surgery, may increase the risk of scleral rupture.[16–18] Scleral thinning may occur after diffuse or nodular anterior scleritis and in necrotizing anterior scleritis. Approximately 50% of all patients with scleritis will have a systemic disease, most commonly a connective tissue disease.[19]

⬥ Pearls on How to Prevent It

To prevent scleral cutout, scleral perforation, and scleral rupture in eyes with thin and friable sclera the following aspects should be considered:

◆ Hold the needle properly when placing the scleral sutures. The proper way to load the needle onto the needle holder is to grasp the middle of the needle in order to have more control of it; spatulated needles are round bodied further up the hilt and tend to rotate when held too far from the tip. Next, pass the needle at a depth of half the thickness of the sclera, always looking at the tip of the needle, to make sure that the bite and the course of the needle run parallel to the scleral surface.

◆ The proper placement of the buckle requires the use of a spatulated needle with 5-0 nonabsorbable suture such as nylon. Braided sutures such as Mersilene could weaken or produce an irregular traumatic effect on the sclera. When suturing encirclements the anterior suture is placed 2 to 3 mm posterior to the muscle insertion, that is, anterior to the posterior margin of the vitreous base. The posterior suture is placed in a position related to the width of the buckle and to an optimal buckling effect. The sutures should be placed 2 mm farther apart than the width of a buckle, so that the band slides freely through the sutures (Fig. 1-1).

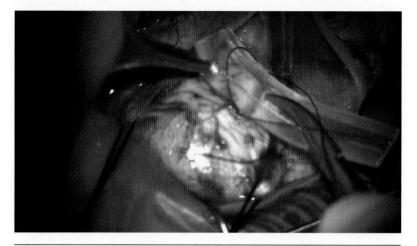

Figure 1-1 After sclerotomy and subretinal fluid drainage is performed, the buckle is placed covering the sclerotomy site and the sutures are closed.

◆ If extreme scleral thinning with visualization of underlying uvea is discovered during examination, the surgeon must avoid this location and choose normal sclera to pass the sutures; even a small area of spared sclera may be helpful. If the area of scleral thinning is localized and small, the explant must be sutured to normal sclera by passing the sutures away from the defect or in a discontinued manner biting normal sclera between abnormal thinned sclera. In addition, the farther apart the bites of the sutures are placed, the greater the height of the buckle. Surgeons must try to avoid areas of thinned sclera because its rupture is associated with an unfavorable anatomic and visual outcome. If the technique chosen is a segmental buckle and the scleral ectasia is at the site the scleral buckle is going to be placed, then the surgeon should try to pass the sutures through normal sclera adjacent to the thinned sclera. It has been described the possibility to place a scleral graft, followed by scleral buckle and vitrectomy if necessary, in fact different grafts have been described and proposed to treat scleral defects: Cartilage, fascia lata, aortic tissue, tibial periosteum, skin, and autologous sclera.[20] However, it is very common to observe spare zones of sclera that can be used in order to pass the sutures with no need to use any of the abovementioned materials.

◆ Some preoperative tests have been considered helpful in patients suspected to have scleral thinning, such as ultrasound biomicroscopy that may identify anterior scleral defects or optical coherence tomography (OCT) for posterior scleral defects.

◆ It may be advisable to use the operating microscope or a magnifying lens (loupes) in order to detect scleral thinning and avoid areas at risk of perforation. This practice is considered an updated way to place scleral buckles.

✤ Pearls on How to Solve It

◆ If partial thickness suture cutout occurs, the suture should be replaced. A different site to place the new bite should be considered. It is important that the surgeon understands why this has happened to prevent occurring again (for instance, if the suture was too superficial, a deeper one should be placed).

◆ If suture cutout occurs and a drainage site is created, then the next step to undertake will depend on whether the eye has maintained good intraocular pressure or not. If hypotony is noted as a result of the drainage of subretinal fluid, air could be injected into the vitreous cavity. Once the intraocular pressure is restored, it is then easier to place a wider suture and tighten the buckle in order to seal the drainage site. Indirect ophthalmoscopy must be done to make sure that a retinal tear/hole has not been created when the eye was entered. If a tear/hole is found, cryotherapy or laser with indirect binocular ophthalmoscope should be undertaken.

◆ If scleral tissue is lost and it is observed that there is "cheese wiring" of the sclera, a patch graft using the abovementioned materials (see Section "How to Prevent It") should be considered.

Scleral Perforation and Inadvertent Drainage of Subretinal Fluid

Scleral perforation occurs more frequently during suture placement and the surgeon notices it because subretinal fluid, blood, or pigment appears through the suture tract. The scleral perforation may be associated with several complications such as retinal incarceration and choroidal or subretinal hemorrhage. This complication causes many difficulties during and after surgery, such as hypotony, distortion of the globe, and the presence of hemorrhage that may interfere with visualization and treatment of retinal breaks. Accidental drainage of subretinal fluid during scleral buckle placement has been reported to happen in 6% of the cases.

Risk Factors

The most important risk factor is high myopia; a study reported that 74% of the cases in which scleral perforation had occurred were myopic eyes.[2] Hypotonic eyes are also considered at greater risk.

Pearls on How to Prevent It

◆ Mattress sutures of 5-0 monofilament nylon have the ideal thickness to prevent erosion of the sclera when passing the suture. Thinner sutures tend to erode out of the sclera.

◆ Make sure that the eye has normal pressure when placing the suture; if the eye is soft it is easier to accidentally penetrate the choroid when placing deep scleral sutures.

◆ The sutures must be placed deep and long enough so that the suture will not cut out of the sclera; the needle can be gently lifted while passing it through the sclera parallel and keeping its depth continuously.

◆ In those patients considered at "high risk" for perforation during scleral buckle surgery, such as high myopes, it may be useful to identify under the operating microscope areas of scleral thinning and avoid them. In addition, in selected patients, it may be useful to have an air line connected to the vitrectomy machine so that, if perforation occurs, air can be injected through the vitrectomy machine to restore intraocular pressure right away which may avoid hypotony and other subsequent problems such as intraocular hemorrhage.

It is better to select the drainage site after placement of scleral sutures. The drainage site must be chosen when possible, just above or below the horizontal meridian in a place where it is safe to enter the subretinal space and drain the fluid. This location avoids the major choroidal vessel and vortex veins; in addition, the horizontal meridian allows easy access to the sclera.

Pearls on How to Solve It

◆ If inadvertent drainage of subretinal fluid occurs, the surgeon must rule out the potential complications associated with it such as hypotony, subretinal and choroidal/suprachoroidal hemorrhage, and retinal incarceration. If intraocular pressure had been raised by tightening the buckle and an accidental drainage happens, then hypotony is more likely to happen.

◆ The procedure to follow after unintended perforation depends upon the amount of subretinal fluid present before perforation and if a drainage procedure was planned to be done. If so, the need for formal drainage is already accomplished. The suture involved in the inadvertent drainage is removed; the surgeon should place the suture more widely to ensure sealing of the drainage site with the scleral buckle (i.e., the site of inadvertent drainage should be covered by the scleral buckle). Next, cryotherapy or laser with indirect binocular ophthalmoscope should be done to treat the tear hole causing retinal detachment as well as the site of inadvertent perforation.

◆ If the eye is hypotonic after the inadvertent drainage, balanced saline solution, air, or an expansile gas should be injected or the assistant may indent the eye with a cotton-tipped applicator to try to keep the intraocular pressure nearly normal until the surgeon adjusts the buckle indentation.

 Expected Outcomes: What Is the Worst-case Scenario

Sudden decompression of the eye can occur as a result of the above complications and can lead to suprachoroidal/subretinal hemorrhage with a subsequent devastating visual outcome if the macula is involved. Failure to attach the retina and development of proliferative vitreoretinopathy can also occur if the above complications take place.

REFERENCES

1. Wilkinson CP, Bradford RH Jr. Complications of draining subretinal fluid. *Retina.* 1984;4:1–4.
2. Brown P, Chignell AH. Accidental drainage of subretinal fluid. *Br J Ophthalmol.* 1982;66:625–626.
3. Tabandeh H, Flaxel C, Sullivan PM, et al. Scleral rupture during retinal detachment surgery: Risk Factors, management options, and outcomes. *Ophthalmology.* 2000;107:848–852.
4. Abdullah AS, Jan S, Qureshi MS, et al. Complications of conventional scleral buckling occurring during and after treatment of rhegmatogenous retinal detachment. *J Coll Physicians Surg Pak.* 2010;20(5):321–326.
5. Fastenberg DM, Perry HD, Donnenfeld ED, et al. Expulsive suprachoroidal hemorrhage with scleral buckling surgery. *Arch Ophthalmol.* 1991;109:323.
6. Tabandeh H, Sullivan PM, Smahliuk P, et al. Suprachoroidal hemorrhage during pars plana vitrectomy. Risk factors and outcomes. *Ophthalmology.* 1999;106:236–242.
7. Speaker MG, Guerriero PN, Met JA, et al. A case-control study of risk factors for intraoperative suprachoroidal expulsive hemorrhage. *Ophthalmology.* 1991;98:202–209.
8. Chu TG, Green RL. Suprachoroidal hemorrhage. *Surv Ophthalmol.* 1999;43(6):471–486.
9. Cantor LB, Katz LJ, Spaeth GL. Complications of surgery in glaucoma. Suprachoroidal expulsive hemorrhage in glaucoma patients undergoing intraocular surgery. *Ophthalmology.* 1985;92:1266–1270.

10. Chu TG, Cano MR, Green RL, et al. Massive suprachoroidal hemorrhage with central retinal apposition. A clinical and echographic study. *Arch Ophthalmol.* 1991; 109:1575–1581.
11. Gressel MG, Parrish RK 2nd, Heuer DK. Delayed nonexpulsive suprachoroidal hemorrhage. *Arch Ophthalmol.* 1984;102:1757–1760.
12. Hawkins WR, Schepens CL. Choroidal detachment and retinal surgery. *Am J Ophthalmol.* 1966;62:813–819.
13. Piper JG, Han DP, Abrams GW, et al. Perioperative choroidal hemorrhage at pars plana vitrectomy. A case-control study. *Ophthalmology.* 1993;100:699–704.
14. Sharma T, Virdi DS, Parikh S, et al. A case-control study of suprachoroidal hemorrhage during pars plana vitrectomy. *Ophthalmic Surg Lasers.* 1997;28:640–644.
15. Wilkinson CP, Rice TA. *Michels Retinal Detachment.* 2nd ed. St. Louis, MO: Mosby; 1997:988–990.
16. Chechelnitsky M, Mannis MJ, Chu TG. Scleromalacia after retinal detachment surgery. *Am J Ophthalmol.* 1995;119:803–804.
17. Mauriello JA Jr, Pokorny K. Use of split-thickness dermal grafts to repair corneal and scleral defects—a study of 10 patients. *Br J Ophthalmol.* 1993;77:327–331.
18. Mamalis N, Johnson MD, Haines JM, et al. Corneal-scleral melt in association with cataract surgery and intraocular lenses: A report of four cases. *J Cataract Refract Surg.* 1990;16:108–115.
19. Lee DA. *Clinical Guide to Comprehensive Ophthalmology.* New York, NY: Thieme Medical Publishers, Inc.; 1999.
20. Sangwan VS, Jain V, Gupta P. Structural and functional outcome of scleral patch graft. *Eye (Lond).* 2007;21(7):930–935.

2

COMPLICATIONS ASSOCIATED with DRAINAGE of SUBRETINAL FLUID

BORJA CORCÓSTEGUI, ALBERTO ARTEAGA,
JUAN DIEGO CARPIO, AND LUCIENNE COLLET

Drainage of subretinal fluid is one of the most challenging decisions of scleral buckling procedures. There are considerable differences in opinion regarding when to drain, and its use depends on the case and also on the surgeon's training. In the majority of cases, the decision is made based upon the characteristics of the retinal detachment and the quantity of subretinal fluid present. Special care must be taken when draining subretinal fluid to avoid complications.

◆ Draining Subretinal Fluid: How to Do It

Selection of the Drainage Site

The ideal subretinal fluid drainage site is where the retinal detachment is more elevated, decreasing the risk of retinal incarceration. The safest place to do the incision/prick on the sclera should be just below the horizontal meridian, between the inferior and lateral rectus muscle or between inferior and medial rectus muscle in retinal detachments involving the inferior quadrants. This approach has the advantage of avoiding choroidal vessels and vortex veins and allows easy access to the sclera.[1,2] If subretinal drainage is done at the superior quadrants, choroidal vessels may be avoided; however, scleral access is more difficult in these quadrants. Subretinal fluid drainage should be done within certain distance from retinal tears, especially when retinal tears are large enough so that vitreous may pass through them and leak out of the eye. The drainage site should be done, a little anterior to the equator, where the buckle will be placed, so that the drainage point will be covered by it. In this manner, the scleral buckle, in its place, will give support to the scleral incision (when a cutdown technique is used to drain subretinal fluid) especially if retinal incarceration happens and at the same time it avoids the need for a scleral suture.[1,2]

The following factors should be considered when draining subretinal fluid:

1. Retinal detachment configuration: Drainage should be done where retinal detachment is more elevated.
2. Characteristics of vitreoretinal traction and the presence of incipient vitreoretinal proliferation (PVR). Drainage should not be done close to zones with PVR (start fold or rigid retina).
3. Retinal tears localization and scleral buckle configuration: Avoid drainage close to large retinal tears.
4. Choroidal vascularization: Drainage should be done away from the vortex veins.
5. Drainage should be done, if possible, in an area where there is good scleral access and it is easier to evaluate intraocular changes using indirect ophthalmoscopy.

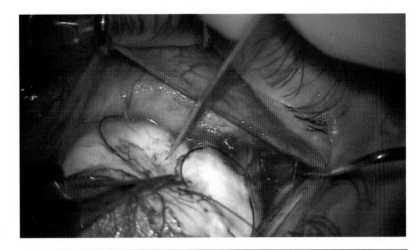

Figure 2-1 The sutures are placed through the sclera, sclerotomy is done under an operating microscope, a 3-mm radial sclerotomy is done, and the choroid is exposed.

Techniques for Subretinal Fluid Drainage

Scleral Cutdown

The eye must be prepared with sutures around each rectus muscle to allow an adequate manipulation of the globe. The drainage site is chosen by indirect ophthalmoscopy, based on the above criteria. Then the eye is placed so that the sclerotomy site is well exposed and should be kept in the same position during subretinal fluid drainage. Under an operating microscope, a 3-mm radial sclerotomy is done in order to expose the choroid **(Fig. 2-1)**. Subtle pressure is then applied just beside the sclerotomy and at the same time a forceps is used to separate the incision; the choroid is herniated and ready for choroidotomy **(Fig. 2-2)**. The choroidotomy is best performed using an 810-nm diode infrared laser for better penetration of the choroidal tissue **(Fig. 2-3)**. The following parameters are used in order to coagulate

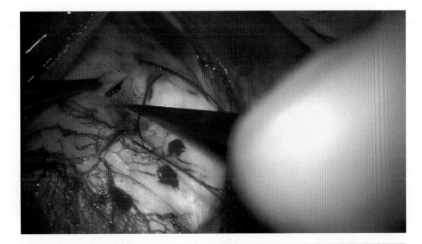

Figure 2-2 Pressure is applied just beside the sclerotomy and at the same time a forceps is used to separate the incision, the choroid is herniated and ready for choroidotomy.

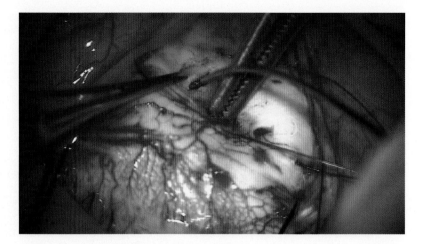

Figure 2-3 An 810-nm diode infrared laser is used to perform choroidotomy. The probe is placed near the choroid.

choroidal vessels and close small vessels: 400 mW followed by a power increase to 800 mW and up to 1 W in order to open completely the choroidal tissues and facilitate the slow drainage of subretinal fluid. Once drainage is completed, the sclera most often does not require suturing.

It is important, at the beginning of the procedure, not to exert external pressure on the globe as subretinal fluid will spontaneously exit the eye. The anterior part of sclerotomy should be depressed then only in a delicate manner to increase intraocular pressure and complete the drainage **(Fig. 2-4)**. If retinal tears are large, then the sclera should be depressed at the same site as the retinal tears in order to allow subretinal fluid egress but with no vitreous passing into the subretinal space.[2] The presence of pigment while draining subretinal fluid indicates the end stage of subretinal fluid drainage. It is very important to perform indirect ophthalmoscopy with careful observation of the sclerotomy site while draining subretinal fluid in order to make an immediate diagnosis of possible complications.

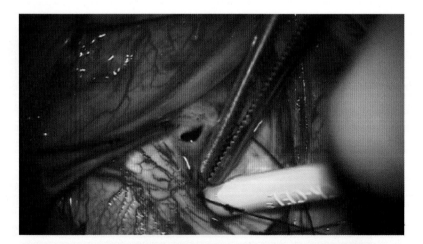

Figure 2-4 The sclera should only be depressed in the same place of retinal tears if retinal tears are too big; this is done in order to tamponade and allow subretinal fluid egress with no vitreous passing into the subretinal space.

It has been suggested that the scleral cutout and laser drainage technique would be useful in cases of shallow retinal detachments,[3] although the need for drainage will have to be considered under these circumstances. In our opinion, laser drainage allows a slow controlled drainage of subretinal fluid, with a low complication rate.[4]

Needle Techniques

Suture Needle Drainage

In this technique, a spatulated needle (5/0 ethibond) held in a needle holder 2 to 3 mm from its tip is used to perforate the sclera–choroid through a single, smooth motion, perpendicular to the scleral surface.[5] The needle is then withdrawn as the globe is simultaneously indented with the tip of a finger. Pressure is maintained to avoid/limit bleeding from the choroidal circulation and facilitate subretinal fluid drainage through the small sclerotomy. After ~2 minutes, the pressure is gradually reduced and the drainage site is explored internally using the indirect ophthalmoscope. If any signs of bleeding are detected, pressure should be applied again.

It is unclear which of the above techniques for subretinal fluid drainage is better. Thus, in a prospective, randomized controlled trial comparing the scleral cutout technique, done in a similar fashion as that described above but using argon laser rather than diode infrared laser, with the suture needle drainage (as described herein) in which 93 patients were included, Aylward and colleagues[5] found a success rate (adequate drainage of subretinal fluid) of 97.9% in the scleral cutout and argon laser drainage group compared with 84.8% in the suture needle drainage group. The incidence of clinically significant subretinal hemorrhage was 4.3% in the former compared with 28.3% in the latter; no differences were found with regards to the occurrence of vitreoretinal incarceration. However, Ibanez and collaborators,[6] in a randomized clinical trial in which 175 patients were included, failed to detect statistically significant differences between both surgical techniques of subretinal fluid drainage.

27G Hypodermic Needle Technique

Pearce and coworkers[7] describe the use of a 27G hypodermic needle, bent 2 mm from the tip, for the purpose of draining subretinal fluid. The needle is used to perforate the sclera and choroid in a single, controlled motion. The bent tip of the needle is introduced perpendicular to the globe and is held in place for few seconds and then removed. Digital pressure is applied immediately with the counter tension provided by pulling on the recti slings. If a large amount of fluid is present and thus drained, air can be injected intravitreally to adjust the intraocular pressure and to prevent the occurrence of intraocular bleeding. This technique is fast, safe, and easy to perform.

Complications of Subretinal Fluid Drainage

The complications of subretinal fluid drainage are secondary to a combination of multiple factors. There are complications that depend upon the characteristics of the retinal detachment; others may depend on the surgical technique used. The surgeon has to evaluate each patient and detect any risk factors for the development of complications; then determine the best surgical approach.

The main complications related to subretinal fluid drainage are choroidal and subretinal hemorrhage, retinal incarceration, iatrogenic retinal tear, and dry tap.

Choroidal/Subretinal Hemorrhage

Choroidal hemorrhage occurs in up to 3% to 4% of the cases and it is considered the most frequent complication associated with subretinal fluid drainage.[2]

Risk Factors

Risk factors for the development of intraoperative choroidal hemorrhage include: High myopia, glaucoma, systemic cardiovascular diseases, and diabetes.

Although there is no firm evidence that the use of warfarin or aspirin is not associated with increased risk of bleeding during subretinal fluid drainage, recent studies appear to suggest that this may be the case.[8,9] With regard to the use of cryotherapy, prospective randomized controlled study ($n = 80$) failed to detect statistically significant differences in the occurrence of intraocular hemorrhage when drainage was performed prior to versus post cryotherapy.[7]

Pathogenesis

Choroidal hemorrhage occurs as a result of bleeding through ruptured choroidal vessels at the site where the choroid is entered. Bleeding would occur if the choroidal (intravessel) pressure exceeds the intraocular pressure and, thus, it tends to occur if hypotony occurs during the procedure (see also Chapter 26C). The risk of bleeding should increase if a large choroidal vessel is punctured/damaged.

Pearls on How to Prevent It

◆ Choroidal blood vessels should be avoided when the site of subretinal fluid drainage is chosen. A good location for subretinal fluid drainage, if possible, would be on either side (above or below) of the rectus muscles.[10]

◆ Care must be taken, when the scleral cutout technique is used, to avoid doing a large choroidotomy manipulating thick choroidal vessels or doing insufficient cauterization. This complication may happen less frequently if choroidotomy is performed with infrared laser or diathermy coagulation, as described before.

◆ As the fluid drains, it is very important to maintain a relatively normal and constant intraocular pressure to prevent choroidal hemorrhage.[11]

Pearls on How to Solve It

◆ In the majority of cases, the choroidal hemorrhage may concentrate in a small area around the choroidotomy site. If such is the case, frequent observation is recommended until the hemorrhage resolves by itself.

◆ Significant hemorrhage should be managed by closing the drainage site, if a scleral cutout technique has been used, as quickly as possible with either the buckle or a sclerotomy suture, and the intraocular pressure (IOP) elevated above the systolic perfusion pressure. This may be done either by raising the scleral buckle or by injecting an air/gas bubble into the vitreous cavity. If the drainage site is temporal, the eye should be positioned to place the located site as inferiorly as possible to prevent gravitation of the subretinal blood to the fovea.[12]

◆ If the hemorrhage is seen to have reached the macula, pars plana vitrectomy may be required.

◆ In cases complicated with vitreous hemorrhage, a pars plana vitrectomy should be considered.

Ineffective Drainage (Dry Tap)

The term "dry tap" refers to the absence of drainage of subretinal fluid through the scleral incision.

Pathogenesis

It may happen after an incorrect drainage site has been chosen and the choroidotomy has been performed in a place where there is none or minimal subretinal fluid. It may occur also as a result of inadequate perforation of the sclera–choroid (inadequate depth) when using needle techniques to drain subretinal fluid; this may happen more often in eyes with thick sclera such as hyperopic eyes.

Pearls on How to Prevent It

◆ Follow the advice given at the beginning of this chapter.

◆ The possibility of subretinal fluid shifting away from the drainage site can be minimized by visualizing the subretinal fluid immediately before drainage.[11]

Pearls on How to Solve It

◆ If no complications have occurred as a result of the first attempt at drainage (this should be confirmed by indirect ophthalmoscopy), another drainage site should be chosen. The most frequent cause of "dry tap" is retinal configuration that may stop subretinal fluid outflow. In addition, retinal incarceration should be ruled out under indirect ophthalmoscopy. This should be taken into account when selecting the new site.

Vitreoretinal Incarceration

Vitreoretinal incarceration occurs when retina, vitreous, or both prolapsed through the sclerotomy site (see also Chapter 1).

Pathogenesis

Vitreoretinal incarceration may be seen in 2% to 3% of the cases, at early stages of drainage, usually after the choroidotomy has been performed and it is associated with a sudden interruption of subretinal fluid outflow. If during a scleral buckle procedure vitreoretinal incarceration occurs or is probable to happen, then the surgeon must immediately release all traction and indirect ophthalmoscopy examination should be performed. Classically, it can be identified as a simple appearance of the retina with radial folds over the sclerotomy (see also Chapter 1).

Risk Factors

Large sclerotomies have the tendency to produce retinal incarceration as well as increased intraocular pressure at the beginning of subretinal fluid drainage. In this case, retinal incarceration may happen as a result of an uncontrolled and rapid subretinal fluid outflow through the incision, if a scleral cutout technique has been used for the drainage; this would lead to a fast flattening of the retinal detachment at the drainage site increasing the risk of retinal incarceration.[1] The surgeon may produce a fast drainage of subretinal fluid if the sclerotomy performed is too large or the surgeon puts pressure on the scleral incision or on the globe to force subretinal fluid outflow.

Pearls on How to Prevent It

◆ If using scleral cutout techniques for drainage, avoid large sclerotomies.

◆ Avoid exerting marked pressure on the globe during drainage when a scleral cutout technique for drainage is used.

◆ As the fluid drains, it is important to maintain a relatively normal and constant IOP. Indentation of the globe at the ora serrata in the meridian of the drainage site facilitates elevation of the retina over the site and allows movement of subretinal fluid to the drainage site. As the fluid drains, the loss of intraocular volume can be compensated for by indentation with cotton-tipped applicators starting 180 degrees away from the drainage site.[11]

 Pearls on How to Solve It

◆ If vitreoretinal incarceration is observed, the drainage site must be closed either by placing the buckle on the sclerotomy or by passing a suture. Repositioning of the vitreous or retinal entrapment may be beneficial in those cases where the tissue herniated is considerable.[13]

REFERENCES

1. Ryan SJ. In: Glaser BM, Michels RG, eds. *Retina*, Vol. 3. Toronto, Baltimore, Philadelphia, St. Louis: C.V Mosby Company; 1989:127–133.
2. Guyer DR, Yannuzzi LA, Chang S, et al. *Retina-Vitreous-Macula*. Philadelphia, London, Montreal, Sydney, Tokyo: W.B. Saunders Company; 1999:1257–1264.
3. Ryan EH Jr, Arribas NP, Olk RJ, et al. External argon laser drainage of subretinal fluid using the endolaser probe. *Retina*. 1991;11:214–218.
4. Fitzpatrick EP, Abbott D. Drainage of subretinal fluid with the argon laser. *Am J Ophthalmol*. 1993;115:755–757.
5. Aylward GW, Orr G, Schwartz SD, et al. Prospective, randomised, controlled trial comparing suture needle drainage and argon laser drainage of subretinal fluid. *Br J Ophthalmol*. 1995;79:724–727.
6. Ibanez HE, Bloom SM, Olk RJ, et al. External argon laser choroidotomy versus needle drainage technique in primary scleral buckle procedures. A prospective randomized study. *Retina*. 1994;14:348–350.
7. Pearce IA, Wong D, McGalliard J, et al. Does cryotherapy before drainage increase the risk of intraocular haemorrhage and affect outcome? A prospective, randomised, controlled study using a needle drainage technique and sustained ocular compression. *Br J Ophthalmol*. 1997;81:563–567.
8. Chandra A, Jazayeri F, Williamson TH. Warfarin in vitreoretinal surgery: a case controlled series. *Br J Ophthalmol*. 2011;95:976–978.
9. Narendran N, Williamson TH. The effects of aspirin and warfarin therapy on haemorrhage in vitreoretinal surgery. *Acta Ophthalmol Scand*. 2003;81:38–40.
10. Brinton DA., Wilkinson CP. *Retinal Detachment: Principles and Practice*. Oxford University Press, USA; 3rd ed. vol 166;Ch 7;2009.
11. Williams GA, Aaberg TM Jr. Techniques of scleral buckling. In: Tansman W, Jaeger EA, eds. *Duane's Ophthalmology*. Philadelphia, Pa: Lippincott Williams & Wilkins;15th ed. vol 6, ch 59;2012.
12. Burton RL, Cairns JD, Campbell WG, et al. Needle drainage of subretinal fluid. A randomized clinical trial. *Retina*. 1993;13:13–16.
13. Michels RG, Wilkinson CP, Rice TA. *Desprendimiento de retina*. Toronto, Baltimore, Philadelphia, St. Louis: C.V Mosby Company; 1990:562–567.

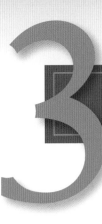

COMPLICATIONS ASSOCIATED with the INJECTION of AIR/GAS

GEORGE WILLIAM AYLWARD

3A Air/Gas Injection Under Tenon's Conjunctiva

❖ The Complication: Definition

The goal of air/gas injection is a single bubble of air/gas in the vitreous cavity (**Fig. 3A-1**). Rarely air/gas may end up in the subconjunctival space, though this is a rare complication. Thus, subconjunctival gas occurred in only three cases of 1,274 in a large series.[1] The consequences of this complication are slight.

❖ Risk Factors

The main risk factor is incorrect positioning of the needle, usually due to excessive withdrawal of the needle once inserted. More commonly, leakage through the needle track, particularly in eyes with thin sclera, can also occur. High pressure in the eye due to injection of too much gas is also a risk factor.

❖ Pathogenesis: Why Does It Occur

In order to prevent the air/gas going under the Tenon's conjunctiva, the tip of the needle should be, when withdrawn prior to the injection of air/gas, just inside the

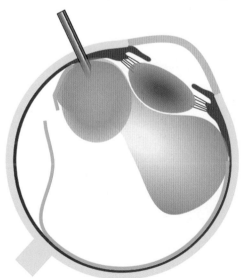

Figure 3A-1 An ideal outcome from injection of gas showing a single bubble forming at the highest point of the eye.

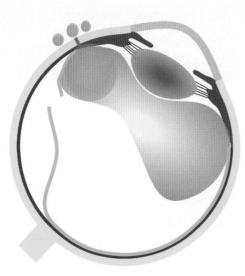

Figure 3A-2 Small bubbles of gas have escaped through the needle track resulting in subconjunctival gas and a smaller intraocular gas bubble than intended.

vitreous cavity. If the needle is withdrawn too far, then the tip may be outside the sclera, so that air/gas will be injected directly into the subconjunctival space.

Air/gas may also leak out through the needle track after injection **(Fig. 3A-2)**,[2] particularly if the sclera is thin, if the needle track is adjacent to the gas bubble at the moment of withdrawal, and if the IOP is high.[3]

Pearls on How to Prevent It

◆ Ensure correct positioning of the needle prior to air/gas injection into the vitreous cavity.

◆ Immediately place a cotton-tip applicator over the injection site following withdrawal of the needle. This closes the needle track and prevents air/gas leaking outside.

◆ Rotate the patient's head immediately after withdrawal of the needle so that the injection site is no longer at the highest position.

Pearls on How to Solve It

◆ Small air/gas bubbles can be ignored.

◆ A large gas bubble can be drained by incising the conjunctiva over the gas bubble, or simply passing a needle on a syringe without a plunger into the bubble.

Expected Outcomes: What Is the Worst-case Scenario

The presence of air/gas in the subconjunctival space per se does not have any serious consequences. However, if the gas originated by leakage from the intraocular bubble, then there will be a smaller bubble than was intended, which may result in inadequate tamponade and failure of treatment.

REFERENCES

1. Hilton GF, Tornambe PE. Pneumatic retinopexy. An analysis of intraoperative and postoperative complications. The Retinal Detachment Study Group. *Retina.* 1991;11: 285–294.
2. Kim RY, D'Amico DJ. Postoperative complications of pneumatic retinopexy. *Int Ophthalmol Clin.* 2000;40:165–173.
3. Wirostko WJ, Han DP, Perkins SL. Complications of pneumatic retinopexy. *Curr Opin Ophthalmol.* 2000;11:195–200.

3B   "Fish-Egg" Air/Gas Bubble Formation

⬩ The Complication: Definition

The goal of an injection of air/gas into the vitreous is the achievement of a single bubble **(Fig. 3B-1)**. However, sometimes the injection results in multiple, small bubbles, which clump together giving an appearance similar to fish eggs **(Fig. 3B-2)**. This is undesirable for several reasons, particularly when the gas injection is being given as part of the treatment of retinal detachment (pneumatic retinopexy).[1] Firstly, the multiple air/fluid interfaces cause a significant degradation of the view, which may prevent application of retinopexy to a retinal break. Secondly, bubbles which are smaller than the retinal break may pass into the subretinal space, delaying retinal reattachment and reducing the chance of success.[2]

⬩ Risk Factors

Risk factors which increase the likelihood of multiple bubbles include the following:

- ◆ Needle not inserted at the highest point of the eye
- ◆ Tip of the needle inserted too far into the vitreous cavity
- ◆ Injection speed too slow

⬩ Pathogenesis: Why Does It Occur

Consider what is happening at the tip of the needle within the eye as air/gas is being injected **(Fig. 3B-1)**. As a bubble forms at the tip of the needle it will be subject to buoyancy forces which will act to move the bubble vertically upward (red arrow). This upward motion will continue until the bubble reaches the highest point of the vitreous cavity. At the same time further injection of gas is enlarging the gas bubble so

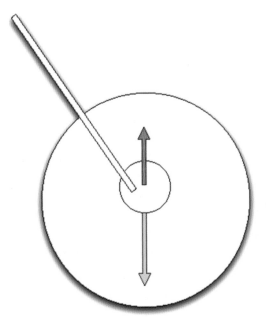

Figure 3B-1 When gas is being injected into the vitreous cavity, buoyancy forces move the bubble vertically upward (*red arrow*), while enlargement of the bubble as additional gas is injected moves the lower border of the bubble downward (*green arrow*). If the speed in the direction of the red arrow exceeds that in the direction of the green arrow, multiple bubbles will result.

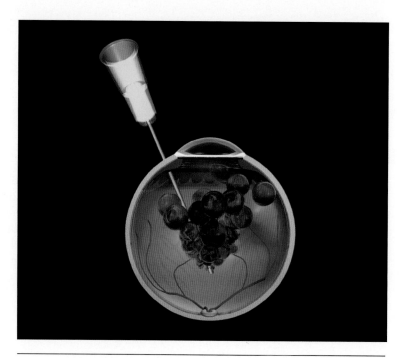

Figure 3B-2 Multiple gas bubbles, or "fish eggs" in the vitreous cavity.

that the lower border is moving downward relative to the centre (green arrow). If the rate of upward movement (red arrow) exceeds the downward movement of the lower border (green arrow), then the bubble will move away from the needle tip, and the whole process will start again, producing a second bubble.[3] By contrast if the bubble is enlarging faster than it is moving upward, the needle tip will remain within the air/gas, and a single bubble will result. Once the bubble has reached the top of the eye, then there is no further upward movement, and a single bubble will remain, irrespective of speed of injection of the gas. An additional factor comes into play if the air/gas is injected very quickly, and that is the momentum of the injected air/gas. Under these circumstances a stream of very small bubbles can form as the momentum carries the nascent bubble away from the needle in the direction of injection.[4]

Pearls on How to Prevent It

◆ Ensure that the needle is inserted into the highest point of the vitreous cavity, and withdraw the needle so that the tip is within, but only just within, the vitreous cavity. Together these two maneuvers will minimize the distance that the bubble can travel vertically, before its continued movement is checked by contact with the superior boundary of the cavity.

◆ Inject sufficiently rapidly so that the lower border of the bubble moves downward at a faster rate than the bubble moves upward.[3]

◆ Ensure that the patient's head is positioned in such a way that any bubbles migrate away from the tear.

Pearls on How to Solve It

◆ It may be possible to carry on with the case if the bubbles are not too numerous, or they can be moved out of the view by positioning the patient.

◆ Waiting a few minutes is often helpful, as bubbles in contact with each other may coalesce, reducing the total number.

♦ Coalescence can be aided by literally "flicking" the eye with the tip of a gloved finger, after giving a suitable explanation to the patient about what is happening.

♦ Small bubbles of gas can be ignored if the gas has been injected at a nonexpansible concentration. If expansible subretinal gas has been injected and persists, then it may be necessary to carry out a vitrectomy.[2]

Expected Outcomes: What Is the Worst-case Scenario

If the fish eggs cannot be resolved, then this may prevent the application of retinopexy at the same sitting. However, the patient may be brought back the following day for retinopexy to be applied. The fish eggs will have usually resolved overnight due to coalescence of the bubbles. If bubbles have entered the subretinal space by passing through the break, then this will prevent reattachment and inhibit the development of a chorioretinal adhesion. This situation should be managed immediately, since it is very difficult to displace the trapped gas from the subretinal space once the bubbles have coalesced and expanded.

REFERENCES

1. Hilton GF, Grizzard WS. Pneumatic retinopexy. A two-step outpatient operation without conjunctival incision. *Ophthalmology.* 1986;93:626–641.
2. McDonald HR, Abrams GW, Irvine AR, et al. The management of subretinal gas following attempted pneumatic retinal reattachment. *Ophthalmology.* 1987;94:319–326.
3. Aylward GW, Lyons CJ. The importance of injection rate in achieving a single intraocular gas bubble. *Eye (Lond).* 1996;10:590–592.
4. Bourla DH, Gupta A, Hubschman JP, et al. The slower the better: On the instability of gas jets in a model of pneumatic retinopexy. *Invest Ophthalmol Vis Sci.* 2007;48:2734–2737.

3C Air/Gas Injection Behind the Lens

The Complication: Definition

The goal of air/gas injection is a single bubble in the vitreous cavity, usually for tamponade of a retinal break and to achieve neuroretina–retinal pigment epithelium apposition and an adequate intraocular pressure during a D-ACE (Drain-Air-Cryo-Explant) procedure. Occasionally however, the air/gas may be injected into the prehyaloid space. This is known as the canal of Petit, and lies between the anterior hyaloid space and the back of the crystalline lens (Fig. 3C-1). The gas collects in a ring shape behind the periphery of the lens, creating an appearance known as the "sausage" or "donut" sign.[1,2]

Risk Factors

This complication is more likely to occur in younger patients with a thicker anterior hyaloid.

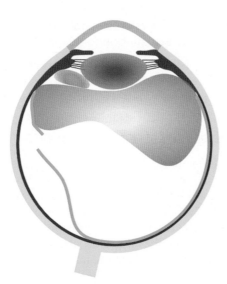

Figure 3C-1 A gas bubble lying within the canal of Petit.

Pathogenesis: Why Does It Occur

If the needle is not advanced into the vitreous cavity before being withdrawn prior to the injection, so that the tip is at the highest point, then there may not be a channel for the gas to penetrate, even with the effect of buoyancy. If the tip is in the canal of Petit, then the gas will be injected there, and remain in that position, despite the patient's positioning.

Pearls on How to Prevent It

◆ Ensure the tip of the needle has penetrated into the anterior hyaloid prior to gas injection.

Pearls on How to Solve It

◆ Small quantities of trapped air/gas will dissipate rapidly.

◆ For larger amounts, positioning the patient face down overnight usually allows the expanding bubble to break free and enter the vitreous cavity.

◆ Take a tuberculin syringe containing saline with the plunger removed, and insert through the pars plana into the trapped gas. The escaping gas can then be seen bubbling through the saline in the syringe.[3]

Expected Outcomes: What Is the Worst-case Scenario

If the gas does not migrate into the vitreous cavity, then there will be insufficient volume for a tamponade effect, and the retina may not reattach.

REFERENCES

1. Steinmetz RL, Kreiger AE, Sidikaro Y. Previtreous space gas sequestration during pneumatic retinopexy. *Am J Ophthalmol*. 1989;107:191–192.
2. Hilton GF, Tornambe PE. Pneumatic retinopexy. An analysis of intraoperative and postoperative complications. The Retinal Detachment Study Group. *Retina*. 1991;11:285–294.
3. Brinton DA, Hilton GF. Pneumatic retinopexy and alternative retinal detachment techniques. In: Ryan SJ, Wilkinson CP, eds. *Retina, vol. 3*. 3rd ed. St. Louis, MO: Mosby Inc; 2001:2047–2062.

3D   Subretinal Injection of Air/Gas

◈ The Complication: Definition

The goal of air/gas injection is a single bubble in the vitreous cavity. In cases of retinal detachment, the aim of the air/gas is to tamponade the retinal break in order to reduce the flow of fluid into the subretinal space, leading to retinal reattachment and to achieve neuroretina–retinal pigment epithelium apposition and an adequate intraocular pressure during a D-ACE (Drain-Air-Cryo-Explant) procedure. The presence of air/gas in the subretinal space **(Fig. 3D-1)** will have the opposite effect, and reduce the likelihood of surgical success.[1]

◈ Risk Factors

Multiple small gas bubbles are a major risk factor for this complication, as is the presence of large retinal breaks.

◈ Pathogenesis: Why Does It Occur

Air/gas can end up in the subretinal space either by direct injection, or much more commonly by passing through a retinal break. Direct injection can occur if the needle is inserted too far back in a meridian with overlying retinal detachment, or if the needle is inserted too deeply so that it passes through the detached retina. The surface tension of a gas bubble in liquid is the reason gas is a good tamponade agent, and therefore it will not pass through a retinal break unless it is either small (see Chapter 3B), or if there is unrelieved traction.

◈ Pearls on How to Prevent It

◆ Direct injection can be easily avoided by taking care to insert the needle through the pars plana, and to ensure that the tip is observed directly with the indirect ophthalmoscope before injecting the gas.

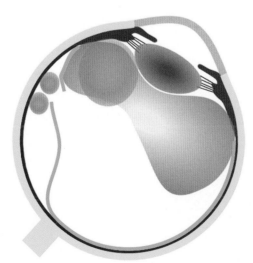

Figure 3D-1 Gas bubbles in the subretinal space.

◆ Avoid fish eggs, and if they occur, immediately position the patient so that any large retinal breaks are at the lowest point.

Pearls on How to Solve It

◆ Position the patient so that the subretinal air/gas is directly below the largest retinal break, and any bubbles that have passed through will pass back into the preretinal space.

◆ Do this quickly, since if there is more than one bubble, and they coalesce to form a bubble larger than the break, it is then unlikely to be maneuvered out by positioning.

◆ If there is a large bubble, or if positioning fails to remove it, the only recourse is to carry out a vitrectomy and directly aspirate the bubble.

Expected Outcomes: What Is the Worst-case Scenario

The worst-case scenario is that the expected treatment effect (e.g., tamponade) fails, so that the retinal detachment persists. An early decision should be made as to whether sufficient air/gas remains in the preretinal space for the procedure to work. If success looks unlikely, then an early vitrectomy, removal of subretinal air/gas, directly fluid/air–gas exchange, and retinopexy are indicated, with a good chance of success. However, this does mean that a more major procedure than that originally planned has become necessary.

REFERENCE

1. Hilton GF, Tornambe PE. Pneumatic retinopexy. An analysis of intraoperative and postoperative complications. The Retinal Detachment Study Group. *Retina.* 1991;11:285–294.

4
COMPLICATIONS of "BUCKLING" the RETINAL BREAK

W̲ILLIAM E. S̲MIDDY

4A Cannot Find Retinal Break

◈ The Complication: Definition

Cannot find a retinal break in an eye with a retinal detachment that appears to be rhegmatogenous.

The appearance of a rhegmatogenous retinal detachment is usually characteristic—bullous with hydration lines and a visible retinal break. The Greek word for a break is *rhegma,* hence the etymology of rhegmatogenous retinal detachment. Building on Gonin's seminal finding proving that sealing the retinal break cures the retinal detachment, closing the retinal break (seen or unseen) by inducing a choroidal retinal scar (with diathermy initially, and currently with cryo treatment or laser) is the critical objective in reattaching a detached retina.[1] While retinal reattachment without creating a retinopexy has been reported, application of permanent retinopexy was shown to improve greatly the success rate.[2] Strategies that might maximize successful treatment even if a retinal break cannot be found will be discussed in this chapter, but such cases generally result in a lower success rate.[2–6]

◈ Risk Factors

A retinal break more commonly eludes detection with suboptimal visualization (corneal, lenticular, or vitreous opacities; small pupil), with small breaks, or when substantial folds or retinal epiretinal membranes are encountered.

Breaks cannot be found in 2% to 4% of phakic retinal detachments.[7,8] The incidence in pseudophakic retinal detachments ranges from 5% to 22.5%.[9–12] Breaks associated with aphakic and pseudophakic retinal detachments are notoriously smaller and more commonly accompanied by some degree of media opacities.

◈ Pearls on How to Prevent It

◆ The first step in seeking an elusive retinal break is to maximize the opportunity to visualize it by minimizing impediments. These may include debridement of edematous, opaque corneal epithelium, washing out a hyphema, attempting further pupillary dilation, performing Neodymium Yttrium Aluminum Garnet (YAG) capsulotomy to remove opacities at the level of the pupil or pseudophakos, using higher magnification examining lenses or indirect ophthalmoscopic lenses with smaller entrance pupil requirements, or allowing a circulating vitreous opacity opportunity to sediment to resolve. Some of these steps

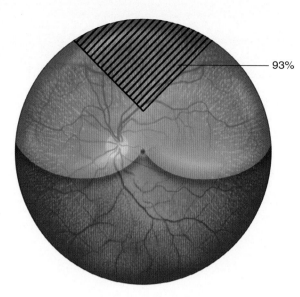

93%

Figure 4A-1 Superior retinal detachments are usually due to retinal breaks located within 1.5 clock hours of the 12 o'clock meridian. (Redrawn from Lincoff H, Gieser R. Finding the retinal hole. *Arch Ophthalmol.* 1971; 85:565–569.)

may be utilized preoperatively and some are specifically valuable intraoperatively, even if pursuing scleral buckling without vitrectomy.

◆ A second important step is to know where the most likely location of the break is so as to focus attention (or treatment) in that narrowed-down location. The landmark study that gives direction in this strategy tabulated the location of the break in large number of retinal detachments with different configurations, and found that with accuracy rates around 90% one can predict within a couple of clock hours the location of a retinal break for a given configuration.[13] Lincoff's rules can be summarized as follows:

◆ The break is usually (93%) within about 1.5 clock hour of the 12 o'clock meridian for a superior or total retinal detachment **(Fig. 4A-1)**.

◆ However, if a detachment spares even a small region superiorly on one side of the 12 o'clock meridian, the break is usually (98%) on the side which extends more superiorly, and usually above the corresponding meridian of highest extent of the opposite side **(Fig. 4A-2)**. If the detachment is distributed only on one side of the eye, the break is most commonly within a clock hour or so of the most superior extent of the detachment.

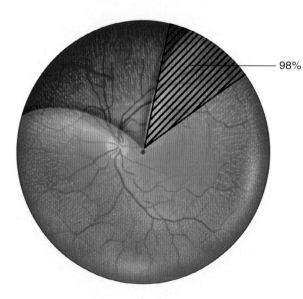

98%

Figure 4A-2 Asymmetric retinal detachment that spare even a small region to one side of the 12 o'clock meridian are usually due to retinal breaks between the edge of the detached area on the highest side and the corresponding meridian to the highest extent on the other side. (Redrawn from Lincoff H, Gieser R. Finding the retinal hole. *Arch Ophthalmol.* 1971;85:565–569.)

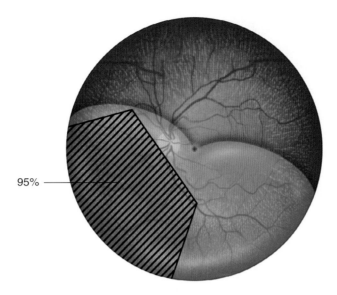

95%

Figure 4A-3 Asymmetric inferior retinal detachments usually harbor a break on the side of the highest extent. (Redrawn from Lincoff H, Gieser R. Finding the retinal hole. *Arch Ophthalmol* 1971;85:565–569.)

◆ The break is usually near the 6 o'clock meridian for a symmetrically distributed inferior detachment.

◆ However, if the inferior detachment is asymmetrically distributed, the break is usually (95%) on the side that rises higher **(Fig. 4A-3)**.

◆ The more posteriorly located a break, the more likely its meridional position will deviate from these rules. In addition, large, irregular breaks, and eyes with previous vitrectomy can yield unusual patterns.

◆ Examination of the peripheral retina is an ongoing learning process that can be humbling. The light brightness and alignment must be optimized. In difficult cases, the beam-splitting (teaching mirror) should be flipped out of the optical path to maximize illumination. Ambient light, which might decrease contrast or increase glare, should be reduced. Techniques to maximize scleral indentation include using a T-shaped depressor and moving it in an anterior to posterior motion, in contrast to the commonly used cotton-tipped applicator rolled circumferentially. Such anterior to posterior motion with a flat depressor may tend to fishmouth a retinal break and betray its presence.

◆ The most anterior extent of the vitreous separation—the posterior margin of the vitreous base—can be an important landmark to refine the most likely location of a break. This might be conveniently highlighted by a thin sediment of vitreous hemorrhage. A retinal break should be at or slightly posterior to, but not anterior to, this landmark. In addition, if there is a small degree of layered hemorrhage, the break (its likely source) is less likely to be below that level, so attention should be focused on meridians above the hemorrhage. Occasionally, a useful strategy may be to look for a subtle discontinuity on the "horizon" formed by the prominence of posterior vitreous base which is often visible even in the absence of hemorrhage. Another clue might be an underlying retinal pigment epithelium (RPE) change corresponding to a break or a previously demarcated region of detachment that "broke through." Occasionally, a break might be found a meridian or two superior to a focus of epiretinal membrane.

◆ Indirect ophthalmoscopy using scleral indentation is the most valuable tool for evaluating the peripheral retina, but in some instances a three-mirror biomicroscopic examination may yield the break.

◆ Other clues can be derived from the character of the detachment. An inferior bullous retinal detachment commonly suggests a more superior break, possibly

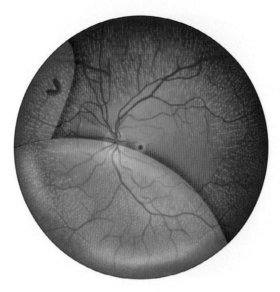

Figure 4A-4 One circumstance to be alert to is if there is bullous retinal detachment that is seen only inferiorly. Since breaks due to inferior retinal detachments are usually inferior, and therefore usually lead only to shallow degrees of subretinal fluid, one should look for the possibility of an inconspicuous superior retinal break that is connected to the inferior fluid via a shallower, exclusively anterior gutter of fluid. (Redrawn from Lincoff H, Gieser R. Finding the retinal hole. *Arch Ophthalmol.* 1971;85:565–569.)

feeding the detachment via a subtle anterior gutter of fluid **(Fig. 4A-4)**.[13] In contrast, shallow, inferior detachments are usually due to inferior breaks.

◆ An intraoperative strategy is to "look" at suspicious areas (that might have been identified as a suspect but could not be confirmed) with retinocryopexy in the hopes that a retinal break will "light up" (remain dark, silhouetted by the whitening of the retina bordering it as it freezes) intraoperatively.[3] Unfortunately, especially small breaks might yield equivocal results or escape detection even with this technique.

◆ If doing a vitrectomy, additional intraoperative clues that might betray the location of the break include the altered appearance with the endoilluminator, the Schlieren phenomenon created when subretinal fluid with a different refractive index egresses from the subretinal space into the vitreous cavity,[14] or the different angle of viewing the break after elevation with a scleral buckle. Others have described the use of wide-angle viewing with meticulous scleral indentation with the finding of elusive retinal breaks in vast majority of cases.[15]

◆ Another thing to bear in mind is that the breaks might be elusive because they are atypical. The classic break is horseshoe shaped and anteriorly located. However, breaks along retinal vessels might be linear and parallel the vessel, escaping detection. Another category of atypia is posteriorly located breaks, for example, an unsuspected macular hole.

◆ A wild card is that almost 50% of cases have multiple breaks.[16] Even though some of the extra breaks represent round holes or not be pathogenic, it is necessary to close them to affect reattachment. A corollary of this principle is that if a hole is found in a location that violates the localization principles, then there is a reasonable possibility that there is another, unseen break. Therefore, therapeutic steps should be taken to anticipate "and cover" such a possibility.

❖ Pearls on How to Solve It

◆ The first strategy when a break can absolutely not be identified is to apply retinopexy over a broader zone.[3] Either this would include treatment throughout the limits of a detachment, or the surgeon may make a calculated "gamble" and treat the areas of most likelihood in accordance with Lincoff's rules and the strategies delineated in the forgoing section.[13]

◆ A related strategy that might facilitate or minimize the adverse consequence of broader application of retinopexy is to combine vitrectomy and scleral buckling techniques, or vitrectomy alone with broad application of laser which may be of less potentially negative consequence.[17–26] While the threshold to do a vitrectomy is lower in a pseudophakic patient, the commitment to a vitrectomy carries somewhat more weight in a phakic patient because the vitrectomy will have the additional side effect of accelerating nuclear sclerosis cataract formation.[27]

◆ Expected Outcomes: What Is the Worst-case Scenario

Simply put, the worst-case scenario is not only that the retina fails to reattach, but that the failure exacerbates features of proliferative vitreoretinopathy, exacerbating the severity of the detachment, forcing an escalation of treatment and poorer prognosis. Studies of results when no break is found are difficult to compare since many have selected out certain cases and managed them in different ways. When such cases are treated with scleral buckling, anatomic success rates of 53% to 85% have been reported.[3,7,28] This contrasts to results in the 85% to 90% range without this limitation.[9] Still, some of these reports excluded cases that were treated additionally with vitrectomy techniques which may or may not yield higher success rates.

REFERENCES

1. Gonin J. The treatment of detached retina by searing the retinal tears. *Arch Ophthalmol.* 1930;4:621–625.
2. Custodis E. Treatment of retinal detachment by circumscribed diathermal coagulation and by scleral depression in the area of tear caused by imbedding of a plastic implant. *Klin Monbl Augenheilkd Augenarztl Fortbild.* 1956;129:476–495.
3. Griffith RD, Ryan EA, Hilton GF. Primary retinal detachments without apparent breaks. *Am J Ophthalmol.* 1976;81:420–427.
4. Wong D, Billington BM, Chignell AH. Pars plana vitrectomy for retinal detachment with unseen retinal holes. *Graefes Arch Clin Exp Ophthalmol.* 1987;225:269–271.
5. Criswick VG, Brockhurst RJ. Retinal detachment. 360 degree scleral buckling as a primary procedure. *Arch Ophthalmol.* 1969;82:641–650.
6. Grizzard WS, Hilton GF, Hammer ME, et al. A multivariate analysis of anatomic success of retinal detachment treated with scleral buckling. *Graefes Arch Clin Exp Ophthalmol.* 1994;232:1–7.
7. Norton EW. Retinal detachment in aphakia. *Am J Ophthalmol.* 1964;58:111–124.
8. Ashrafzadeh MT, Schepens CL, Elzeneiny II, et al. Aphakic and phakic retinal detachment. I. Preoperative findings. *Arch Ophthalmol.* 1973;89:476–483.
9. Cousins S, Boniuk I, Okun E, et al. Pseudophakic retinal detachment in the presence of various IOL types. *Ophthalmology.* 1986;93:1198–1208.
10. Vatne HO, Syrdalen P. Retinal detachment after intraocular lens implantation. *Acta Ophthalmol (Copenh).* 1986;64:544–546.
11. McHugh D, Wong D, Chignell A, et al. Pseudophakic retinal detachment. *Graefes Arch Clin Exp Ophthalmol.* 1991;229:521–525.
12. Bradford JD, Wilkinson CP, Fransen SR. Pseudophakic retinal detachments. The relationships between retinal tears and the times following cataract surgery at which they occur. *Retina.* 1989;9:181–186.
13. Lincoff H, Gieser R. Finding the retinal hole. *Arch Ophthalmol.* 1971;85:565–569.
14. Friberg TR, Tano Y, Machemer R. Streaks (schlieren) as a sign of rhegmatogenous detachment in vitreous surgery. *Am J Ophthalmol.* 1979;88:943–944.
15. Rosen PH, Wong HC, McLeod D. Indentation microsurgery: Internal searching for retinal breaks. *Eye (Lond).* 1989;3:277–281.
16. Lincoff H, Kreissig I. Extraocular repeat surgery of retinal detachment. A minimal approach. *Ophthalmology.* 1996;103:1586–1592.

17. Desai UR, Strassman IB. Combined pars plana vitrectomy and scleral buckling for pseudophakic and aphakic retinal detachments in which a break is not seen preoperatively. *Ophthalmic Surg Lasers.* 1997;28:718–722.

18. Devenyi RG, de Carvalho Nakamura H. Combined scleral buckle and pars plana vitrectomy as a primary procedure for pseudophakic retinal detachments. *Ophthalmic Surg Lasers.* 1999;30:615–618.

19. Brazitikos PD, D'Amico DJ, Tsinopoulos IT, et al. Primary vitrectomy with perfluoron-octane use in the treatment of pseudophakic retinal detachment with undetected retinal breaks. *Retina.* 1999;19:103–109.

20. Tewari HK, Kedar S, Kumar A, et al. Comparison of scleral buckling with combined scleral buckling and pars plana vitrectomy in the management of rhegmatogenous retinal detachment with unseen retinal breaks. *Clin Experiment Ophthalmol.* 2003;31:403–407.

21. Hakin KN, Lavin MJ, Leaver PK. Primary vitrectomy for rhegmatogenous retinal detachment. *Graefes Arch Clin Exp Ophthalmol.* 1993;231:344–346.

22. Hassan TS, Sarrafizadeh R, Ruby AJ, et al. The effect of duration of macular detachment on results after the scleral buckle repair of primary, macula-off retinal detachments. *Ophthalmology.* 2002;109:146–152.

23. Escoffery RF, Olk RJ, Grand MG, et al. Vitrectomy without scleral buckling for primary rhegmatogenous retinal detachment. *Am J Ophthalmol.* 1985;99:275–281.

24. Campo RV, Sipperley JO, Sneed SR, et al. Pars plana vitrectomy without scleral buckle for pseudophakic retinal detachments. *Ophthalmology.* 1999;106:1811–1815.

25. Oshima Y, Emi K, Motokura M, et al. Survey of surgical indications and results of primary pars plana vitrectomy for rhegmatogenous retinal detachments. *Jpn J Ophthalmol.* 1999;43:120–126.

26. Heimann H, Hellmich M, Bornfeld N, et al. Scleral buckling versus primary vitrectomy in rhegmatogenous retinal detachment (SPR Study): Design issues and implications. SPR Study report no.1. *Graefes Arch Clin Exp Ophthalmol.* 2001;239:567–574.

27. de Bustros S, Thompson JT, Michels RG, et al. Nuclear sclerosis after vitrectomy for idiopathic epiretinal membranes. *Am J Ophthalmol.* 1988;105:160–164.

28. Salicone A, Smiddy WE, Venkatraman A, et al. Management of retinal detachment when no break is found. *Ophthalmology.* 2006;113:398–403.

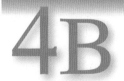 Inability to Close the Retinal Break on the Buckle

The Complication: Definition

The retinal break is not properly positioned on the scleral buckle effect.

Historically, it has been felt to be imperative to support a retinal break on a scleral buckle. With the advent of vitrectomy technique (and pneumatic retinopexy) it has been demonstrated that at least in some cases or to some degree when vitreous traction is relieved internally, this is not as important. Nevertheless, the traction must be relieved enough to allow application of effective retinopexy at the break.

Risk Factors

Generally, the main reason why a break cannot be incorporated on a standard buckle is because it is more posterior in its extent or it is large or irregularly shaped so as to defy support by the usual scleral buckling configurations.

Exceptional cases more commonly involve trauma or high myopia. In the latter instance, the surgeon must be alert to the finding of abnormally posterior persistent vitreous attachment zones, and also that the ora serrata is somewhat more posteriorly located relative to the corresponding location of the line of the rectus muscle insertions.[1] Crafting an atypically configured scleral buckle effect requires customization. Some such breaks may be incorporated either by extending radially oriented buckling elements or by using broader encircling elements. Smaller breaks can be supported with a radial element to surprisingly posterior distances. Circumferential elements can be shifted posteriorly to some degree. However, if encircling elements are shifted too far posteriorly behind the equator, they may have a tendency to ride "downhill" and migrate excessively posteriorly.

✛ Pearls on How to Prevent It

If one's intention is to perform scleral buckling and support the break then there are several maneuvers that might be considered to prevent insufficient support of the break on the indentation.

◆ Recognizing the eye to be myopic or the recipient of blunt trauma will allow planning to decide upon the scleral buckling elements—to anticipate the need for more posteriorly located element—or to commit to vitrectomy techniques ahead of time.

◆ A surgical technique principle to avoid an insufficient indentation effect at the break is to localize the break properly. Basic technique involves avoiding errors from parallax that might be more common with particularly bullous detachments **(Fig. 4B-1)**.[2] Usually the error introduced by parallax results in localizing the break posteriorly. This is of less consequence as long as the indentation effect extends sufficiently anteriorly. Less commonly, the scleral buckle effect also is positioned too posteriorly, and the anterior portion of the break—the more important margin, since it is where any residual vitreous traction might still be operative—is left unsupported. Parallax errors at the localization step are more consequential if they lead to marking the break in the wrong meridian when a radially oriented element is used.

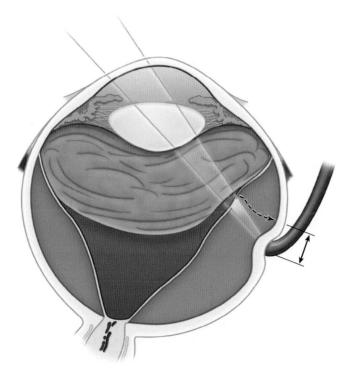

Figure 4B-1 When localizing a retinal break one must be aware that especially when the break is in highly bullously detached retina, the phenomenon of parallax will make the putative corresponding scleral localizing indent appear to be more posterior (*dotted arrow*) than it really is (*double arrow*). (Redrawn from Michel RG, Wilkinson CP, Rice TA. *Retinal Detachment.* St. Louis, MO: CV Mosby Company; 1990:541.)

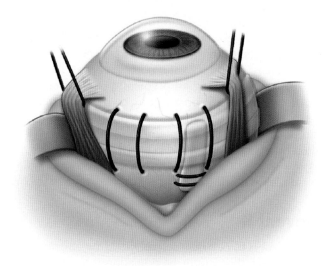

Figure 4B-2 When the retinal break is especially posteriorly located it is difficult, if not counterproductive, to position even a broad circumferential to support it. In such cases, a radial element either alone or in combination with a circumferential element may be more conveniently positioned to cover more posterior pathology. (Redrawn from Smiddy WE, Glaser BM, Michels RG, et al. Scleral buckle revision to treat recurrent rhegmatogenous retinal detachment. *Ophthalmic Surg.* 1990;21:716–720.)

◆ A second basic technique principle is to secure elements in such a way as to generate the appropriate amount of indentation. For example, the suture bed must be slightly larger than the element (generally about 3 mm wider than a sponge element and 25% wider than a solid silicone element). If the sutures are too close together there is not enough scleral arc length for indentation. Another rule of thumb is to position the element in the proper anterior to posterior location to support the break by placing tunnels or sutures at least 2 mm posterior to the external mark of the localization.

◆ A radial element can be more conveniently extended more posteriorly than a circumferential one, but it must be positioned more precisely in the proper meridian **(Fig. 4B-2)**. A particularly vulnerable situation to avoid with a radial element, however, is if a retinal break is left at the junction between a radial and circumferential element. In such instances transverse traction between the two perpendicular indentation "peaks" may prevent an edge of the break from properly settling into the crevice.

◆ Another circumstance to be alert to avoid is when the retinal break falls on the down slope of a buckle, especially when this occurs inferiorly. Probably the same factors of transverse traction sufficient to prevent settlement and to prevent formation of a water-tight seal are the factors. This is notorious in cases of proliferative vitreoretinopathy (PVR). Adjusting by placing the episcleral sutures more posteriorly may alleviate this circumstance **(Fig. 4B-3)**. Especially large breaks are best treated by using larger elements or resorting to combined scleral buckle-vitrectomy or primary vitrectomy with retinotomy if needed.

Pearls on How to Solve It

◆ Avoid the circumstance by ascertaining that the break is more posterior than normal preoperatively to formulate a proper surgical plan. For example, it might lead to the decision to perform vitrectomy or to replace or augment the scleral buckling. Internal relief of traction on the flap (especially when present superiorly) may partially or even wholly substitute for external neutralization, obviating the need to shift or design a scleral buckle configuration in a way that might be difficult or even hazardous.

◆ Once faced with a surgical failure, or even if faced with an insufficient buckle placement intraoperatively, another option besides adding vitrectomy is to reposition the scleral buckle as described in the section above. This can be

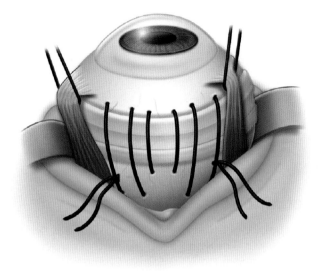

Figure 4B-3 If the circumferential indentation effect is seen to be insufficiently posterior as to support the break, the element can be moved posteriorly by shifting the episcleral sutures more posteriorly. (Redrawn from Smiddy WE, Glaser BM, Michels RG, et al. Scleral buckle revision to treat recurrent rhegmatogenous retinal detachment. *Ophthalmic Surg.* 1990;21:716–720.)

especially challenging and time consuming in a previously operated eye or an eye with thinned sclera, and a decision to avoid such efforts may be self rationalized incorrectly. In the instance of the element being properly located, but simply too low, tightening a band through an existing sleeve or suture might yield enough indentation to support the break. The height of the buckle must be a judgment call and probably is most important to be higher to neutralize more substantial degrees of vitreous base traction than the actual break. Such eyes are most commonly treated with a vitrectomy, and less broad scleral buckle elements are increasingly being utilized for this purpose.

◆ In the instance of a fishmouthed retinal break, if the circumferential element is loosened, it may allow the retina to settle better. Alternatively, a supplemental radial element may be helpful. In addition, or instead, an intraocular gas bubble is likely to facilitate reapproximation to the RPE at the margins of the retinal break.

◆ Expected Outcomes: What Is the Worst-case Scenario

The worst-case scenario is that the reattachment attempt fails and PVR intervenes.[3] This would entail not just a reoperation but, commonly, an escalation of therapy to include vitrectomy, membrane peeling, and possibly retinotomy or silicone oil techniques with their attendant poorer visual prognosis. Furthermore, reoperations may engender other complications such as corneal decompensation, hypotony, and additional cellular proliferations and retinal foreshortening.

REFERENCES

1. Gallogly P, Smiddy WE, Feuer WJ. The effect of myopia on the position of the ora serrata. *Ophthalmic Surg Lasers Imaging.* 2007;38:518–519.
2. Michel RG, Wilkinson CP, Rice TA. *Retinal Detachment.* St. Louis, MO: CV Mosby Company; 1990:541.
3. Smiddy WE, Glaser BM, Michels RG, et al. Scleral buckle revision to treat recurrent rhegmatogenous retinal detachment. *Ophthalmic Surg.* 1990;21:716–720.

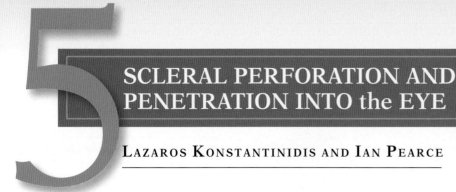

SCLERAL PERFORATION AND PENETRATION INTO the EYE

LAZAROS KONSTANTINIDIS AND IAN PEARCE

The Complication: Definition

Inadvertent rupture of the sclera is a rare potentially serious complication of scleral buckling surgery.[1–5] The complication can occur acutely during surgery through inadvertent suture perforation (see also Chapter 1), direct perforation of the indentor during scleral depression, or direct perforation of the sclera as the explant height is raised. Another reason for scleral rupture is the forceful removal of the cryoprobe, whilst it is still adherent to thin sclera by the ice-ball. The thin sclera in these cases forms part of the ice-ball and can literally fracture or crack. The cryoprobe acts like a lever to cause the rupture.

Scleral rupture can rapidly result in secondary intraoperative complications such as hypotony, retinal incarceration, and hemorrhage into the choroidal, subretinal, and vitreous spaces.[6] These secondary complications can significantly compromise the final anatomic and functional outcome.[4]

Data on the incidence of inadvertent scleral perforation during scleral depression for identifying breaks in the course of buckle surgery for retinal detachment are very limited. Tabandeh et al.[4] reported 15 cases of scleral perforation over an estimated 5,000 cases of retinal detachment (RD) surgery that corresponds to an estimated incidence of 0.3%. Five of these cases occurred during external scleral buckle surgery (estimated incidence of about 0.1%) and four occurred during scleral depression for identifying breaks (estimated incidence of about 0.08%).

Risk Factors

The main risk factor for rupture of the sclera during scleral buckling surgery is the presence of thin sclera. This thin sclera can be associated with myopia,[7] secondary to inflammatory scleritis/collagen tissue disorders or as a result of previous surgical trauma.

The full extent of scleral thinning in a myopic retinal detachment patient is not always appreciated until the conjunctiva and Tenon's tissue are recessed. It is not unusual to find the thinnest area of sclera is directly overlying the retinal breaks, particularly, if these are close to muscle insertions.

Localized areas of scleromalacia are often encountered in patients with rheumatoid arthritis.[8] Severe thinning of the sclera can occur following necrotizing scleritis which may be secondary to rheumatoid arthritis, Wegener's granulomatosis, or systemic lupus erythematosus (SLE).[9]

Other underlying diseases that have been associated with thin sclera include Marfan syndrome[10] and rare forms of abnormal collagen synthesis, such as osteogenesis imperfecta with generalized scleral thinning[11] and fragility of the sclera.[12]

Scleral inflammation, thinning and necrosis, and consequently weakening of the sclera may also be associated with previous ocular surgery. The implicated surgeries not only include vitreoretinal procedures but also anterior segment surgery and glaucoma surgery.[1,4,13,14] The adjunctive use of mitomycin C and beta irradiation in ocular surgery have also been associated with severe scleral necrosis.[10,15]

Cases involving areas of previous cryotherapy or scleral buckling are particularly prone to localized thinning of the sclera. In such cases, scleral depression over these sites or adjacent sites may result in rupture.[4]

Tabandeh et al.[4] reported that scleral rupture during RD surgery was associated with previously failed RD surgery in 71% of cases and with a pre-existing scleral pathologic condition in 29%. Furthermore, according to that study, the site of rupture was in the bed of the previous scleral buckle in all cases of buckle revision surgery.

◈ Pathogenesis: Why Does It Occur

Conventional scleral buckling surgery causes wide fluctuations in intraocular pressure (IOP).

It has been demonstrated that during scleral buckling surgery for rhegmatogenous retinal detachments, intraocular pressure increases to a mean of 116 mm Hg and may rise up to 210 mm Hg, during scleral depression and cryopexy.[16] Thus, it has been hypothesized that eyes with predisposing significant scleral thinning are more susceptible to develop scleral perforation during surgical maneuvers that increase intraocular pressure. It has been reported that scleral rupture was related to scleral depression for cryotherapy, laser photocoagulation, or identification of breaks in 64% of scleral rupture cases during RD surgery.[4]

The sclera can rarely be perforated during the dissection for the exposure of the sclera, extraocular muscle, or a previously placed scleral explant. The dissection is more hazardous in eyes that have undergone multiple previous surgeries, resulting in extensive fibrosis of the tissues around the buckle and scleral thinning under the buckle.[4]

◈ Pearls on How to Prevent It

- ◆ Identify possible risk factors of abnormal scleral thinning.

- ◆ Preoperative assessment: Identify possible visible focal areas of scleral thinning that are identifiable by the bluish tinge from the uvea seen through the thin sclera. Ultrasound examination and ocular coherence tomography could be used in selected cases for the evaluation of posterior sclera. Identify and record the retinal breaks thoroughly at preoperative assessment to aid rapid localization of breaks intraoperatively.

- ◆ Avoid disturbing/removing original scleral explant material unless completely necessary.

- ◆ In the presence of risk factors, avoid any forcible scleral depression and consider indirect laser photocoagulation without indentation in areas of retinal breaks in flat retina. Consider scleral depression and retinopexy only after drainage of subretinal fluid or following anterior segment paracentesis.[1]

- ◆ If significant scleral thinning is identified during surgery in areas where scleral depression and cryopexy are necessary to achieve adequate treatment, consider abandoning the intended buckle surgery and performing a pars plana vitrectomy.[2] During the vitrectomy procedure, lower the intraocular pressure to allow minimal force during scleral depression.

- ◆ When placing scleral sutures in thin sclera, make long suture tracts to prevent sutures cutting through thin sclera and thus further compromising the integrity of the sclera (see also Chapter 1).

- ◆ Consider paracentesis prior to raising the height of the buckle to prevent high IOP occurring during this maneuver.

◆ Alert the assistant to avoid pressing too firmly on the scleral explant whilst the suture knots are tied.

◆ As scleral rupture occurs at least partly as a result of marked and sudden increase in the IOP, maneuvers that lead to this event should be avoided. For instance, care should be taken when undergoing scleral depression or when raising the buckle to press on the eye gently and slowly so that the IOP gradually falls (rather than increase) as a result of outflow increase. One should take time with scleral depression; this allows the IOP to adjust such that a high indent can be achieved without pressing hard.

◆ Make sure to only remove the cryoprobe when the ice-ball has completely disappeared and complete thaw has taken place.

Pearls on How to Solve It

When scleral rupture occurs, the immediate management should focus on the restoration of intraocular pressure, avoidance of intraocular hemorrhage, and prevention of vitreoretinal incarceration.

◆ Immediate digital compression over the site of perforation whilst pulling on the recti slings can restore IOP and prevent hypotony and intraocular hemorrhage.

◆ Having an air line available during high-risk cases can prove useful to restore IOP. The airline pressure should be set at 40 mm Hg and have continuous flow and attached to a 27G needle. The flow can be checked by allowing the air to bubble through a pot of sterile fluid. The firm digital pressure over the perforation site should be maintained whilst the needle with attached airline is inserted 3.5/4 mm from the limbus through the pars plana. If possible the eye should be rotated, whilst maintaining firm digital compression and control of the muscle slings, into a position that the needle is at the most dependent position (i.e., hub of needle pointing to the ceiling). At this point the digital pressure on the eye should be swiftly removed to allow a single air bubble expansion within the eye. Once the air bubble has fully expanded and IOP is temporarily restored, further maneuvers can be performed to repair the perforation. The above should only be considered if the scleral rupture is small. If the rupture is large, air infusion (at 40 mm Hg) may result in vitreous and retinal incarceration in the rupture site. This method relies on the fact that the surface tension prevents air coming out even at an IOP of 40 mm Hg in the presence of a small scleral wound.

◆ In the case of a very limited perforation such as that might occur during suture placement, no further action specific to the perforation apart from examining the posterior segment, to confirm that no inadvertent retinal damage or incarceration has occurred, would be needed (see Chapter 1). Direct repair of the scleral rupture through suturing is commonly required unless the rupture is very small and it is going to be covered by the buckle.

◆ If the site of scleral rupture is more extensive then a patch graft over the affected area may be required. A number of graft materials are currently available, including allograft materials such as lyophilized donor scleral material or cadaveric dura mater, autologous grafting with fascia lata, or periosteum.[1,4,5]

◆ After restoration of the globe integrity, check for secondary intraoperative complications such as choroidal, subretinal, and vitreous hemorrhage, and retinal incarceration that may require further management. Most of these complications along with the treatment of the RD itself may require converting to pars plana vitrectomy.

◆ When scleral perforation results in subretinal hemorrhage, immediate pressure over the perforation site, as described above, may be applied and the eye positioned to prevent gravitation of the blood beneath the fovea. If massive subretinal bleeding occurs, immediate vitrectomy with internal drainage of subretinal fluid and removal of subretinal blood should be considered (see also Chapter 28).[17] Subretinal drainage can be managed using an extrusion needle or intraocular forceps for clotted blood.[18] Alternatively, liquid blood can be displaced anteriorly, through a retinal break or drainage retinotomy, into the vitreous cavity by perfluorocarbon liquids.[19] Smaller subretinal hemorrhages can be displaced from the macula by injecting 0.3 to 0.5 cc of 100% C3F8 gas and positioning the patient face-down postoperatively. The bubble will displace the blood from the macula to the periphery.[17]

✦ Expected Outcomes: What Is the Worst-case Scenario

Intraocular hemorrhage, postoperative hypotony, and development of proliferative vitreoretinopathy will all compromise final anatomic and visual outcome.[1,4]

Tabandeh et al.[4] reported that 43% of eyes with scleral rupture during RD surgery needed further surgical retinal detachment repair while 36% of cases needed long-term retinal tamponade with silicone oil. Ultimately, they reported that 71% of these eyes developed PVR (grade $\geq$ C).

REFERENCES

1. Carpineto P, Ciancaglini M, Scaramucci S, et al. Management of scleral rupture during retinal detachment surgery: a case report. *Eur J Ophthalmol.* 2002;12: 553–555.
2. Kuchenbecker J, Schmitz K, Behrens-Baumann W. Inadvertent scleral perforation in eye muscle versus retinal detachment buckle surgery. *Strabismus.* 2006;14:163–166.
3. Schwartz PL, Fastenberg DM, Maris PJ. Scleral ruptures during retinal detachment surgery. *Ophthalmic Surg.* 1984;15:402–405.
4. Tabandeh H, Flaxel C, Sullivan PM, et al. Scleral rupture during retinal detachment surgery: Risk factors, management options, and outcomes. *Ophthalmology.* 2000;107:848–852.
5. Yu YS, Chang BL. Scleral perforation after scleral buckling surgery for retinopathy of prematurity. *Korean J Ophthalmol.* 1999;13:49–51.
6. Sternberg P Jr., Tiedeman J, Prensky JG. Sutureless scleral buckle for retinal detachment with thin sclera. *Retina.* 1988;8:247–249.
7. Rada JA, Shelton S, Norton TT. The sclera and myopia. *Exp Eye Res.* 2006;82:185–200.
8. Fleming A, Dodman S, Crown JM, et al. Extra-articular features in early rheumatoid disease. *Br Med J.* 1976;1:1241–1243.
9. Okhravi N, Odufuwa B, McCluskey P, et al. Scleritis. *Surv Ophthalmol.* 2005;50:351–363.
10. Deramo VA, Haupert CL, Fekrat S, et al. Hypotony caused by scleral buckle erosion in Marfan syndrome. *Am J Ophthalmol.* 2001;132:429–431.
11. Ruedemann AD Jr. Osteogenesis imperfecta congenita and blue sclerotics; a clinico-pathologic study. *AMA Arch Ophthalmol.* 1953;49:6–16.
12. Chan CC, Green WR, de la Cruz ZC, et al. Ocular findings in osteogenesis imperfecta congenita. *Arch Ophthalmol.* 1982;100:1458–1463.
13. Chechelnitsky M, Mannis MJ, Chu TG. Scleromalacia after retinal detachment surgery. *Am J Ophthalmol.* 1995;119:803–804.
14. Mamalis N, Johnson MD, Haines JM, et al. Corneal-scleral melt in association with cataract surgery and intraocular lenses: A report of four cases. *J Cataract Refract Surg.* 1990;16:108–115.
15. Moriarty AP, Crawford GJ, McAllister IL, et al. Severe corneoscleral infection. A complication of beta irradiation scleral necrosis following pterygium excision. *Arch Ophthalmol.* 1993;111:947–951.

16. Gardner TW, Quillen DA, Blankenship GW, et al. Intraocular pressure fluctuations during scleral buckling surgery. *Ophthalmology*. 1993;100:1050–1054.

17. Rubsamen PE, Flynn HW Jr., Civantos JM, et al. Treatment of massive subretinal hemorrhage from complications of scleral buckling procedures. *Am J Ophthalmol*. 1994;118:299–303.

18. Flynn HW Jr., Davis JL, Parel JM, et al. Applications of a cannulated extrusion needle during vitreoretinal microsurgery. *Retina*. 1988;8:42–49.

19. Chang S, Reppucci V, Zimmerman NJ, et al. Perfluorocarbon liquids in the management of traumatic retinal detachments. *Ophthalmology*. 1989;96:785–791; discussion 791–792.

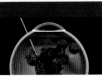

EXPOSURE AND INFECTION of the SCLERAL BUCKLE

MARIO R. ROMANO, JOHN B. CHRISTOFORIDIS, AND JOSE LUIS VALLEJO-GARCIA

✦ The Complication: Definition

Exposure of the scleral buckle (SB) is defined as the absence of tissue, Tenon's capsule, and conjunctiva, which leaves the buckle material in contact with the external environment and ocular surface bacterial flora. This exposure may occur in the immediate postoperative period if conjunctival sutures loosen, or it may be delayed for months or years if slow erosion of the overlying tissues occurs.

Extrusion is the process of disengagement of the SB from the implant site. It can occur in a quiet as well as in an inflamed eye, with conjunctival thinning or dehiscence.

Infection of the SB is characterized by an inflamed culture-positive eye with or without buckle extrusion. The infection can be acute, usually occurring in the first few days postoperatively or it may be delayed up to the first postoperative month, or even later, if a virulent germ colonizes the buckle. Chronic infections are more difficult to identify, as many cases are asymptomatic or do not cause a serious disturbance to the patient. They are usually only diagnosed when a positive culture is obtained after removal of an exposed buckle.

It is important to differentiate a scleral *implant*, which involves dissection of the scleral bed and placement of a silicone tire within the scleral layers, from a scleral *explant*, which involves placement of a silicone tire over the entire, full-thickness of the sclera.[1] Since implants are no longer commonly used in retinal detachment repair, in this chapter we will focus on complications of scleral explants, such as exposure and infection.

Incidence

Causes of implant removal include extrusion, infection, pain, diplopia, and scleritis. The incidence of removal varies from 1.3% to 24%.[2–5] Extrusion, followed by infection, is the most common reason for removal of SB.[5] The rate of positive culture of a buckle in removal surgery varies from 38% to 83.3%.[3,6–8] The incidence of SB infection is 0.5% to 5.6% of all cases and is often presumed to be due to contamination at the time of surgery.[9–13] More recent statistics have shown a reduction in maximum incidence from 24.4%[10] to approximately 1%.[14] The reported incidence might be underestimated since exposed buckles that may be colonized are often not sent for cultures when removed if there are no clinical symptoms

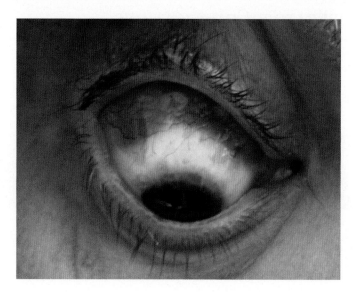

Figure 6-1 Hemolacria and mucous secretions without pain that were associated to chronic infection without buckle exposure.

of acute or chronic infection. One study revealed the rate of silent infection to be 27%.[15] In this same series, buckles removed due to other causes and without exposure were all bacteria free.[15]

How to Recognize Exposure

Exposure of SB is easily recognized by slit lamp examination or under direct examination; full retraction of the eyelids may be necessary to visualize explants located posteriorly. The patient usually complains of increased ocular mucous secretion, local redness, and foreign body sensation.

When chronic exposure occurs and microbiologic cultures are positive for more indolent bacteria, the initial event is more difficult to identify, leading us to the key question: Which was the cause and which the effect: The chicken or the egg? Was it colonized at the moment of surgery by nonvirulent bacteria that has taken months or years to expose the buckle or was it colonized after exposure?

Acute infection is easy to identify: Pain, secretion, focal hyperemia, and buckle extrusion are almost always seen. More rarely, a transpalpebral extrusion can be seen.[16] Signs of chronic infection are the same as for buckle exposure and conjunctival fistulas are frequently observed.[6] Recurrent hemolacria may also indicate a chronic infection, as described by Mukkala et al.[17] (**Fig. 6-1**).

Infection of the SB must not be viewed only as an external infection of the eye since it can indicate the presence of infectious scleral necrosis, vitritis, cystoid macular edema, localized or diffuse exudative retinal detachments, and/or frank endophthalmitis in the case of severe infection.[18–20]

Orbital computed tomography and brain magnetic resonance imaging have been reported to assist in the early diagnosis and management of SB infections.[21] Diffuse scleral thickening and preseptal soft tissue swelling are often observed in acute SB infections. In the chronically infected SB, the sclera can be thickened around the buckle, with scleral melt under the buckle.[21] Whenever infection does occur, surgical buckle removal is the definitive treatment.

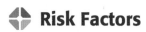 **Risk Factors**

A review of the literature revealed several common factors in SB exposure and/or infection, aside from the SB material itself.

Patient Characteristics

◆ Age: Lindsey et al.[3] demonstrated a significant risk for SB removal in older patients, that is, in the subgroup who underwent primary retinal detachment surgery between 71 and 80 years of age.

◆ Systemic disease comorbidity.

  ◆ *Diabetes:* Covert et al.[22] found that diabetic patients had an increased risk for SB removal for any reason; this is most likely due to the compromised wound healing and predisposition to infection that characterize these patients.

  ◆ *Atopic dermatitis:* Oshima et al.[20] reported an acute infection rate after SB procedures of 7/293 patients, six of whom were affected by atopic dermatitis. Overall, the infection rate in the subgroup affected by atopic dermatitis was 18.8% (6/32), including three patients with suspected endophthalmitis, whereas in patients not affected by this condition, the rate was 0.4% (1/261). In all cultures, methicillin-resistant *staphylococcus aureus* was identified. The authors proposed that a higher *S. aureus* colonization of the skin and conjunctival sac occurs in atopic dermatitis patients, making them susceptible to SB infection. In addition, chronic treatment of dermatitis with antibiotics and steroids favors the development of resistance. Contamination from skin can also occur due to the inherent difficulty in correctly isolating the surgical area when applying the adhesive surgical drapes to the periorbital skin.

◆ Ocular conditions

  ◆ Covert et al.[22] reported that chronic ocular topical therapy, glaucoma, and/or prior ocular procedures increase the risk for SB removal. A traumatic origin of retinal detachment, with perforating or penetrating trauma at the time of SB placement, was also demonstrated to increase the risk of SB removal. The authors proposed that alterations in the ocular surface and prior contamination of the wound are probably responsible for this increased risk.

  ◆ Retinal detachment due to retinal dialysis was found to result in higher rates of SB removal (46.4%) than other causes of retinal detachment. James et al.[23] suggested that this might be due to the anterior positioning of the buckle.

Buckle Material

Since 1937, when Jess performed the first scleral indentation procedure with a gauze pad, many different materials and techniques have been used with varying success. In addition to failure of retinal attachment, the same problem has been encountered frequently: Extrusion and/or infection of the SB material. In this section, we will very briefly summarize the most popular materials used historically and the principal problems associated with them.

In 1953, Custodis promoted the use of polyviol, a mixture of Arabic gum, polyvinyl alcohol, and Congo red that was soon abandoned because of high rates of infection and inflammation. A few years later, in 1957, Schepens[24] started to use polyethylene tubing as an intrascleral device to encircle the equator of the ocular globe. Its disadvantages were many: A small area of indentation, a too narrow tube since bigger tubes were difficult to handle, chronic infection due to the nonabsorbable sutures in the tube's lumen, and lastly, material precipitation and hardening with time, causing erosion into the adjacent tissues, sclera, choroid, and retina, and ultimate penetration into the vitreous cavity. This finding was also observed with the use of encircling sutures for indentation. When solid silicone rubber started to be used in 1960, it was found to be a safe material leading to fewer complications. In 1967, Lincoff and Mclean promoted the use of silicone sponges. These had several advantages over rubber but also had a significantly higher rate of extrusion and infection.

Hydrogels were initially used in 1970, with the most popular, the MIRAgel or Mai gel, introduced in 1980 by Refojo and used into the mid-1990s (MIRA, Waltham, Mass). While the MIRAgel buckles showed very low complication rates in initial studies, long-term follow-up revealed a characteristic disadvantage that ultimately led to its discontinuation: Swelling and fragmentation causing pain, discomfort, diplopia, and orbital inflammation.[22,24] In most studies in which MIRAgel buckles were included, the material itself was responsible for buckle removal.[22,25-27] Nevertheless, MIRAgel buckles have been shown to be statistically less prone to infection than silicone, solid, and/or sponge explants.[25]

Currently, silicone is used, either in its rubber or sponge form. When analyzing silicone buckles, sponges have a higher rate of complications leading to SB removal than solid explants.[6,9] The latter has a removal rate of 0.6% while sponge removal varies from 3.5% to 9.6% and as high as 24.4%.[6,9,10] The problem with sponges is most likely due to their segmental–radial cut edge, which lies directly under the conjunctiva and can promote its erosion.[28] In addition, its larger volume results in greater eyelid friction. However, Brown et al.[28] reported a 0.7% rate of SB removal, similar to solid silicone, when sponges are used as a circumferential buckle. The authors propose that this difference lies in the use of a smooth oval silicone sponge rather than a sharp-edged sponge that may chronically irritate the conjunctiva.

Intraoperative Characteristics

◆ Multiple SB implants: The number of explant buckles is thought to be related to a higher probability of SB removal surgery; however, literature regarding this is not clear. Only one article, that of Roldan-Pallares,[6] has actually reported this association.

◆ Concurrent pars plana vitrectomy (PPV) has been identified as a risk factor for SB removal in a series reported by Covert and Brown.[22,28] They proposed that increased surgical time and manipulation, complexity of the cases and the use of silicone–gas could play an important role in removal rates. In a study by Brown et al.,[28] with the exception of one patient who necessitated SB removal due to diplopia, all patients who required removal of buckles had also undergone PPV.

Postoperative Events

Secondary trauma to the ocular surface integrity, such as an additional surgical procedure, may cause disruption and inflammation, and was demonstrated to favor SB removal in the studies of Ulrich and Covert.[11,22] In particular, cataract surgery increased the risk of SB removal due to infection.

◆ Pathogenesis: Why Does It Occur

Extrusion of the explant depends on its material, shape, and location. Friction created between the eyelid and conjunctiva overlying the buckle and loosening of sutures can facilitate exposure, allowing a previously fixed buckle to move and thereby contribute to erosion (**Fig. 6-2**). When analyzing hydrogel buckles (MIRAgel),[29] extrusion and infection rates were very low.[5] Ho et al.[30] hypothesized that the degree of swelling of an explant could be altered by varying its state of hydration. He proposed that its softness and elasticity were protective against erosion (**Fig. 6-3**). It was also less prone to infection because of the lack of dead space and the material's ability to initially absorb and then gradually release the subconjunctivally placed antibiotics.[25,31] This hydration is now well known to cause the swelling and fragmentation of the buckle with subsequent symptoms.[22]

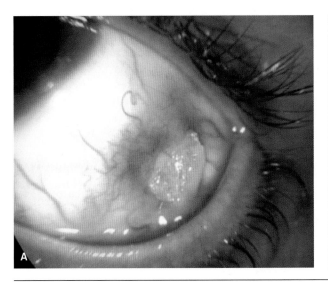
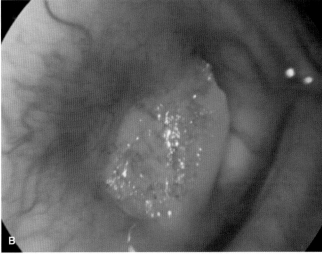

Figure 6-2 A 37-year-old man with previously placed sponge radial element for retinal detachment 30 years earlier. The sponge was found to be protruding from the temporal conjunctiva but did not appear grossly purulent. **A:** The exposed buckle can be seen after removal of conjunctiva and Tenon's capsule. **B:** Forceps were used to gently pull the sponge forward and away from sclera. Gram stain and culture of the removed material were negative for any organisms. (Courtesy of Frederick Davidorf, MD and Ahmad Tarabishy, MD.)

Infection begins when bacteria manage to colonize the buckle. This can happen during the surgical procedure or after a subsequent ocular surface disruption, such as a new surgical procedure, or with extrusion of the device.

Free-floating bacteria begin to form biofilms by attaching to surfaces. They then synthesize an extracellular polymeric matrix composed of extracellular DNA, proteins, and polysaccharides in various configurations, by which cells adhere to each other and/or to a surface. The biofilm is held together and protected by a matrix of extracellular polymeric substances or exopolysaccharide.[32] The biofilm may give an aggregate cell colony or colonies an increased resistance to detergents

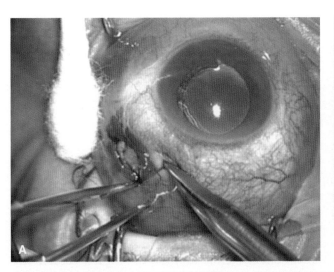
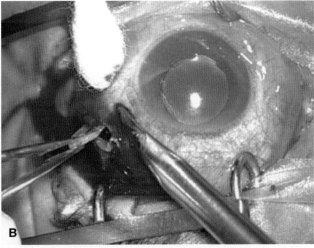

Figure 6-3 This patient had been operated 10 years previously with an encircling band for rhegmatogenous retina detachment in his left eye. The patient complained of recurrent conjunctivitis on–off for the past 4 years. **A:** Examination showed exposure of the encircling band. **B:** During the surgery it was found that under the band, the sclera was completely eroded in the superior temporal quadrant with exposure of the uvea. (Courtesy of Joaquin Marticorena, MD.)

and antibiotics, since the dense extracellular matrix and the outer layer of the cells protect the interior of the colony. Biofilms have a leading role in most infections, such as those of the urinary tract, catheter, and middle ear, and they encourage the formation of dental plaque and subsequently gingivitis. Biofilms are also responsible for endocarditis, infections in cystic fibrosis, joint prostheses and heart valves, and coating contact lenses. They will in all cases perpetuate the infection if the substrate is not definitively removed.[32]

Etiology

The bacteria most responsible for infecting SBs are staphylococcus species. Most studies identify coagulase-negative *staphylococcus* (epidermidis) as the most frequent pathogen,[8] but others find *S. aureus* to be the most common agent.[3,20] Methicillin-resistant *S. aureus* has been found to be predisposed for infecting SBs in patients with atopic dermatitis.[20] Other bacteria isolated from SBs include *mycobacterium* spp., *proteus* spp., *corynebacterium* spp., *proteus mirabilis,* and *pseudomonas aeruginosa.* While fungal species are a rare cause of infection, Pathengay et al.[8] reported the largest series of fungal isolates after SB removal in the Indian population, finding aspergillus to be responsible for most infectious cases.

Pearls on How to Prevent It

♦ Prevention of infection begins with meticulous surgery and aseptic procedures minimizing contamination of the surgical area and buckle material.

♦ It is important that Tenon's space is reached, as this ensures **complete exposure of the underlying sclera**.

♦ The size and location of the explant are directly correlated with the rate of exposure/infection. Thus, **smaller scleral explants** should be used, paying particular attention, as much as possible, to prevent a very anterior fixation of the buckle.

♦ Solid silicone buckles must be kept **under liquid** until use, as their electrostatic charge attracts dust particles. While there is still conflicting evidence as to the benefits of antibiotic soaking, we prefer to conserve silicone sponges in this manner until immediately before fixation.[14,33]

♦ When cutting the buckles, the surface must be **as smooth as possible**.

♦ The buckle and sutures must be tight, with the **knot as posterior as possible**.

♦ In young patients, when Tenon's capsule is present, it should be secured directly to the episclera with absorbable sutures; in older patients it is not necessary to suture it as the Tenon's capsule is thinner, and it is enough to ensure that the buckle is covered and the capsule returns to its natural position.

Pearls on How to Solve It

If extrusion or infection occurs, **removal of the buckle** is ultimately the only definitive solution. Covering the buckle with conjunctival flaps and/or sclera or other tissue patches are only temporary solutions for exposed buckles. When a buckle erodes through tissues, it is a sign that its fixation is compromised, and it will likely erode the patched tissue repetitively. Indication for removal is even more obvious when the buckle is infected. Topical and systemic antibiotics will not resolve this complication since the biofilm acts as a bacterial reservoir on the buckle, making the infection impossible to completely eradicate if the buckle is not removed. Some studies have successfully used autologous fascial grafts to re-cover the exposed explants, but they did not perform cultures to verify whether these long term results were because the buckles were not infected. We do not recommend this treatment, as it does not resolve the problem of a potentially infected or malpositioned buckle that can erode surrounding tissues.

◆ Radial silicone sponges that are exposed, not infected, can be more easily removed through a small conjunctival opening or even through the erosion at the slit-lamp.

◆ The conjunctiva should be **opened 360 degrees** in cases in which the **infection is severe**, the material used is unknown, or there is suspicion of necrosis or fragility of adhesion to the sclera.

◆ Rectus muscles should be hooked or isolated with a silk suture in order to **correctly expose the buckle** and the underlying sclera in search for necrosis or scleral thinning.

◆ The sutures and segmentation of the encircling buckle should be cut in every quadrant in order to **gently extract** it in its entirety.

◆ **Cryoprobes** can be helpful when the buckle is made of hydrogel material. These buckles can be very difficult to remove due to their fragmentation. When hydrated, the hydrogel material becomes gel-like and is difficult to grasp with forceps. With a simple cryoprobe, less time is needed to fully remove the buckle and less fragmentation occurs. When the water inside is frozen, it creates an adhesion that allows for gentle traction in the removal of large fragments of hydrogel. The use of cryoprobes also prevents excessive manipulation or traction of areas with thin or necrotized sclera.[25]

◆ In the presence of scleral necrosis, segmentation of the buckle prior to its removal and a scleral patch is recommended.

When scleral necrosis is found under the buckle, it must be removed with great care. In some cases, it is preferable to cut the buckle in order to **leave the smallest buckle piece over the dangerous zone rather than to remove it entirely and risk globe perforation**. If scleral thinning is severe, a patch of sclera should be sutured over the dangerous zone with antibiotic rinsing of the area in cases of scleral abscess.

✦ Expected Outcomes: What Is the Worst-case Scenario

Re-detachment after SB Removal

Modern rates of re-detachment for any reason vary from 0% to 8.8%.[5,25,26,34] Most reports agree that the critical period lies in the first 6 postoperative months, with the highest number in the first month and most occurring in the first 90 days.[3]

Risk Factors for Re-detachment

◆ Gender: Male gender was curiously found to be a significant risk factor by Deokule et al, although they had a small number of patients and could not eliminate confounding factors.[34]

◆ Original detachment: The extent of the original detachment and the presence of vitreous traction (retinal tears, vitreous bands, and retinal folds present at the original surgery) were found to be significant risk factors by Lindsey et al.[3]

◆ Infection: Studies from the 1970s found that infected buckles accounted for between 30% and 40% of the re-detachments.[2,3,10,11] More recent studies report much lower rates, with no association of infection with re-detachment.[5,20,26,34] Similarly, immediate postoperative infection of the buckle with subsequent removal has not been shown to facilitate re-detachment.[20]

◆ Surprisingly, the length the explant has been in position (from the time of the surgery to being explanted) has not been shown to be a risk factor.[3,6,26,34]

Rupture of the Globe

This grave complication can eventually lead to phthisis bulbi.[3] When performing SB removal, extreme care must be taken since the underlying sclera may be necrotic or extremely thin due to continuous erosion of the buckle, intrinsic characteristics of the patient, myopia, or senile scleral thinning. A full conjunctival peritomy with isolation and tagging of the four rectus muscles to correctly explore the entire buckle is mandatory. Segmental extraction is recommended. If removal of certain sections of the buckle compromises globe integrity, these remnants must be left in place, cutting them into the smallest pieces possible.[29]

If the eye becomes hypotonic during the procedure, scleral rupture must be suspected, even if vitreous loss or an open scleral defect is not seen. In these cases, the sclera must be carefully explored to locate the site of rupture and repair the defect with a scleral patch graft and/or tissue glue to ensure a watertight wound closure. Due to the risk of retinal extrusion through a scleral defect, infusion into the vitreous cavity must not be performed until the sclera is repaired. Even when a concurrent vitrectomy is performed with SB removal, infusion should not be opened before assuring the integrity of the globe. Then, a vitrectomy can be safely performed with endolaser over the original tear and the patched zone.

REFERENCES

1. Gopal L, D'Souza CM, Bhende M, et al. Scleral buckling: Implant versus explant. *Retina.* 2003;23:636–640.
2. Schwartz PL, Pruett RC. Factors influencing retinal redetachment after removal of buckling elements. *Arch Ophthalmol.* 1977;95:804–807.
3. Lindsey PS, Pierce LH, Welch RB. Removal of scleral buckling elements. Causes and complications. *Arch Ophthalmol.* 1983;101:570–573.
4. Hilton GF, Wallyn RH. The removal of scleral buckles. *Arch Ophthalmol.* 1978;96: 2061–2063.
5. Deutsch J, Aggarwal RK, Eagling EM. Removal of scleral explant elements: A 10-year retrospective study. *Eye (Lond).* 1992;6 (Pt 6):570–573.
6. Roldan-Pallares M, del Castillo Sanz JL, Awad-El Susi S, et al. Long-term complications of silicone and hydrogel explants in retinal reattachment surgery. *Arch Ophthalmol.* 1999;117:197–201.
7. Smiddy WE, Miller D, Flynn HW Jr. Scleral buckle removal following retinal reattachment surgery: Clinical and microbiologic aspects. *Ophthalmic Surg.* 1993;24: 440–445.
8. Pathengay A, Karosekar S, Raju B, et al. Microbiologic spectrum and susceptibility of isolates in scleral buckle infection in India. *Am J Ophthalmol.* 2004;138:663–664.
9. Lincoff H, Nadel A, O'Connor P. The changing character of the infected scleral implant. *Arch Ophthalmol.* 1970;84:421–423 passim.
10. Russo CE, Ruiz RS. Silicone sponge rejection. Early and late complications in retinal detachment surgery. *Arch Ophthalmol.* 1971;85:647–650.
11. Ulrich RA, Burton TC. Infections following scleral buckling procedures. *Arch Ophthalmol.* 1974;92:213–215.
12. Hahn YS, Lincoff A, Lincoff H, et al. Infection after sponge implantation for scleral buckling. *Am J Ophthalmol.* 1979;87:180–185.
13. Folk JC, Cutkomp J, Koontz FP. Bacterial scleral abscesses after retinal buckling operations. Pathogenesis, management, and laboratory investigations. *Ophthalmology.* 1987;94:1148–1154.
14. Lorenzano D, Calabrese A, Fiormonte F. Extrusion and infection incidence in scleral buckling surgery with the use of silicone sponge: To soak or not to soak? An 11-year retrospective analysis. *Eur J Ophthalmol.* 2007;17:399–403.
15. Wirostko WJ, Covert DJ, Han DP, et al. Microbiological spectrum of organisms isolated from explanted scleral buckles. *Ophthalmic Surg Lasers Imaging.* 2009;40:201–202.

16. Khan AA. Transpalpebral extrusion of solid silicone buckle. *Oman J Ophthalmol.* 2009; 2:89–90.

17. Mukkamala K, Gentile RC, Rao L, et al. Recurrent hemolacria: A sign of scleral buckle infection. *Retina.* 2010;30:1250–1253.

18. Oz O, Lee DH, Smetana SM, et al. A case of infected scleral buckle with Mycobacterium chelonae associated with chronic intraocular inflammation. *Ocul Immunol Inflamm.* 2004;12:65–67.

19. Dev S, Mieler WF, Mittra RA, et al. Acute macular edema associated with an infected scleral buckle. *Arch Ophthalmol.* 1998;116:1117–1119.

20. Oshima Y, Ohji M, Inoue Y, et al. Methicillin-resistant Staphylococcus aureus infections after scleral buckling procedures for retinal detachments associated with atopic dermatitis. *Ophthalmology.* 1999;106:142–147.

21. Mansour AM, Han DP, Kim JE, et al. Radiologic findings in infected and noninfected scleral buckles. *Eur J Ophthalmol.* 2007;17:804–811.

22. Covert DJ, Wirostko WJ, Han DP, et al. Risk factors for scleral buckle removal: A matched, case-control study. *Am J Ophthalmol.* 2008;146:434–439.

23. James M, O'Doherty M, Beatty S. Buckle-related complications following surgical repair of retinal dialysis. *Eye (Lond).* 2008;22:485–490.

24. Schepens CL, Acosta F. Scleral implants: An historical perspective. *Surv Ophthalmol.* 1991;35:447–453.

25. Le Rouic JF, Bettembourg O, D'Hermies F, et al. Late swelling and removal of Miragel buckles: A comparison with silicone indentations. *Retina.* 2003;23:641–646.

26. Nuzzi G, Rossi S. Buckle removal in retinal detachment surgery: A consecutive case series. *Acta Biomed.* 2008;79:128–132.

27. Yu SY, Viola F, Christoforidis JB, et al. Dystrophic calcification of the fibrous capsule around a hydrogel explant 13 years after scleral buckling surgery: capsular calcification of a hydrogel explant. *Retina.* 2005;25:1104–1107.

28. Brown DM, Beardsley RM, Fish RH, et al. Long-term stability of circumferential silicone sponge scleral buckling exoplants. *Retina.* 2006;26:645–649.

29. Kearney JJ, Lahey JM, Borirakchanyavat S, et al. Complications of hydrogel explants used in scleral buckling surgery. *Am J Ophthalmol.* 2004;137:96–100.

30. Ho PC, Chan IM, Refojo MF, et al. The MAI hydrophilic implant for scleral buckling: A review. *Ophthalmic Surg.* 1984;15:511–515.

31. Hwang KI, Lim JI. Hydrogel exoplant fragmentation 10 years after scleral buckling surgery. *Arch Ophthalmol.* 1997;115:1205–1206.

32. Holland SP, Pulido JS, Miller D, et al. Biofilm and scleral buckle-associated infections. A mechanism for persistence. *Ophthalmology.* 1991;98:933–938.

33. Arribas NP, Olk RJ, Schertzer M, et al. Preoperative antibiotic soaking of silicone sponges. Does it make a difference? *Ophthalmology.* 1984;91:1684–1689.

34. Deokule S, Reginald A, Callear A. Scleral explant removal: The last decade. *Eye (Lond).* 2003;17:697–700.

MIGRATION of the SCLERAL BUCKLE

CHRISTOS HARITOGLOU

✛ The Complication: Definition

The aim of a scleral buckling procedure for the treatment of retinal detachment is to close the causative retinal break and relieve tractional forces by an indentation of the sclera in the area of the retinal break. Today, most surgeons use silicone rubber or sponges as a buckling material and suture them on the surface of the sclera (explant). A great variety of different kinds, shapes, and sizes are nowadays available and can be placed either radially, parallel to the limbus as a segmental buckle, or as encircling bands. Sometimes, an encircling band may also be combined with other radially orientated solid silicone rubber or sponge buckles.

The explant is usually fixed with nonabsorbable sutures (e.g., 5 polyester suture) with each bite being approximately half the scleral thickness in depth. Scleral buckling materials constitute foreign bodies and therefore carry the risk of infection and are at risk for extrusion. Under certain circumstances and as a late complication following scleral buckling surgery, the explant may migrate from its original site. It may either penetrate externally and become exposed and visible trough the conjunctiva (extrusion), or may erode through the sclera and choroid and rest in the subretinal space and finally penetrate (intrude) into the vitreous cavity. These conditions can become a very serious complication during the postoperative course and were more frequently seen when the technique was in its infancy and in association with specific materials used (such as polyethylene tube hardware). Therefore, removal of the material was part of the treatment plan in these days.

Today, following improvements of material and design of scleral explants, they are well tolerated by the patient and usually left in situ. However, even today extrusion of the scleral buckle still is one of the major indications for removal of the explant followed by pain, infection, redness, and diplopia.[1,2] The present chapter will give an overview on potential pathomechanisms, underlying conditions, complications, and treatment options in cases of scleral buckle migration.

✛ Risk Factors and Pathogenesis of External Migration

The main reasons for external migration include infection, mechanical forces, and tissue loss.

Infection (see also Chapter 6)

Explant infection is an infrequent complication occurring in approximately 1% of cases[3,4] and is associated with an exposure of the buckle in almost all cases.[3] In clinically symptomatic infections, patients present with purulent discharge, injection of the conjunctiva, ocular pain, and epiphora (Fig. 7-1). The most common infecting organisms are coagulase-negative staphylococcus species in 70% to 90%, but other organisms such as methicillin-resistant *Staphylococcus aureus*, *Pseudomonas*

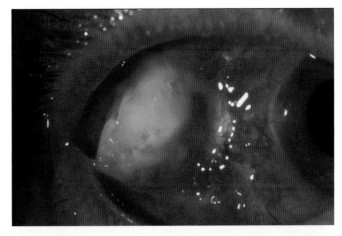

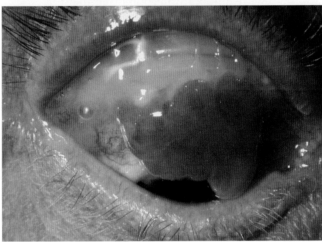

Figure 7-1 Infection of the scleral bed. Note the discharge, conjunctival injection, erosion, and tissue loss over the buckle. (Courtesy of Carsten Meyer, Olten **(Upper Panel)** and B. Aylward, London **(Lower Panel)**.)

aeruginosa, Mycobacterium abscessus, or *Corynebacterium pseudotuberculosis* have been described.[3,5,6] In chronic subclinical infections, other organisms are identified including commensal skin flora such as *Staphylococcus epidermidis.*[3,7] The risk for scleral buckle infection and extrusion is positively correlated with the number of sponges/explants sutured on the sclera[8,9] and the number of reoperations.[4,10] The increased incidence after subsequent surgical interventions is probably related to shrinkage of the conjunctiva and thickness of the Tenon's layer as a result of repeated surgery.[11]

It has been mentioned in the literature in a study including 921 scleral buckling procedures using episcleral sponges, that preoperative soaking of 30 minutes with antibiotics may significantly decrease the risk of infection and extrusion especially when soft silicone sponges are used for scleral buckling.[10] Some surgeons treat patients with systemic antibiotics for prevention, others limit the use of antibiotics to reoperations. However, the value of either strategy is unproven.[11]

On the other hand, infection may not always necessarily be the cause for exposure, but also be the consequence of the latter. Therefore simple measures may help to prevent this complication including carefully cutting off the edges of the buckle in order to prevent sharp edges, rotating the knots of the suture posteriorly, and carefully choosing the scleral buckle material and its preparation. As sponges seem to be associated with higher incidences of exposure,[12] probably due to the rough texture of the material and edges, some authors suggested cutting a cylindrical sponge lengthwise and suturing it to the sclera with the convex side facing the globe in order to avoid excessive bulging toward the conjunctiva and Tenon's capsule and ensure sufficient coverage of the buckle.[13] Others suggest a separate closure of conjunctiva and Tenon's capsule to cover the buckle material.

In order to maintain vision, prompt removal of infected buckles and treatment with broad-spectrum topical antibiotics are mandatory. Topical and systemic antibiotics occasionally result in symptomatic improvement, but they are rarely curative. In patients with combinations of encircling bands and radial sponges, the encircling band may be left in place if all additional soft sponges and their fixation sutures are removed.[10] In some cases, scleral buckle infections tend to be persistent as well as resistant to antimicrobial treatment. It was suggested that infecting organisms may be able to persist on scleral buckles by elaborating a glycocalyx matrix or biofilm that offers protection against host defenses and antimicrobial treatment.[14] This biofilm was demonstrated on the surfaces and ends of solid silicon elements and extended into the matrix of silicone sponges. The authors concluded that bacterial production of biofilm explains for the persistence of scleral buckle infections and their ability to withstand antimicrobial treatment.[14]

Mechanical Forces

Intrascleral fixation sutures are not only placed to keep the explant in place, but also to create the scleral indentation in segmental radial or circumferential buckles. Despite the effort to fixate the explant to the sclera, the material may loosen and migrate. Anterior migration has especially been described for encircling elements. In theory, migration might occur predominantly in cases where the explant is placed too tightly, too anteriorly, and where fixation sutures are inadequately placed to keep the buckling material in its location, for example, if the sutures are not placed deep enough within the sclera. In these cases, the tensile strength of the fixation suture may be exceeded by the anterior force vector.[11] In a case series of five patients with anterior movement of a solid encircling silicone element, Lanigan and coworkers[15] described this uncommon complication, namely the anterior migration of the explant through the rectus muscle insertions. Of note, none of the muscles had been disinserted temporarily during surgery, and motility dysfunction was very rare indicating that there was some reattachment of the muscle sheath or fibers closely behind the explant.[15] The authors suggested that the underlying pathomechanism may be related to local tissue necrosis and/or ischemia resulting in a "cheesewiring" through the muscle insertion.[15] Large subconjunctival hemorrhages from newly formed fibrovascular membranes around the explant may indicate progressive mechanical stress to the buckling element and repeated buckle movement[15,16] and may therefore contribute to scleral buckle migration. The time interval between surgery and anterior migration of the explant can be very variable.[15] Besides the anterior migration as described, hydrogel scleral buckling material was also found to migrate into the upper lid requiring surgical removal[17] or even to simulate an orbital tumor or orbital cyst.[18] The use of hydrogel explants has been discontinued due to their now well-established long-term complications which are the result of a progressive swelling and fragmentation of the material.[19]

Tissue Loss

Extrusion may also be related to insufficient coverage of the explant. This aspect is especially relevant in cases of repeated surgery where not enough may be available due to progressive scarring, shrinkage, and thinning of the conjunctiva and Tenon's layer.[11] There is a greater risk for extrusion of scleral buckles placed in the superior temporal quadrant probably due to mechanical stress as a result of upper eyelid movement. Interestingly, the exposure mostly begins at the anterior part of the buckle since mechanical forces are most predominant in that area (**Fig. 7-2**) and conjunctival shrinkage would also expose the anterior part in the first place.[11]

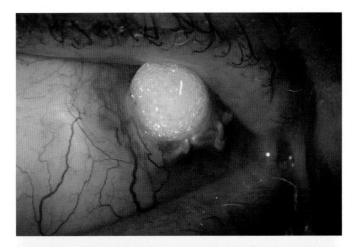

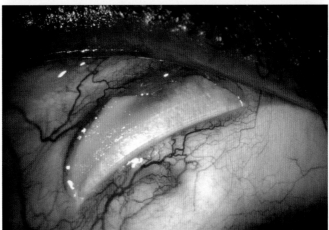

Figure 7-2 Upper Panel: Extrusion without infection of the anterior part of a radial silicone sponge in the upper temporal quadrant. Not the loosened green fixation suture. **Lower Panel:** Extrusion and anterior displacement of an encircling element. (Courtesy of Bill Aylward, London.)

Prominent suture knots may be associated with loosened end of the explants (Fig. 7-3), discomfort, and conjunctival hyperemia and also represent a predisposition to tissue thinning, fistulation, or laceration. In order to prevent exposure of the sutures, some surgeons rotate the fixation knots posteriorly and also place the suture as deep within the sclera as possible in order to prevent loosening of and irritation especially when placing the buckle in the temporal upper quadrant where the sclera is known to be thicker compared to other locations. Independently from the location of the scleral buckle, the surgeon should pay attention to cover the material carefully. Nowadays, as most surgeons use a limbal peritomy to gain access to the sclera, it appears easy to avoid direct contact between the anterior portion of the buckle as seen in posterior peritomies, and to reliably approximate both conjunctiva and Tenon's layer when closing the wound at the end of the procedure by placing limbal sutures.

In cases of explant exposure, there are four possible treatment options available:

1. Observation with topical antibiotic treatment
2. Removal of the explant
3. Conjunctivoplasty
4. Patch grafts

Removal of the explant may result in a re-detachment of the retina, as discussed later on in this chapter. Conjunctivoplasty has been used to cover exposed buckling material, but appears to be the least effective treatment and should not be considered a permanent solution due to the complications such as shortening of the

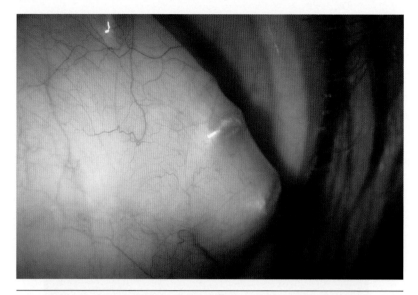

Figure 7-3 Prominent and partially loosened suture knots associated with a prominent end of the silicone buckle causing severe discomfort.

fornix, conjunctival thinning, or tissue dissolving over the wound associated with this approach.[11] Scleral patch grafts represent more viable alternatives.[20]

Risk Factors and Pathogenesis of Erosion and Internal Migration

Erosion refers to an inward migration of the explant through the sclera and choroid **(Figs. 7-4** and **7-5)**. Finally, the explant may be seen within the vitreous cavity, which is called intrusion **(Fig. 7-5)**. Both erosion and intrusion were commonly seen when encircling polyethylene tubes were used for scleral buckling surgery.[21] As polyethylene tubes have been replaced by silicone rubber and soft silicone encircling elements, both erosion and intrusion nowadays occur infrequently following

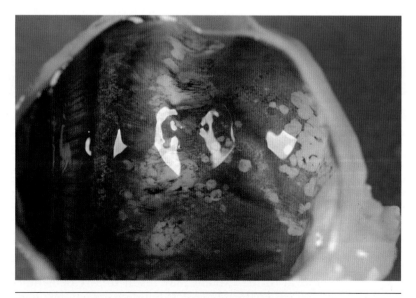

Figure 7-4 Gross section of an enucleated painful eye. Note the encircling band and the erosion of the suture knot through the sclera.

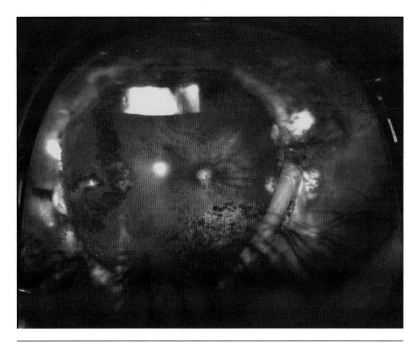

Figure 7-5 Intrusion of an encircling buckling material. The material has intruded partially under the choroid and retina

scleral buckling surgery. This is explained by the greater softness of the material, which is also maintained over years after fixation, and the longer radius of the curvature created.[22] Nevertheless, one recent study reported four cases out of an estimated number of 4,400 scleral buckling procedures using silicone rubber performed within a period of 20 years.[22] It has been reported that erosion is more frequent after intrascleral placement but can also occur following an episcleral fixation.[23] Recent research on the development of myopia[24,25] underlined that the sclera is a rather dynamic tissue, which is capable of altering extracellular matrix composition and changing its biomechanical properties. The fact that all patients in this case series were myopic (approximately –7.5 diopters) emphasizes the role of a thin sclera and the associated changes in the biomechanical properties as a potential pathomechanism. Besides the scleral weakening in myopic patients, a thinning of the sclera predisposing to erosion and intrusion of an explant may be secondary to other conditions such as intensive treatment using cryotherapy, diathermy, or photocoagulation or a crushing effect of a severely tightened encircling band.[22] Intrusion may also be associated with specific buckle material such as hydrogel, used as a supplemental buckle element under a solid silicone implant in a dissected scleral bed.[26] The complications were likely related to chemical changes within the polymer of the hydrogel implant, which changed from a soft, spongy, whitish material to a friable, gel-like, cream-colored material.[26,27]

Pearls on How to Prevent It

External Migration

Infection

◆ Solid silicone material should be the preferred buckle material.

◆ If silicone sponges are used, they should be split lengthwise and soaked in antibiotics.

♦ The edges of the buckle material should be carefully trimmed to avoid exposure.

♦ Exposed suture knots should be avoided.

♦ The explant should be covered carefully by separately closing conjunctiva and Tenon's layer at the limbus.

♦ The value of systemic antibiotics after surgery is unproven, but may be considered in reoperations.

Excessive Mechanical Forces

♦ Encircling bands should not be placed too anteriorly.

♦ Encircling bands should not be pulled too tight.

Tissue Loss

♦ A limbal peritomy should be preferred to a posterior peritomy.

♦ Fixation suture knots could be rotated posteriorly and should be placed closed enough to the sclera rather than on top of the buckle.

♦ Careful closure and approximation of both the conjunctiva and Tenon's layer should be achieved.

♦ In cases with postoperative exposure of the explant associated with tissue loss in the wound area and situations where a removal of the explant seems impossible, one might consider to cover the area of exposure with scleral patch grafts (which should be preferred to conjunctivoplasty, see above).

Erosion and Intrusion

♦ Solid silicone rubber and soft silicone encircling material should be the preferred material.

♦ Preoperatively thin sclera in highly myopic eyes and following potential pretreatments such as cryotherapy should be considered when planning the approach. If a buckling procedure seems not possible or advisable, a switch to vitrectomy should be performed, which may require scleral sutures even if performed as a transconjunctival small-gauge vitrectomy. In some cases with appropriate localization of the retinal break and limited extent of the retinal detachment, one may consider pneumatic retinopexy.

♦ Encircling bands should not be pulled too tight.

Pearls on How to Solve It

External Migration

♦ Extruded scleral buckling material without evidence of infection usually requires removal of the buckle element.

♦ In cases of infection, the explant has to be removed and the scleral bed should be irrigated with antibiotics.

♦ In cases where a removal is undesirable, scleral patch grafts or processed human donor pericardium may be considered to cover the exposed scleral buckling material and allow for a conjunctival re-epithelialization over the element.[20,28]

♦ Topical antibiotics should be applied in cases of exposed explants to prevent infection. In cases where a removal of the buckling material is felt to be associated with a high risk of re-detachment, observation may be appropriate with this regimen.

Erosion and Intrusion

◆ A removal of an intruding band is not always necessary if the patient is otherwise asymptomatic.

◆ It may be enough to observe the patient[26] or to partially remove the explant or even just to divide it.

◆ However, it is important to judge the individual risk or benefit from removing the buckle for each patient as such a surgery may be complicated by perforation of the sclera, vitreous hemorrhage, or re-detachment of the retina.

◆ If surgical intervention is indicated, successful cases of complex surgical procedures combining removal of the swollen intruded implant, repair of the scleral defect using a scleral graft, and vitrectomy to repair the retinal detachment have been reported.[27]

✦ Expected Outcomes: What Is the Worst-case Scenario

If a removal of the explant is indicated for the reasons discussed above, symptomatic relief can be achieved in the vast majority of patients.[2] However, there is a risk for re-detachment of the retina associated with this approach. In the literature, the re-detachment risk varies between 4% and 33%.[2,9,29] A study published in 1977 by Schwartz and Pruett[30] reported that a short duration of buckling and the presence of retinal tears, as opposed to holes, appeared to predispose to recurrence; in addition, a significantly higher re-detachment rate was found when buckles were removed for infection, which was attributed to the short duration of buckling and the associated inflammatory reaction found in these eyes. Re-detachments after removal of the buckle are related to the extent of vitreoretinal traction still present in the area of the original detachment and its extent. There is evidence that the risk for re-detachment is correlated to the timeframe between scleral buckle surgery and its removal with a decreased incidence seen in eyes with the buckle having been in place for a longer duration. Re-detachment rates were reported to be 39% in eyes in which the buckle was removed within 6 months after surgery, 21.4% after removal between 6 and 12 months, and 5.8% in eyes treated more than a year before removal of the explant.[30] Others found re-detachment rates of 47% after removal within a month after retinal detachment surgery.[31] It is somehow obvious that the presence of proliferative vitreoretinopathy at the time of buckle removal predisposes to a re-detachment of the retina.[31] In cases where scleral buckle removal is scheduled, a laser photocoagulation around the breaks and the areas of assumed traction may be considered but is not mandatory. Scleral buckle removal may be considered in eyes where vitrectomy is performed to reattach the retina, as scleral buckle removal may provide a more favorable retinal profile and improve the contact of the tamponade with the retinal surface.[32]

REFERENCES

1. Deutsch J, Aggarwal R, Eagling E. Removal of scleral buckling elements: A 10-year retrospective study. *Eye.* 1992;6:570–573.
2. Deokule S, Reginald A, Callaear A. Scleral explant removal: The last decade. *Eye.* 2003;17:697–700.
3. Smiddy WE, Miller D, Flynn HW Jr. Scleral buckle removal following retinal detachment surgery: Clinical and microbiologic aspects. *Ophthalmic Surg.* 1993;24:440–445.
4. Wiznia RA. Removal of solid silicone rubber exoplants after retinal detachment surgery. *Am J Ophthalmol.* 1983;95:495–497.

5. Wirostko WJ, Covert DJ, Han DP, et al. Microbiological spectrum of organisms isolated from explanted scleral buckles. *Ophthalmic Surg Lasers Imaging.* 2009;40(2): 201–202.

6. Liu DT, Chan WM, Fan DS, et al. An infected hydrogel buckle with Corynebacterium pseudotuberculosis. *Br J Ophthalmol.* 2005;89(2):245–246.

7. Ulrich RA, Burton TC. Infections following scleral buckling procedures. *Arch Ophthalmol.* 1974;92(3):213–215.

8. Buettner H, Goldstein BG, Anhalt JP. Infection prophylaxis with silastic sponge explants in retinal detachment surgery. *Dev Ophthalmol.* 1981;2:71.

9. Russo CE, Ruiz RS. Silicone sponge rejection. Early and late complications in retinal detachment surgery. *Arch Ophthalmol.* 1971;85:647–650.

10. Arribas NP, Olk RJ, Shertzer M, et al. Preoperative antibiotic soaking of silicone sponges. Does it make a difference? *Ophthalmology.* 1984;91:1684–1689.

11. Kittredge KL, Conway BP. Management of the exposed scleral explant. *Seminars in Ophthalmology.* 1995;10:53–60.

12. Roldán-Pallarés M, del Castillo Sanz JL, Awad-El Susi S, et al. Long-term complications of silicone and hydrogel explants in retinal reattachment surgery. *Arch Ophthalmol.* 1999;117(2):197–201.

13. Kishore K. Technique of scleral buckling for retinal detachment repair. In: Peyman GA, Meffert SA, Conway MD, eds. *Vitreoretinal Surgical Techniques.* Martin Dunitz, London, 3rd ed. 74.

14. Holland SP, Pulido JS, Miller D, et al. Biofilm and scleral buckle associated infections. A mechanism for persistence. *Ophthalmology.* 1991;98:933–938.

15. Lanigan LP, Wilson-Holt N, Gregor ZJ. Migrating scleral explants. *Eye.* 1992;6:317–321.

16. Russo CE, Ruiz RS. Silicone sponge rejection. Early and late complications in retinal detachment surgery. *Arch Ophthalmol.* 1971;85:647–650.

17. Shah CP, Garg SJ, Penne RB. Extrusion of hydrogel exoplant into upper eyelid 16 years after a scleral buckle procedure. *Indian J Ophthalmol.* 2011;59:238–239.

18. Shields CL, Demirci H, Marr BP, et al. Expanding MIRAgel scleral buckle simulating an orbital tumor in four cases. *Ophthal Plast Reconstr Surg.* 2005;21(1):32–38.

19. Le Rouic J, Bettembourg O, D'Hermies F, et al. Late swelling and removal of Miragel buckles: A comparison with silicone indentations. *Retina.* 2003;23:641–646.

20. Dresner SC, Boyer DS, Feinfeld RD. Autogenous fascial grafts for exposed retinal buckles. *Arch Ophthalmol.* 1991;109:288–289.

21. Regan C, Schepens CL. Erosion of the ocular wall by circling polyethylene tubing: a late complication of scleral buckling. *Trans Am Acad Ophthalmol Otolaryngol.* 1963; 67:335–341.

22. Nguyen QD, Lashkari K, Hirose T, et al. Erosion and intrusion of silicone rubber scleral buckle. Presentation and management. *Am J Ophthalmol.* 2001;21:214–220.

23. Urrets-Zavalia A Jr. Acute scleral necrosis: A hitherto unrecognized complication of retinal detachment surgery. *Trans Am Acad Ophthalmol Otolaryngol.* 1971;75:1035–1046.

24. McBrien NA, Jobling AI, Gentle A. Biomechanics of the sclera in myopia: Extracellular and cellular factors. *Optom Vis Sci.* 2009;86(1):E23–E30.

25. Rada JA, Shelton S, Norton TT. The sclera and myopia. *Exp Eye Res.* 2006;2(2):185–200.

26. Marin JF, Tolentino FI, Refojo MF, et al. Long-term complications of the MAI hydrogel intrascleral buckling implant. *Arch Ophthalmol.* 1992;110:86–88.

27. Kokame GT, Germar GG. Successful management of intruded hydrogel buckle with buckle removal, scleral patch graft, and vitrectomy. *Retina.* 2003;23(4):536–538.

28. Weissgold DJ, Millary RH, Bochow TA. Rescue of exposed scleral buckles with cadaveric pericardial patch grafts. *Ophthalmology.* 2001;108:753–758.

29. Hilton GF, Wallyn RH. The removal of scleral buckles. *Arch Ophthalmol.* 1978;96: 2061–2063.

30. Schwartz PL, Pruett RC. Factors influencing retinal redetachment after removal of buckling elements. *Arch Ophthalmol.* 1977;95(5):804–807.

31. Lindsey PS, Pierce LH, Welch RB. Removal of scleral buckling elements. Causes and complications. *Arch Ophthalmol.* 1983;101:570–573.

32. Rossi T, Boccassini B, Iossa M, et al. Scleral buckle removal associated with pars plana vitrectomy for recurrent retinal detachment. *Eur J Ophthalmol.* 2009;19(6):1050–1054.

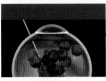

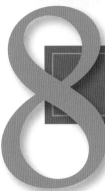

MISSED AND NEW RETINAL BREAKS

PAUL E. TORNAMBE

Most pneumatic retinopexy (PR) failures are due to new or missed retinal breaks. For the purpose of this chapter, I will not address other reasons for failure such as a break which fails to close, a break that re-opens, delayed resolution of subretinal fluid which is misdiagnosed as a failed procedure, subretinal gas (see Chapter 3), an inadequate size gas bubble (see Chapter 3), anterior hyaloid gas (see Chapter 3), or proliferative vitreoretinopathy (PVR) which collectively makes up about 10% of failed cases.

◆ The Complication

In the PR trial,[1] the initial failure rate from all causes was 27%, and the incidence of new or missed retinal breaks was 13%. Most new retinal breaks were located within 3 clock hours of the original break. The development of a new retinal break(s) does not usually doom the final prognosis.[2,3] Actually, we found that eyes which developed new breaks that were treated with another pneumatic procedure attained higher levels of vision than eyes successfully treated with one scleral buckling procedure.[1] Furthermore, initial failure did not diminish the overall retinal attachment rate.

Some misconceptions about the surgical success of PR relate to complications/outcomes associated with the use of heavy cryopexy or initially failed cases in which a rescue operation is performed long after the initial failed PR. This (waiting between failure and reoperation) would facilitate the development of PVR negatively affecting the outcome of future surgery. If gentle cryopexy is used and failed cases are re-operated within several days, outcomes are, in my personal experience, good.

PR does not directly address vitreous traction. Injection of the gas bubble, simply by taking up space and pushing the vitreous aside, may even aggravate vitreous traction. It is therefore not surprising that some eyes develop new breaks. Also, the natural history of posterior vitreous separation may result in subsequent new break formation. Interestingly, the incidence of new break formation after cryopexy or laser alone to treat a retinal break, not associated with a retinal detachment, has been reported to be ~14%.[4] This is comparable to the 13% incidence of new (or missed) retinal breaks observed in the PR clinical trial. PR deals with vitreous traction in two ways: (1) Laser applied to the retinal break will create an adhesion which will hopefully exceed vitreous tractional forces; (2) 360-degree laser photocoagulation cerclage performed between the posterior insertion of the vitreous base (which is not necessarily the equator) and the ora, although it will not prevent subsequent new break formation, it will prevent a new break from detaching the retina. I recommend 360-degree laser in all pseudophakic eyes following PR and in phakic cases which might be prone to new break formation (such as those with associated lattice degeneration, multiple retinal tears, mild vitreous hemorrhage, etc; see below).

One cannot separate the surgeon from the surgery. A trained surgeon, who finds all retinal breaks present, will have the best outcomes following PR. PR is, on the surface, a seductively simple operation to perform. However, success is largely determined by case selection and a good preoperative examination. "New" breaks may be more common in a busy teaching clinic where one assumes that all breaks are found in a pseudophakic eye with mild capsular clouding and a total bullous retinal detachment, or, in the patient where the superior half of the retina is detached but a mild hemorrhage limits a crisp view of the retina inferiorly making it difficult to be absolutely sure there are no round holes present in attached retina. The bubble is injected, the subretinal fluid is displaced inferiorly, and voila, the missed previously invisible flat hole is now elevated! The surgeon determines the operation failed from a "new" break.

Some feel new/missed retinal breaks occur more frequently in pseudophakic eyes treated with PR, and believe that pseudophakia is a relative contraindication for this procedure. Although new/missed breaks might occur more frequently in pseudophakic eyes treated with PR, in my experience, these eyes usually ultimately do well. To evaluate this issue, I reviewed 51 consecutive pseudophakic retinal detachments (unpublished data) that I personally operated upon (Tables 8-1 and 8-2). I defined a new break as positively a break that could not have been missed prior to the gas bubble injection. I defined missed breaks as subtle breaks, which were found at the time of re-operation. Certainly it is possible that a pinpoint hole could have developed when the gas bubble was injected, but I assumed not. Forty (78%) of these pseudophakic eyes were attached with a single pneumatic procedure, eleven (22%) failed. Of the 42 eyes I treated with 360-degree laser, 40 (95%) were attached with one operation. Obviously if the subretinal fluid did not resolve after the pneumatic operation, 360-degree laser could not be performed. Anatomical and visual results on this series of 51 pseudophakic eyes have been summarized in Table 8-2. Of the 11 eyes which failed initially to a single PR but which all ultimately attached, 82% (9/11) achieved ≥20/50 visual acuity, 64% (7/11) attained ≥20/40, and 18% (2/11) had a visual acuity of ≤20/400 or worse.

This study suggests that pseudophakic eyes may be successfully managed with PR with excellent overall visual acuity results, including eyes which failed the first

Table 8-1 • Pseudophakic Retinal Detachment Repair			
Author:	**Greven**[a]	**Ranta**[b]	**Tornambe**
Procedure	SB	SB +/− PPV	PR[c]
Single-op Success	77%	74%	78%
Missed Breaks	8%	22%	18%
New Breaks	10%	9%	4%

[a]Greven CM, Sanders RJ, Brown GC, et al. Pseudophakic retinal detachments. Anatomic and visual results. *Ophthalmology.* 1992;99(2):257–262.
[b]Ranta P, Kivelä T. Functional and anatomic outcome of retinal detachment surgery in pseudophakic eyes. *Ophthalmology.* 2002;109(8):1432–1440.
[c]Unpublished data.
SB, scleral buckle; PPV, pars plana vitrectomy.

Table 8-2 • Anatomical and Visual Outcomes of Pneumatic Retinopexy in a Consecutive Series of 51 Pseudophakic Retinal Detachments

Anatomical Outcomes	n (%)
Retina attached with a single PR	40/51 (78%)
Initial failure	11/51 (22%)
due to "new" breaks	2/51 (4%)
due to "missed" breaks	9/51 (18%)
PVR	2/51 (4%)
Retina attached at last follow-up[a]	51/51 (100%)
Functional Outcomes	
In "macula on" cases (22/51, 43%)	—
≥20/40	22/22 (100%)
≥20/25	19/22 (86%)
In "macula off" cases (29/51, 57%)	—
≥20/50	25/29 (86%)

[a]Further surgery (repeated PR, scleral buckling, or pars plana vitrectomy) was required to attach the retina following initial PR failure.

PR, pneumatic retinopexy; PVR, proliferative vitreoretinopathy

pneumatic attempt. This study compares favorably with other studies of pseudophakic detachments treated with scleral buckling or scleral buckling and vitrectomy (Table 8-1). Although higher initial failure rates are expected in pseudophakic eyes when compared with phakic eyes following PR, success can be achieved in many cases with this minimally invasive procedure and, even if initially unsuccessful, PR does not seem to negatively affect final outcomes.

Pathogenesis

The retina may detach following the occurrence of a retinal tear(s) before there is complete vitreous separation. True new retinal breaks can occur because the vitreous, which is only partially detached, continues to separate from the retina where it was previously attached at the vitreous base or elsewhere. If an operation is performed which does not address the attached vitreous at the vitreous base or elsewhere, when this attached vitreous separates, a new break may be created. This may happen as a result of the natural history of the vitreous separation from the retina or as a result of the vitreous being "forced" to separate by the expanding gas bubble, which occupies space, displaces the vitreous, and may facilitate the occurrence of vitreoretinal traction. As noted previously, eyes treated with cryopexy alone, and no gas bubble, have been reported to be associated with new breaks in ~14% of cases.

Risk Factors

The occurrence of multiple breaks, particularly at different distances from the ora serrata suggests abnormal vitreoretinal relationships. Eyes with vitreous blood or vitreous haze (uveitis) may be more prone to new breaks. If PR is attempted on these eyes, new breaks may be more likely. These factors can usually be determined preoperatively and these may not be the ideal eyes to undergo a pneumatic operation. If a larger than usual gas bubble is injected, more vitreous may be displaced and may result in a new retinal break. If excessive cryopexy is used or if cryotherapy is applied to the bare retinal pigment epithelium (RPE) beneath a large retinal tear/hole and RPE cells are liberated, new breaks may be more likely to occur as a result of PVR. It may be useful to check the number of pigmented cells present in the anterior vitreous prior to the PR and compare them with those seen following this procedure, as eyes with considerably higher number of pigmented cells following the pneumatic operation may be prone to develop new retinal breaks.

Pearls on How to Prevent It

◆ The larger the gas bubble the more likely vitreous traction will be adversely affected. Similarly, the longer the bubble is in the eye, the greater the chance the bubble will adversely affect the outcome. The bubble is your friend when the retina is detached but becomes your enemy once the retina attaches. I, therefore, almost always (95% of cases) inject a short-acting 0.5-cc SF6 bubble, which expands to about 1 cc, subtends 3 clock hours and lasts less than 2 weeks. I limit the patient's activity for the entire time the bubble is in the eye. I limit reading, exercise, and anything that might agitate the bubble. I reserve larger, longer-acting bubbles (C3F8) in cases where the eye is large, the break is large and/or posterior, or there is significant traction on the break mandating that the bubble be in contact with the break until the laser or cryopexy adhesion is mature, which takes about 17 days.

◆ Which eyes are prone to new breaks? The presence of several retinal breaks suggests a broader area of abnormal vitreoretinal traction. If incomplete vitreous separation is present, which may be detected clinically or ultrasonographically, the bubble of gas could also facilitate the occurrence of vitreoretinal traction and break formation. These are not ideal cases for PR, and new breaks can be expected. Eyes with active uveitis are also more likely to develop new breaks. These eyes may be hypotonous and are sometimes associated with choroidal detachment. PR may be tried in these cases; the success rate is lower in these PVR-prone eyes but sometimes gas insertion will raise the intraocular pressure (IOP) and resolve the choroidal detachment, making subsequent surgery safer. The pneumatic may sometimes even cure the detachment permanently.

◆ Can missed breaks be avoided? Certainly an experienced surgeon with a trained eye will miss fewer breaks. George Hilton was a master with the indirect ophthalmoscope; a break rarely missed his eye. The first pneumatic paper he and Sandy Grizzard[5] published revealed a single operation success rate of 80%. A recent review of Medicare patients treated with PR[6] reported about a 60% pneumatic success rate. The PR Clinical Trial 6-month results[7] showed wide variability between the seven participating centers, which included only fellowship-trained vitreoretinal specialists who were experienced with PR. For example, one center in the trial reported a single operation success rate of 100% for sclera buckle surgery, and 83% for PR. Another center reported a single operation success rate of 57% for sclera buckle surgery, and 67% for PR. One cannot separate the surgeon from the surgery. All surgeons do not get the same results, even trained vitreoretinal specialists.

◆ I advice doing a paracentesis before the bubble of gas is injected for two reasons: It prevents a sudden high pressure rise which is less traumatic to the retinal circulation and circulation to the optic nerve, and may make more room for the bubble to move around the vitreous gel with less force. It will also prevent prolapsing gas through sometimes damaged zonules into the anterior chamber. I also advice avoiding excessive cryopexy.

◆ I advice 360-degree laser photocoagulation in all pseudophakic eyes following PR and in phakic eyes which might be prone to new retinal break formation such as eyes with predisposing lesions such as associated lattice degeneration, multiple tears, mild vitreous hemorrhage, etc. Close follow-up is important for the first month when most new breaks develop. If a new break is diagnosed early, focal laser may be all that is necessary to prevent re-detachment. A 360-degree laser barrier to attached retina between the insertion of the vitreous base and the ora will minimize the chances of re-detachment from a new break in pseudophakic eyes and in phakic eyes prone to new breaks. It is important to apply the laser posterior to the insertion of the vitreous base. This area usually can be determined by noting the most posterior location of the most posterior retinal break. Unless a break is located directly over the long posterior ciliary nerves at 3 and 9 o'clock, I try to avoid retinopexy over these nerves which can result in a dilated pupil. I have done this treatment for several decades and have observed no long-term complications.

In conclusion, new breaks will develop even in the hands of experienced surgeons using the best techniques. This is the natural history of a posterior vitreous detachment. Most new breaks are likely missed breaks. A meticulous fundus examination by an experienced surgeon will minimize the chances of overlooking a break, and perhaps result in selecting a different operation if the break is inferiorly located. Smaller volume, shorter-acting gas bubbles are less likely to create new breaks. Minimal cryopexy incites less inflammation and is less likely to displace RPE cells, which should minimize the PVR rate.[8]

◆ Pearls on How to Solve It

◆ A new break, which re-detaches the retina or prevents the retina from initially attaching, is not a catastrophic event. If these eyes are re-operated promptly, within several days of the initial procedure, the outcomes are still very good. I prefer PR for it gives the best visual outcome, has the least morbidity, and remains the most cost effective means to reattach the retina even when re-operations are factored in.[9]

◆ In cases of failed PR and given that, based on my extensive experience, failure usually relates to the presence of abnormal vitreoretinal traction, I often prefer to perform pars plana vitrectomy for it is the only way to completely address vitreous traction and will remove inflammatory cytokines liberated by cryopexy. I will sometimes (~15%) use a buckle in addition to the vitrectomy. Re-intervention should be done very soon following the initial failure.

◆ Expected Outcomes: What Is the Worst-case Scenario

All operations carry some degree of risk, and the surgeon cannot be separated from the surgery. There is no disease in the human body that cannot be made worse by the doctor. However, PR if properly performed, even if initially unsuccessful, managed promptly would have very little downside. The worst-case scenario would be that the retina does not attach and a vitrectomy must be performed. The most common reason eyes are lost to retinal detachment is PVR. The pneumatic clinical trial proved that the PVR risk was not higher with PR than with a scleral buckle. Almost all intraoperative complications are avoidable. Some of these surgical misadventures include striking the crystalline lens during a paracentesis, closing the central retinal artery by injecting too much gas, injecting a gas bubble beneath the retina, incarcerating vitreous into the injection site with secondary tear formation, creating a new break during injection of gas, injecting gas into the space of Petit, and incarcerating iris into the paracentesis wound or vitreous hemorrhage. Immediate postoperative worst-case scenario includes endophthalmitis (which I have personally never seen even though I perform a paracentesis prior to gas bubble insertion on every case), new break formation, subretinal gas migration, failure of the retina to attach, choroidal detachment (never significant), and macular hole formation.

REFERENCES

1. Tornambe PE, Hilton GF, Brinton DA, et al. Pneumatic retinopexy. A two-year follow-up study of the multicenter clinical trial comparing pneumatic retinopexy with scleral buckling. *Ophthalmol.* 1991;98:1115–1123.
2. Ambler JS, Meyers SM, Zegarra H, et al. Reoperations and visual results after failed pneumatic retinopexy. *Ophthalmology.* 1990;97:786–790.
3. Boker T, Schmitt C, Mougharbel M. Results and prognostic factors in pneumatic retinopexy. *Ger J Ophthalmol.* 1994;3:73–78.
4. Verdaguer J, Vaisman M. Treatment of symptomatic retinal breaks. *Am J Ophthalmol.* 1979;87(6):783–788.
5. Hilton GF, Grizzard WS. Pneumatic retinopexy. A two-step outpatient operation without conjunctival incision. *Ophthalmology.* 1986;93:626–641.
6. Day S, Grossman DS, Mruthyunjaya P, et al. One-Year outcomes after retinal detachment surgery among medicare beneficiaries. *Am J Ophthalmol.* 2010;150(3): 338–345.
7. Tornambe PE, Hilton GF. Pneumatic retinopexy. A multicenter randomized controlled clinical trial comparing pneumatic retinopexy with scleral buckling. The Retinal Detachment Study Group. *Ophthalmology.* 1989;96:772–783.
8. Singh AK, Michels RG, Glaser BM. Scleral indentation following cryotherapy and repeat cryotherapy enhance release of viable retinal pigment epithelial cells. *Retina.* 1986;6:176–178.
9. Tornambe PE. Pneumatic retinopexy: The evolution of case selection and surgical technique. A twelve-year study of 302 eyes. *Trans Am Ophthalmol Soc.* 1997;95: 551–578.

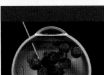
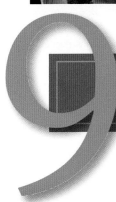

COMPLICATIONS RELATED TO the SETTING UP, MAINTAINING, AND CLOSING OFF the PORTS

JOSE GARCIA ARUMI AND MIGUEL ANGEL ZAPATA

9A Subconjunctival Hemorrhage, Marked Chemosis

A thorough understanding of how to set up and maintain the ports during surgery is crucial to the final surgical outcome. In addition, special care must be taken when closing the ports. Intraoperative problems related to the ports can lead to severe postoperative complications.

In small-gauge vitrectomy, the sclerotomy incisions are made with a trocar.[1] Microcannulas are hollow tubes mounted on the trocars before insertion to provide a port for passing instruments into the vitreal cavity. The trocar is removed once the microcannula is in place. These concepts are not always clear in the literature, where the terms trocar and microcannula are used interchangeably, and they are important to understand this chapter. The microcannulas are removed at closure of the sclerotomy sites.

SUBCONJUNCTIVAL HEMORRHAGE, MARKED CHEMOSIS

Subconjunctival hemorrhage and chemosis are usually innocuous complications, but their presence can hinder surgery and lengthen the operating time. These events are easily prevented and should be avoided to facilitate the procedure.

⬥ Risk Factors

Patients receiving antiplatelet or anticoagulation drugs.

⬥ How and When Does It Occur

During anesthesia, chemosis can occur when an excessive amount of anesthetic is instilled in the peribulbar space.

In conventional surgery, subconjunctival hemorrhage can occur when the conjunctiva is dissected. Profuse bleeding can obstruct the sclerotomy sites and hinder entry of instruments through the ports. Sometimes the bleeding stains the back of the wide-angle lens and compromises visibility.

In small-bore surgery, subconjunctival hemorrhage can occur on inserting or withdrawing the trocars. Although it is not a significant surgical risk, it can make location of the sclerotomies difficult, especially if they must be lengthened or sutured.

Pearls on How to Prevent It

◆ Correct Tenon dissection and diathermy are essential to prevent bleeding. In patients receiving antiplatelet or anticoagulant medication, treatment should be interrupted before surgery, if possible.

Pearls on How to Solve It

◆ In conventional surgery, chemosis does not create much of a problem as it can be easily corrected with proper dissection of the conjunctiva and use of a microsponge.

◆ When performing small-bore surgery, chemosis due to filtering around the microcannulas should be avoided, as it may change the degree of inclination of the trocars. To prevent this, trocar entries should be clean, and excessive manipulation of the microcannulas during surgery should be avoided. Chemosis can also occur when removing the microcannulas. If the wound leaks, fluid from the vitreous cavity can pass to the subconjunctival space producing a bleb. This does not imply an added risk, but makes it more difficult to locate the sclerotomies; in these cases, we advise suturing the sclerotomy. If the sclerotomy is easily located, a direct transconjunctival suture can be performed, using a loop suture. This is removed the following day to avoid granuloma formation and suture-related discomfort.

REFERENCE

1. Fujii GY, de Juan E Jr, Humayun MS, et al. A new 25-gauge instrument system for transconjunctival sutureless vitrectomy surgery. *Ophthalmology.* 2002;109:1807–1812.

9B Difficulties Related to the Location/Size of Sclerostomies

The location of the sclerostomies is very important, especially in patients who have undergone previous vitrectomy. In naive patients, the choice of sclerotomy sites is at the surgeon's discretion. Generally, we place the infusion in an inferotemporal location and perform a sclerotomy at 2 o'clock and 10 o'clock for the light and vitrectomy probe, respectively.[1] In patients with high myopia, these should be spaced further apart (3- and 9 o'clock); otherwise the instruments will be too vertical when accessing the macular area because of the increased anteroposterior diameter of the eye. In this way, it is easier to reach the entire retina with greater comfort for the surgeon.

DIFFICULTIES ESTABLISHING PORT SITES IN EYES WITH PREVIOUS VITRECTOMY

In patients who have undergone previous vitrectomy, it is helpful to know the location of previous sclerotomies and whether they were made radial or parallel to the limbus. With this information, the surgeon will be more confident when choosing sites for the new ports. We should avoid making new sclerotomies close to or perpendicular to previous incisions. We can use transillumination to find them.

It is important to check the condition and mobility of the conjunctiva over the area where the sclerotomy is planned. Usually, the conjunctiva and sclera are in a better state when the previous procedure was small-bore surgery. If the conjunctiva is scarred and immobile, a direct entry is preferable, with dissection of the adjacent conjunctiva at the end of the surgery to cover the sclerotomy.

If the first surgery was a 20G procedure performed less than 2 weeks before, an attempt can be made to use the same sites by removing the sutures and reopening the sclerotomies. When more than 2 weeks have passed, new port sites should be chosen. In small-bore surgery, we recommend not to use the tunnels made during the previous vitrectomy, because a double track can easily occur. If new entries are required, the infusion cannula should be placed on the side opposite to its previous location. The surgeon should remember not to compromise hand positioning when making these new sclerotomies.

ENLARGEMENT OF SCLEROTOMIES IN EYES WITH THIN SCLERA AND/OR PREVIOUS SURGERIES

✢ Risk Factors

Enlargement of the sclerotomies is more common in conventional surgery, particularly when performing vitrectomy in highly myopic eyes, those with thin sclera, or in children.[2,3]

✢ How and When Does It Occur

It occurs in thin and elastic scleras.

✢ Pearls on How to Prevent It

This event should be expected in at-risk cases and acted upon accordingly. As has been mentioned, it is more common in 20G vitrectomy and very uncommon with microcannula use. In small-bore vitrectomy in pediatric patients, patients with thin scleras, and highly myopic patients, the creation of the ports is similar to the technique used in conventional patients, but it is advisable to suture the sclerotomies.

✢ Pearls on How to Solve It

The following considerations should be kept in mind when large sclerotomies are used:

◆ The wounds are difficult to close and often need several sutures. Cross-stitching or U-shaped sutures are recommended in these cases.

◆ In large sclerotomies, vitreous incarceration easily occurs, and there is a higher risk of iatrogenic retinal breaks. The use of valved microcannulas can avoid this risk. At the end of the surgery, extraction of the microcannula with the light probe inside the instrument can also minimize vitreous incarceration.

If the enlarged sclerotomies are radial to the limbus, they may include the retina or ciliary body, which should be carefully checked after suturing.

REFERENCES

1. Michels RG. *Vitreous Surgery.* St Louis, MO: CV Mosby Co; 1981:114–118.
2. Zauberman H, Hemo I. The use of a silicone strip over the sclerotomy in vitreous surgery. *Ophthalmic Surg.* 1995;26(4):360–361.
3. Corcostegui B, Adan A, Garcia-Arumi J, et al. Cirugía Vitreorretiniana. Indicaciones y Técnicas. LXXV Official Lecture of the Spanish Society of Ophthalmology, Madrid. *Tecnimedia.* 1999:47.

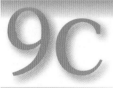

"Losing" the Tunnels During Trocar Insertion in Small-Bore Vitrectomy

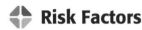

Risk Factors

Scleral tunnels may be "lost" on accidental withdrawal of the microcannulas. This usually occurs as the instruments are being removed and is more common with curved instruments, such as laser probes or forceps.

How and When Does It Occur

Removal of instruments drags the microcannula out of the sclera.

Pearls on How to Prevent It

◆ The most important measure is extreme care when removing the instruments, and awareness that they may be twisted and run aground when we remove them.

Pearls on How to Solve It

◆ If a microcannula is accidentally withdrawn, the first thing to do is return it to the trocar, locate the conjunctival wound, and, if possible, the scleral wound, and reinsert it. This is a difficult maneuver because chemosis quickly forms from the passage of fluid into the subconjunctival space and it becomes difficult to locate the entry. In such cases, it is helpful to dissect the conjunctiva and Tenon to achieve direct access to the sclera.

◆ When the scleral tunnel cannot be located, the area can be dried with micro-sponges to detect the leak. Another technique is to instill a topical dye (brilliant blue or diluted iodine solution) to expose the sclerotomy. The dye can be instilled over the conjunctiva or over the sclera if conjunctival dissection has been performed. Washing of the dye shows the leakage.

◆ If we still cannot locate the incision, the following can be done: Air exchange is performed and while the suspected area is continually irrigated with saline, the surgeon gently presses on the sclera to open the lip of the incision, where bubbles will be observed at the sclerotomy site. In rare cases, diathermy can be performed on suspected areas to show up the incision. The final option would be to create additional sclerotomies.

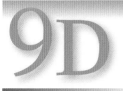

Suprachoroidal and Subretinal Infusion

Suprachoroidal and subretinal infusion are intraoperative complications that can have serious consequences. Their diagnosis and quick resolution are important for successful surgery.

SUPRACHOROIDAL AND SUBRETINAL INFUSION IN CONVENTIONAL 20G SURGERY

Risk Factors

Risk factors for suprachoroidal or subretinal infusion include media opacities, such as vitreous hemorrhage, and factors that make it difficult to reach the vitreous cavity, such as bullous retinal detachment or previous choroidal detachment. This complication occurs more commonly in reoperations, recent cataract surgery, and trauma.[1–3]

How and When Does It Occur

In conventional surgery without trocars, the infusion cannulas are usually 4 mm long and in some cases, the cannula does not reach the vitreous cavity.

Pearls on How to Prevent It

◆ Surgeons should take particular care in at-risk patients. Six-millimeter cannulas can be used in cases where difficulty reaching the vitreous cavity is expected.

Pearls on How to Solve It

◆ The infusion is closed at entry, and once the cannula is in place, it should be checked to ensure that it is within the vitreous cavity. It is advisable to perform this maneuver while indenting the infusion with forceps and illuminating with the light probe from outside the eye. If there is choroidal tissue on the cannula, it should be removed before opening the infusion. A contralateral sclerotomy is made, and the light probe is inserted. Since this is a blunt instrument, it can be used to gently rub against the edge of the infusion cannula, thereby opening the pars plana, and enabling access of the infusion to the vitreous cavity. The light probe will also let us see when the cannula is freed. This maneuver has also described with the use of a needle or 20G lancet.[1,4] We believe the light probe is safer because there is less risk of choroidal injury or bleeding than when the maneuver is done with a needle.

SUPRACHOROIDAL AND SUBRETINAL INFUSION IN SMALL-BORE SURGERY

✥ Risk Factors

Suprachoroidal or subretinal infusion has become a less common complication with the use of trocars and microcannulas. Usually the microcannulas are about 6 mm in length, and the trocars can be observed through the visual axis as they enter the vitreous cavity. Nonetheless, bullous retinal detachment, previous choroidal detachment, re-operations, recent cataract surgery, and trauma are risk factors for this complication.

✥ How and When Does It Occur

Suprachoroidal placement of the infusion may occur if highly angled incisions (about 5 or 8 degrees) with large scleral tunnels are performed.

✥ Pearls on How to Prevent It

◆ When the trocar is removed and the infusion line is in place, it must be checked to ensure that it is inside the vitreous cavity before opening the infusion. The same steps are followed as in conventional surgery. To check whether the infusion is within the vitreous cavity, the infusion line is held with an Adson forceps and the sclera is depressed. With direct visualization outside the microscope, we attempt to illuminate the metal cannula inside the eye with the handheld light probe. If the cannula is not visible, we can open a second port, insert the cutter, and do a bit of core vitrectomy to reduce pressure, thereby allowing easier scleral depression to see the cannula.

✥ Pearls on How to Solve It

◆ In small-bore vitrectomy involving a suprachoroidal or subretinal infusion, we can place a plug, open another port, and act in the same way as in conventional surgery, that is, attempt to remove choroidal tissue from the cannula before opening it.

CHOROIDAL DETACHMENT, CHOROIDAL HEMORRHAGE, RETINAL DETACHMENT

✥ Risk Factors

These complications are usually restricted to the beginning of the learning curve, and were more common in the first publications on small-bore surgery than they are today.[5]

✥ How and When Does It Occur

If the infusion line is opened when it is outside the vitreous cavity, retinal detachment, choroidal detachment, or suprachoroidal hemorrhage can occur.

✥ Pearls on How to Prevent It

◆ The position of the line should always be checked before it is opened, and checked again if we believe it has been accidentally moved during surgery.

Pearls on How to Solve It

◆ If the infusion is misdirected, the line should be closed as soon as possible. In pseudophakic patients, we may choose to place the infusion line in the anterior chamber. In this maneuver, the posterior capsule is respected because fluid is passing through the zonules. This temporary infusion is very useful in cases of hypotony or vitreous bleeding until another posterior infusion is established. In phakic patients, we recommend that a new infusion line be placed in the contralateral sclera. Proper positioning of the new line is verified before it is opened. Once the new infusion is established, it is advisable to remove the first infusion line so that subretinal or subchoroidal fluid can drain through the sclerotomy. When the surgeon is working with microcannulas, this complication can be resolved by changing the infusion to another microcannula at an entry site where there is no choroidal or retinal detachment. In some cases, the pars plana pigmented epithelium can be cut down with the vitrectomy probe to reveal the infusion. In phakic patients, it is advisable to perform this maneuver through the ipsilateral sclerotomy and in pseudophakic patients, through the contralateral sclerotomy. The epithelium is cut and pushed to the sclera.

REFERENCES

1. Michels RG. *Vitreous Surgery*. St Louis, MO: CV Mosby Co; 1981:114–118.
2. Corcostegui B, Adan A, Garcia-Arumi J, et al. Cirugía Vitreorretiniana. Indicaciones y Técnicas. LXXV Official Lecture of the Spanish Society of Ophthalmology, Madrid. *Tecnimedia*. 1999:47.
3. Charles S. *Vitreous Microsurgery*. Baltimore, MD: Williams & Wilkins; 1981:59.
4. de Juan E Jr, Landers MB 3rd. New technique for visualization of infusion cannula during vitreous surgery. *Am J Ophthalmol*. 1984;97(5):657–658.
5. Wimpissinger B, Kellner L, Brannath W, et al. 23-Gauge versus 20-gauge system for pars plana vitrectomy: A prospective randomized clinical trial. *Br J Ophthalmol*. 2008;92(11):1483–1487.

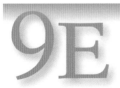 ## Accidental Intraoperative Removal of the Infusion Port

 ## Risk Factors

Nonfixed infusion, infusion fixed with Vicryl.

 ## How and When Does It Occur

Accidental removal of the infusion line is uncommon during conventional surgery because it is usually sutured with 5-0 or 6-0 nylon. Some surgeons prefer not to fix the infusion port or to fix the line with 6-0 or 7-0 Vicryl. The same Vicryl is used to close the sclerotomy at completion of surgery. In these cases, the strand is unstable and the infusion line can move easily.

✥ Pearls on How to Prevent It

◆ Accidental removal of the infusion line is uncommon during conventional surgery if suturing was done with 5-0 or 6-0 nylon. If Vicryl is preferred, the surgeon must be cautious during the procedure to avoid moving the line. It is advisable to put tape or a sterile strip on the cannula and drape to reduce the risk of pull-out. Experienced assistants minimize this risk.

✥ Pearls on How to Solve It

◆ If the infusion is accidentally removed, it is of utmost importance to reinfuse volume into the cavity to avoid hypotony and severe associated complications, such as choroidal hemorrhage.

◆ If accidental removal of the infusion line occurs during conventional surgery, the instruments are withdrawn and another infusion line is quickly placed through another sclerotomy to increase intraocular pressure. We should check to ensure that removal of the infusion cannula has not caused choroidal or retinal detachment, and again place the infusion line in the original port. If there is choroidal or retinal detachment at the original sclerotomy, another port can be used as the permanent infusion line.

◆ In small-bore vitrectomy, there are two infusion-related scenarios:

Accidental removal of the infusion line: The line is closed, it is reinserted in the microcannula, positioning is verified, and it is opened.

Accidental removal of the infusion line and microcannula: The infusion line is inserted through another microcannula and the procedure described in the section *"Losing the tunnels"* is followed. As was mentioned, it is very important to avoid hypotony.

◆ In small-gauge vitrectomy, some surgeons prefer to place the infusion in an inferior position. This is suggested to be a safer location, where accidental removal by the surgeon's assistant would be more difficult.

9F   Vitreoretinal Incarceration at the Sclerotomy

✥ Risk Factors

Wide sclerotomies and inadequate vitrectomy at the ports are risk factors for this complication.

✥ How and When Does It Occur

Differences in pressure from inside to outside pull the vitreous through the sclerotomy.

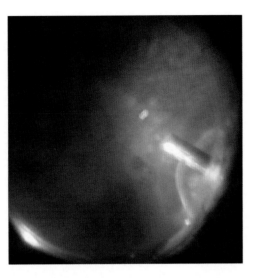

Figure 9F-1 Verification by scleral indentation just posterior to the entry site.

✦ Pearls on How to Prevent It

Vitreoretinal incarceration during surgery can lead to iatrogenic breaks and retinal detachment (see also Chapter 15). Certain precautions can help to prevent incarceration.

◆ Do not open the infusion line until the instruments are inside the eye.

◆ Perform conscientious vitrectomy at the ports.

◆ Check all sclerotomies before completing the surgery.

Use of an accessory light, such as a Chandelier or Torpedo, enables sclera indentation to be performed with one hand and shaving of the vitreous around the port with the other.

At the end of surgery, the sclerotomy and microcannula are checked with the wide-field lens and scleral indentation just posterior to the entry site **(Fig. 9F-1)**. Use of valved microcannulas averts exit of fluid when the instruments are removed, and decreases the risk of vitreous incarceration **(Fig. 9F-2)**.

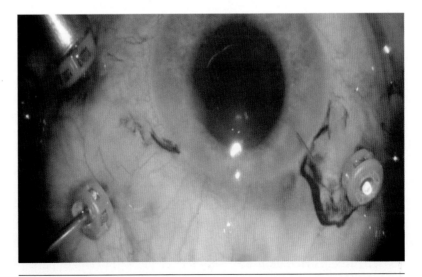

Figure 9F-2 Use of valved cannulas avoids exit of fluid when instruments are removed from the vitreous cavity and decreases the risk of vitreous incarcerations.

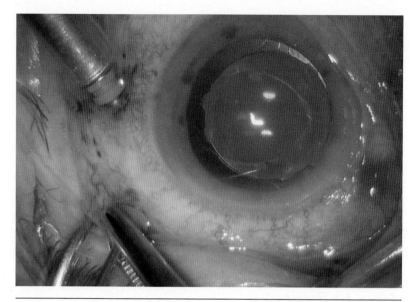

Figure 9F-3 Removal of the microcannulas with the light inside to decrease the risk of vitreous incarceration.

In small-bore vitrectomy, there is always some vitreous incarceration, usually at the time the microcannula is inserted.[1] Some authors have suggested that this could be a method for closing the sclerotomy.[2] The scleral tunnel is longer in small-bore surgery than in conventional surgery, and internal vitreous incarceration may not be accompanied by vitreous prolapse at the external sclera. Although there is some concern that vitreous plug vitrectomy during small-bore surgery might result in peripheral vitreous and retinal traction, the incidence of retinal detachment following 25G vitrectomy surgery does not seem to be higher than that of standard 20G surgery.[2–4] This may be because the intraocular portion of the microcannula protects the vitreous base around the sclerotomy during instrument insertion, withdrawal, or exchange, and the amount of vitreous that plugs the sclerotomy is likely not large enough to induce clinically significant traction.[2]

To prevent vitreous incarceration when using microcannulas, the microcannula should be removed while the light probe is inside **(Fig. 9F-3)**. Thus, the vitreous can be pushed back into the cavity before the light and its cannula are removed.[5]

New instruments have been created to prevent vitreous incarceration, such as an illuminated, curved 25G vitrectomy probe for removing vitreous from the sclerotomy sites.[6]

Pearls on How to Solve It

- Extensive vitreous base cleaning with scleral indentation is recommended when there are incarcerations or breaks near the sclerotomy.[7]

REFERENCES

1. Koch FH, Luloh KP, Singh P, et al. 'Mini-Gauge' pars plana vitrectomy: 'Inside-Out view' with the GRIN solid. rod endoscope. *Ophthalmologica*. 2007;221: 356–362.
2. de Juan E Jr, Fujii GY. 25-Gauge transconjunctival sutureless vitrectomy. Chapter 156. *Retina*. Philadelphia, PA: Elsevier Inc; 2006.

3. Recchia FM, Scott IU, Brown GC, et al. Small-gauge pars plana vitrectomy: A report by the American Academy of Ophthalmology. *Ophthalmology.* 2010;117(9): 1851–1857.

4. Scartozzi R, Bessa AS, Gupta OP, et al. Intraoperative sclerotomy-related retinal breaks for macular surgery, 20- vs 25-gauge vitrectomy systems. *Am J Ophthalmol.* 2007;143(1):155–156.

5. Rizzo S, Belting C, Genovesi-Ebert F, et al. Incidence of retinal detachment after small-incision, sutureless pars plana vitrectomy compared with conventional 20-gauge vitrectomy in macular hole and epiretinal membrane surgery. *Retina.* 2010;30(7): 1065–1071.

6. Chalam KV, Shah GY, Agarwal S, et al. Illuminated curved 25-gauge vitrectomy probe for removal of subsclerotomy vitreous in vitreoretinal surgery. *Indian J Ophthalmol.* 2008;56(4):331–334.

7. Wimpissinger B, Binder S. Entry-site-related retinal detachment after pars plana vitrectomy. *Acta Ophthalmol Scand.* 2007;85(7):782–785.

9G Leaking Ports at the End of Surgery

In conventional surgery, all sclerotomies must be sutured. Some authors use 6-0 or 7-0 nylon or silk.[1] We prefer an absorbable suture such as 7-0 Vicryl. Leaking ports are more common in small-bore vitrectomy.

Risk Factors

The angle of the incision and the bevelled effect created are important factors in sclerotomy closure. Over-angled sclerotomies make longer tunnels, but the microcannula may be accidentally placed in the suprachoroidal space. Under-angled sclerotomies make shorter tunnels that are less self-sealing.[2–4] Hypotony may influence the angle of the incisions, and special attention should be paid to this possible circumstance. In addition, significant manipulation of the sclerotomies during surgery can change the wound architecture from its original construction and thus make it relatively unstable and unpredictable.[5] Self-sealing may also depend on the shape and bevel direction of the trocars.[4] The shape of the incision can differ between different brands of trocars, but there are no studies to date comparing intraoperative complications between the various types.

How and When Does It Occur

Correct small-bore wound construction is critical to achieve self-sealing sclerotomies and avoid wound leakage and related complications. Oblique or bevelled incisions have been suggested to decrease wound leakage by creating an internal lip that presses against the external lip, which, with the aid of intraocular pressure, helps to close the wound.[6–9] Also, a small vitreous plug on the internal side of the port and the Tenon on the external side may help to close the sclerotomy.[10]

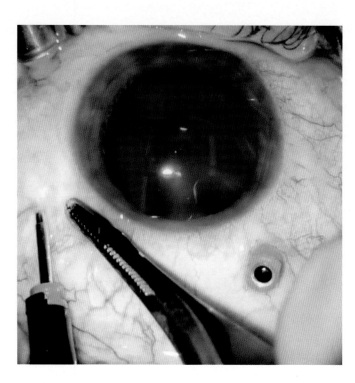

Figure 9G-1 Over-angled sclerotomies make longer tunnels and decrease the risk of leakage.

◆ Pearls on How to Prevent It

◆ We recommend initiating the sclerotomy at 5 degrees from the sclera, and at the midpoint of the maneuver, changing the angle to 30 degrees to finish entry (Fig. 9G-1).

◆ Pearls on How to Solve It

◆ Leaking sclerotomies can increase the risk of endophthalmitis and lead to post-operative hypotony. Some authors have described normalization of intraocular pressure during the first week.[10] Nevertheless, hypotonic eyes are at higher risk in proliferative diabetic retinopathy because vitreous hemorrhage and inflammation can occur. In pediatric patients, considerable inflammation can arise due to postoperative hypotony.

In the study by Woo et al.[11] including 322 eyes, the risk of leakage in 23G sclerotomies was 11.2%. In the same study, the following risk factors were cited for intraoperative sclerotomy leakage after 23G transconjunctival sutureless vitrectomy:

◆ Prior vitrectomy and vitreous base dissection, probably related to peripheral vitreous contraction,[10] and absence of the vitreous plug in the sclerotomy.

◆ Young age at operation: In patients younger than 40 years, leaking sclerotomies occurred in over 60% of cases. High elasticity of the sclera is related to leaking ports. In infants younger than 1 year of age, suturing sclerotomies is mandatory.[12]

In Woo's study, the risk of leakage had no correlation with sex, use of gas, or combo surgery. There were no statistical differences between the three sclerotomies.

The sclerotomies should be meticulously reviewed. We recommend sutures in highly myopic patients, and children, re-operations, and in those with silicone oil in the vitreous cavity. In young people, leaking through the sclerotomies is also more frequent; under these circumstances we recommend exhaustive revision and suturing if sclerotomies leak. Although the sclerotomies are usually self-sealing, they should all be checked to prevent postoperative endophthalmitis.[10] In a recent report, use of hydrogel polymer over the wound was proposed to seal the entries.[13]

When working with microcannulas, the presence of a leaking port during infusion of fluid into the vitreous cavity can lead to rapid chemosis or development of a subconjunctival bleb at the entry site. It is useful to dry the area with a microsponge to enable visualization of the leak. This can be helped by using a drop of topical colorant, such as brilliant blue, or a small drop of diluted iodine solution. If air is infused, saline solution irrigation over the conjunctiva will show up air bubbles. For suturing small-gauge wounds, some surgeons prefer direct transconjunctival suture. This is not possible when there is chemosis or a large bleb over the wound, however, and in these cases, dissection of the conjunctiva is mandatory.[10] We prefer absorbable 7-0 Vicryl for suturing the sclera and conjunctiva.

REFERENCES

1. Charles S. *Vitreous Microsurgery*. Baltimore, MD: Williams & Wilkins; 1981:59.
2. Witte V, Berger E, Guthoff R, et al. Three-dimensional visualization of sclerotomies with ultrasound biomicroscopy. Comparison of 20 and 23 gauge incisions on the porcine eyeball. *Ophthalmologe*. 2011;108:658, 660–664.
3. Gupta OP, Maguire JI, Eagle RC Jr, et al. The competency of pars plana vitrectomy incisions: A comparative histologic and spectrophotometric analysis. *Am J Ophthalmol*. 2009;147(2):243.e1–250.e1.
4. Choi KS, Kim HD, Lee SJ. Sclerotomy site leakage according to wound shape in 23-gauge microincisional vitrectomy surgery. *Curr Eye Res*. 2010;35(6):499–504.
5. Chen D, Lian Y, Cui L, et al. Sutureless vitrectomy incision architecture in the immediate postoperative period evaluated in vivo using optical coherence tomography. *Ophthalmology*. 2010;117(10):2003–2009.
6. Eckardt C. Transconjunctival sutureless 23-gauge vitrectomy. *Retina*. 2005;25:208–211.
7. Singh RP, Bando H, Brasil OF, et al. Evaluation of wound closure using different incision techniques with 23-gauge and 25-gauge microincision vitrectomy systems. *Retina*. 2008;28:242–248.
8. López-Guajardo L, Pareja-Esteban J, Teus-Guezala MA. Oblique sclerotomy technique for prevention of incompetent wound closure in transconjunctival 25-gauge vitrectomy. *Am J Ophthalmol*. 2006;141(6):1154–1156.
9. Taban M, Sharma S, Ventura AA, et al. Evaluation of wound closure in oblique 23-gauge sutureless sclerotomies with visante optical coherence tomography. *Am J Ophthalmol*. 2009;147(1):101.e1–107.e1.
10. de Juan E Jr, Fujii GY. 25-gauge transconjunctival sutureless vitrectomy. Chapter 156. *Retina*. Philadelphia, PA: Elsevier Inc; 2006.
11. Woo SJ, Park KH, Hwang JM, et al. Risk factors associated with sclerotomy leakage and postoperative hypotony after 23-gauge transconjunctival sutureless vitrectomy. *Retina*. 2009;29(4):456–463.
12. Gonzales CR, Singh S, Schwartz SD. 25-Gauge vitrectomy for paediatric vitreoretinal conditions. *Br J Ophthalmol*. 2009;93(6):787–790.
13. Singh A, Hosseini M, Hariprasad SM. Polyethylene glycol hydrogel polymer sealant for closure of sutureless sclerotomies: a histologic study. *Am J Ophthalmol*. 2010; 150(3):346.e2–351.e2.

9H   Difficulties Suturing and Closing the Sclerotomies

Risk Factors

Difficulties in suturing often depend on the size of the sclerotomy and particularly, the state of the sclera. Greater difficulties are encountered in patients with thin sclera, those with previous vitreoretinal surgery, and cases in which a double track is created on insertion of the instruments or trocars.

How and When Does It Occur

Large or double track sclerotomies usually need more than one suture. Difficulties in suturing the sclerotomy usually occur when previous and current sclerotomies are made close to each other and are not aligned. Under these circumstances, the tightening of the sutures in the recent sclerotomy may lead to leaking of the previously performed one.

Pearls on How to Prevent It

- Surgeons must be cautious in at-risk cases, taking care not to enlarge the sclerotomies or establish double tracks. We believe it is imperative to sufficiently dissect the conjunctiva and Tenon over the incision and use only thin forceps with small teeth so as to not harm the lips of the sclerotomy.

Pearls on How to Solve It

- Surgeons must concentrate when suturing, although it is at the end of surgery. Cross-stitching or U-shaped sutures are sometimes advisable. In some cases, such as highly myopic eyes or following multiple surgeries, a patch of dura mater or similar material can be used to close intractable ports. This is exceptional in small-bore surgery.

10 COMPLICATIONS RELATED to the CRYSTALLINE LENS

MARTIN S. SPITZER AND PETER SZURMAN

10A Development of Cataract Intraoperatively (Not Related to Lens Touch)

⬥ The Complication: Definition

The development of cataract is the most frequent complication associated with pars plana vitrectomy. While the formation of lens opacities frequently occurs postoperatively, especially following long-term tamponade, it may also occur intraoperatively and interfere with adequate fundus visualization.[1]

The typical intraoperative (or early postoperative) feathered subcapsular opacification will disappear within days,[2] but may hinder the surgeon's view at the end of the procedure or during long cases.

It should be noted that a relatively sudden poor view of the fundus is not always necessarily related to lens opacification. Particularly in complicated cases, there are many reasons that may explain poor visualization of the fundus mimicking increased lens opacity, as follows: (1) Vitreous hemorrhage may adhere to the retrolental vitreous which is difficult to remove; (2) anterior chamber erythrocytes can sediment on top of the lens capsule and remain unrecognized; (3) triamcinolone or emulsified silicone oil particles can be easily entrapped in the retrolental vitreous remnants; (4) dyes, especially trypan blue, are well recognized for their staining capacity of the lens capsule leading to a darker fundus view for several minutes; (5) perfluorocarbon liquid (PFCL) tends to stick to the posterior capsule if filled up too anteriorly; (6) this is also true for some heavy silicone oils (Densiron 68). In many cases a meticulous irrigation of the anterior and posterior chamber or a fluid–air exchange will solve the problem by removing the obscuring material from the lens.

⬥ Risk Factors

The precise causes of intraoperative cataract formation or progression during vitrectomy are unknown. But several risk factors have been identified and comprise extensive surgical manipulation, high fluid flow during the procedure, and repetitive fluid–air/gas exchanges.[3] Of interest, duration of vitrectomy does not seem to be among them. Cheng and colleagues could show that the development of cataract was independent of surgical time.[4]

One of the most important risk factors for intraoperative (and postoperative) lens opacification is age. If lens opacification occurs during vitrectomy, it is most likely that a pre-existing cataract has deteriorated intraoperatively (Fig. 10A-1).

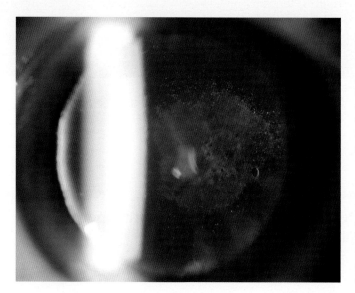

Figure 10A-1 Slit-lamp photography (day 2) of a preoperatively unrecognized subcapsular cataract which dramatically deteriorated that impaired fundus view during vitrectomy. Note the fluid vacuoles (around the pre-existing fibrosis) that correspond to multilocular subcapsular fluid accumulation. Postoperatively, the vacuoles completely resolved, while the fibrotic part remained, but did not show relevant progression.

Elder lenses are obviously more prone to cataract progression.[5–7] This vulnerability of the lens is due to a "weaker" capsule which withstands less to an intraoperative fluid ingress (short-term "lens feathering") and the lower concentration of protective antioxidant substances within the lens in elderly people (long-term progression of nuclear sclerosis).[8]

Intraoperative cataract rarely develops in juvenile, healthy eyes. If so, it is either due to an intraoperative trauma [lens touch (see Chapter 10B), high fluid flow, and working under air] or due to a pre-existing (unrecognized) damage to the lens capsule. A rare but rather worrisome complication is the inadvertent intralenticular injection of air or gas during vitrectomy. This may necessitate early cataract surgery or even lensectomy during vitrectomy.

Pathogenesis: Why Does It Occur

The crystalline lens can opacify during surgery especially in complicated cases, which makes retinal manipulations later on in the procedure extremely challenging. As stated above, intraoperative opacification rarely happens in a clear and juvenile lens and it is more likely that a pre-existing cataract deteriorates intraoperatively. Hence, there is an increasing trend toward combined surgery with phacoemulsification, intraocular lens (IOL) implantation, and vitrectomy in patients over 60 years.

The precise mechanisms that are responsible for intraoperative cataract development are unknown. However, it is likely that the underlying pathophysiology is similar to the mechanisms of postoperative cataract formation:

In many eyes a transient posterior subcapsular cataract ("lens feathering") may be observed within 24 hours after vitreoretinal surgery commonly when gas is inserted **(Fig. 10A-2)**. It is hypothesized that high fluid flow during the procedure and repetitive fluid/air exchange cause acute damage in the permeability of the posterior capsule. This facilitates accumulation of fluid in the posterior subcapsular lens fibers. This fluid collection usually resolves within a few days thereafter and normally results in no permanent lens opacification.[8]

A similar mechanism may be responsible for an intraoperative lens opacification. Extensive manipulation in the retrolental space and high fluid flow may weaken the lens capsule (microruptures) and allow water ingress and fluid accumulation in the subcapsular space. This particularly happens when the infusion cannula is pointing directly at the lens.

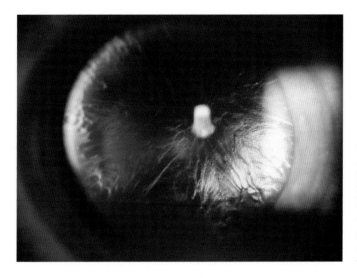

Figure 10A-2 Slit-lamp photography (day 1) of a transient posterior subcapsular cataract ("lens feathering") after vitreoretinal surgery with gas tamponade. It disappeared after 3 days.

If a clear lens spontaneously clouds during vitrectomy, it is most probably a sign for the above mentioned microruptures of the posterior capsule. However, it may also hint at a pre-existing weakness of the lens capsule: A typical situation is vitreoretinal surgery in trauma cases where the lens seems to be uninjured but rapidly becomes intumescent during constant irrigation. This is similar in vitrectomy for endophthalmitis, where the lens capsule may also be invisibly damaged due to bacteria toxins and intravitreal antibiotics. Finally, one should also consider a subtle lens touch with or without a capsular breach having remained unrecognized (see Chapter 10B).

Another factor for capsular weakening and consecutive water ingress is the transient dehydration of the posterior capsule during the filling of the vitreous cavity with air or gas. This is of special importance if working under air for a longer time (e.g., laser photocoagulation under air in retinal detachment surgery). Albeit transient, this may lead to a progressively obscured view making further vitreoretinal maneuvers difficult **(Fig. 10A-3)**. Unfortunately, switching to balanced salt solution (BSS) rarely improves the situation, but rather deteriorates it due to increased water ingress.

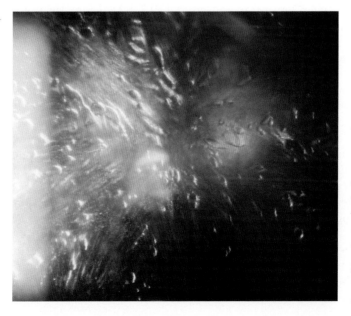

Figure 10A-3 Slit-lamp photography (day 1) of subcapsular fluid accumulation that developed during vitrectomy. Intraoperatively, visualization rapidly obscured after 20-minutes surgical time during endophotocoagulation under air. Note the similarity to the "classic" postoperative lens feathering.

Harlan and colleagues proposed the use of humidified air or gas to delay or to prevent dehydration of the lens capsule.[9] They confirmed their hypothesis in a rabbit vitrectomy model testing the intravitreal instillation of humidified versus room air.

One of the most important factors for intraoperative and early postoperative cataract formation is the excessively high oxygen tension during vitrectomy and postoperative gas tamponade which is responsible for the classic "lens feathering." The increased oxygen tension leads to oxidative stress to the vulnerable lens fibers. The irrigation solution provides an excessively high oxygen level that interferes with the electrolyte balance within the lens fibres and leads to fluid inflow into the subcapsular space. Of interest, even the irrigation solution (without any use of air) provides an excessively high oxygen level. It has been shown that balanced salt solution shortly after opening the bottle had an oxygen tension of 70 mm Hg that increased further due to the irrigation tubing and room air to 160 mm Hg before entering the eye.[10] Breathing oxygen during general anesthesia may increase the intravitreal oxygen tension even further.[11] The oxygen level remains increased even long after vitrectomy due to the removal of the vitreous gel itself.

On the other hand a high oxygen tension albeit possibly damaging to the lens may be protective for the retina during and after vitrectomy. Thus, attempts to lower the oxygen tension during vitrectomy might not be helpful. For cataract prevention one should rather consider irrigation solutions with added antioxidants such as glutathione[12] or taurine[13]; however, these newer irrigation solutions have not been evaluated in this respect to date.

Why does oxygen promote cataract formation? Reactive oxygen species (ROS) are known to inhibit most enzymes through oxidation.[14] This is especially true for the Na^+-K^+-ATPase which is most important for the fluid equilibrium within the lens fibres. The fluid and electrolyte balance is mainly maintained through potassium-selective ion channels and the Na^+-K^+-ATPase on the lens basement membrane and on the outer lens fibers. A disturbance of these channels may cause fluid inflow into the lens especially in the posterior subcapsular part causing "lens feathering" intraoperatively or in the early postoperative period.

Physiologically, oxygen concentration in the human lens is much lower (around 2.5 mm Hg) than that in the anterior chamber or the vitreous.[15,16] The pressure gradient has been best shown in a rabbit model: In nonvitrectomized eyes the lowest oxygen partial pressure has been found inside the lens (10.4 ± 3 mm Hg) and in the central vitreous behind the lens (12.7 ± 3.2 mm Hg), whereas the highest was found directly over the retina at the retinal vessels (40 to 60 mm Hg). Immediately after vitrectomy the oxygen tension increased to 119.3 ± 18.9 mm Hg in the central vitreous. Thirty minutes after the end of surgery oxygen tension decreased to 28.9 ± 12.2 mm Hg.[17] Of interest, even months after vitrectomy the oxygen tension remained elevated in the lens.[10]

Similar results have been found in humans.[10] Obviously the vitreous is protective against cataract development.[18] This has also been shown in young patients with Stickler syndrome or high myopia with a liquefied vitreous who develop cataracts much earlier than age-matched controls.[19] The presence of liquefaction of the vitreous prior to vitrectomy also seems to hasten cataract development. Patients younger than 50 years without vitreous liquefaction develop far less cataracts than patients above the age of 50 years with a liquefied vitreous.[7] Vitreoretinal procedures without vitreous gel removal such as membrane peeling without vitrectomy, pneumatic retinopexy, or repetitive intravitreal injections hardly cause cataract progression.[17,20]

Of interest, due to the syncytium physiology of the lens fibres, the intraoperative breakdown of the fluid and electrolyte balance in the subcapsular region will also have an impact on the inner lens fibres in the nucleus. While the initial subcapsular fluid is rapidly resolved the nuclear sclerotic lens opacification like in age-related cataract slowly proceeds.[3]

Pearls on How to Prevent It

◆ Perform biometry prior to vitrectomy whenever rapid cataract development must be expected. To be on the safe side, try to generally establish biometry as part of the routine preoperative assessment in all cases of phakic patients undergoing pars plana vitrectomy. This will enable you to perform unplanned phacoemulsification and IOL implantation if needed.

◆ When silicone oil tamponade is planned, select the IOL for the refractive status after silicone oil removal unless long-term silicone oil filling is desired.

◆ Perform slit-lamp evaluation of the lens status preoperatively in all vitrectomy patients. When the lens opacification is pronounced combined cataract extraction and vitrectomy may be considered.

◆ When placing the infusion cannula care should be taken that the tip and the fluid stream is directed away from the crystalline lens.

◆ During indentation avoid pushing the infusion port into the lens equator. Indent the infusion port toward the center of the eye, not anteriorly, toward the lens.

◆ Meticulously avoid any maneuvers risking an intraoperative lens touch (for more details on avoiding and management of lens touch see Chapter 10B).

◆ The use of humidified air may prevent or delay lens feathering.

◆ One might assume that transconjunctival small-gauge vitrectomy using trocars especially with valves may contribute to a lower rate of intraoperative lens opacities due to their considerably lower fluid convection, infusion volumes, and intraoperative pressure changes.

◆ Use only balanced salt solution for intravitreal irrigation that contains the appropriate bicarbonate, pH, and ionic composition necessary for the maintenance of normal cell physiology [e.g., PuriProtect (Zeiss) or BSS Plus (Alcon)].[21]

◆ Consider the use of balanced salt solution with added antioxidants such as glutathione or taurine for surgery with a long intraocular perfusion time.

◆ Try to limit all factors that may increase the oxygen tension of the irrigating solution used before entering the eye (both long tubing and long-standing contact of the bottled salt solution to room air increase oxygenation).[10]

 ## Pearls on How to Solve It

◆ Make sure that there is no other reason for obscured fundus view mimicking a lens opacification.

◆ To remove adhering PFCL drops from the lens it is often sufficient to tilt the globe and the "heavy" liquid will flow out.

◆ In long-lasting vitreoretinal surgery, be aware that corneal edema is more likely to develop than an intraoperative cataract. In these cases a corneal abrasion may improve the view to the posterior pole sufficiently enough to finish the vitreoretinal surgery.

◆ A transient lens feathering after fluid/air exchange rarely improves even if BSS is inserted again into the vitreous cavity. It rather worsens the situation due to rapid water ingress through the weakened capsule.

◆ A significant opacification, that develops during vitrectomy is rarely reversible and has to be managed by phacoemulsification with IOL implantation in most cases. Certain aspects should be taken into account when performing cataract surgery during vitrectomy:

◆ If at all possible try to identify high-risk cases (trauma eyes, senile cataract) for intraoperative opacification prior to vitrectomy and consider in doubt a combined approach with completing phacoemulsification and IOL implantation first before starting with vitrectomy.

◆ If an intraoperative opacification of the lens occurs obscuring the view to the posterior pole an unplanned cataract surgery has to be performed. Phacoemulsification can be done at any time point of vitrectomy except after fluid/air exchange. The vitreous cavity can be filled with BSS, PFCL, or in rare cases with silicone oil, but not with air or gas. The latter exerts high pressure to the lens capsule making cortex aspiration and IOL implantation difficult. An anterior approach with clear cornea incision may be preferable for simultaneous cataract surgery. During phacoemulsification, the infusion is closed. In these cases the use of trocars with valves is advantageous to maintain a pressurized globe. If not available, all sclerotomies have to be temporarily sutured or closed with plugs. Special attention should be given to a meticulous capsular rhexis to ensure that the edge of the rhexis circularly covers the IOL, as the optic can easily dislocate during vitrectomy and especially after gas tamponade.[22,23] If you have the suspicion of a subtle capsular breach, especially in trauma eyes, avoid any kind of hydrodissection and use a low infusion pressure (low bottle height). Both may deteriorate a pre-existing capsular breach with inadvertent nucleus drop to the posterior pole. The IOL is usually implanted before the vitrectomy is continued. Place a 10-0 nylon suture at the tunnel in all cases, not only if the tunnel is unstable. Constant scleral depression has the capacity to reopen even meticulously prepared self-sealing tunnel incisions.

◆ If preferred, IOL implantation can be delayed to the end of vitrectomy. However, the IOL should be implanted prior to gas or silicone oil instillation.

◆ If an IOL is placed, try to avoid posterior capsulotomy, if working under air is intended. Air humidity may condense on the IOL surface obscuring the view within seconds. Placement of hydroxypropyl–methylcellulose gel may help solving this problem **(Fig. 10A-4)**.

◆ When capsular bag implantation is not feasible in combined procedures with gas or silicone oil filling, alternative fixation techniques of the IOL (sulcus

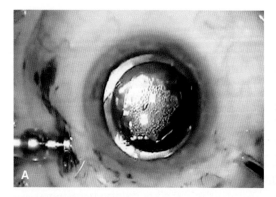
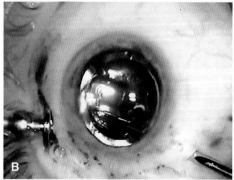

Figure 10A-4 A: Intraoperative photography of condensing air humidity on the posterior surface of an IOL immediately after posterior capulotomy. **B:** After placing hydroxypropyl–methylcellulose gel the fundus view improved.

placement, transscleral or iris fixation) should be postponed to the time point of silicone oil removal or gas resolution.

 ## Expected Outcomes: What Is the Worst-case Scenario

An inadvertent injection of an air or gas bubble into the lens may lead to acute lens opacification and a large capsular breach. Albeit uncommon, this leads to an immediate and complete loss of fundus visualization. This makes endophacoemulsification via pars plana impossible (see Chapter 12B). Alternatively, the limbal approach is also difficult because anterior chamber irrigation in the presence of a large capsular defect often leads to a nucleus drop.

REFERENCES

1. Petermeier K, Szurman P, Bartz-Schmidt UK, et al. [Pathophysiology of cataract formation after vitrectomy]. *Klin Monbl Augenheilkd.* 2010;227:175–180.
2. Hsuan JD, Brown NA, Bron AJ, et al. Posterior subcapsular and nuclear cataract after vitrectomy. *J Cataract Refract Surg.* 2001;27:437–444.
3. Panozzo G, Parolini B. Cataracts associated with posterior segment surgery. *Ophthalmol Clin North Am.* 2004;17:557–568, vi.
4. Cheng L, Azen SP, El-Bradey MH, et al. Duration of vitrectomy and postoperative cataract in the vitrectomy for macular hole study. *Am J Ophthalmol.* 2001;132: 881–887.
5. Cherfan GM, Michels RG, de Bustros S, et al. Nuclear sclerotic cataract after vitrectomy for idiopathic epiretinal membranes causing macular pucker. *Am J Ophthalmol.* 1991;111:434–438.
6. Melberg NS, Thomas MA. Nuclear sclerotic cataract after vitrectomy in patients younger than 50 years of age. *Ophthalmology.* 1995;102:1466–1471.
7. Thompson JT. The role of patient age and intraocular gas use in cataract progression after vitrectomy for macular holes and epiretinal membranes. *Am J Ophthalmol.* 2004;137:250–257.
8. Petermeier K. Cataract formation. *Klin Monbl Augenheilkd.* 2010;227:175–180.
9. Harlan JB Jr, Lee ET, Jensen PS, et al. Effect of humidity on posterior lens opacification during fluid-air exchange. *Arch Ophthalmol.* 1999;117:802–804.
10. Barbazetto IA, Liang J, Chang S, et al. Oxygen tension in the rabbit lens and vitreous before and after vitrectomy. *Exp Eye Res.* 2004;78:917–924.
11. Holekamp NM, Shui YB, Beebe DC. Vitrectomy surgery increases oxygen exposure to the lens: a possible mechanism for nuclear cataract formation. *Am J Ophthalmol.* 2005;139:302–310.
12. Araie M, Shirasawa E, Hikita M. Effect of oxidized glutathione on the barrier function of the corneal endothelium. *Invest Ophthalmol Vis Sci.* 1988;29:1884–1887.
13. Schultheiss M, Ruschenburg H, Warga M, et al. Neuroprotective effects of a taurine-containing irrigation solution for vitrectomy. *Retina.* 2012;32:1343–1349.
14. Delamere NA, Tamiya S. Expression, regulation and function of Na,K-ATPase in the lens. *Prog Retin Eye Res.* 2004;23:593–615.
15. Helbig H, Hinz JP, Kellner U, et al. Oxygen in the anterior chamber of the human eye. *Ger J Ophthalmol.* 1993;2:161–164.
16. Shui YB, Fu JJ, Garcia C, et al. Oxygen distribution in the rabbit eye and oxygen consumption by the lens. *Invest Ophthalmol Vis Sci.* 2006;47:1571–1580.
17. Saito Y, Lewis JM, Park I, et al. Nonvitrectomizing vitreous surgery: a strategy to prevent postoperative nuclear sclerosis. *Ophthalmology.* 1999;106:1541–1545.
18. Holekamp NM, Harocopos GJ, Shui YB, et al. Myopia and axial length contribute to vitreous liquefaction and nuclear cataract. *Arch Ophthalmol.* 2008;126:744;author reply 744.

19. Harocopos GJ, Shui YB, McKinnon M, et al. Importance of vitreous liquefaction in age-related cataract. *Invest Ophthalmol Vis Sci.* 2004;45:77–85.
20. Mougharbel M, Koch FH, Boker T, et al. No cataract two years after pneumatic retinopexy. *Ophthalmology.* 1994;101:1191–1194.
21. Winkler BS, Simson V, Benner J. Importance of bicarbonate in retinal function. *Invest Ophthalmol Vis Sci.* 1977;16:766–768.
22. Girard LJ, Canizales R, Esnaola N, et al. Subluxated (ectopic) lenses in adults. Long-term results of pars plana lensectomy-vitrectomy by ultrasonic fragmentation with and without a phacoprosthesis. *Ophthalmology.* 1990;97:462–465.
23. Rahman R, Rosen PH. Pupillary capture after combined management of cataract and vitreoretinal pathology. *J Cataract Refract Surg.* 2002;28:1607–1612.

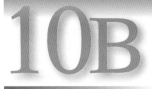

Lens Touch with or without Capsular Breach

 ## The Complication: Definition

A lens touch during pars plana vitrectomy is a serious complication. It nearly always results in rapid cataract formation and bears the potential of capsular damage during phacoemulsification. The extent of lens touch can be quite variable which may have very different consequences (depending on the severity of lens touch). The vitreoretinal surgeon has to be able to manage this problem appropriately.

A mild touch of the lens happens **(Fig. 10B-1)** quite commonly and often stays unnoticed if located peripherally at the lens equator. A circumscribed mild lenticular touch most likely will result later in sectorial or generalized lens opacity; however, it will not interfere with the intraoperative course during vitrectomy. The

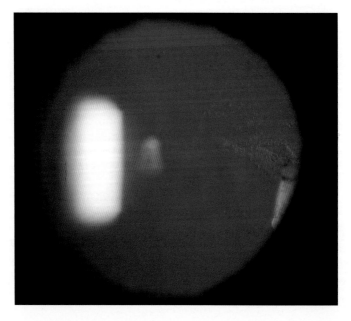

Figure 10B-1 Slit-lamp photography of a lens touch without capsular breach.

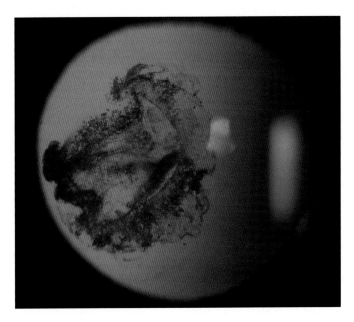

Figure 10B-2 Slit-lamp photography of a lens touch with capsular breach.

vitreoretinal surgeon can proceed as planned and the problem can be approached later at the time of cataract surgery, which often may be more complicated than in "untouched" lenses.

In more severe cases of lens touch an opacity that interferes with fundus visualization may develop during vitrectomy. In such cases the vitreoretinal surgeon must decide whether to perform an unplanned phacoemulsification with or without intraocular lens (IOL) implantation. Apart from the general dangers associated with an unplanned procedure, one must make a judgment whether a sufficiently stable iris–lens diaphragm can be achieved, if the use of a tamponade is planned.

In extreme cases lens touch may lead to a capsular breach **(Fig. 10B-2)** with dropping of lens fragments or even the entire nucleus. In such (fortunately rare) circumstances the surgeon has to deal with two problems: On the one hand lens removal via pars plana with the phacofragmatome or the vitreous cutter is more difficult and is known to bear a considerable risk for intraoperative retinal breaks and cellular damage to the retina. On the other hand, pronounced capsular damage mostly makes preserving a stable iris–lens diaphragm by IOL implantation difficult or impossible.

The most important question the surgeon has to answer after identifying lens touch is whether managing this problem can be delayed to a time point after vitrectomy or whether it should be addressed intraoperatively. Basis for the decision should be the following two considerations: (1) Is intraoperative view to the fundus sufficient to complete vitrectomy safely? (2) Can the iris–lens diaphragm be sufficiently preserved or restored?

An intraoperative lens touch is a good example that modern intraocular surgery is nowadays less suitable for rigid subspecialization. If possible, vitreoretinal surgeons should learn and master cataract surgery to be capable to solve complex situations including anterior segment problems like lens touch or a dislocated lens.

⬥ Risk Factors

Although a lens touch may happen to any vitreoretinal surgeon at any time, less-experienced surgeons are more likely to touch the crystalline lens accidentally. Often it results from wrong judgment of the spatial distance to the posterior lens surface. There are typical situations and risky maneuvers which predispose to a consecutive lens touch.[1] A fundamental working knowledge of these risk factors as well as the correct anatomy of the pars plana and the position of the lens help to prevent many unfavorable situations.

First, one should bear in mind that there is only little space peripheral to the crystalline lens in phakic eyes and the convex anatomy of the lens should be kept in mind when vitrectomy close to the lens is performed. Access to the vitreous base is limited and too much ambition in trimming the vitreous base may cause trouble.

One should remember that the eye is basically a sphere with the lens extending spherically behind the pars plana. The posterior margin of the lens is nearly at the same level (height) as the sclerotomies. This means that only a consequent perpendicular direction of the surgical instruments introduced via the pars plana is safe. Therefore, the correct positioning of the sclerotomies is an important step to prevent lens touch. It typically occurs at the lens periphery at the 2- or 10 o'clock position, hence adjacent to the working sclerotomies.

With the advent of small-gauge surgery the incidence of lens touch seems to have decreased (although unproven), because trocars allow for a smoother insertion of the instruments compared to 20G surgery where often a resistance during instrument introduction through the sclerotomy is encountered.

The use of trocars may avoid this specific problem, but also a too anteriorly selected location of the trocars bears the risk for a lens touch. In phakic eyes it is recommended to create sclerotomies at 4 mm posterior to the limbus (in adults with normal axial length). However, problems may occur if this rule is followed in hyperopic eyes with a short axial length or children, in whom the pars plana is shorter.[2]

Another maneuver with risk for lens touch is the introduction of the infusion cannula. It is mandatory to examine the inner opening of the infusion cannula to verify its intravitreal position with a free orifice before starting the infusion. However, during this maneuver the surgeon must be careful not to touch the lens in phakic patients.

Another potential danger of small-gauge vitrectomy systems is that the infusion cannula is more mobile than with 20G system. The latter is usually secured with a scleral suture. A mobile infusion port can easily be angled or displaced during small-gauge vitrectomy. Therefore, the loop of the infusion tubing should be secured either to the drape or better to a special clamp attached to the lid speculum to avoid unintentional displacement of the infusion cannula.

The presence of the natural lens makes working in the area of the vitreous base and the retrolental space challenging. The surgeon must be aware that the access to the vitreous base in phakic eyes is limited. A common mistake is the attempt to cross the midline with the instruments to trim the opposite vitreous base. In phakic eyes, you can cross the midline only when working at the posterior pole to the midperiphery. In elderly patients even greater care has to be taken before attempting to cross the midline because of the lens thickness with increasing age.

It is a general rule of vitreoretinal surgery that the position of the working ports should be chosen wisely according to the lens status and the pathology addressed. In phakic eyes it is recommended to move the working ports closer to the 3- and 9 o'clock positions allowing for a better angle to trim the vitreous base with a lower risk for lens touch.

Of interest, lens touch frequently is not due to movements made with the cutter but is rather caused by the light pipe. This is either due to trying to focus the light beam on the peripheral vitreous during trimming of the vitreous base or simply by a lack of attention. Selective attention is a mistake made more frequently (but not exclusively) by beginners: One focuses on the orifice of the working instrument (e.g., the vitreous cutter) but forgets the other intraocular instrument (mostly light pipe).

A great proportion of intraoperative lens touch is also caused by the tip of the endolaser. In earlier days, the laser probe was rigid and a lens touch mostly occurred when treating the retinal periphery on the opposite side. Today, curved laser probes that can be advanced and retracted through a mechanism within the

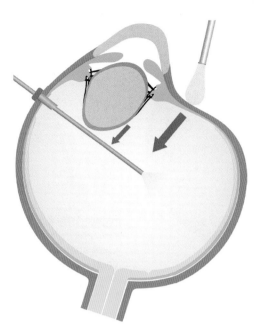

Figure 10B-3 Schematic drawing of deep scleral depression. Note the lens being pushed posteriorly with potential contact to a surgical instrument.

handpiece are available and allow for crossing the midline to reach any part of the retina. However, this requires some training before operating safely within the eye, and many lens touches occur while trying to retract the flexible part of the probe before removing the instrument.

Also, extensive scleral depression is a frequent mistake and should be minimized in phakic eyes. Deep scleral depression may push the lens posteriorly and provoke contact to a surgical instrument **(Fig. 10B-3)**.

Some rare events, mostly sudden and inadvertent, like a soft globe situation (e.g., empty bottle, dislocated infusion line) or hypertony (e.g., during silicone oil filling the infusion port, the light pipe, or other instruments may bounce on the lens if the eye is overfilled with silicone oil) are situations with the risk for an uncontrolled lens touch.

Pathogenesis: Why Does It Occur

Anterior segment surgeons who start training in vitreoretinal surgery often are surprised how much space is present in the vitreous cavity. More difficulties are encountered at the borders of the vitreous body and the vitreoretinal interface: On the one hand beginners may find it difficult to induce a posterior vitreous detachment; on the other hand they have difficulties in judging the spatial distances at the vitreous base and the retrolental space; both areas with limited room in phakic eyes.

A common beginner's mistake is to work too anteriorly out of the fear to get too close to the retina. However, indeed it is more difficult to judge the spatial distance to the posterior capsule than to the retina. We are used to estimate the distance to the retina by the instrument's shadow (shadow effect of the cutter illuminated by the focused light of a hand-held light pipe). However, such a mode of indirect orientation is missing in respect to the lens capsule.

Another not negligible factor is lack of attention. Often the surgeon dedicates all his concentration on one instrument ignoring the second instrument or the light pipe. One has to bear in mind that vitreoretinal surgery is bimanual surgery. Both instruments should be orchestrated together and one should be aware of their position and distance to the neighboring tissue at any time.[3]

An important factor remains crossing the midline with the instruments. Every surgeon is aware that crossing the midline has to be done with caution. However,

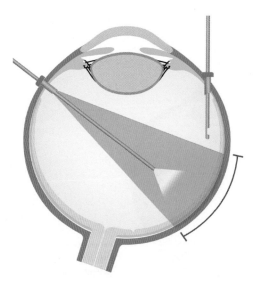

Figure 10B-4 Schematic drawing of the "danger zone" for instruments crossing the midline. Clear anatomical landmarks are lacking. Further, great interindividual variety exists.

clear anatomical landmarks are lacking. The "danger zone" begins somewhere between the vascular arcades and the equator **(Fig. 10B-4)**.

The estimation of the limit to move is made even more difficult by the fact that great difference among patients may exist. In hyperopic eyes (due to the shorter axial length) and in elderly people (due to thicker lens) it is wise to stay more centrally, while myopic eyes and younger patients allow for more peripheral maneuvers. However, in children again the situation is different with a shorter pars plana.

Unfortunately, in certain situations it is necessary to work in close proximity to the lens. Particularly in retinal detachment surgery the vitreous must be removed as completely as possible. Here, residual vitreous may continue to exert traction on the retina and cause postoperative redetachment. Only a fundamental knowledge of the anatomy, scleral depression techniques to visualize the peripheral vitreous, the use of various chandelier lights, and consequent bimanual working from both sides may spare the lens.[4] It is also legitimate to consider a prophylactic phacoemulsification (prior to vitrectomy or combined) to guarantee an unhindered access to the vitreous base in complicated cases.[5] On the other hand, in cases of macular surgery without the need for complete vitrectomy you should limit your ambition to remove the vitreous at the vitreal base completely. In contrast, working too aggressively in this area may cause more harm by inducing retinal breaks or lens touch.

In case of a lens touch a localized opacification develops after a variable time period. The basic principle is the same for a lens touch with or without a capsular breach: Similar to any kind of mechanical lens trauma a lens touch induces shearing forces and mechanical rupture of lens fibers, disturbance of the lens syncytium, consecutive water ingress, and conformational changes of structural lens proteins (see Chapter 12A). These changes are mostly irreversible and lead to a change of the refractive index and scattering of light.[6] The macroscopic picture frequently resembles a contusion rosette with a flower peddle or feather shape underneath the posterior capsule. A rapid opacification may be an important sign for a capsular breach which can otherwise not always been verified.

✜ Pearls on How to Prevent It

◆ Perform a detailed preoperative slit-lamp examination to evaluate the anterior segment anatomy and the status of the crystalline lens.

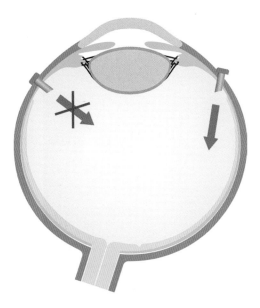

Figure 10B-5 Schematic drawing of different trocar placement. Horizontal sclerotomies (from above pointing to the posterior pole) may provide a safer access to the vitreous cavity directly pointing to the posterior pole (right). In contrast, instruments having been introduced through vertical sclerotomies (parallel-to-the-limbus trocars) directly point to the lens (left).

◆ Manipulation at the vitreous base is significantly easier to perform in pseudo-phakic patients. Therefore, in complex cases where vitreous base manipulation will be necessary, you should rather prefer a combined approach with phaco-emulsification prior to vitrectomy. This is of particular importance in retinal detachment cases.

◆ Mark the incision site with a scleral marker to be sure about the correct positioning of the trocars. Create sclerotomies in phakic eyes at 4 mm rather than at 3.5 mm from the limbus (in adults with normal axial length).

◆ For best placement of the trocars consider horizontal sclerotomies (from above pointing to the posterior pole, external penetration site 3 mm, internal 4 mm) rather than parallel-to-the-limbus sclerotomies. Using this approach the trocars point to the posterior pole and not to the lens **(Figs. 10B-5** and **10B-6).**[7]

◆ Position the working ports closer to the 3- and 9 o'clock positions (instead of 2- and 10 o'clock). This allows a better angle to trim the vitreous base with a lower risk for lens touch.

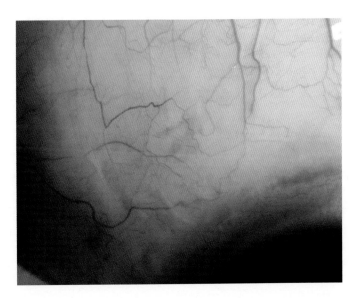

Figure 10B-6 Slit-lamp photography of a horizontal sclerotomy 1 day postoperatively.

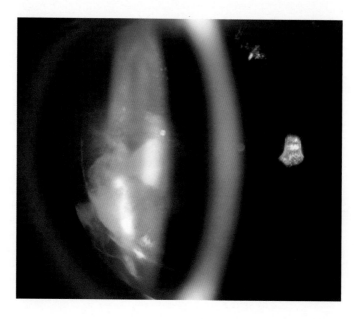

Figure 10B-7 Slit-lamp photography of a peripheral lens touch at the site of the infusion trocar due to scleral indentation.

◆ Avoid pushing the infusion port into the lens equator during indentation **(Fig. 10B-7)** by taking extra care in this area. Indent the infusion port toward the center of the eye, not anteriorly, toward the lens.

◆ Always secure a loop of the infusion tubing either to the drape or better to a special clamp at the lid speculum to avoid unintentional displacement of the infusion cannula.

◆ Introduce the instruments perpendicularly (almost vertically toward the macula). Start vitrectomy in the mid-vitreous and at the posterior pole. Perform calm and slow movements of cutter and light pipe working simultaneously at a constant distance.

◆ Use a wide-angle viewing system to ensure viewing the entire retinal periphery over 360° up to the ora serrata. This helps to estimate the distance to the posterior lens capsule.

◆ For beginners, staining of the vitreous with triamcinolone helps visualizing the vitreous and the spatial distance to the posterior lens surface.

◆ Avoid extensive removal of retrolental vitreous. In cases of dense vitreous hemorrhage the retrolental vitreous may also be cloudy and will need to be removed to enable a good intraoperative view. This can sometimes be difficult without touching the crystalline lens. Decide preoperatively if a combined approach may be preferable.

◆ Be aware that the crystalline lens is thicker in elderly patients.

◆ Do not try to remove small air bubbles that may be accidentally trapped in the retrolental vitreous. They may even help to better demarcate the posterior lens capsule.

◆ In phakic eyes, you should cross the midline only when working at the posterior pole to mid-periphery.

◆ Vitreous is recognized best in the light cone of a hand-held light pipe which provides a more focused and brighter light and a helpful shadow effect to estimate the vicinity of the retina. In pseudophakic (or aphakic) eyes working in the far periphery is easier because you can move cutter and light pipe simultaneously at a constant distance assuring good visualization of the peripheral vitreous and the vitreous cutter. Be aware that illumination of the periphery is completely different in phakic eyes. The light pipe cannot follow beyond the mid-periphery, hence any direct illumination of the vitreous and the vitreous cutter is not possible during vitreous base trimming. In these cases a chandelier light may be helpful to provide a wide angle illumination.

◆ Use of a chandelier light also enables bimanual surgery and allows you to use a scleral depressor for bimanual trimming of the vitreous base.

◆ If using scleral depression for indenting the peripheral retina, use it only with extreme caution because scleral depression may push the lens equator posteriorly and induce a lens touch.

◆ Pearls on How to Solve It

◆ Try to establish biometry as part of the routine preoperative assessment in all cases of phakic patients undergoing pars plana vitrectomy. IOL calculation should include the calculation for capsular bag IOL, sulcus IOL, and either transsclerally fixated or iris-fixated IOL, the latter according to your preference. This will enable you to perform unplanned phacoemulsification and IOL implantation in all cases of intraoperative lens damage if needed.

◆ Look actively for a possible lens touch at the end of each vitrectomy as it is sometimes subtle. If noticed, clearly document it in your surgical notes. It is important to know this if you are planning to perform cataract surgery at a later stage. A pre-existing lens touch is known to bear a considerable risk for a capsular rupture, zonulolysis, and nuclear loss.

◆ The presence of a capsular breach does not preclude proceeding with vitrectomy if safe implantation of an IOL in the bag can still be performed, however it is advisable to remove the lens as soon as possible once a capsular break has occurred because the lens may become cloudy during vitrectomy and lens particles may predispose to intraocular inflammation and cystoid macular edema. Depending on the kind and extend of the capsular break you can remove the lens with one of the techniques mentioned below. After managing the lens the vitrectomy should be completed. Depending on the capsular remnants, the stability of the iris–lens diaphragm, the kind of tamponade needed, the surgically induced inflammation, and your personal experience, you should finally consider either postponing or choosing an appropriate IOL implantation technique:

(1) In simple cases of lens damage an anterior approach with clear cornea (or corneoscleral if preferred) incision may be preferable for simultaneous cataract surgery. During phacoemulsification, the pars plana infusion is closed. In these cases the use of trocars with valves is advantageous to maintain a pressurized globe. If not available, all sclerotomies have to be temporarily closed. Special attention should be given to a meticulous capsulorhexis to ensure that the edge of the rhexis circularly covers the IOL, as the optic can easily dislocate during vitrectomy and especially after gas instillation.[8] There are two important variations compared to standard phacoemulsification to be aware of: (a) Avoid any kind of hydrodissection and (b) perform phacoemulsification with a low infusion pressure (low bottle height) to avoid a high pressure gradient in the anterior chamber. Both may deteriorate a pre-existing capsular break with inadvertent nucleus drop to the posterior pole. The IOL is usually implanted before the vitrectomy is continued. Place a 10-0 nylon suture at the tunnel in all cases, not only if the tunnel is unstable. Constant scleral depression has the capacity to reopen even

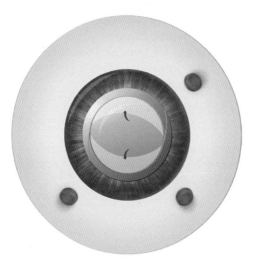

Figure 10B-8 Schematic drawing of button holing. The IOL is implanted into the sulcus, and then the optic is enclavated behind the anterior capsule.

meticulously constructed self-sealing tunnel incisions, and the elevated intraocular pressure given by the infusion line may lead to rapid prolapse of intraocular tissue.

(2) In more severe cases with a visible capsular breach the risk of nucleus drop is too high to proceed with a limbal approach. Nevertheless, even cases with pars plana lensectomy are recommended to be started with an anterior (!) capsulorhexis to achieve perfect rhexis circularity due to the same reasons as mentioned above. The viscoelastics should be temporarily left during lensectomy to stabilize the anterior chamber. There are two basic techniques for lens removal via the pars plana.[9] In the (rare) case of a soft, juvenile lens the vitreous cutter can be used for lensectomy. In most cases of denser lens opacification the use of a fragmatome is preferred for endophacoemulsification. The latter is available in 23G but is used without a trocar cannula. The infusion line remains open during the procedure. Of interest, the lens fragments can mostly be removed without drop of relevant lens fragments (without hydrodissection the lens material sticks to the capsule). With a previously formed anterior capsulorhexis (and a break in the posterior capsule) an implanted sulcus IOL can be securely enclavated with posterior button holing (haptic in the sulcus, optics in the bag).[10] With a perfect rhexis size an IOL even withstands the pressure exerted from a gas tamponade **(Fig. 10B-8)**.

(3) The most serious scenario of a spontaneous nucleus drop; it is quite rare after a lens touch. Normally, the lens material sticks to the capsule and will only drop if the consecutive phacoemulsification is done in a wrong manner (e.g., performing hydrodissection or working with a high pressure gradient in the anterior chamber). If a nucleus drop occurs pars plana endophacoemulsification with perfluorocarbon liquid protecting the macula is performed in the same manner like in cases with complete lens dislocation (see Chapter 12C).

◆ The basic principle of IOL implantation is to achieve a stable iris–lens diaphragm. This minimizes the risk of tamponade prolapse into the anterior chamber.

◆ Use transsclerally or iris-fixated IOLs only if the need for a tamponade like gas or oil can be excluded because neither of these IOLs will prevent a tamponade prolapse into the anterior chamber. Even worse, it may entrap the tamponade material within the anterior chamber. Therefore, those types of IOL fixation should be rather considered for a secondary IOL implantation at a later stage. In cases of silicone oil surgery and a capsular breach it may be advisable to leave the eye aphakic and plan secondary IOL implantation at the time of silicone oil removal. In those cases do not forget the inferior (Ando) iridectomy.

◆ Never forget to remove the viscoelastics placed in the anterior chamber at the end of the case as this may cause undesirable increases of intraocular pressure.

Expected Outcomes: What Is the Worst-case Scenario

The worst-case is not a lens touch, but a lens capsule aspiration. This happens not with active aspiration by the cutter, but mostly with a flute needle in situations of inadvertently high intraocular pressure. The typical situation occurs at the end of an active silicone oil filling (air/silicone oil exchange), where the flute needle is used to remove remaining air from the vitreous base and at the retrolental vitreous cavity. If the cannula is stuck with silicone oil the pressure rises rapidly and an inadvertent proximity to the crystalline lens may result in a sudden lens capsule aspiration (also possible in pseudophakic eyes). The same can happen in active silicone oil removal via vacuum syringes or an active silicone oil aspiration system. Both situations have the potential of high pressure aspiration of the lens capsule often resulting in extensive capsular breaches and zonulolysis. In those situations a stabile iris–lens diaphragm can rarely be restituted. Temporary aphakia with secondary sulcus or iris-fixated IOL implantation a few months later may be preferred then.

REFERENCES

1. Hoerauf H, Roider J, Herboth T, et al. Outcome after vitrectomy in rhegmatogenous retinal detachment and dense vitreous opacities. *Klin Monbl Augenheilkd.* 1997;211:369–374.
2. Lemley CA, Han DP. An age-based method for planning sclerotomy placement during pediatric vitrectomy: a 12-year experience. *Retina.* 2007;27:974–977.
3. Hubschman JP, Son J, Allen B, et al. Evaluation of the motion of surgical instruments during intraocular surgery. *Eye (Lond).* 2011;25:947–953.
4. Chalam KV, Shah VA, Gupta SK, et al. Evaluation and comparison of lens and peripheral retinal relationships with the use of endolaser probe and newly designed curved vitrectomy probe. *Retina.* 2003;23:815–819.
5. Ogino N, Kumagai K. Advantage of combined procedure in vitreous surgery. *Semin Ophthalmol.* 2001;16:137–138.
6. Pau H. Cortical and subcapsular cataracts: significance of physical forces. *Ophthalmologica.* 2006;220:1–5.
7. Sawada T, Kakinoki M, Sawada O, et al. Closure of sclerotomies after 25- and 23-gauge transconjunctival sutureless pars plana vitrectomy evaluated by optical coherence tomography. *Ophthalmic Res.* 2011;45:122–128.
8. Kim SW, Oh J, Song JS, et al. Risk factors of iris posterior synechia formation after phacovitrectomy with three-piece acrylic IOL or single-piece acrylic IOL. *Ophthalmologica.* 2009;223:222–227.
9. Sourdille P. Lensectomy-vitrectomy indications and techniques in cataract surgery. *Curr Opin Ophthalmol.* 1997;8:56–59.
10. Menapace R. Posterior capsulorhexis combined with optic buttonholing: an alternative to standard in-the-bag implantation of sharp-edged intraocular lenses? A critical analysis of 1000 consecutive cases. *Graefes Arch Clin Exp Ophthalmol.* 2008; 246:787–801.

10C Crystalline Lens Subluxation and Luxation

❖ The Complication: Definition

The term *subluxation* refers to a partial dislocation **(Fig. 10C-1)**, whereas *luxation* refers to a total displacement of the crystalline lens **(Fig. 10C-2)**. It most often occurs as a consequence of weakness of the zonular fibers leading to a separation of the lens from its zonular attachments, allowing displacement into the anterior chamber or occasionally into the vitreous. Crystalline lens dislocation is caused by trauma, most commonly, preceding ocular surgery, hereditary systemic diseases, or primary ocular disorders.

The extent of lens displacement can be quite variable—ranging from a hardly noticeable subluxation to a complete luxation of the lens into the vitreous cavity. In the case of trauma, extensive additional damage to the anterior and posterior segment may coexist, which has to be addressed separately.

The hallmark of the subluxated or totally luxated lens is the usually intact lens capsule. This often implies special challenges and distinguishes the surgical approach from that in retained lens fragments and a dropped nucleus after complicated phacoemulsification or phacovitrectomy.

Today, basically every type of lens luxation or subluxation can be successfully treated. The management of subluxated and dislocated lenses has been improved dramatically with the development of modern vitreoretinal microsurgical techniques. From a surgical stand point it is crucial whether a lens subluxation or luxation is present preoperatively or whether it develops during surgery. To recognize a pre-existing zonular dialysis is of great importance in order to plan the surgical procedure accordingly. If the vitreoretinal surgeon is surprised by lens subluxation due to zonular weakness during surgery, great intraoperative difficulties may be encountered.

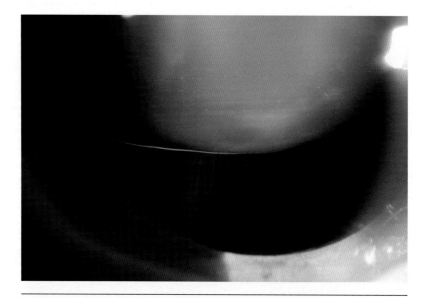

Figure 10C-1 Slit-lamp photography of a subluxated lens.

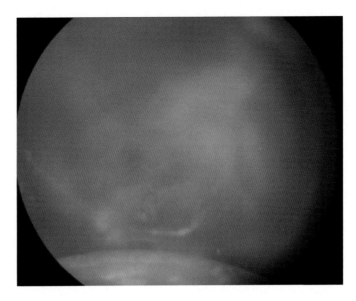

Figure 10C-2 Fundus photography of a totally luxated lens into the vitreous cavity.

Especially in trauma eyes with extensive hyphema or hemophthalmos it may be difficult to evaluate the anterior segment anatomy. In these cases, ultrasound examination and a meticulous history may be helpful.

⬥ Risk Factors

The most common cause for lens subluxation or dislocation is trauma with a frequency slightly above 50% of all cases of complete lens displacement.[1] Eyes with a significant blunt trauma to the eye or head are prone to develop lens dislocation.

However, there are other ocular and systemic conditions that can cause crystalline lens luxation. Absence of a trauma history should evoke suspicion for concomitant hereditary systemic disease or associated ocular disorders.[2]

Hereditary systemic conditions commonly associated with lens dislocation are homocystinuria, Marfan syndrome, Weill-Marchesani syndrome, and hyperlysinemia.[3,4] Other systemic conditions like Sturge–Weber syndrome or Ehlers–Danlos syndrome are reported to be rarely associated, but still show a higher incidence of lens dislocation.[5] Although these systemic diseases are rare, one should take into account that most of these conditions are prone to retinal detachment or other retinal disorders and often need vitreoretinal surgery. Therefore, vitreoretinal surgeons are more often confronted with a simultaneous lens dislocation than assumed. This is also true for hereditary conditions without systemic manifestation like isolated ectopia lentis or ectopia lentis et pupillae. Both conditions show an elevated risk for associated retinal detachment and consecutive need for vitreoretinal surgery.[6]

Primary ocular disorders can also be associated with crystalline lens dislocation. This comprises high myopia, pseudoexfoliation, hypermature cataract, chronic uveitis, ciliary body tumors, and retinitis pigmentosa. Causative is an acquired weakening or degeneration of the zonules.[7,8] Also, these eyes frequently develop retinal diseases and need to undergo vitreoretinal surgery more often.

Preceding eye surgery may also lead to weakening of the zonules. Therefore, every kind of repeat vitreoretinal surgery is suspicious for subclinical lens dislocation. Several influencing factors should be considered: First, all buckling procedures, especially the use of an encircling band or a circumferential segmental buckle have an impact on the zonular tension. Also, vitrectomy itself may lead to zonular weakening due to varying pressure gradients between anterior and posterior chambers. Especially multiple fluid–air exchanges have the potential to overstretch the zonular fibers. Finally, the type of tamponade agent and the duration of the tamponade are relevant factors for a slow but probably relevant zonular degeneration. Repetitive surgery with silicone oil is of high risk for lens dislocation intra- or postoperatively.

Pathogenesis: Why Does It Occur

If planning a vitreoretinal surgery, a concomitant dislocation of the crystalline lens is not an isolated anterior segment problem. In contrast, it is of high importance for the success of vitreoretinal surgery because many vitreoretinal strategies base on a stable iris–lens diaphragm. A preoperatively not visible, but intraoperatively relevant zonular dialysis may interfere with this important compartmentalization.

An impaired lens–iris diaphragm may be especially bothersome during fluid–air exchange and when gas or silicone oil instillation is planned. Decompartmentalization can make both maneuvers difficult. The first sign encountered often is a small air bubble in the anterior chamber during fluid–air exchange. This not only interferes profoundly with fundus visualization, but also points to the threat of overspill of gas or silicone oil into the anterior chamber, which may damage the corneal endothelium. In addition, unwanted intracameral gas or silicone oil may lead to underfilling in the vitreous cavity resulting in an increased risk for a recurrent retinal detachment.

Further, eyes with lens dislocation are at a higher risk for developing secondary angle closure glaucoma. In one series of lens dislocation, 56% had a preoperative elevation of intraocular pressure.[9] This frequent complication is significantly increased with the use of a gas tamponade which exerts further pressure on the lens. Another complication is vitreous prolapse around the lens and into the anterior chamber that has the potential to exert traction onto the vitreous base and consecutive tearing of the retina.

Hence, a working knowledge of the causes of a lens dislocation and the associated systemic and ocular conditions is paramount. The most important cause is a pre-existing damage to the zonules. The risk factors which lead to a hereditary or acquired weakening or degeneration of the zonules are mentioned in Table 10C-1.

Despite the detailed description of causes of lens dislocation in the literature, in most cases the exact etiology of zonular weakness remains unknown or idiopathic.[10] In some cases, a preceding trauma or pseudoexfoliation can be identified, but the vast majority remains unclear.

Therefore, a meticulous preoperative examination of the anterior segment is mandatory prior to any kind of vitreoretinal surgery. Early slit-lamp signs of lens subluxation are shallowing of the anterior chamber, increased iris convexity, and crowding of the angle.[2]

In trauma cases, not only posterior but also anterior segment abnormalities can be expected, for example, corneal scars, conjunctival scarring, or scleral thinning. The greater the extent of lens damage, the poorer the visual prognosis in eyes with penetrating injuries. The prognosis is especially bad if the lens is displaced or expelled.[11]

Pearls on How to Prevent It

- ◆ In eyes with a pre-existing damage of the zonules, such as eyes with pseudoexfoliation or trauma, lens luxation may be difficult to avoid if vitrectomy combined with cataract surgery is planned. In these cases, a thorough preoperative examination is paramount. Lens subluxation may occasionally be subtle. Zonular dehiscence is marked by the presence of iridodonesis and phacodonesis. Examine the anterior chamber carefully for the presence of vitreous. Keep in mind that in pseudoexfoliation the dilation of the pupil is often poor: Detection of mild subluxation may be difficult in these cases preoperatively.

Table 10C-1 • Specific Causes for Crystalline Lens Luxation/Subluxation

- Trauma (Most Common Cause)
- **Surgical**
  Repetitive eye surgery
  Encircling band or circumferential segmental buckle
  Previous silicone oil tamponade
  Multiple fluid–air exchange
- **Hereditary conditions without systemic manifestation**
  Isolated ectopia lentis
  Ectopia lentis et pupillae
- **Systemic conditions commonly associated with lens luxation**
  Homocystinuria
  Marfan syndrome
  Weill-Marchesani syndrome
  Hyperlysinemia
- **Systemic conditions rarely associated with lens luxation**
  Sturge–Weber syndrome
  Ehlers–Danlos syndrome
- **Primary ocular disorders associated with lens luxation**
  High myopia
  Pseudoexfoliation
  Hypermature cataract
  Chronic uveitis
  Ciliary body tumor
  Retinitis pigmentosa

◆ You can minimize deterioration of a pre-existing zonular weakness by very careful surgical maneuvers.

◆ Carefully weigh the pros and cons of adjunctive buckles to decrease the risk of lens luxation during vitrectomy in eyes with compromised zonules. Be aware that placement of encircling bands or large scleral buckles often can cause weakening of the zonules.

◆ Try to avoid high-pressure gradients between the anterior and the posterior segment during fluid–air exchange. Intraoperative pressure changes during vitrectomy may cause an overexpansion of the zonules.

◆ When air gets into the anterior chamber during fluid–air exchange medical miosis of the pupil (e.g., with acetylcholine) may be helpful. If the retinal situation allows it, short-acting gases or air should be used. Advise the patient to remain in a prone position after surgery for some time to prevent overspill of gas or oil into the anterior chamber.

◆ Be aware that the previous use of long-term vitreous substitutes especially silicone oils is a risk factor for zonular weakness. It is unknown how silicone oil interacts with the zonules; however, eyes with silicone oil filling that need to undergo repeat vitrectomy seem to have a higher incidence of zonular dialysis. Use long-term vitreous substitutes only when warranted by the retinal situation.

◆ If long-term tamponade is needed and lens dislocation is significant, do not hesitate to perform endophacoemulsification by using one of the techniques mentioned below.

✦ Pearls on How to Solve It

◆ Performing preoperative biometry is wise prior to vitreoretinal surgery in phakic eyes.

◆ ***Subtle to moderate lens subluxation; phacoemulsification with capsular tension ring:*** In selected cases with subtle lens subluxation and zonular dialysis (extending up to 3 clock hours) a standard phacoemulsification with or without implantation of a capsular tension ring may be sufficient to stabilize the iris–lens diaphragm prior to vitrectomy.

◆ ***Phacoemulsification in moderate lens subluxation:*** In cases with moderate lens subluxation (4–8 hours of zonular dialysis), performing a curvilinear capsulorhexis in the usual fashion and hooking the rhexis with one or two iris retractors to stabilize the capsular bag may allow standard phacoemulsification **(Fig. 10C-3)**. After hooking the capsular bag with iris retractors placing capsular tension segments may further stabilize the lens capsular bag **(Fig. 10C-4)**. If the zonular weakness extends beyond 6 hours the capsular tension segments should be suture fixated to the sclera—for example, by using Cionni-modified capsular tension rings. The pars plana infusion should be stopped while the phacoemulsification is done and the irrigation be performed through the anterior chamber as usually done in phacoemulsification surgery. In some cases of a moderately subluxated lens, the capsule may be damaged during lens removal or zonular support is inadequate to support placement of a posterior chamber intraocular lens. Removal of the empty capsular bag can be achieved with an intraocular forceps by grasping the capsule from under the iris.

◆ ***Pronounced lens subluxation:*** In cases of pronounced lens subluxation, phacoemulsification often is not feasible any more. In such situations rather combine vitrectomy with lensectomy via the pars plana either with the vitreous cutter or endophacoemulsification. Before performing lensectomy in the vitreous cavity, a near complete vitrectomy is very advisable. However, when this is not possible, for example, because of poor fundus visualization at least a core vitrectomy and clearing of the vitreous base should precede lens removal in order to avoid traction on the retina. Moreover, of special importance is a meticulous anterior vitrectomy behind the plane of the iris and in the anterior chamber to reduce the chance of transpupillary anterior traction on the vitreous base, creating retinal tears, or even worse inducing a retinal detachment **(Fig. 10C-5)**. A posterior vitreous detachment can be performed at a later stage of the procedure. Various techniques of endophacoemulsification are possible:

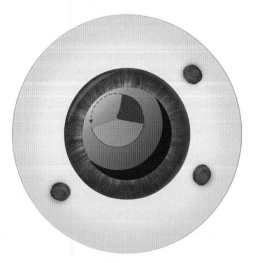

Figure 10C-3 Schematic drawing of phacoemulsification in a subluxated lens. Capsulorhexis, although sometimes difficult, should be centered in the lens, not in the pupil. In some cases the rhexis has to be partially done under the iris.

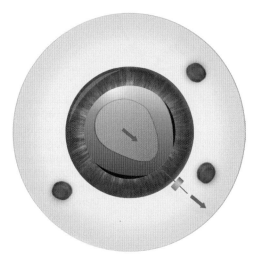

Figure 10C-4 Schematic drawing of phacoemulsification in a subluxated lens. By hooking the capsular bag with an iris retractor it can be pulled and centered in the pupil.

◆ *Bimanual endophacoemulsification in pronounced lens subluxation:* In cases in which the lens is considerably subluxated, the lens is best removed by intracapsular endophacoemulsification **(Fig. 10C-6)**. If possible, phacofragmentation should be performed in the pupillary plane, because this allows direct visualization without the need for wide angle viewing system. In addition, emulsification is performed at a safe distance away from the retina. Some aspects need to be considered for phacofragmentation in the pupillary plane: (1) The crystalline lens must be securely stabilized in the pupillary plane during the endophacoemulsification procedure. (2) The capsular bag should be pressurized, for example, using intracapsular irrigation (from bimanual irrigation/aspiration handpieces for cataract surgery) in order to avoid collapse and damage of the capsule during aspiration. Both can be achieved best with bimanual phacofragmentation. A 23G microvitreoretinal blade is introduced through the sclerotomy, penetrating directly behind the equator of the lens. Keep in mind that the currently available phacofragmatomes are 23G, but are used without a trocar. If small-gauge surgery is performed, one trocar needs to be removed and the conjunctiva opened for introduction of the endophacoemulsification tip. Alternatively, you can create separate sclerotomies for the endophaco procedure. The phacofragmatome and the irrigation handpiece are introduced in opposite positions. This allows inflating

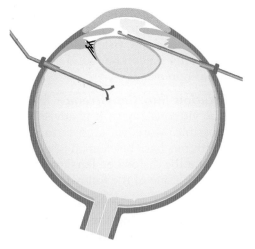

Figure 10C-5 Schematic drawing of cleaning anterior vitreous via pars plana to reduce the chance of transpupillary anterior traction on the vitreous base.

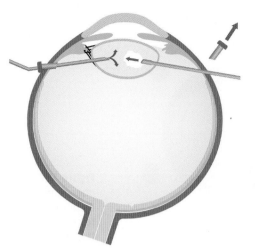

Figure 10C-6 Schematic drawing of endo-phacoemulsification in a subluxated lens. The phacofragmatome and the irrigation handpiece are introduced in opposite positions near the lens equator. The capsular bag is inflated and stabilized, while phacofragmentation is performed in a linear mode. This allows for removing the complete lens material without losing the fragments posteriorly.

and stabilizing the capsular bag during the procedure. For that the irrigation has to be disconnected from the infusion port for a while and attached to the irrigation cannula; alternatively, use a second bottle for irrigation. Perform phacofragmentation without prior hydrodissection or nuclear fragmentation (no chopping) to reduce the risk of losing the fragments posteriorly. Use a linear phaco mode and activate phaco energy and aspiration only when the tip is moved in a forward direction. The aim is to aspirate the entire lens material within the capsular bag without damaging the capsular bag. Thereafter, the irrigation is reconnected with the infusion port and the empty capsular bag can be removed with an intraocular serrated forceps introduced through the pars plana. You can employ gentle scleral depression to ease visualization and removal of peripheral capsular or lenticular remnants. After all lens material has been removed, vitrectomy can be completed.

◆ *Bimanual lensectomy with vitreous cutter in pronounced lens subluxation:* One might assume that using a cutter instead of a phacofragmatome is less difficult. In selected cases of a soft, juvenile lens a simple aspiration with the vitreous cutter might work. But in most cases the viscosity and durability of a senile lens is underestimated especially if using a 23G cutter **(Fig. 10C-7)**.

◆ *Visco-assisted endophacoemulsification:* It is advisable to use a syringe with an ophthalmic viscosurgical device (OVD) (delivered via a flute needle) instead of an irrigation handpiece to stabilize and to inflate the capsular bag. The intracapsular OVD may stabilize the capsular bag much better than intracapsular BSS irrigation. It allows you to keep the capsular bag constantly pressurized without the risk of encountering hypotony. Moreover, fluid irrigation of the capsular bag encompasses the risk of flushing lens particles into the vitreous cavity which often later on can be found adhering to the vitreous base where they are difficult to remove.

◆ **Complete lens luxation into the vitreous:** In cases in which the entire lens is displaced into the vitreous cavity, it is advisable first to remove the vitreous as completely as possible. Moreover a posterior vitreous detachment should be attempted and the vitreous base be cleaned prior to lens removal. Simply removing the vitreous around the dislocated lens may not be sufficient. Thereafter the lens can be removed with one of the following methods:

◆ *Lensectomy with the vitrectomy probe:* Soft lenses without a significant nuclear sclerosis can be removed using the vitrectomy cutter alone. However, this may be quite time consuming and may cause small lens fragments to float

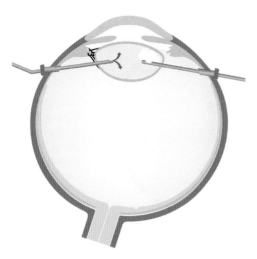

Figure 10C-7 Schematic drawing of intracapsular lensectomy in a soft lens situation by simple aspiration with the vitreous cutter.

into the vitreous cavity. A small amount of perfluorocarbon liquid (PFCL) may be injected beneath the lens to protect the macula from the impact of the lens or lens fragments during the fragmentation maneuvers.

◆ *Intravitreal endophacoemulsification:* Many vitreoretinal surgeons prefer to remove the nucleus within the vitreous cavity using a phacofragmatome **(Fig. 10C-8)**. Under these circumstances it is again advisable to protect the posterior pole with a PFCL bubble. However, it must be considered that although PFCL protects the macula from the impact of descending lens fragments or instrument manipulation it hardly shields the posterior pole from the ultrasound energy transmitted from the fragmentation probe. In contrast the ultrasound waves may even be transmitted to the macula by the PFCL bubble. That is why the dropped lens at first should be aspirated and lifted in the mid-vitreous before phacofragmentation is started. As every phacoemulsification procedure induces some rebound the lens may bounce back into the direction of the macula once in a while during the operation. With a PFCL bubble in place the posterior pole should be sufficiently protected. However, the lens must be repeatedly aspirated by the phacofragmatome to engage and draw the lens into the mid-vitreous cavity. Increase the phaco power setting proportionally with increasing lens nucleus density. It is crucial not to activate the ultrasound before the fragment is elevated. Furthermore, the ultrasound has a tendency to bounce the lens fragment away from the aspirating needle tip. It is important to use PULSED MODE, rather than continuous ultrasound. It

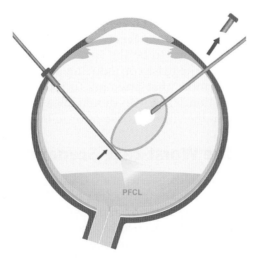

Figure 10C-8 Schematic drawing of endophacoemulsification of a totally luxated lens. After protecting the macula with a PFCL bubble the nucleus can be aspirated and lifted in the mid-vitreous before phacofragmentation. Stay away from the retina during phaco mode. The shaft should be carefully cooled to avoid scleral burn, but be aware that vaporized water may condense on the fundus loupe impairing view.

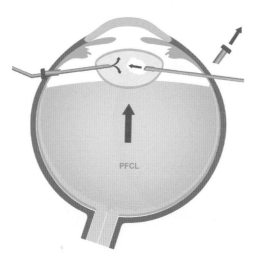

PFCL

Figure 10C-9 Schematic drawing of endophacoemulsification in the pupillary plane. Phacofragmentation within the pupillary plane is more controlled and can be performed under direct visualization using the microscope red reflex. This is achieved by filling almost the entire vitreous cavity with PFCL, the lens is then floating in the pupillary plane.

is important that the minimum effective power should be employed, because heat from the fragmentation unit is transmitted all along the shaft of the frag-matome and can cause retinal/scleral burns and retinal breaks. To avoid these complications, the shaft should be constantly cooled by watering the scle-rotomy. The most common complication to occur during this procedure is the formation of retinal breaks from instrument manipulations near the retina or from the heat produced by the phacofragmatome unit itself. Another disad-vantage of lens removal within the vitreous cavity is the difficult view through the wide angle viewing system. Water that has been vaporized by the ultra-sound energy rapidly condensates on the fundus loupe and often interferes with fundus visualization.

◆ *Endophacoemulsification in the pupillary plane:* Whenever feasible the phaco-fragmentation of the lens within the pupillary plane is the method of choice, which allows lens removal under the advantageous view of the microscope red reflex **(Fig. 10C-9)**. This can be achieved by floating the lens into the pupil-lary plane by filling almost the entire vitreous cavity with PFCL (use decaline instead of octaline). Thereafter, the lens can be removed by endophacoemulsifi-cation in analogy to the procedure used for a subluxated lens (see above).

◆ *Intracapsular cataract extraction:* In the rare case of a very hard black nucleus, it may be necessary to deliver it via a corneoscleral section. In this case, the infusion should be placed before enlarging the incision to avoid transient hypotony.

◆ In principle all techniques mentioned above are appropriate and may be used according to the situation present and according to the preference and per-sonal experience of the surgeon. Safety and surgical outcome of the various approaches have been shown to be the same.[12] However, you should note that all techniques pose a marked risk for inducing a retinal detachment (intra- and postoperatively). Remember that attempts to retrieve dislocated lens material may create retinal traction. Thus, you should always release all vitreous traction and meticulously clean the vitreous base prior to lens removal.

✦ Expected Outcomes: What Is the Worst-case Scenario

The worst-case scenario most likely is a severe trauma case with lens luxation, dam-age to the vitreous base, significant intraocular bleeding, and other serious trauma-related tissue alterations of the anterior and posterior segment. In such a case the problems present need to be approached in a consecutive manner. The abovemen-tioned principles for management of a luxated lens apply here too.

More clinically relevant for the vitreoretinal surgeon are commonly subtle lens subluxations, which have little (or even no) significance prior to vitrectomy, but may cause great problems intra- and postoperatively. In such circumstances, a complete and stable tamponade with gas or silicone oil may be difficult to achieve. Gas or silicone oil may get into the anterior chamber and not only become hazardous to the cornea, but also put the patient at risk for re-detachment because of underfilling within the vitreous cavity.

One example might be a young myopic patient who is suffering from repetitive retinal detachments that have been treated by vitrectomy. In such a patient invisible zonular weakness may cause air to get into the anterior chamber during fluid–air exchange. This air bubble may be removed from the anterior chamber by injecting BSS or an OVD.

However, the gas or silicone oil likely still will re-appear in the anterior chamber even with the use of OVDs. This is especially with silicone oil which poses the cornea at risk for decompensation and may increase intraocular pressure. Thus, in such patients the surgeon often is forced to opt for a shorter-lasting tamponade or an early removal of silicone oil, which again puts the retina at risk for recurrence of the pathology. Such situations pose a dilemma, for which there is no optimal solution. Sometimes, cataract surgery with placement of a capsular tension ring may be helpful under such circumstances. However, often the surgeon may have to decide leaving a patient aphakic with an inferior iridectomy (Ando-iridectomy) which will keep the silicone oil behind the iris plane.

REFERENCES

1. Choi DY, Kim JG, Song BJ. Surgical management of crystalline lens dislocation into the anterior chamber with corneal touch and secondary glaucoma. *J Cataract Refract Surg.* 2004;30:718–721.
2. Willoughby CE, Wishart PK. Lensectomy in the management of glaucoma in spherophakia. *J Cataract Refract Surg.* 2002;28:1061–1064.
3. Ganesh A, Smith C, Chan W, et al. Immunohistochemical evaluation of conjunctival fibrillin-1 in Marfan syndrome. *Arch Ophthalmol.* 2006;124:205–209.
4. Wentzloff JN, Kaldawy RM, Chen TC. Weill-Marchesani syndrome. *J Pediatr Ophthalmol Strabismus.* 2006;43:192.
5. Nelson L. Ectopia lentis in childhood. *J Pediatr Ophthalmol Strabismus.* 2008;45:12.
6. Dagi LR, Walton DS. Anterior axial lens subluxation, progressive myopia, and angle-closure glaucoma: Recognition and treatment of atypical presentation of ectopia lentis. *J AAPOS.* 2006;10:345–350.
7. Eid TM. Retinitis pigmentosa associated with ectopia lentis and acute angle-closure glaucoma. *Can J Ophthalmol.* 2008;43:726–727.
8. Dureau P. Pathophysiology of zonular diseases. *Curr Opin Ophthalmol.* 2008;19:27–30.
9. Rosenbaum LJ, Podos SM. Traumatic ectopia lentis. Some relationships to syphilis and glaucoma. *Am J Ophthalmol.* 1967;64:1095–1098.
10. Kawashima M, Kawakita T, Shimazaki J. Complete spontaneous crystalline lens dislocation into the anterior chamber with severe corneal endothelial cell loss. *Cornea.* 2007;26:487–489.
11. Sternberg P Jr, de Juan E Jr, Michels RG, et al. Multivariate analysis of prognostic factors in penetrating ocular injuries. *Am J Ophthalmol.* 1984;98:467–472.
12. Hakin KN, Jacobs M, Rosen P, et al. Management of the subluxated crystalline lens. *Ophthalmology.* 1992;99:542–545.

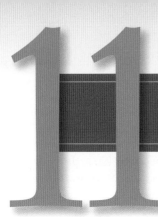

11

COMPLICATIONS DURING PHACO-VITROECTOMY

KEVIN K. SUK AND TIMOTHY G. MURRAY

11A Continuous Flattening of the Anterior Chamber

 The Complication: Definition

Phacoemulsification occurs entirely within the limited surgical space of the anterior chamber. When the anterior chamber flattens, the lens and iris move forward, which decreases the working space and destabilizes the surgical environment. This can make surgical maneuvers difficult and increase the risk of complications. Moreover, a flattening anterior chamber can also herald the development of a severe complication such as a suprachoroidal hemorrhage.

Risk Factors

Both ocular and systemic factors can contribute to flattening of the anterior chamber.
Weak zonules and a flaccid posterior capsule may allow the lens–iris diaphragm to move excessively and cause the anterior chamber to flatten, particularly in the presence of positive vitreous pressure.

Excessive Mobility of the Lens–Iris Diaphragm Can be Seen With:

◆ Age: The zonules may be weaker with age,[1] allowing the lens to move forward.

◆ Mature cataract: The posterior capsule in white and brunescent cataracts is flaccid and more mobile.[2,3] The intumescent lens may also cause the zonules to be lax.

◆ Previous vitrectomy: Previously vitrectomized eyes have weakened zonules[4–7] and loss of vitreous support[6,8] which results in an unstable posterior capsule that is unusually mobile and flaccid.[4–6,9]

◆ Pseudoexfoliation (PXF): This systemic disease causes instability and weakness of the zonules[10] which can manifest as decreased anterior chamber depth as well as iridodonesis and phacodonesis.[10–14]

◆ High myopia: Loss of scleral rigidity and laxity of the zonules in high myopia[15] may contribute to flattening of the anterior chamber.

Increased Positive Vitreous Pressure Can be Seen With:

◆ Elevated venous pressure: Positive vitreous pressure can occur in patients with chronic obstructive pulmonary disease, obesity, and in anxious patients who may be performing valsalva.[16]

◆ Posterior capsule rupture/zonulodialysis: A defect in the posterior capsule or zonules can allow fluid to reach posteriorly to hydrate the vitreous which, in turn, can increase positive vitreous pressure. The risk factors for posterior capsule rupture and zonulodialysis are discussed later.

◆ Vitreous hydration: Some surgeons prefer to insert the cannulae, including the posterior infusion cannula, prior to phacoemulsification. If the posterior infusion is inadvertently left on, the vitreous can become hydrated. The expanded volume of the vitreous can then increase positive vitreous pressure and cause the anterior chamber to shallow.

◆ Suprachoroidal hemorrhage: Hemorrhage into the potential space between the sclera and choroid can displace the vitreous forward and cause the anterior chamber to shallow and, in severe cases, expulsion of the intraocular contents.[17,18] Risk factors include glaucoma, aphakia, high myopia, hypertension, diabetes, and advanced age.[18] For further information on this intraoperative complication, see also Chapter 26C.

◆ Pathogenesis: Why Does It Occur

Anatomy

The crystalline lens measures approximately 9 to 10 mm in diameter[19,20] and is largely unaffected by age. The thickness of the lens, however, increases from approximately 3.6 mm at age 20 to 5 mm at age 80.[19,20] The distance from the lens to the cornea, the anterior chamber depth, measures approximately 3.5 mm and varies with age and refractive status.[21,22] Thus, the working space from the cornea to the posterior capsule ranges from approximately 7.1 to 8.5 mm, an important relation to remember considering that the phaco needle measures approximately 1 mm in diameter (**Fig. 11A-1**).

The anterior chamber depth is maintained by a balance of inflow and outflow. An imbalance in the fluidics of the eye, along with an excessively mobile lens–iris diaphragm, can cause the anterior chamber to flatten.

Inflow: Inadequate flow into the anterior chamber can decrease the volume of the anterior chamber and cause it to flatten.

Outflow: Outflow of fluid from the anterior chamber, in excess of inflow decreases anterior chamber volume and depth.

◆ The corneal incision may be too wide or unstable with leakage of fluid through the wound.

◆ Excessive vacuum or ultrasound power, especially with soft nuclei, can cause the anterior chamber to collapse. Vacuum builds up in the aspiration tubing with occlusion of the phaco tip. When the occlusion breaks after the piece of nucleus is

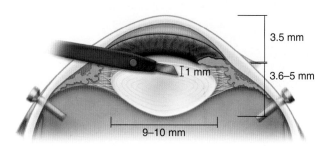

3.5 mm

1 mm

3.6–5 mm

9–10 mm

Figure 11A-1 Anterior chamber dimensions.

aspirated, the elastic tubing collapses, then rebounds back into shape,[23] creating a surge of vacuum. Since the anterior chamber has a volume of approximately 175 μL,[24] any small surge can cause the anterior chamber to flatten.

Positive vitreous pressure: The iris and lens can be pushed forward by positive vitreous pressure, causing the anterior chamber to flatten. Several mechanisms contribute to the pathogenesis.

Misdirection of the infusion fluid posteriorly into the retrolenticular space or along the vitreoretinal interface can push the lens and iris forward, flattening the anterior chamber.

If the posterior capsule is ruptured or there is zonular dehiscence, infusion fluid can move posteriorly and hydrate the vitreous, causing forward displacement of the anterior vitreous and the lens. The entire vitreous body can be pushed forward in the case of a suprachoroidal hemorrhage. In addition, an air bubble from the posterior infusion can push the posterior capsule and iris forward during nuclear removal.

✥ Pearls on How to Prevent It

Flattening of the anterior chamber is problematic for several reasons. When the anterior chamber shallows, particularly with positive vitreous pressure, the iris tends to prolapse through the corneal incision. This makes it difficult to insert any instrument through the wound, while iris manipulation and trauma can cause the pupil to constrict. A smaller surgical space places the corneal endothelium and the posterior capsule closer to the surgical instruments including the phacoemulsification tip, which can increase the risk of damage to these structures.

To prevent anterior chamber flattening:

◆ Air in the posterior infusion should be avoided. If a small-gauge trocar system is used, the following steps can prevent air bubbles. Once the first microcannula is inserted, confirm that it is in the vitreous space before inserting the infusion line. Once the position is confirmed, insert the infusion cannula while fluid is running and turn the infusion off once the infusion cannula is connected and in the eye. This prevents air from entering the infusion line which can occur from the negative pressure created from pinching the tubing during insertion **(Fig. 11A-2)**. Alternatively, phacoemulsification can be completed before inserting the infusion cannula.

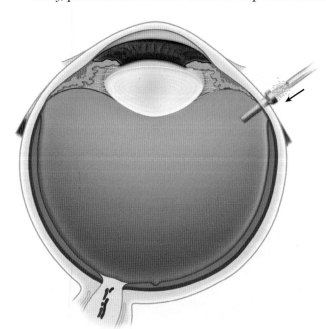

Figure 11A-2 After inserting the microcannula and confirming its position in the vitreous cavity, the infusion line is inserted while the fluid is running. This helps prevent air bubbles from entering the vitreous cavity from the posterior infusion.

◆ Wound construction is important. The paracentesis should be small and the corneal incision should be beveled, self-sealing, and not too wide. The incisions should be placed slightly anterior to the limbus, away from the iris root.

◆ Keep vacuum and ultrasound power proportional to the hardness of the nucleus to prevent surges in vacuum.

◆ Anterior chamber flattening during vitrectomy: We prefer to insert the intraocular lens prior to vitrectomy to stabilize the bag. A suture is placed across the corneal incision prior to vitrectomy and the viscoelastic is left in the anterior chamber after intraocular lens insertion. This stabilizes the anterior chamber during vitrectomy.

Pearls on How to Solve It

When the anterior chamber continues to flatten:

◆ First, raise the infusion bottle to increase inflow.

◆ Then, check the corneal incision and paracentesis. If the wound is too large and leaking irrigation fluid, place a suture across the wound.

◆ Lower the aspiration rate.

◆ Check to make sure the posterior infusion is not turned on during phacoemulsification.

◆ Inspect the red reflex and examine the fundus if there is any suspicion of a suprachoroidal hemorrhage. In the case of a suprachoroidal hemorrhage, stop and suture all incisions and increase the intraocular pressure. The surgery may need to be postponed.

◆ If iris prolapse prevents insertion of the phacoemulsification tip or other instrument, the paracentesis should be utilized to inject a cohesive viscoelastic between the iris and the corneal incision while gently sweeping the iris out of the wound and into the eye. It is easier to pull the iris into the eye than to push it in from externally. Once a barrier of viscoelastic is placed between the incision and the iris, the anterior chamber can be further deepened with viscoelastic **(Fig. 11A-3)**. Entry into the eye with the phacoemulsification instrument should be with the infusion off to avoid disturbing the viscoelastic barrier and the iris.

◆ If the anterior chamber continues to flatten despite these measures, perform a limited anterior vitrectomy while keeping the posterior infusion off. The vitrector

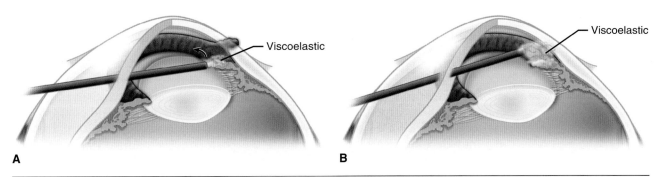

A   **B**

Figure 11A-3 When the iris prolapses through the main incision, **(A)** the paracentesis is utilized to inject a cohesive viscoelastic between the iris and the corneal incision while gently sweeping the iris back into the eye. **B:** This creates space between the iris and the incision and acts as a barrier to prevent further prolapse of the iris.

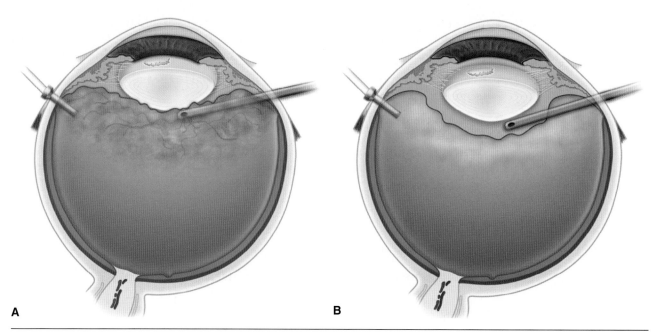

A **B**

Figure 11-4 A: Positive vitreous pressure displaces the lens anteriorly. **B:** Removal of a small amount of anterior vitreous increases space, relieves misdirection of infusion fluid, and reduces positive vitreous pressure. It is important to keep the posterior infusion off and to direct the vitrector port laterally, away from the lens capsule.

should be visualized behind the lens and the port directed to the side, away from the posterior capsule. Removal of a small amount of the anterior vitreous can increase space, relieve misdirection of infusion fluid and reduce the positive vitreous pressure **(Fig. 11A-4)**.

◆ If the anterior chamber flattens during vitrectomy, first check the wound and place a suture as necessary. The anterior chamber should be filled with viscoelastic prior to vitrectomy to maintain stability and volume. Lowering the posterior infusion pressure can be helpful.

⬥ Expected Outcomes: What Is the Worst-case Scenario

Continuous flattening of the anterior chamber can make the surgery more challenging and time consuming, and can lead to complications with possible adverse outcomes.

When the anterior chamber flattens, the iris has a propensity to prolapse through the corneal wound. Manipulation of the iris can then cause the pupil to constrict, making the cataract surgery more difficult and interfering with the subsequent vitrectomy.

The close proximity of the phacoemulsification tip and other instruments to the endothelium and posterior capsule in a shallow anterior chamber can cause damage to these structures. The cornea may become edematous and compromise the surgical view for both phacoemulsification and vitrectomy. In addition, the cornea may decompensate and complicate the postoperative course. Damage to the posterior capsule or zonules can lead to multiple problems, which are discussed in greater detail below.

If the cause of anterior chamber flattening is a suprachoroidal hemorrhage, untimely management can lead to progression to an expulsive hemorrhage, with extrusion of the intraocular contents and loss of the eye.

REFERENCES

1. Assia EI, Apple DJ, Morgan RC, et al. The relationship between the stretching capability of the anterior capsule and zonules. *Invest Ophthalmol Vis Sci.* 1991;32:2835–2839.
2. Ermiş SS, Oztürk F, Inan UU. Comparing the efficacy and safety of phacoemulsification in white mature and other types of senile cataracts. *Br J Ophthalmol.* 2003; 87:1356–1359.
3. Vajpayee RB, Bansal A, Sharma N, et al. Phacoemulsification of white hypermature cataract. *J Cataract Refract Surg.* 1999;25:1157–1160.
4. Díaz Lacalle V, Orbegozo Gárate FJ, Martinez Alday N, et al. Phacoemulsification cataract surgery in vitrectomized eyes. *J Cataract Refract Surg.* 1998;24:806–809.
5. Pinter SM, Sugar A. Phacoemulsification in eyes with past pars plana vitrectomy: Case-control study. *J Cataract Refract Surg.* 1999;25:556–561.
6. Smiddy WE, Stark WJ, Michels RG, et al. Cataract extraction after vitrectomy. *Ophthalmology.* 1987;94:483–487.
7. Biró Z, Kovacs B. Results of cataract surgery in previously vitrectomized eyes. *J Cataract Refract Surg.* 2002;28:1003–1006.
8. Sneed S, Parrish RK 2nd, Mandelbaum S, et al. Technical problems of extracapsular cataract extractions after vitrectomy. *Arch Ophthalmol.* 1986;104:1126–1127.
9. McDermott ML, Puklin JE, Abrams GW, et al. Phacoemulsification for cataract following pars plana vitrectomy. *Ophthalmic Surg Lasers.* 1997;28:558–564.
10. Schlötzer-Schrehardt U, Naumann GO. Ocular and systemic pseudoexfoliation syndrome. *Am J Ophthalmol.* 2006;141:921–937.
11. Shingleton BJ, Marvin AC, Heier JS, et al. Pseudoexfoliation: High risk factors for zonule weakness and concurrent vitrectomy during phacoemulsification. *J Cataract Refract Surg.* 2010;36:1261–1269.
12. Schlötzer-Schrehardt U, Naumann GO. A histopathologic study of zonular instability in pseudoexfoliation syndrome. *Am J Ophthalmol.* 1994;118:730–743.
13. Shingleton BJ, Crandall AS, Ahmed II. Pseudoexfoliation and the cataract surgeon: Preoperative, intraoperative, and postoperative issues related to intraocular pressure, cataract, and intraocular lenses. *J Cataract Refract Surg.* 2009;35:1101–1120.
14. Küchle M, Viestenz A, Martus P, et al. Anterior chamber depth and complications during cataract surgery in eyes with pseudoexfoliation syndrome. *Am J Ophthalmol.* 2000;129:281–285.
15. McBrien NA, Gentle A. Role of the sclera in the development and pathological complications of myopia. *Prog Retin Eye Res.* 2003;22:307–338.
16. Khng C, Osher RH. Surgical options in the face of positive pressure. *J Cataract Refract Surg.* 2006;32:1423–1425.
17. Wong KK, Saleh TA, Gray RH. Suprachoroidal hemorrhage during cataract surgery in a vitrectomized eye. *J Cataract Refract Surg.* 2005;31:1242–1243.
18. Lakhanpal V. Experimental and clinical observations on massive suprachoroidal hemorrhage. *Trans Am Ophthalmol Soc.* 1993;91:545–652.
19. Pierscionek BK, Weale RA. The optics of the eye-lens and lenticular senescence. A review. *Doc Ophthalmol.* 1995;89:321–335.
20. Jones CE, Atchison DA, Pope JM. Changes in lens dimensions and refractive index with age and accommodation. *Optom Vis Sci.* 2007;84:990–995.
21. Huang J, Pesudovs K, Wen D, et al. Comparison of anterior segment measurements with rotating Scheimpflug photography and partial coherence reflectometry. *J Cataract Refract Surg.* 2011;37:341–348.
22. Yan PS, Lin HT, Wang QL, et al. Anterior segment variations with age and accommodation demonstrated by slit-lamp-adapted optical coherence tomography. *Ophthalmology.* 2010;117:2301–2307.
23. Devgan U. Phaco fluidics and phaco ultrasound power modulations. *Ophthalmol Clin North Am.* 2006;19:457–468.
24. Chen Y, Bao YZ, Pei XT. Morphologic changes in the anterior chamber in patients with cortical or nuclear age-related cataract. *J Cataract Refract Surg.* 2011;37:77–82.

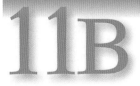

Posterior Capsule Rupture (Can I Insert a Lens? Can I Preserve the Capsular Bag?) and Zonulodyalysis

 ## The Complication: Definition

Posterior capsule rupture and zonulodialysis are important complications of cataract surgery. Loss of these structures can make insertion of an intraocular lens challenging and can interfere with the outcome of the vitreoretinal procedure.

The posterior capsule ruptures at a rate of 0.82% to 2.1% during combined phaco-vitrectomy.[1–4] This is similar to the rate seen with cataract surgery alone (0.29–2.7%).[5–10] Zonulodialysis occurs at a rate of 1.75% during phaco-vitrectomy[11] and 0.29% to 0.9%[6,8] during cataract surgery.

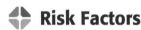 ## Risk Factors

Age: The risk of posterior capsule rupture and zonulodialysis may increase with age.[5,12,13] The mechanical strength and extensibility of the posterior capsule and zonules decrease with increasing age.[14] A higher incidence of posterior capsule plaques and dense cataracts is also seen[15] and may contribute to a higher risk of capsular and zonular complications.

Mature cataract: Several factors contribute to the increased risk of posterior capsule rupture and zonulodialysis in eyes with mature cataracts. A poor red reflex through an opaque, hydrated cortex and dense nucleus can make the capsulorhexis more challenging. The anterior capsule may also be lax and is often calcified.[16,17] Also, the high intracapsular pressure from liquefied cortical material tends to cause the capsulorhexis to extend radially. Nuclear removal can also be difficult. Lens to posterior capsule adhesions[18,19] and posterior capsule plaques[16–21] can make it difficult to rotate and mobilize the nucleus,[18,19] and cause the posterior capsule to tear during these maneuvers. The dense nucleus may also take longer to phacoemulsify, requiring more power or manipulation.[17,18] Brunescent cataracts tend to have very cohesive lens fibers that make division of the nucleus difficult.[19] Moreover, the posterior capsule is not only weak, but flaccid, making if prone to rupture during phacoemulsification; the problem is worsened by the absence of any epinucleus to protect the posterior capsule.[16,17]

Pseudoexfoliation (PXF): This systemic disorder can have several ocular findings that can contribute to posterior capsule rupture and zonulodialysis. The pupil may dilate poorly and the zonules may be compromised, which can manifest as phacodonesis, iridodonesis, lens subluxation, and decreased anterior chamber depth.[22–26] Though the lens capsule is involved in PXF, the lens capsule thickness and elasticity do not appear to be different from that in eyes without PXF.[27]

Alpha antagonist use: The use of alpha antagonists, particularly tamsulosin, has been shown to cause intraoperative floppy iris syndrome.[28–31] It is characterized by a fluttering and billowing iris that has a propensity to prolapse through the cataract incisions, along with progressive pupillary miosis.[31]

Previous vitrectomy: Cataract surgery in a previously vitrectomized eye has unique challenges. Poor mydriasis is not uncommon[32] and weakened zonules[33–36] and loss of vitreous support[35,37] result in an unstable posterior capsule that is unusually mobile and flaccid.[33,35,38] Posterior capsule plaques are also frequently encountered during surgery in post-vitrectomy eyes and can be difficult to remove.[34,36,39,40] A cataract developing within weeks of the vitrectomy should raise suspicion for damage to the posterior capsule during surgery.[36,41]

Others: Other possible risk factors for posterior capsule rupture and zonulo-dialysis include:

Previous trauma,[12] surgeon experience,[5,12,42–45] myopia,[5,46,47] posterior polar cataract,[20,48–50] poor visibility to the fundus,[5,12] fellow eye with complicated surgery,[5,51,52] glaucoma,[5,53] and diabetic retinopathy.[5]

✣ Pathogenesis

Anatomy

The lens capsule is the thickest basement membrane in the body[14] and completely envelops the crystalline lens. The posterior capsule is thinner than the anterior capsule and measures between 2 and 9 μm,[54] and is the thinnest at its center. It is composed mostly of type IV collagen and has a laminar structure[14] that contributes to its elasticity.[14,55] The zonules morphologically resemble the microfibrils of elastic tissue[56,57] and are capable of stretching before they are torn. In one study of postmortem eyes, the zonules were able to be stretched a mean of 3.82 mm before breaking.[58] The elastic properties and mechanical strength of the capsule and zonules allow the cataract to be removed in situ, but nonetheless, posterior capsule rupture and zonulodialysis can occur at any stage of surgery. Surgical trauma is the most common cause[17] and the mechanisms include direct damage by the surgical instruments and excessive stress or strain on the zonules and capsule. The pathogenesis of posterior capsule rupture and zonulodialysis varies with the stage of the surgery.

Microvitreoretinal (MVR) blade/Trocar insertion: The posterior capsule or zonules can be damaged during entry of the MVR blade or with insertion of the small-gauge trocar system if it is angled toward the lens or inserted anteriorly.

Capsulorhexis: A tear in the anterior capsule can extend peripherally around the equator to cause a rupture of the posterior capsule. However, radial tears of the anterior capsule usually do not extend posteriorly unless the zonules bridging the tear are severed or force is applied to the bag.[58]

Hydrodissection: The posterior capsule can rupture from excessive pressure in the capsular bag during hydrodissection, particularly if the injection of fluid is over-vigorous. Strong equatorial cortical adhesions to the lens capsule can allow fluid to accumulate posteriorly such that the excessive hydrostatic pressure overwhelms the extensibility of the posterior capsule. Any weakness of the posterior capsule such as from a posterior polar[48,49] or mature cataract[16] can increase the risk.

Nuclear management: The posterior capsule can be damaged during nuclear management through several mechanisms. Direct mechanical trauma, whereby the phaco tip or the second instrument directly punctures the capsule is one mechanism. This usually occurs during chopping maneuvers or during phacoemulsification, if high vacuum settings lead to vacuum surges, especially in the presence of an excessively mobile posterior capsule.[16,17,33–35,38] Sculpting too deeply can also directly puncture the capsule, when steep angulation of the phaco tip is necessary in deep anterior chambers. With dense cataracts, the irregular and hard surfaces of the nuclear fragments can perforate the capsule.[16,18] The tear resulting from direct mechanical damage is usually limited in size and has well-defined borders.[59]

Another mechanism by which the capsule is damaged is excessive mechanical stress during manipulation of the nucleus, especially when posterior capsule plaques or other adhesions make mobilization of the nucleus difficult.[18,19,34,36,39,40] In this case, the forces applied to the capsule exceed its mechanical strength. The tears created in this manner tend to be large with poorly defined borders.[50]

The zonules can be torn or disinserted if the forces transmitted to these structures exceed its elastic capacity. Insufficient phaco power during sculpting and aggressive manipulation of the lens during nuclear removal can place undue stress on the zonules and cause dialysis. Zonular weakness from PXF,[22,24,51] myopia, or trauma can contribute to the pathogenesis.

As mentioned above, a tear in the anterior capsule can extend posteriorly from the forces applied to the bag during manipulation of the nucleus.[60,61] When posterior capsule rupture occurs, it develops during nuclear management in 40% to 50% of cases.[51,59,62,63] Half of zonulodialysis also occurs during this stage.[51]

Irrigation/Aspiration (I/A): The posterior capsule can be directly damaged during I/A by excessive vacuum, aspiration with the port close to the posterior capsule or aspiration within a shallow or fluctuating anterior chamber.[7,16,17,33,40,64,65] The zonules can also disinsert or rupture if the capsule is inadvertently aspirated and pulled away, particularly if the zonules are weak.[37]

Intraocular lens insertion: The posterior capsule can rupture during this stage if excessive pressure is placed on the capsule by the distal loop of the intraocular lens or if the intraocular lens is rotated at an incorrect angle.[66] Also, if a posterior capsule tear is already present, manipulation of the intraocular lens can cause extension of the tear toward the equator.[67]

◆ Pearls on How to Prevent It

Each step of cataract surgery is dependent on the successful completion of the prior step, making every step important in preventing complications such as zonulodialysis and posterior capsule rupture.

- ◆ MVR/Trocar entry:

    - ◆ Angle the MVR or trocar blade away from the lens and toward the center of the eye. Use a second instrument (forceps or cotton-tip applicator) to stabilize the eye to maintain primary position during entry. It may be difficult to judge the angle of entry if the eye is rotated.

    - ◆ Avoid air bubbles in the infusion line (see "How to Prevent It" in the Section above). An air bubble can push the posterior capsule forward and increase the risk of posterior capsule rupture during phacoemulsification and I/A.

- ◆ Capsulorhexis: When an anterior capsule tear begins to extend to the equator:

    - ◆ Flatten the anterior capsule with a high molecular weight viscoelastic, using it to simultaneously elevate the flap to expose the leading edge. Grasp the flap at the edge and pull centripetally toward the lens center (Fig. 11B-1).

    - ◆ If the above maneuver fails to prevent equatorial extension of the rhexis, complete the capsulorhexis from the opposite direction. Avoid excessive hydrodissection, as the hydrostatic pressure can extend the tear posteriorly.

- ◆ Hydrodissection

    - ◆ Inject with moderate pressure and decompress the capsular bag after each injection with a gentle downward push on the nucleus with the cannula.

    - ◆ Establish mobility of the nucleus to ensure all lenticular–capsular adhesions are broken. This minimizes stress on the zonules and the posterior capsule during nuclear management.

- ◆ Nuclear management

    - ◆ Keep the posterior infusion off. This will prevent hydration of the vitreous and forward pressure on the posterior capsule.

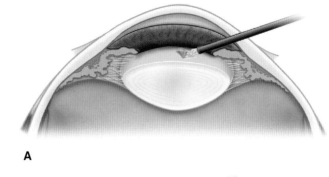

A

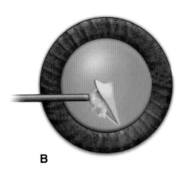

B

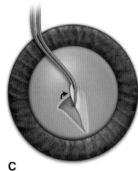

C

Figure 11B-1 **A:** When an anterior capsule tear begins to extend radially, a high molecular weight viscoelastic is used to flatten the anterior chamber. **B:** The viscoelastic concurrently elevates the flap. **C:** The edge of the flap is then grasped and pulled centripetally.

◆ Use sufficient ultrasound power to minimize stress on the zonules. If the nucleus moves forward during sculpting, increase the power.

◆ Only use ultrasound in the center of the pupil. Do not chase nuclear fragments.

◆ A second instrument under the phaco tip can prevent inadvertent damage to the posterior capsule, particularly when it is excessively mobile.

◆ When there is zonular weakness, use chopping maneuvers to minimize stress. Use a dispersive viscoelastic to protect the endothelium if phacoemulsification occurs in the anterior chamber.

◆ Avoid fluctuation of anterior chamber depth. This can extend an anterior capsule tear posteriorly and can also bring the posterior capsule in contact with nuclear fragments.

◆ Engage nuclear quadrants or chopped fragments at the apex, particularly with a hard nucleus, to keep the sharp edges away from the posterior capsule.

◆ If there is a posterior capsule plaque resistant to removal, a primary posterior capsulotomy can be performed later with the vitrector after the intraocular lens is placed in the bag.

◆ Irrigation/Aspiration

  ◆ Use low flow and moderate aspiration, with high aspiration only after cortical material is in the port. Pull tangentially and peel in a slow and deliberate fashion rather than pulling centripetally and attempting to remove en bloc. Stop and reflux if there are any striae in the posterior capsule as this may indicate that the capsule has been aspirated into the port.

◆ Intraocular lens insertion

  ◆ After deepening the anterior chamber and filling the capsular bag with viscoelastic, inject additional viscoelastic into the capsular bag across from the site of intraocular lens entry to ensure that there is adequate space. This will prevent the intraocular lens haptic from snagging the posterior capsule.

Pearls on How to Solve It

The first step in managing the complication is to recognize the problem. The signs may be subtle. A sudden change in anterior chamber depth or pupil size may indicate a sudden movement of fluid through a posterior capsule defect. Loss of the ability to attract and hold cataract fragments (followability) and phaco efficiency, a peaked pupil or abnormal pupil movement may signal the presence of vitreous. Once recognized, the management strategy depends on whether vitreous is present in the anterior chamber and if the nucleus has fallen posteriorly into the vitreous.

◆ Once there is suspicion of a posterior capsule rupture or zonulodialysis, stop, lower the bottle, and assess without removing the instruments from the eye. Do not allow the anterior chamber to collapse.

◆ Stabilize the anterior chamber with viscoelastic injected through the paracentesis before removing any instruments. A fluctuating anterior chamber may extend the tear (**Fig. 11B-2**).

◆ Posterior capsule rupture/zonulodialysis with an intact hyaloid face:

   ◆ Inject a dispersive viscoelastic between the nucleus and the posterior capsule defect or zonulodialysis to lift the nucleus and to serve as a barrier between the nucleus and the vitreous.

   ◆ The remaining nuclear material can then be removed. Use low flow to avoid washing out the viscoelastic and to limit hydration of the vitreous. The vacuum should be moderate to high and the ultrasound power should be low to provide followability and to minimize turbulence and chatter. Reinject viscoelastic as necessary.

   ◆ After nuclear removal, if the hyaloid face is still intact, the I/A handpiece can be used under low flow to remove the residual cortex. Otherwise a vitrectomy should be performed.

◆ Posterior capsule rupture/zonulodialysis with disruption of the hyaloid face:

   If there is vitreous in the anterior chamber, a vitrectomy should be performed. Phacoemulsification is inefficient and dangerous when cataract has mixed with vitreous. Vitreous displaces the nucleus and is preferentially attracted to the phaco tip. Aspiration of the anterior vitreous in this setting transmits tractional forces to the peripheral retina.

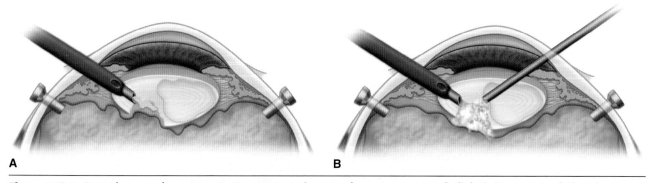

A   B

Figure 11B-2 Posterior capsule rupture. **A:** Once a posterior capsule rupture or zonulodialysis is recognized, the phaco-emulsification instrument should not be removed from the eye. **B:** Viscoelastic is injected through the paracentesis to stabilize the anterior chamber before removing the instrument.

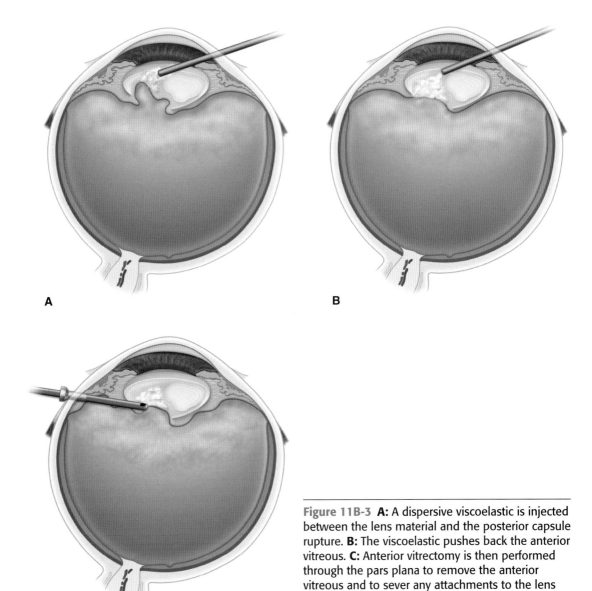

A

B

C

Figure 11B-3 A: A dispersive viscoelastic is injected between the lens material and the posterior capsule rupture. **B:** The viscoelastic pushes back the anterior vitreous. **C:** Anterior vitrectomy is then performed through the pars plana to remove the anterior vitreous and to sever any attachments to the lens material.

◆ Inject a dispersive viscoelastic between the nucleus and the posterior capsule rupture/zonulodialysis **(Fig. 11B-3).**

◆ Perform an anterior vitrectomy through the pars plana. Use high cutting speeds and low to moderate aspiration to minimize vitreoretinal traction.

◆ The goal of anterior vitrectomy is to remove the anterior hyaloid and to sever any attachments to the vitreous in the anterior chamber. The vitreous should be separated from the nuclear material **(Fig. 11B-3).** Diluted preservative-free triamcinolone acetonide can be used to highlight the vitreous.

◆ The vitrector should be used through the opening of the posterior capsule rupture to preserve as much of the posterior capsule as possible. If the anterior capsulotomy is intact, avoid damaging the rhexis **(Fig. 11B-3).** In the case of zonulodialysis, the vitrector should be used through the area of dehiscence while keeping the port away from the capsule to preserve the bag.

◆ Alternatively, if the zonulodialysis is small (1–3 clock hours) or if its location makes it difficult to maneuver the vitrector from a posterior approach, the anterior vitrectomy may be performed through the paracentesis with a small-gauge vitrector.

◆ After the vitrectomy, if the remaining nucleus is soft, the fragments can be removed with the vitrector, using a second instrument to feed the vitrector port. If the nucleus is hard, inject a dispersive viscoelastic over the posterior capsule rupture/zonulodialysis, then remove with phacoemulsification using low flow and high vacuum.

◆ If the zonulodialysis is less than 6 clock hours an endocapsular ring can be used to stabilize the capsular bag. Alternatively, iris hooks can be used to hold the edge of the rhexis in place. A dispersive viscoelastic can then be used to keep the bag formed during nuclear removal.

◆ After the vitreous and nucleus have been cleared, the cortex can be removed with the vitrector set to vacuum. The cutter can be used if any residual vitreous is present. Gently engage the peripheral cortex and pull tangentially to remove the cortex.

◆ Posterior capsule rupture/zonulodialysis with disruption of the hyaloid and displacement of the nucleus into the vitreous:

◆ Perform an anterior vitrectomy and remove all nuclear fragments and cortex that remain in the anterior chamber.

◆ A core vitrectomy should then be performed. Diluted preservative-free triamcinolone acetonide can be helpful in ensuring that the nuclear fragments are free of vitreous. Depending on the density of the nuclear piece, either the vitrector or the fragmatome can be used to remove the nucleus.

◆ If there is a concomitant retinal detachment, perfluorocarbon liquid can be used to flatten the retina and float the nucleus forward.

◆ Can I preserve the capsular bag? Can I insert an intraocular lens?

◆ The intraocular lens can be implanted in the bag if the zonulodialysis is limited to 3 clock hours or less. The haptic should be placed to support the area of zonulodialysis.

◆ If less than 6 clock hours of zonular support remain, the sulcus cannot be used for intraocular lens placement, unless the intraocular lens is sutured. In this case, the entire capsule should be removed and an anterior chamber intraocular lens used.

◆ The intraocular lens should be implanted into the bag only if the posterior tear is limited with defined borders and has been converted to a posterior capsulorhexis.

◆ If the anterior capsulorhexis is intact, the intraocular lens can be placed in the sulcus and the optic captured.[68] The intraocular lens is placed in the sulcus with the haptics situated 90 degrees from the posterior capsule rupture. Next, one side of the optic, 90 degrees away from the optic–haptic junction, is pushed behind the anterior capsulorhexis with a lens manipulator such as a Sinskey hook. Once that side of the optic is placed under the anterior capsule, the other side is similarly pushed under the rhexis to capture the optic. This provides more stability to the intraocular lens, compartmentalizes the anterior chamber, and places the intraocular lens in the plane of the bag. Compartmentalization of the anterior chamber from the vitreous cavity is especially important when a tamponade agent such as gas or silicone oil is to be used. Capturing the optic prevents migration of air, gas, or silicone oil into the anterior chamber and also stabilizes the intraocular lens.

◆ If the anterior capsulorhexis is not intact, the intraocular lens can be placed in the sulcus if there is adequate posterior capsule support 180 degrees apart. It is surprising how little residual capsule is needed to support a posterior chamber intraocular lens.

Expected Outcomes: What Is the Worst-case Scenario

When there is inadequate or questionable support for a posterior chamber intraocular lens, an anterior chamber intraocular lens may need to be used. Alternatively, the patient can be left aphakic and a secondary intraocular lens inserted at a later time. Time spent on the anterior segment should be kept minimal, as surgical trauma to the endothelium may cause the cornea to decompensate, compromising the view and the subsequent vitreoretinal portion of the surgery.

In addition, the peripheral retina is weak and has strong adhesions to the vitreous base. Traction on the anterior vitreous can cause retinal tears and possible retinal detachment, complicating the subsequent vitreoretinal procedure and clinical outcome.

REFERENCES

1. Mochizuki Y, Kubota T, Hata Y, et al. Surgical results of combined pars plana vitrectomy, phacoemulsification, and intraocular lens implantation. *Eur J Ophthalmol.* 2006;16:279–286.
2. Demetriades AM, Gottsch JD, Thomsen R, et al. Combined phacoemulsification, intraocular lens implantation, and vitrectomy for eyes with coexisting cataract and vitreoretinal pathology. *Am J Ophthalmol.* 2003;135:291–296.
3. Jun Z, Pavlovic S, Jacobi KW. Results of combined vitreoretinal surgery and phacoemulsification with intraocular lens implantation. *Clin Experiment Ophthalmol.* 2001; 29:307–311.
4. Wensheng L, Wu R, Wang X, et al. Clinical complications of combined phacoemulsification and vitrectomy for eyes with coexisting cataract and vitreoretinal diseases. *Eur J Ophthalmol.* 2009;19:37–45.
5. Narendran N, Jaycock P, Johnston RL, et al. The Cataract National Dataset electronic multicentre audit of 55,567 operations: Risk stratification for posterior capsule rupture and vitreous loss. *Eye (Lond).* 2009;23:31–37.
6. Muhtaseb M, Kalhoro A, Ionides A. A system for preoperative stratification of cataract patients according to risk of intraoperative complications: A prospective analysis of 1441 cases. *Br J Ophthalmol.* 2004;88:1242–1246.
7. Misra A, Burton RL. Incidence of intraoperative complications during phacoemulsification in vitrectomized and nonvitrectomized eyes: Prospective study. *J Cataract Refract Surg.* 2005;31:1011–1014.
8. Agrawal V, Upadhyay J. Validation of scoring system for preoperative stratification of intra-operative risks of complications during cataract surgery: Indian multicentric study. *Indian J Ophthalmol.* 2009;57:213–215.
9. Ang GS, Whyte IF. Effect and outcomes of posterior capsule rupture in a district general hospital setting. *J Cataract Refract Surg.* 2006;32:623–627.
10. Zaidi FH, Corbett MC, Burton BJ, et al. Raising the benchmark for the 21st century—the 1000 cataract operations audit and survey: Outcomes, consultant-supervised training and sourcing NHS choice. *Br J Ophthalmol.* 2007;91:731–736.
11. Sisk RA, Murray TG. Combined phacoemulsification and sutureless 23-gauge pars plana vitrectomy for complex vitreoretinal diseases. *Br J Ophthalmol.* 2010;94: 1028–1032.

12. Artzén D, Lundström M, Behndig A, et al. Capsule complication during cataract surgery: Case-control study of preoperative and intraoperative risk factors: Swedish Capsule Rupture Study Group report 2. *J Cataract Refract Surg.* 2009;35:1688–1693.

13. Robbie SJ, Muhtaseb M, Qureshi K, et al. Intraoperative complications of cataract surgery in the very old. *Br J Ophthalmol.* 2006;90:1516–1518.

14. Krag S, Andreassen TT. Mechanical properties of the human lens capsule. *Prog Retin Eye Res.* 2003;22:749–767.

15. Syam PP, Eleftheriadis H, Casswell AG, et al. Clinical outcome following cataract surgery in very elderly patients. *Eye (Lond).* 2004;18:59–62.

16. Ermiş SS, Oztürk F, Inan UU. Comparing the efficacy and safety of phacoemulsification in white mature and other types of senile cataracts. *Br J Ophthalmol.* 2003; 87:1356–1359.

17. Vajpayee RB, Bansal A, Sharma N, et al. Phacoemulsification of white hypermature cataract. *J Cataract Refract Surg.* 1999;25:1157–1160.

18. Brazitikos PD, Tsinopoulos IT, Papadopoulos NT, et al. Ultrasonographic classification and phacoemulsification of white senile cataracts. *Ophthalmology.* 1999;106: 2178–2183.

19. Singh R, Vasavada AR, Janaswamy G. Phacoemulsification of brunescent and black cataracts. *J Cataract Refract Surg.* 2001;27:1762–1769.

20. Vasavada AR, Chauhan H, Shah G. Incidence of posterior capsular plaque in cataract surgery. *J Cataract Refract Surg.* 1997;23:798–802.

21. Vasavada A, Singh R, Desai J. Phacoemulsification of white mature cataracts. *J Cataract Refract Surg.* 1998;24:270–277.

22. Schlötzer-Schrehardt U, Naumann GO. Ocular and systemic pseudoexfoliation syndrome. *Am J Ophthalmol.* 2006;141:921–937.

23. Shingleton BJ, Marvin AC, Heier JS, et al. Pseudoexfoliation: High risk factors for zonule weakness and concurrent vitrectomy during phacoemulsification. *J Cataract Refract Surg.* 2010;36:1261–1269.

24. Schlötzer-Schrehardt U, Naumann GO. A histopathologic study of zonular instability in pseudoexfoliation syndrome. *Am J Ophthalmol.* 1994;118:730–743.

25. Shingleton BJ, Crandall AS, Ahmed II. Pseudoexfoliation and the cataract surgeon: Preoperative, intraoperative, and postoperative issues related to intraocular pressure, cataract, and intraocular lenses. *J Cataract Refract Surg.* 2009;35: 1101–1120.

26. Küchle M, Viestenz A, Martus P, et al. Anterior chamber depth and complications during cataract surgery in eyes with pseudoexfoliation syndrome. *Am J Ophthalmol.* 2000;129:281–285.

27. Bergmanson JP, Jones WL, Chu LW. Ultrastructural observations on (pseudo-) exfoliation of the lens capsule: A re-examination of the involvement of the lens epithelium. *Br J Ophthalmol.* 1984;68:118–123.

28. Chang DF, Campbell JR. Intraoperative floppy iris syndrome associated with tamsulosin. *J Cataract Refract Surg.* 2005;31:664–673.

29. Chang DF, Osher RH, Wang L, et al. Prospective multicenter evaluation of cataract surgery in patients taking tamsulosin (Flomax). *Ophthalmology.* 2007;114:957–964.

30. Neff KD, Sandoval HP, Fernández de Castro LE, et al. Factors associated with intraoperative floppy iris syndrome. *Ophthalmology,* 2009;116:658–663.

31. Storr-Paulsen A, Nørregaard JC, Børme KK, et al. Intraoperative floppy iris syndrome (IFIS): A practical approach to medical and surgical considerations in cataract extractions. *Acta Ophthalmol.* 2009;87:704–708.

32. Braunstein RE, Airiani S. Cataract surgery results after pars plana vitrectomy. *Curr Opin Ophthalmol.* 2003;14:150–154.

33. Díaz Lacalle V, Orbegozo Gárate FJ, Martinez Alday N, et al. Phacoemulsification cataract surgery in vitrectomized eyes. *J Cataract Refract Surg.* 1998;24:806–809.

34. Pinter SM, Sugar A. Phacoemulsification in eyes with past pars plana vitrectomy: Case-control study. *J Cataract Refract Surg.* 1999;25:556–561.

35. Smiddy WE, Stark WJ, Michels RG, et al. Cataract extraction after vitrectomy. *Ophthalmology.* 1987;94:483–487.

36. Biró Z, Kovacs B. Results of cataract surgery in previously vitrectomized eyes. *J Cataract Refract Surg.* 2002;28:1003–1006.
37. Sneed S, Parrish RK 2nd, Mandelbaum S, et al. Technical problems of extracapsular cataract extractions after vitrectomy. *Arch Ophthalmol.* 1986;104:1126–1127.
38. McDermott ML, Puklin JE, Abrams GW, et al. Phacoemulsification for cataract following pars plana vitrectomy. *Ophthalmic Surg Lasers.* 1997;28:558–564.
39. Chang MA, Parides MK, Chang S, et al. Outcome of phacoemulsification after pars plana vitrectomy. *Ophthalmology.* 2002;109:948–954.
40. Grusha YO, Masket S, Miller KM. Phacoemulsification and lens implantation after pars plana vitrectomy. *Ophthalmology.* 1998;105:287–294.
41. Pardo-Muñoz A, Muriel-Herrero A, Abraira V, et al. Phacoemulsification in previously vitrectomized patients: An analysis of the surgical results in 100 eyes as well as the factors contributing to the cataract formation. *Eur J Ophthalmol.* 2006;16:52–59.
42. Rutar T, Porco TC, Naseri A. Risk factors for intraoperative complications in resident-performed phacoemulsification surgery. *Ophthalmology.* 2009;116:431–436.
43. Randleman JB, Wolfe JD, Woodward M, et al. The resident surgeon phacoemulsification learning curve. *Arch Ophthalmol.* 2007;125:1215–1219.
44. Bhagat N, Nissirios N, Potdevin L, et al. Complications in resident-performed phacoemulsification cataract surgery at New Jersey Medical School. *Br J Ophthalmol.* 2007;91:1315–1317.
45. Blomquist PH, Rugwani RM. Visual outcomes after vitreous loss during cataract surgery performed by residents. *J Cataract Refract Surg.* 2002;28:847–852.
46. Kora Y, Nishimura E, Kitazato T, et al. Analysis of preoperative factors predictive of visual acuity in axial myopia. *J Cataract Refract Surg.* 1998;24:834–839.
47. Ochi T, Gon A, Kora Y, et al. Intraocular lens implantation and high myopia. *J Cataract Refract Surg.* 1988;14:403–408.
48. Das S, Khanna R, Mohiuddin SM, et al. Surgical and visual outcomes for posterior polar cataract. *Br J Ophthalmol.* 2008;92:1476–1478.
49. Hayashi K, Hayashi H, Nakao F, et al. Outcomes of surgery for posterior polar cataract. *J Cataract Refract Surg.* 2003;29:45–49.
50. Osher RH, Yu BC, Koch DD. Posterior polar cataracts: a predisposition to intraoperative posterior capsular rupture. *J Cataract Refract Surg.* 1990;16:157–162.
51. Mulhern M, Kelly G, Barry P. Effects of posterior capsular disruption on the outcome of phacoemulsification surgery. *Br J Ophthalmol.* 1995;79:1133–1137.
52. Androudi S, Ahmed M, Fiore T, et al. Combined pars plana vitrectomy and phacoemulsification to restore visual acuity in patients with chronic uveitis. *J Cataract Refract Surg.* 2005;31:472–478.
53. Abbasoğlu OE, Hoşal B, Tekeli O, et al. Risk factors for vitreous loss in cataract surgery. *Eur J Ophthalmol.* 2000;10:227–232.
54. Ziebarth NM, Manns F, Uhlhorn SR, et al. Noncontact optical measurement of lens capsule thickness in human, monkey, and rabbit postmortem eyes. *Invest Ophthalmol Vis Sci.* 2005;46:1690–1697.
55. Assia EI, Apple DJ, Tsai JC, et al. The elastic properties of the lens capsule in capsulorhexis. *Am J Ophthalmol.* 1991;111:628–632.
56. Streeten BW, Licari PA, Marucci AA, et al. Immunohistochemical comparison of ocular zonules and the microfibrils of elastic tissue. *Invest Ophthalmol Vis Sci.* 1981;21:130–135.
57. Streeten BW, Licari PA. The zonules and the elastic microfibrillar system in the ciliary body. *Invest Ophthalmol Vis Sci.* 1983;24:667–681.
58. Assia EI, Apple DJ, Morgan RC, et al. The relationship between the stretching capability of the anterior capsule and zonules. *Invest Ophthalmol Vis Sci.* 1991;32:2835–2839.
59. Osher RH, Cionni RJ. The torn posterior capsule: its intraoperative behavior, surgical management, and long-term consequences. *J Cataract Refract Surg.* 1990;16:490–494.
60. Assia EI, Apple DJ, Tsai JC, et al. Mechanism of radial tear formation and extension after anterior capsulectomy. *Ophthalmology.* 1991;98:432–437.

61. Marques FF, Marques DM, Osher RH, et al. Fate of anterior capsule tears during cataract surgery. *J Cataract Refract Surg.* 2006;32:1638–1642.
62. Gimbel HV, Sun R, Ferensowicz M, et al. Intraoperative management of posterior capsule tears in phacoemulsification and intraocular lens implantation. *Ophthalmology.* 2001;108:2186–2189.
63. Ang GS, Whyte IF. Effect and outcomes of posterior capsule rupture in a district general hospital setting. *J Cataract Refract Surg.* 2006;32:623–627.
64. NOW Buratto L. *Phacoemulsification: Principles and Techniques.* New Jersey: Slack; 1998:211–262.
65. Ahfat FG, Yuen CH, Groenewald CP. Phacoemulsification and intraocular lens implantation following pars plana vitrectomy: A prospective study. *Eye (Lond).* 2003; 17:16–20.
66. Koch PS. *Mastering phacoemulsification,* 4th ed. New Jersey, NJ: Slack; 1994:67–77.
67. Castaneda VE, Legler UF, Tsai JC, et al. Posterior continuous curvilinear capsulorhexis. An experimental study with clinical applications. *Ophthalmology.* 1992; 99:45–50.
68. Neuhann T. "The Rhexis-Fixated Lens," film presented at the ASCRS Symposium on Cataract, IOL and Refractive Surgery, Boston, Massachusetts, USA, 1991.

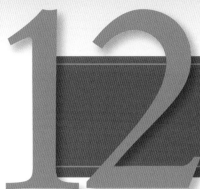

12

COMPLICATIONS RELATED to the INDUCTION of a POSTERIOR VITREOUS DETACHMENT

Tom Williamson

12A I Cannot Detach the Vitreous in an Eye with an Attached Retina

Surgical Steps

1. Remove the core vitreous with the vitrectomy cutter.
2. Shave the cortical gel off the optic nerve head.
3. Aspirate the posterior hyaloid membrane (PHM) into the vitrectomy cutter orifice.
4. Apply traction to the PHM.
5. Watch for separation of the PHM from the surface of the retina.
6. Create a dome of elevation of the PHM.
7. Cut a hole in the PHM at the apex of the dome.
8. Insert the cutter to elevate the PHM in each quadrant.
9. Complete the removal of the vitreous.

Macular Hole

The most common indication for detachment of the PHM is during macular hole surgery.

Detachment of the PHM is facilitated in this condition by partial detachment as seen on optical coherence tomography (OCT), that is, there is a virtual space already **(Fig. 12A-1)**.

In this case the site of highest "occult" posterior vitreous detachment (PVD) is supero-temporal to the disc and away from blood vessels.

The PHM is a much stiffer material than the cortical vitreous; therefore it is important to shave the vitreous off the optic nerve head to allow suction of the cutter to engage the PHM.

Aspirating the cortex only shreds the cortical gel and does not achieve traction on the PHM over the disc.

Aspirating the PHM itself, because of the relative inelasticity of the PHM, allows a good "grip" to be achieved on the membrane thereby allowing the surgeon to overcome the adhesion of the PHM to the optic nerve head by engaging the membrane and applying traction on it.

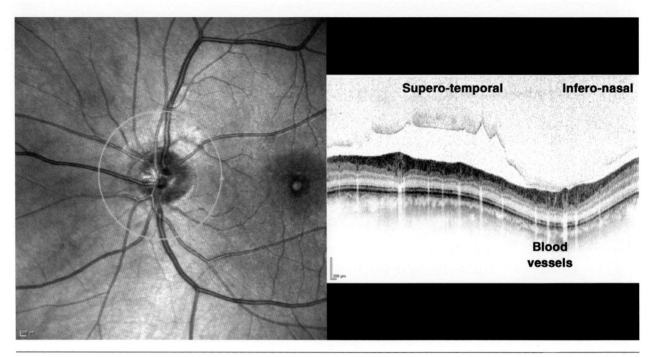

Figure 12A-1 The vitreous tends to more detached temporally and superiorly and away from large blood vessels. This helps to choose a site to aspirate during surgical detachment of the PHM.

Starting at the optic disc edge and moving tangentially over the temporal margin engages the partially detached vitreous over the papillomacular bundle.

The toughest attachment of the vitreous is at the disc; once this is separated the detachment of the remaining PHM is easier.

Watch just around the optic disc for the tell-tale sign of a dark circular line at the edge of adhesion of the PHM to the retina **(Fig. 12A-2)**.

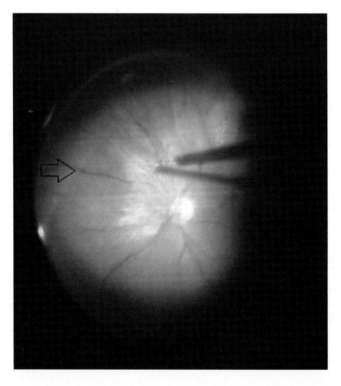

Figure 12A-2 The edge of the posterior hyaloid *(arrow)* peeling off the retina can be observed during PVD induction and is a good guide to the extent of PVD produced.

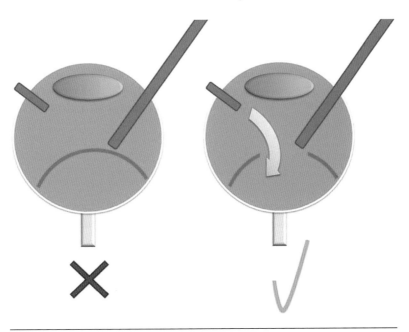

Figure 12A-3 Creating a hole in the PHM during lifting of the membrane allows fluid to enter and removes the negative pressure build up posterior to the PHM if no hole is present.

This line advances peripherally as the PHM detaches.

Once you have created a dome of detachment, use the cutter to create a hole in the PHM to allow fluid to enter behind the membrane. This obliterates the negative pressure which builds in the virtual space behind the PHM if no communication with the fluid-filled vitreous cavity is created **(Fig. 12A-3)**.

Through this hole, extend the cutter under the PHM in each quadrant whilst aspirating, lift the PHM anteriorly in each quadrant thereby extending the elevation of the PHM without causing traction on the vitreous base which might tear the retina **(Fig. 12A-4)**.

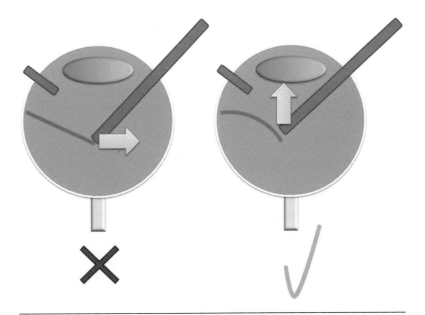

Figure 12A-4 Lift the PHM anteriorly not tangentially to avoid traction at the vitreous base.

As long as you move anteriorly there will be minimal chance of tearing the retina at its adhesion to the vitreous base, because the cord length of the PHM is longer than the radius of the sphere of the eye.

The PHM can be allowed to passively elevate during removal of the remainder of the vitreous with the cutter, but this can leave a segment of vitreous attached in the periphery, requiring repeat peel and vitrectomy at a later stage of the procedure.

Other Conditions

Some conditions do not have an "occult" PVD, for example, asteroid hyalosis, some ERMs, uveitis, and some dropped nuclei. In these cases commencement of the PHM peel can be more difficult.

Younger patents are less likely to have an occult separation.

If the adhesion cannot be broken, stain the vitreous with dye (trypan blue) or steroid (triamcinolone). The visualization of the vitreous allows closer shaving of the vitreous and easier determination of the movement of the PHM once it starts to separate.

Other methods can be tried.

◆ Increase the vacuum pressure from 150 mm Hg to 300 mm Hg with 20 g, or from 300 mm Hg to 450 mm Hg with 23 g.

◆ Try to elevate the PHM from a site away from the disc and move over to separate the disc once the detachment has been started.

◆ Rarely, if the Weiss ring can be seen to partially separate but it will not completely come off, use forceps to pull off the Weiss by grasping its edge.

◆ If the Weiss is very adherent, the optic nerve head may bleed and there is a risk of retinal nerve fiber layer damage and visual field loss.

Do not pull through lattice degeneration or some chorioretinal scars as this will tear the retina. Pull up to the adhesion and around it if it is posterior and trim the vitreous around the site.

Safe to pull PHM through or over:

◆ Idiopathic epiretinal membrane (often separates with the PHM).

◆ Choroidal neovascular membrane.

◆ Myelinated nerve fibers (the myelin comes away with the PHM).

◆ White without pressure.

◆ Cobblestone degeneration.

◆ Reticular degeneration.

◆ Chorioretinal atrophy.

◆ "New" chorioretinal infiltration, for example, infection.

Unsafe to pull through:

◆ Lattice degeneration.

◆ Snail track degeneration.

◆ Neovascular membranes.

Take care:

◆ "Old" chorioretinal scars, for example, toxoplasmosis.

◆ Macroaneurysms.

Damage to the surface of the macula from PHM peel can stimulate epiretinal membrane formation.

Damage to the optic nerve head surface can lead to visual field loss.

12B I Cannot Detach the Vitreous in an Eye with a Detached Retina

 ## Possible Additional Surgical Steps

◆ Elevate the PHM over flat retina first.

◆ Insert heavy liquid to splint the retina.

◆ Apply traction to the PHM parralel to the surface of the detached retina.

◆ Drain subretinal fluid through any retinal breaks.

The surgeon may need to do this in operations for retinoschisis-related rhegmatogenous retinal detachment (RRD), trauma, or in round hole or dialysis-related RRD if the surgeon has chosen to perform pars plana vitrectomy (PPV) in those cases.

There are additional problems in detaching the vitreous in an eye with detached retina.

◆ There is less space to allow movement of the PHM (Fig. 12B-1).

◆ The retina may move with the force applied to detach the PHM preventing separation of the PHM from the retinal surface.

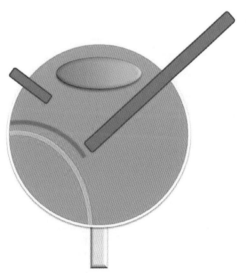

Figure 12B-1 There is less space to manipulate the PHM in an eye with RD.

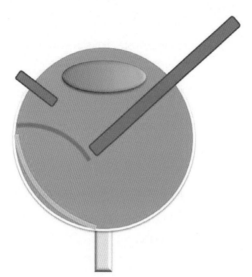

Figure 12B-2 Drain any subretinal fluid (SRF) to create some space.

Luckily, the vitreous is usually contracted and of reduced volume if RD is present.

Commence the PHM peel at the optic nerve head which of course cannot move and the forces can be applied to separate the PHM from its surface.

Extend the PHM peel over the attached retina first thereby establishing the separation and allowing fluid currents to act to separate the PHM off the detached retina.

If a retinal hole is present drain the SRF to achieve space in the vitreous cavity to maneuver the PHM. This will only work temporally as fluid will re-accumulate in the SR space **(Fig. 12B-2)**.

"Splint" the retina with a small bubble of heavy liquid (inserted through a hole in the PHM), once the PHM elevation has been started. This stabilses the retina preventing its movement whilst the surgeon pulls off the PHM. Note that putting heavy liquid on top of the PHM will make elevation of the PHM more difficult **(Fig. 12B-3)**.

In practice, if the PHM is elevated relatively quickly the SRF space does not have time to expand (either by accumulation of fluid from the vitreous cavity through a retinal hole in an RRD or by extravasation of fluid from the choroid in an exudative RD).

Note: If choroidal effusions are present in a hypotonous eye, merely restoring the intraocular pressure by inserting the infusion can cause rapid resolution of the effusions.

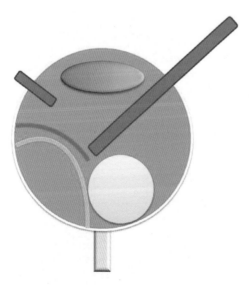

Figure 12B-3 Use a bubble of heavy liquid to splint the retina.

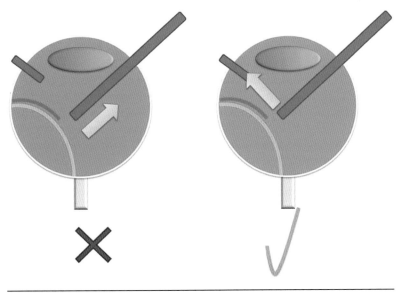

Figure 12B-4 Peel parallel to the surface of the RD not perpendicular.

By elevating the PHM from a point of contact close to the elevated retina, the force to elevate the PHM can be applied parralel to the surface of the RD. This is prefered to pulling the PHM perpendicular to the surface of the detached retina which causes the retina to move with the PHM centrally **(Fig. 12B-4)**.

Again do not pull through lattice degeneration or vitreoretinal adhesions.

Even thin diaphenous retina as in XL retinoschisis will stay intact during PHM peel, possibly due to the presence of the relatively tough ILM.

If a total RD is present the SRF will need to be drained either through a retinotomy or by external drain in which case a 26G needle can be inserted transconjunctivally under internal observation. Look for the indentation of the tip of the needle on the sclera to identify its location to check that it is under a bulla of RD before applying pressure to penetrate the sclera.

Once flattened, the PHM can be peeled and the vitreous removed.

12C Detaching the Vitreous in the Presence of Neovascularization

◆ Possible Additional Surgical Steps

- ◆ Search for vitreoschisis.
- ◆ Delaminate neovascular membranes.
- ◆ Segment neovascular membranes.
- ◆ Use bimanual surgery.

Diabetic Retinopathy

The commonest condition requiring detachment of the vitreous with neovascularization is diabetic retinopathy with tractional retinal detachment.

The natural course of the vitreous in proliferative diabetic retinopathy is to shrink and stiffen, held back from a complete separation from the retina by the adhesion of the neovascular membranes to the surface of the retina.

The PHM in mild tractional retinal detachment (TRD) may be intact to the vitreous base; however, in severe TRD with gliotic membranes, often the PHM has atrophied in the mid-peripheral fundus.

Attachment of the PHM to the retina is by diffuse weak attachments (as seen in other conditions such as macular hole surgery) and strong attachments in the neovascular membranes. The latter are characterized usually by pegs of attachments (small foci of attachment) which may be multiple within the membranous area.

The diffuse weak attachment can be released by tractional elevation of the PHM as in macular hole surgery.

Pegs in the strong membranous attachment are usually best dealt with by cutting with scissors.

Note: Scissors squash the tissue as they cut creating an S-shaped cut in the tissue. The squashing may contribute to the reduced bleeding seen with scissors compared with pulling and avulsing the pegs off the retina or cutting of pegs with the guillotine vitrectomy cutter.

The dissection of the PHM therefore involves:

◆ Identification of the PHM.

◆ Tractional elevation of the PHM where possible.

◆ Cutting of pegs of attachment in neovascular membranes.

In mild TRD, areas of pre-existing elevation of the PHM may be seen and can be incised allowing scissors to be inserted to gain access to the correct plane for surgical dissection. With the scissors closed use the upper edge to elevate the PHM from detached PHM to attached PHM. Watch for any traction on pegs which if found should be cut. If there are any larger areas of attachment elevate the PHM 360 degrees round the attachment before dissection.

Severe TRD may demonstrate vitreoschisis, namely a splitting of the cortical vitreous into an inner and an outer layer (the outer layer having the residual PHM). This can deceive the surgeon into leaving the outer layer of vitreous on the retina and consequently allows membrane reproliferation postoperatively. In addition, the absence of recognition of the outer layer results in difficult dissection through the cortical gel rather than easier dissection under the PHM (Fig. 12C-1).

In severe TRD, try to find the edge of the PHM where it has atrophied, for example, on the slope of the TRD. Once detected lift the PHM with scissors toward the membrane, lift the membrane gently to identify pegs and cut them. Trim the edge of the elevated membrane from time to time to allow a view of the pegs.

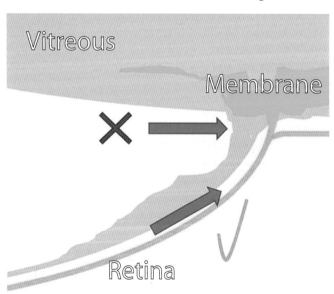

Figure 12C-1 It is important to dissect under the outer layer of a vitreoschisis which is easier than cutting through the vitreous to get to pegs of membranous attachment and avoids leaving vitreous on the retina.

✠ Innovations

◆ Modern small-gauge cutters have the cutting orifice near the tip of the shaft of the cutter and high cut rates which allow the abscission of small bites of membranes near the surface of the retina. For this reason they can be used close to the surface of the retina to remove TRD membranes with little risk of cutting the retina itself.

◆ Use of chandelier illumination allows the surgeon to grasp the PHM with his second hand, facilitating elevation of the edge of adherent PHM to membrane. The pegs can then be easily seen and cut. Often the illumination needs to be directed to the membrane by a surgical assistant, otherwise illumination is poor.

◆ Staining of vitreous gel with intravitreal triamcinolone or trypan blue dye is helpful to identify residual gel on the surface of the retina.

◆ Preoperative intravitreal antiVEGF injection stiffens the membranes and reduces their vascularity. The stiffness eases dissection and the avascularity reduces peroperative bleeding. Give the injection, for example, 1.25 mg bevacizumab 3 to 7 days before the vitrectomy for best effect.

The key elements in deciding between PHM detachment by active traction or sharp dissection of the PHM by the incision of attachments are the nature of any attachment of the PHM to the retina. With practice, the surgeon must make a judgment on the balance of forces at play. If a surgeon chooses to pull a membrane off the retina, he or she must decide if the force required to overcome the attachment of the membrane to the retina is less than the force required to disrupt the integrity of the retina (i.e., the force which will tear the retina). Diabetic retina is usually ischemic and weakened. Therefore although some attachments can be pulled off many will require cutting. In addition, pulling new vessels and rupturing them rather than cutting is associated with increased bleeding **(Fig. 12C-2)**.

Some areas of membrane are so embedded in the retina that dissection and elevation of the membrane is too risky. Often these areas are indicated by the presence of schitic retina. Segmentation of the membrane in these areas can be used, that is, the surgeon removes the attachments around the membrane but leaves the established membrane on the retina. This requires the surgeon to make a "judgment call" on the nature of the adhesion which is not an easy proposition.

Removing the PHM and membranes is a technical challenge which is reflected in the high rate of iatrogenic breaks in TRD surgery (30%). These can be from:

◆ Traction

◆ Direct injury from a sharp instrument.

◆ Incision from vitrectomy cutter.

A combination of the innovations mentioned above may reduce the complication rate of retinal tear formation:

◆ Preoperative antiVEGF

◆ Bimanual surgery

◆ Shaving of simple membranes with cutters

◆ Selective segmentation

Normal

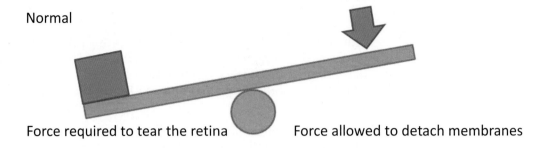

Force required to tear the retina   Force allowed to detach membranes

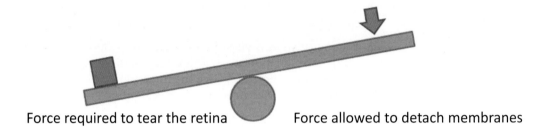

Force required to tear the retina   Force allowed to detach membranes

Diabetic

Figure 12C-2 The balancing act between pulling on an epiretinal membrane (ERM) and avoiding a retinal tear. In the normal eye a large force is required before the retina tears, so that a relatively large force can be applied to pull off an ERM. In the ischemic diabetic retina a small force may tear the retina; therefore only a small force can be applied to ERM to remove it.

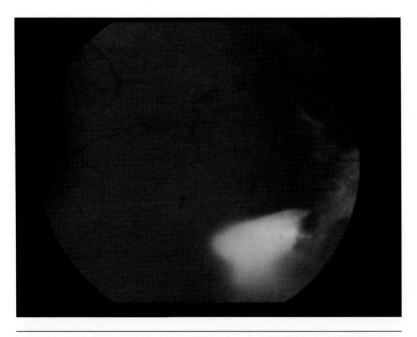

Figure 12C-3 A sea fan complex with thick membrane and blood. These do not dissect off the retina and should be segmented.

Other Conditions

Neovascularization in retinal vein occlusion is only occasionally associated with gliosis requiring delamination, otherwise the new vessels can be trimmed with the cutter.

Choroidal neovascularization remains subretinal and intraretinal; therefore the PHM can be peeled off the surface with traction. Watch out for mild vitreomacular traction over the choroidal neovascularisation (CNV).

Sickle cell retinopathy can result in a number of conditions requiring removal of the vitreous. The PHM can be peeled as usual but do not try to peel through the sea fan complexes. These are best left in place with trimming of gel and membranes around the sea fan complex (segmentation) **(Fig. 12C-3)**.

12D   Detaching the Vitreous in "Friable" Retina

Various Conditions

Conditions which may present with friable retina include severe diabetic retinopathy, retinal vein occlusion, trauma, uveitis, and acute retinal necrosis (ARN). The last is a classical presentation with moth-eaten retina **(Fig. 12D-1)** although a variety of retinal tears may be seen. Extremely thin retina can be found in retinoschisis-related RRD and especially in XL retinoschisis **(Fig. 12D-2)**.

The high rate of retinal detachment in ARN is such that the vitreoretinal surgeon will be required to operate on these patients.

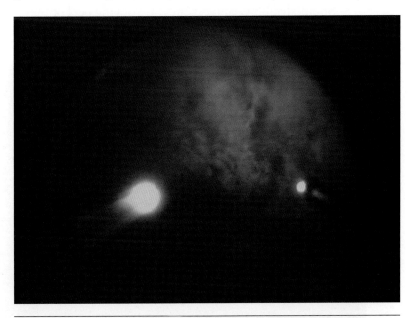

Figure 12D-1 In this patient, a retinal detachment has followed after acute retinal necrosis. Sometimes discrete tears are identifiable, but often the retina is "moth eaten" and the exact location of breaks is difficult.

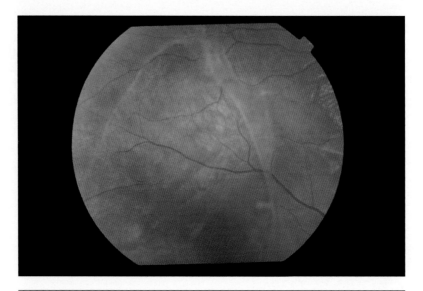

Figure 12D-2 XL retinoschisis has a very diaphanous inner layer. Occasionally, these patients develop retinal detachment as shown here.

Despite the apparent weakness of the retina it is usually possible to peel the PHM off the damaged retina and tearing of the retina is unlikely unless pre-existing abnormal adhesion is present.

The retina in a moth-eaten ARN has to be searched afterward for breaks from disintegration of the retina from the uveitic process.

One presentation of RD in trauma creates a ragged atrophic break in retina affected by commotio retinae. If the surgeon is required to treat such a break by PPV then the vitreous will usually detach from the edges of the break without further tearing. Later in the pathologic process (after weeks) it is possible that vitreoretinal adhesion will develop on the friable edge of the tear; however, usually the retina has proceeded to surgery early or has stabilized without surgery **(Fig. 12D-3)**.

Should friable retina disintegrate during peel of the PHM a broad retinectomy can be created **(Fig. 12D-4)**; however, this must be done sparingly in cases which are primed for PVR such as ARN, trauma, or cases with ischemic retina.

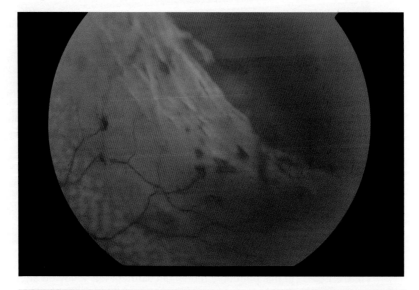

Figure 12D-3 This eye was struck by a soccer football and suffered a contusion injury with a ragged tear from disintegration of the retina in an eye with vitreous attached. The edge was lasered and the retina monitored for extension of the SRF. However, after 1 week the SRF spread and he required PPV.

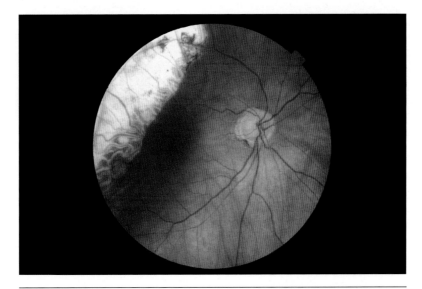

Figure 12D-4 The coloboma from deroofing of a retinoschisis RRD 10 years after the surgery.

Often we extrapolate the management of rare cases from our knowledge of common presentations. As we have seen, however, this is not always correct, for example, sickle retinopathy is best treated using segmentation and no laser is required, in contrast to our usual management of diabetic cases. Similarly we tend to believe that full PHM and vitreous detachment is required because of our management of macular hole. Although desirable, this may not always be true, for example, PPV for RRD in posterior PVD-related breaks without anterior vitreous peel is successful. There may be circumstances in patients with extensive friable retina in which the vitreous or portions of it can be left in place without detriment; however, this is poorly understood and the worry is formation of late postoperative vitreous detachment, retinal tear, and retinal detachment.

SUGGESTED READINGS

Chu TG, Lopez PF, Cano MR, et al. Posterior vitreoschisis. An echographic finding in proliferative diabetic retinopathy. *Ophthalmology.* 1996;103(2):315–322.

Chung SE, Kim KH, Kang SW. Retinal breaks associated with the induction of posterior vitreous detachment. *Am J Ophthalmol.* 2009;147(6):1012–1016.

Dogramaci M, Lee EJ, Williamson TH. The incidence and the risk factors for iatrogenic retinal breaks during pars plana vitrectomy. *Eye (Lond).* 2012;26(5):718–722.

Farah ME, Maia M, Rodrigues EB. Dyes in ocular surgery: principles for use in chromo-vitrectomy. *Am J Ophthalmol.* 2009;148(3):332–340.

Grigoropoulos VG, Williamson TH, Kirkby GR, et al. Outcomes of surgery for progressive symptomatic retinal detachment complicating retinoschisis. *Retina.* 2006;26(1):37–43.

Gupta B, Wong R, Sivaprasad S, et al. Surgical and visual outcome following 20-gauge vitrectomy in proliferative diabetic retinopathy over a 10-year period, evidence for change in practice. *Eye (Lond).* 2012;26(4):576–582.

Sakamoto T, Ishibashi T. Visualizing vitreous in vitrectomy by triamcinolone. *Graefes Arch Clin Exp Ophthalmol.* 2009;247(9):1153–1163.

Schwatz SD, Alexander R, Hiscott P, et al. Recognition of vitreoschisis in proliferative diabetic retinopathy. A useful landmark in vitrectomy for diabetic traction retinal detachment. *Ophthalmology.* 1996;103(2):323–328.

Williamson TH, Rajput R, Laidlaw DA, et al. Vitreoretinal management of the complications of sickle cell retinopathy by observation or pars plana vitrectomy. *Eye.* 2009;23(6):1314–1320.

Wu WC, Drenser KA, Capone A, et al. Plasmin enzyme-assisted vitreoretinal surgery in congenital X-linked retinoschisis: surgical techniques based on a new classification system. *Retina.* 2007;27(8):1079–1085.

13

COMPLICATIONS RELATED TO the INTRAOPERATIVE USE of TAMPONADE AGENTS

13A — Small Bubble Formation when Inserting Perfluorocarbon Liquid

SUSANNE BINDER

◆ The Complication

Perfluorocarbon liquids (PFCLs) consist of a hydrocarbon molecule in which hydrogen atoms are replaced by fluorine atoms. The main advantage of PFCLs in general is that they are immiscible in water and body fluids such as vitreous and blood. They have several characteristics which have made them suitable tools in vitreoretinal surgery. Perfluoro-n octane (C8F18) is mainly chosen because of its slightly better visibility in the eye, but also perfluoro-n dexane (C10F18) is used. In Ophthalmology, PFCLs serve as additional intraoperative tools because of their high specific gravity (1.7) that is almost twice as heavy as water and a refractive index of 1.27 that allows formation of a visible interface with balanced salt solution. Its high vapor pressure (50 mm Hg) minimizes the residual amount of perfluorocarbon liquid (PCL) left in the vitreous cavity after a fluid–air exchange has been performed.[1] Because of all these qualities, PFCLs are used during surgery mainly to reattach a detached retina but also to control bleeding. After vitreous removal and relaxation of the retina PFCLs are carefully injected into the vitreous cavity. Its weight will cause the PFCL to sink posteriorly to the area of the optic nerve, slowly reattaching the detached retina while the PFCL bubble size increases. Once the retina is pushed back against the retinal pigment epithelium all retinal holes can be treated by endophotocoagulation or cryotherapy so that a retinal detachment can be sealed on the operating table. PFCLs allow direct PFCL gas exchange or PFCL–fluid–gas or silicone exchange.

PFCLs were used in human eyes by Stanley Chang in 1988 to facilitate the cure of giant retinal tears but also in complicated retinal detachments with proliferative vitreoretinopathy (PVR), diabetic retinopathy and in eyes with luxated nucleae or lens implants.[2–7] As vitreous surgery is used in primary retinal detachment repair with increasing frequency PFCLs' use is combined with vitrectomy in much higher frequency today. Many studies have shown that PFCLs are only suitable for intraoperative use because of its weight and a possible toxic effect on the retina.[8,9] If turbulences between fluid and PFCLs occur during surgery small bubble formation is very likely to occur.

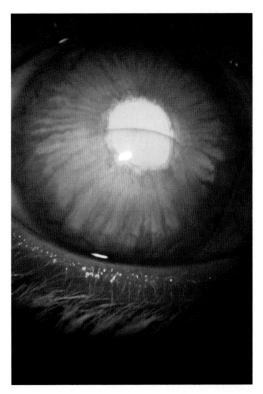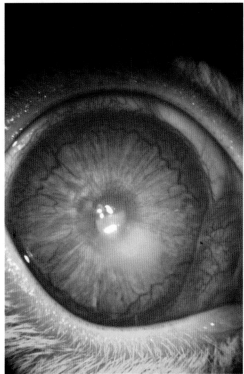

Figure 13A-1 Images of the anterior segment of a rabbit eye in which perfluorocarbon liquid was left in the anterior chamber **(Left panel)**. Anterior chamber inflammation, iris neovascularization and keratopathy developed over a period of 2 weeks **(Right panel)**.

Risk Factors and Pathogenesis

Small bubble formation may worsen the view during the intravitreal insertion of PFCLs and facilitate the displacement of these small bubbles (fish eggs) from the vitreous cavity into other tissues in or in close proximity, such as actually the subretinal space, ciliary body, and/or anterior chamber.

Permanent PFCL bubbles left in the anterior chamber create inflammation, keratopathy, and chronic pain **(Figure 13A-1)**. If PFCL remains under the retina, a local scotoma will develop over time which can be devastating for the patient's vision if the PFCL is located under the fovea.

Small PFCL bubble formation may occur as a result of the following:

a. Small bubble formation in the posterior part of the vitreous cavity may occur if:

◆ The injection of PFCL into the vitreous cavity is done too rapidly.

◆ The end tip of the cannula is not kept within the enlarging PFCL bubble.

b. Small bubble formation in the anterior part of the vitreous cavity: If the level of PFCL is raised up to the level of the pars plana, such as the infusion cannula becomes immersed in the PFCL bubble, then small bubble of PFCL will form. Turbulences on the interface BSS–PFCL will be generated by the jet of balance salt solution (BSS) infused through the infusion cannula giving rise to a high number of small PFCL bubbles.

c. Presence of residual membranes: If PFCL is injected in areas were residual vitreoretinal membranes or areas of vitreoretinal traction are still present they can split the PFCL bubble into several small bubbles. If there are tears under traction in close proximity, there would be a high risk for these small bubbles of PFCL to go under the retina.

d. Small bubbles of PFCL can also occur if PFCL is injected, then aspirated into a syringe and reinjected again. The reason for this is that during the aspiration, there is an admixture of PFCL and BSS.

Pearls on How to Prevent It

◆ Check if PFCL filled cannula is not occluded before entering with this cannula into the eye, otherwise you might inject with high pressure and speed once the occlusion is overcome, which may create either several small PFCL bubbles or damage the retina, vessels, or optic nerve.

◆ Check the eye pressure and the outflow possibilities before you start injecting PFCL.

◆ Inject PFCL only in a soft eye.

◆ Start the injection in the area over the optic nerve head. Keep the end tip of the cannula into the PFCL bubble already injected (into the enlarging PFCL bubble). While injecting, slowly lift the cannula more anteriorly as the bubble size increases.

◆ Inject slowly but continuously.

◆ Prevent high intraocular pressure by controlling simultaneous passive outflow of the intraocular fluid while injecting PFCL. This can be achieved by using a dual bore PFCL cannula.

◆ Observe. If smaller bubbles separate from the central PFCL bubble while the level of PFCL is raised, it is likely that it is occurring because there residual tissue is left anteriorly which separates the PFCL into several bubbles. This would indicate the need to do more vitrectomy and release this traction.

◆ If PFCL previously injected in the vitreous cavity is removed into a syringe, it will contain an admixture of BSS and PFCL and small bubbles of PFCL will form if reinjected. If more PFCL is again needed during the procedure, use new PFCL. Alternative, it would be possible to use the PFCL that had been previously aspirated from the vitreous cavity provided that the BSS from the BSS–PFCL mixture is removed. To do this, hold the syringe upright, let the BSS and PFCL separate, and then expel the BSS from the syringe and inject the PFCL which will remain in the lower part of the syringe.

◆ When raising the level of PFCL up to the pars plana, above the infusion cannula, do not only stop the infusion line but disconnect it to allow passive outflow of fluid while injecting PFCL.

Pearls on How to Solve It

◆ Some bubbles of PFCL may merge with the larger PFCL bubble if you touch them with the cannula or may be removed with the flute needle (back flush cannula).

◆ As explained above, sometimes small bubble formation indicates the presence of residual vitreous; in these cases completion of the vitrectomy is required.

◆ Use a contact lens for better depth perception to remove residual small PCL bubbles over the fovea or macular area.

◆ If a PFCL bubble traveled subretinally and is large—remove PFCL from the vitreous first and then remove the subretinal PFCL (for information on how to do this, see Chapter 19C).

◆ Occasionally, very small single PFCL bubbles can be left under the retina if they are in a safe distance from the fovea. Under these circumstances, some laser around the bubble might prevent traveling of this bubble into the fovea later on.

◆ Anterior chamber PFCL bubbles can be removed under topical anesthesia via a paracentesis on the slit lamp.

Expected Outcomes: What Is the Worst-case Scenario

Decompensation of the cornea and irreversible keratopathy can develop if the anterior chamber is filled with more than a quarter of PFCL.[10] Besides chronic pain and corneal neovascularization can occur as well as secondary glaucoma.[11]

Subretinal PCL hinders reattachment of the retina and can accelerate subretinal fibrosis and strand formation. Over time, the retina will become atrophic and even if repeated surgery is done retinal function cannot be restored in the areas were the PFCL once was.[12]

REFERENCES

1. Chang S, Sparrow JR. Vitreous substitutes. In: Guyer DR, Yanuzzi La, Chang S, Shields JA, Green WR, eds. *Retina-Vitreous-Macula*. Philadelphia, PA: WB Saunders; 1999:1320–1321.

2. Chang S, Lincoff H, Zimmermann NJ, et al. Giant retinal tears. Surgical techniques and results using perfluorocarbon liquids. *Arch Ophthalmol*. 1989;107: 761–766.

3. Chang S, Ozmert E, Zimmerman NJ. Intraoperative perfluorocarbon liquids in the management of proliferative vitreoretinopathy. *Am J Ophthalmol*. 1988;106:668–674.

4. Stolba U, Binder S, Velikay M, et al. Use of perfluorocarbon liquids in proliferative vitreoretinopathy: Results and complications. *Br J Ophthalmol*. 1995;79:1106–1110.

5. Mathis A, Pagot V, David JL. The use of perfluorodecalin in diabetic vitrectomy. *Fortschr Ophthalmol*. 1991;88:148–150.

6. Banker AS, Freeman WR, Vander JF, et al. Use of perflubron as a new temporary vitreous substitute and manipulation agent for vitreoretinal surgery. Wills Eye Hospital Perflubron Study Group. *Retina*. 1996;16:285–291.

7. Lewis H, Blumenkranz Ms, Chang S. Treatment of dislocated crystalline lens and retinal detachment with perfluorocarbon liquids. *Retina*. 1992;12:299–304.

8. Stolba U, Krepler K, Pflug R, et al. Experimental vitreous and aqueous replacement with perfluorophenanthrene. *Retina*. 1997;17:146.

9. Lee GA, Finnegan SJ, Bourke RD. Subretinal perfluorodecalin toxicity. *Aust N Z J Ophthalmol*. 1998;26:57–60.

10. Weinberger D, Goldenberg Cohen N, Axel-Siegel R, et al. Long term follow–up of perfluorocarbon liquid in the anterior chamber. *Retina*. 1998;18:233–237.

11. Stolba U, Binder S, Krepler K, et al. Anterior segment changes after experimental perfluorocarbon tamponade in the rabbit eye. *Graefes Arch Klin Exp Ophthalmol*. 1999;237–243.

12. Batman C, Cekic O. Effects of the long term use of perfluoroperhydrophenanthrene on the retina. *Ophthalmic Surg Lasers*. 1989;29:144–146.

13B | Intraoperative Displacement of Tamponade Agents

SUSANNE BINDER

◆ The Complication

In vitreoretinal surgery gases and silicone oil are the main tamponades used postoperatively. Perfluorocarbon liquid (PFCL) is used nearly exclusively as an intraoperative tool. In this chapter, complications related to the intraoperative displacement of gas/silicone oil/PFCL from the vitreous cavity to the subconjunctival space, anterior chamber, or subretinal/suprachoroidal space will be discussed.

Tamponades are usually calculated to fill the vitreous cavity in a certain percentage and its expansion rate and surface tension is supposed to flatten the retina against the retinal pigment epithelium to support and facilitate permanent retinal reattachment once retinal holes are closed. As a general rule, tamponades of the shortest duration should be used if a successful outcome can be achieved. In short, if air as the shortest-acting and cheapest gas is sufficient it should be preferred to longer-acting gases. Silicone oil as the longest-acting tamponade should be reserved for very complex pathologies and removed between 6 weeks and 6 months postoperatively.[1] For example, gases are needed in eyes with primary retinal detachment repair or macular hole surgery; silicone oil is mostly used for severe cases of proliferative vitreoretinopathy (PVR), diabetic vitreoretinopathy (DVR), and posterior segment trauma. If tamponades are used during vitreoretinal surgery, knowledge about their physical properties, expandance rates, and maintenance in the eye is mandatory. Many chapters and articles deal with the physical properties of gases or silicone oil; here two are cited.[2,3]

Displacement of gas/silicone oil/PFCL can occur to **(a)** the anterior chamber, **(b)** under the retina or choroid, and **(c)** subconjunctivally.

a. If air enters the anterior chamber intraoperatively, this would most often occur either at the time of staining of membranes, if the surgeon decides to stain under air, or at the end of the procedure, when a fluid–air exchange is done. PFCL may enter the anterior chamber intraoperatively, when the level is being raised to completely flatten the retina in phakic/pseudophakic/aphakic eyes or when they are used to float a posteriorly dislocated lens/IOL with the purpose of removing it from the anterior segment in aphakic eyes. The presence of air or PFCL in the anterior chamber will impair the view of the fundus intraoperatively; postoperatively PFCL will lead to further complications (see also Chapter 19A). Gas/silicone oil may enter the anterior chamber at the end of the surgery, and, if left there, may also cause problems postoperatively. Thus, the presence of gas postoperatively in the anterior chamber can cause keratopathy, secondary glaucoma, as well as rapid cataract development[4,5] (see also Chapters 19A and 19B). Silicone oil may lead to either bullous or band-shaped keratopathy if it remains in contact with the endothelium of the cornea for more than several weeks (see also Chapter 19A). In the silicone oil study the incidence of keratopathy was 27% after 2 years. Interestingly, this percentage did not differ significantly between long-acting gases (C3F8) and silicone oil.[6] This silicone oil-induced keratopathy may be irreversible even after the silicone oil is removed. It can lead to chronic pain if band keratopathy develops and is not only visually impairing for the patient but makes reoperations only possible with the use of a temporary keratoprosthesis followed by a full thickness corneal transplant. The patient is confronted not only with an almost blind eye but also cosmetically impaired.

Secondary glaucoma can also occur and visual function as well as proper judgment of the fundus will be compromised in these cases.[7]

b. Air/gas/silicone oil/PFCL can enter the subretinal space intraoperatively, preventing flattening of the retina. Postoperatively, they will hinder a retina from reattachment. Whilst air will absorb rather quickly and might not hinder the healing course longer-acting gases, silicone oil, and PFCL will do so and, thus, they need to be removed unless, exceptionally, very small amounts have been trapped subretinally.[8] Silicone oil and PFCL will remain permanently, create damage to the retinal tissues, and subretinal fibrosis unless they are surgically removed.

c. Subconjunctival gas is usually a sign of leaking sclerotomies, but will absorb on its own (see also Chapter 19A). Clearly, its tamponade effect in the vitreous will be reduced by the reduced amount of tamponade that will remain in the vitreous cavity. In contrast to this, subconjunctival silicone oil—a complication seen more commonly with the use of sutureless vitreous surgery—will not only remain but also form deposits of different sizes under the conjunctiva and in Tenon's capsule which can cause chronic foreign body sensation, redness, and pain. If massive, it can also compromise ocular motility and will need careful removal.

Inadequate insertion of the tamponade agent into the vitreous cavity may also lead to forward displacement of the iris–lens/IOL with shallowing/flattening of the anterior chamber which may lead to irido-corneal and lens/IOL-corneal touch.

Pathogenesis and Risk Factors

Intraoperative Displacement of the Tamponade Agent

a. To the anterior chamber:

◆ Differential pressure between vitreous cavity and anterior chamber: If the pressure in the vitreous cavity increases (for instance, as a result of increasing the infusion pressure) or the anterior chamber pressure decreases (for instance, as a result of a leaking corneal would when doing combined phaco-vitrectomy) the tamponade agent inserted into the vitreous cavity could migrate into the anterior chamber.

◆ Overfilling of the vitreous cavity with the tamponade agent: Overfilling with silicone oil is more likely to occur in reoperations.

◆ Previous vitrectomy surgery: Eyes that have had prior vitrectomy(ies) and anterior vitreous shaving have higher chance to have anterior migration of the tamponade because the zonules are also compromised and the iris–plane barrier is weaker.

◆ Presence of weak zonules, zonulodyalysis, or posterior capsulotomy/capsulectomy.

b. To the subretinal or suprachoroidal space:

◆ Presence of persistent traction around large retinal tears when the tamponade agent is inserted.

◆ Infusion cannula through which the tamponade agent is being inserted not correctly positioned inside the vitreous cavity.

◆ Continuous infusion of the tamponade agent when the cannula is being removed and no longer in the vitreous cavity—this can lead also to insertion of the tamponade in the suprachoroidal space.

◆ In case of PFCL, the presence of "fish eggs" formation may facilitate the PFCL to go through retinal breaks into the subretinal space (see Chapter 13A).

c. To the subconjunctival space:

◆ Sclerostomies not properly closed, which may occur more often in highly myopic eyes.

◆ Continuous infusion of the tamponade after the cannula used to insert it has been withdrawn from the vitreous cavity.

✦ Pearls on How to Prevent It

a. Preventing displacement of the tamponade agent into the anterior chamber:

◆ Insert viscoelastic material into the anterior chamber during surgery to prevent the tamponade agent to prolapse anteriorly intraoperatively in high risk cases (weak zonules, capsulotomy/capsulectomy, eyes undergoing repeated surgery).

◆ Insert air/viscoelastic material in the anterior chamber toward the end of the procedure before completing the tamponade fill of the vitreous cavity in high risk cases. If viscoelastic is used, it would be probably better to leave it in the eye rather than removing it at the very end of the surgery since if this is done migration of the tamponade could still occur. Antiglaucoma and anti-inflammatory medications will be needed to prevent high intraocular pressure postoperatively in these cases.

◆ Avoid overfilling.

◆ Surgery under local anesthesia may allow preventing prolonged supine (face up) position, as the patient can be postured face down right at the end of the surgery, and valsalva maneuvers in the immediate postoperative period which may facilitate anterior displacement of the tamponade agent.

b. Preventing displacement of the tamponade agent into the subretinal and supra-choroidal space:

◆ Avoid raising the level of PFCL above areas of persistent traction if retinal tears/holes, especially if large, are in close proximity.

◆ Maintain the eye in primary position (straight ahead) when working with PFCL if areas of vitreoretinal traction are still present in close proximity to retinal tears/holes.

◆ Avoid inserting silicone oil or gas in the vitreous cavity if the retina is not sufficiently relaxed.

◆ If a reoperation is planned on an eye with subretinal silicone oil and large tears/holes and vitreoretinal traction, it may be possible to do a laser barrier just posterior to these areas, if the retina is flat under the oil. It is likely that in 24 hours there will be an increased adhesion between the neuroretina and pigment epithelium which may help preventing the displacement of the tamponade agent intraoperatively when subsequent surgery is performed.[9]

c. Preventing displacement of the tamponade agent into the subconjunctival space:

◆ Check that the sclerostomies are well closed at the end of surgery. In small-gauge vitrectomy, add sutures if needed.

◆ Always consider suturing of sclerotomies if silicone oil is used.

Pearls on How to Solve It

a. Tamponade agent into the anterior chamber:

◆ If the vitreous cavity is completely filled with gas/oil and a large gas bubble has entered the anterior chamber, constrict the pupil to prevent further gas/ oil moving forward and remove it via paracentesis. If in doubt that adequate gas/oil fill remains in the vitreous cavity, fill the anterior chamber with air or viscoelastic material and insert further gas/oil in the vitreous cavity. If the infusion cannula has been already removed, use a 30G needle for the purpose of injecting gas; reopen a sclerostomy port and inject further silicone oil if a reduced fill is felt to compromise the postoperative success of the surgery. Position the patient face down as soon as possible.

◆ In aphakic eyes an inadequate 6 o'clock iridectomy can prevent the silicone oil from moving back to the vitreous cavity. In such cases patency of the iridectomy needs to be checked and enlargement considered.

b. Tamponade agent into the subretinal and suprachoroidal space:

◆ If during surgery the tamponade agent (gas, silicone oil, or PFCL) is displaced inadvertently under the retina it needs immediate removal.

◆ If silicone oil is present in the suprachoroidal space and noted quickly by the surgeon, an immediate change of the infusion line to a superior sclerostomy is needed to avoid hypotony and further complications. Oil may reflux out of the suprachoroidal space when the infusion is removed; this may be facilitated by making this sclerostomy the highest point. Once the eye is stabilized a different sclerostomy or a new one could be created, preferably at the 12 o'clock position, to safely continue the silicone insertion.

◆ If gas is injected into the suprachoroidal space, careful aspiration might be attempted. This can be achieved by slow aspiration via the infusion line. If this is not possible removal of the infusion line is recommended to allow for passive outflow through an open sclerostomy while surgery is continued and the eye pressure maintained via a new infusion line.

c. Tamponade agent in the subconjunctival space:

◆ Subconjunctival silicone oil can be easily removed by doing a small cut in the conjunctiva/Tenon's or by using the small slit in the conjunctiva created when introducing the trocars when small-gauge vitrectomy is used. Reinspection of the sclerotomies will be needed as well as judging whether further tamponade filling is required.

What Is the Worst-case Scenario

Persistence of the tamponade agent in the anterior chamber postoperatively causes keratopathy, cataract, and secondary glaucoma (see Chapter 19A). Each of these three complications alone can compromise vision either temporarily or permanently.

The presence of a tamponade in the subretinal space will prevent retinal reattachment. If left there postoperatively, it will lead to anatomical and functional failure, retinal atrophy, and subretinal fibrosis (see also Chapters 13C and 19C). Loss of vision in these eyes is very likely, if the tamponade is not removed in time.

Subconjunctival displacement of tamponades indicates most often inadequate closure of the sclerotomies. If not addressed intraoperatively, the subsequent reduced intravitreal tamponade volume will reduce its tamponade effect on the retina and might prevent a retina from reattachment or a macular hole from closing. Hypotony may also ensue.

Subconjunctival silicone deposits will not threaten the patient's vision but may cause discomfort and, as mentioned above, may lead to insufficient intravitreal tamponade.

REFERENCES

1. Falkner CI, Binder S, Kruger A. Outcome after silicone oil removal. *Brit J Ophthalmol.* 2001;85:1324–1327.
2. Chang S. Intraocular gases. In: Ryan S, Wilkinson P, eds. *Retina.* Mosby: St Louis, Missouri. 3rd ed. 1994;3:Ch 129: 2147–2161.
3. Mohamed S, Lai T. Intraocular gases in vitreoretinal surgery. In: Saxena S, Meyer Ch, Ohji M, Akduman L, eds. *Vitreoretinal surgery.* Jaypee Highlights Medical Publishers. 2012;8:84–93.
4. Gedde SJ. Management of glaucoma after retinal detachment surgery. *Curr Opin Ophthalmol.* 2002;13:103–109.
5. Lee DA, Wilson MR, Yoshizumi MO, et al. The ocular effect of gases when injected into the anterior chamber of rabbit eyes. *Arch ophthalmol.* 1991;109:571–575.
6. Abrams GW, Azen SP, Barr CC, et al. The incidence of corneal abnormalities in the Silicone Study. Silicone Study Report 7. *Arch Ophthalmol.* 1995;113:764–769.
7. Federmann JL, Schubert HD. Complications associated with the use of silicone oil in 150 eyes after retina-vitreous surgery. *Ophthalmology.* 1988;95:870–876.
8. Blumenkranz M, Gardner T, Blankenship G. Fluid-gas exchange and photocoagulation after vitrectomy. *Arch Ophthalmol.* 1986;104:291–296.
9. Yoon YH, Marmor MF. Rapid enhancement of retinal adhesion by laser photocoagulation. *Ophthalmology.* 1988;95(10):1385–1388.

13C Difficulties Removing Tamponade Agents After Short- and Long-Term Tamponade

STANISLAO RIZZO AND FEDERICA GENOVESI EBERT

Silicone oil (SO) has been used for more than 20 years as a long-term retinal tamponade in the surgical management of patients with complex retinal detachments. The insertion and removal of SO are usually straightforward: It is usually removed after 3 months if the retina is attached. Patients are monitored routinely for intraocular pressure check, to evaluate whether there is oil emulsification, and, importantly, to assess the retinal status before a decision concerning the oil removal is taken. Whilst SO removal is mandatory, the factors of timing or decision making regarding SO removal technique are still not very clear and are usually dependent on the individual surgeon's approach.

Conventional Removal Techniques for SO in Phakic–Pseudophakic Patients

The removal can be performed with a three-port approach using active aspiration through the pump used for injection which is connected to a 19G cannula: The tip is immersed in the SO bubble and observed through the microscope. Active aspiration can be done also using a 20G short beveled needle, such as a Peyman's needle, attached to a 10-mL syringe and manual aspiration.

Another method of removal of SO is passive removal, in which one of the ports is kept open after opening the infusion line, allowing for the passive egress of the SO: Oil mixed with balanced salt solution escapes slowly.

Conventional Removal Technique for SO in Aphakic Patients

Removal in aphakic patients can also be carried out using a limbal approach with two ports: One for infusion that can be an anterior chamber maintainer or a pars plana infusion and one for extraction via the limbus through a small 20G or 23G opening made in the clear cornea near the limbus in the superior sector[1]: Disadvantages may be corneal damage and the lack of opportunity to check the status of the retina.

Removal of SO in a Minimally Invasive System

The most up-to-date technique for SO removal is a three-port approach that can currently be easily performed with a 23G system by using active aspiration through an aspiration pump equipped with a syringe with a silicone soft cannula inserted on the guide of one of the two superior sclerostomy sites, while the other is closed with a plug **(Fig. 13C-1)**. This third sclerostomy site will then be used to pass the light probe to check on the status of the retina once the SO has been removed.

Heavy Oil Removal

In 2003, the first "heavy" SO (Oxane HD) for the surgical treatment of inferior parts of the retina was introduced into the market.[2]

For this commercially available heavy silicone oil (HSO) a mixture of 5,000-millipascal second viscosity SO and a partially fluorinated olefin [perfluorooctyl-5-methyl-hex-2-ene (RMN3)] was used. The addition of 10.8% RMN3 (specific density 1.45 g/mL) enhances the specific density of the SO to 1.02 g/mL and reduces the viscosity from 5,000 to 3,500 millipascal seconds. The other current commercially available heavy oil is Densiron 68 that is composed of a mixture of 69.5% polydimethylsiloxane (CH3)3SiO-(Si(CH3)2O)n-Si(CH3)3 and 30.5% ultrapure

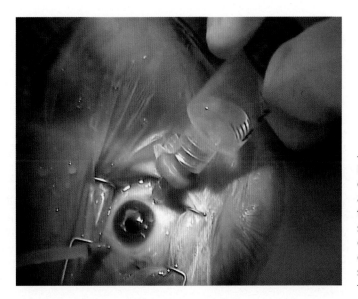

Figure 13C-1 23G silicone oil removal with active aspiration through an aspiration pump equipped with a syringe with a silicone soft cannula inserted on the guide of one of the two superior sclerotomies.

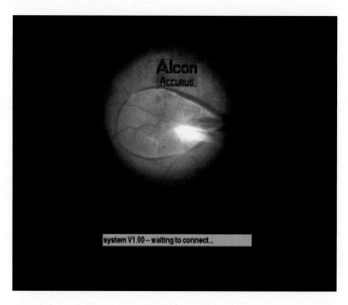

Figure 13C-2 Heavy silicone oil removal.

perfluorohexyloctane (F6H8). Physical properties are viscosity 1,400 millipascal seconds and density 1.06 g/cm^3.

Heavy silicone oil (HSO) removal can be challenging and differs considerably from conventional oil as it requires special attention and the use of an elevated vacuum relatively close to the retina. Traditionally, strong active aspiration had to be applied through a long 18G needle, just above the optic disc. If the needle was momentarily emptied of the viscous oil, there would be a sudden increase in flow, and the needle tip could damage the retina as hypotony causes the eye to suddenly collapse.

To avoid such complication "tubeless siphoning" allows the use of small-gauge short needles at a greater distance from the retina.[3] The idea of a tubeless siphon is that some viscoelastic fluid can flow upward even without a tube, driven by suction of the syringe and by the stored energy of extensional flow. However, the surgeon must be careful to make sure that the needle stays inside the bubble of HSO at all times because if the fluid were to be interrupted (as in a siphoning effect), it would not be possible to pick up the bubble again and resume flow, thus requiring the use of a long cannula **(Fig. 13C-2)**.

Currently, HSO removal can be performed easily with a 23G system by using a 23G short cannula.[4]

Difficulties and Complications Removing Tamponade Agents

There have been anecdotal reports of difficulties removing conventional as well as HSO from the vitreous cavity at the end of the tamponade time. These difficulties can be due to a change in its properties ("sticky" SO), emulsification, or the presence of subretinal SO.

"STICKY" SILICONE OIL

Friberg presented at the Club Jules Gonin meeting in 2000 (Sicily) a number of cases in which the perfluorocarbon liquid (PFCL) had apparently interacted with the conventional SO, forming a viscous gel-like substance that adhered to the retina and was difficult to aspirate. The occurrence of "sticky" SO was first reported in the Netherlands in 2000 in Utrecht (University Medical Centre Utrecht) and Rotterdam (The Rotterdam Eye Hospital).

Definition of the Complication

Veckeneer[5] described a phenomenon occurring during conventional SO oil removal: Patches of SO-like material remained "glued" to the retina ("sticky" SO), usually near or within the posterior pole, after the bulk of the SO had been removed.

In 2003, Van Meurs et al.[6] reported on an "epidemic" of "sticky" SO. Of 95 conventional SO removals, 22 were difficult due to adherence to the retina.

Risk Factors

In 2007, Veckeneer[5] performed a chart review to identify possible patient or procedural factors that could predispose to the formation of "sticky" SO. The use of perfluoro-octane (PFO) rather than perfluorodecalin (PFD) seemed to be associated with this phenomenon ($P < 0.001$). Indeed, gas chromatography and mass spectroscopy analysis revealed a significant presence of PFO in samples of "sticky" SO.

Pathogenesis: Why Does It Occur

In order to elucidate the phenomenon of stickiness of conventional SO, Dresp[7] analyzed samples of HSO that have been explanted either uneventfully or with reported "stickiness," as well as the results of a laboratory experiment. Dresp's experiments showed that the cohesion of the SO was lower than the adhesion between SO and Perfluorocarbon liquid (PFCL). Therefore the aspiration of SO from the vitreous cavity after a PFCL/SO exchange could be extremely difficult.

Winter et al.[8] demonstrated that total removal of PFCL during surgery is almost impossible. Thus, if intraoperatively PFCL is used and SO tamponade inserted, at the time of SO removal the following materials would interact with each other: SO, PFCL (remnants), aqueous, the retina itself, and the material of the cannula used to remove the SO. All these materials, at their interfaces, have to be in a special energetic condition to allow for an uncomplicated removal. In the in vitro set-up, the three phases (SO, aqueous, PFCL) arrange themselves in such a way as to reach the lowest total energy possible. To separate these phases in order to aspirate the SO, energy has to be applied until the adhesion force between the SO and its direct contact material is exceeded.

The adherence of the SO to the material of the cannula in combination with the suction force should be stronger than the adherence of the SO to the aqueous material and to the PFCL layer, and/or stronger than the adherence of the PFCL layer to the underlying retina.

However, PFCL concentration seems not to be the only cause for stickiness.

Wong et al.[9] demonstrated that the two phases can adhere to each other due to their nonpolar nature, as PFCL dissolves in SO by diffusion and by convection processes.

Despite the fact that PFO and PFD are very similar in their surface behaviors, the solubility of these two substances in SO differs significantly. Indeed, the solubility of PFD in SO (5.1 m%) is much higher than the solubility of PFO (3.2 m%). As mentioned above, the complete removal of PFCL during surgery is not possible and remnants always remain on the retina and during SO filling. On the other hand, residual PFCL can dissolve in SO over time. The smaller the solubility of the PFCL used, the higher the amount of PFCL left over the retina and present at the time of SO removal; it is the adhesion of the SO to the PFCL remnants that can lead to the "sticky" behavior of SO. The effect should be concentrated where small droplets of PFCL are located. In other words, the precondition for stickiness is a certain amount of PFCL, which is high enough to form small droplets.

There are anecdotal reports of sticky SO associated with heavy tamponades, although this is a complication that is often discussed as a potential complication of heavy tamponades. Recent publications of the second-generation heavy tamponades Oxane HD, Densiron 68, and HWS 46-3000, however, reported no cases of sticky SO.[2,10,11]

Pearls on How to Prevent It

- Achieve complete removal of PFCL when used. As explained above, the so-called stickiness of SO appears to relate to the presence of trace amounts of PFCL. Moreover, stickiness is not primarily related to viscosity, type or brand of SO used, type of PFCL used, and probably tamponade duration. The results of Veckeneer et al.,[5] chemical analysis of sticky SO specimens, showing the presence of a partially fluorinated (chlorine-containing) fraction in the PFO, as well as short chains in the SO, could be important. Polar components like 1H-PFO and chlorine-containing compounds dissolved in PFCL can be accumulated on the surface, functioning as simple surfactants and changing the interactions with surrounding media.[12] It was reported by Prather et al.[13] that polar impurities in PFCL (especially chlorine-containing compounds; 500 μg/mL) lead to an absorption of proteins on the surface. It has to be considered, then, that cells and other organic compounds are able to form a coating on the surface of the PFCL and function in combination with surface-active components in the PFCL as a primer, improving the interaction between all phases (retina, PFCL, and SO) involved in the sticky behavior. Dresp et al.[14] demonstrated in their in vitro experiments that the purity of PFCL and SO is essential. The impurities found in sticky SO, PFCL, and in SO straight from the vial could in fact contribute to an increased interaction between the different phases involved, and impurities from other sources such as tubing, sterilization, solutions etc. might also be significant, even if a causative relationship between the impurities found and the sticky oil phenomenon could not be drawn. Veckeneer et al.[5] concluded that avoiding direct contact between the different components required for sticky oil development seems crucial. In a recent paper on the interaction between ocular endotamponades,[3] the importance of meticulous PFCL removal was emphasized. Fluid (PFCL) to air exchange to prevent direct contact between PFCL and SO could be useful in this regard. Taking into account the information provided in the previous section, it seems reasonable that, if PFD is used, and all small droplets of residual PFCL carefully removed at the time of SO insertion, the occurrence of "sticky" SO at the time of its removal would be very unlikely.

- The transparent nature of the PFCL, especially PFO, makes its complete removal very difficult during direct exchange with SO and especially when PFCL–air exchange is undertaken. A colored PFCL that facilitates its visualization and, thus, its removal may prevent or, at least, reduce many of these problems.[15]

- In addition, a saline rinse after PFCL exchange (see also Chapter 19C) can be performed to reduce the occurrence of "sticky" SO, as it has been reported that this maneuver may help to collect the microscopic PFCL layer (residual after macroscopic removal of PFCL) on the retinal surface posteriorly.[8] In addition, performing a saline rinse gives extra time of contact with an air phase, during which PFCL could evaporate further.[8] On the other hand, direct PFCL–silicone exchange, even if it allows a better PFCL visualization, does not provide for a saline rinse, and can therefore lead to a higher possibility of stickiness developing.

- Joussen and Wong[16] reported that "sticky" SO is mostly seen in patients with posterior vitreous remnants that allow for adhesion of the SO to the retinal surface. Complete removal of the vitreous by using triamcinolone acetonide as vitreous highlighter may be also helpful to reduce the possibility for this complication to occur.

◆ Pearls on How to Solve It

◆ Sticky conventional SO as well as sticky HSO can be removed from the retina with the use of semifluorinated alkanes (SFAs) or PFCL.

SFAs are heavier-than-water transparent liquids that are tolerated by the retina. Perfluorohexyloctane (F6H8) has gained attention as a long-term vitreous substitute. SFAs can dissolve in SO, a strategy that is used, for example, to create HSO. The solubility of SFAs in SO can be used to remove SO remnants: F6H8 is able to dissolve SO from the surface of silicone intraocular lenses (IOLs) and from the vitreous cavity.

PFCL is helpful in the removal of sticky SO. Adhesion of HSO to PFCL is greater than the adhesion of HSO to the retina. Therefore PFCL can be used to collect HSO from the surface of the retina like a sticky tape. Finally, the conglomerate of PFCL and HSO can be removed from the eye via the flute needle.[17]

◆ Another reason why "sticky SO" may occur is given by Dresp[7] in his in vitro study using gas chromatography. The reduced surface tension of the surrounding aqueous material and/or the contamination of SO with PFCL, create interruption of the material flow, giving the impression of adherence of the SO to the retina. It has to be considered that cells and other organic materials are able to form a coating on the surface of PFCL and act in combination with surface-active components in PFCL as a trigger, improving the interaction between all phases involved in sticky behaviors. The significant lowering of the interfacial tension of the water-containing part of the explants is a hint that water-soluble components with surface-active characteristics participate in the formation of stickiness, too. Removal is difficult if the cohesion of the substance to be removed is smaller than its adhesion to the underlying surface. If suction is applied, it depends on the interfacial tension of the SO, whether a constant material flow into the cannula can be achieved, or if the tear off of the SO thread gives the impression of sticking to the underlying surface. The effect of impurities in the endotamponade media can be a simple enhancement of adhesions but can also activate surface-active components such as inflammatory mediators.

◆ Heating the balanced salt solution used for infusion may also facilitate the "sticky" remnant to be removed.

◆ If the "sticky" oil is a heavy tamponade such as Oxane HD[18] (or O62[19] not commercially available), the removal can be more difficult. It requires special attention and the use of high vacuum relatively close to the retina. To avoid complications like inadvertent touching of the retina or sudden pressure loss, "tubeless siphoning" allows the use of small-gauge short needles in a greater distance from the retina.[20]

◆ If a film of oil remains on the retina, a long 20G polyurethane cannula (Venflon) is required to aspirate the liquid close to the retinal surface, but it must be taken into account that the aspiration pressure at the tip of a long needle would be low once completely filled with the high-viscosity oil.

◆ As we have mentioned above, "sticky" oil remnants lying on the surface of the retina may be difficult to remove. Veckeneer[5] showed that, on rare occasions, they could cause postoperative visual disturbances (relative scotomata). These symptoms, however, may be temporary (from 2 to 4 weeks) since the "sticky" SO bubble can spontaneously unglue and migrate upward to the 12 o'clock position. On the contrary, forceful attempts to remove the "sticky" SO may lead to complications such as choroidal hemorrhages and peripheral retinal tears. Therefore, while the presence of SO remnants on the retina might not cause lasting side effects, forceful attempts at its removal can lead to complications; thus, the surgeon would need to decide how aggressive he/she should be in the removal of "sticky" conventional SO and HSO.

SILICONE OIL EMULSIFICATION

The Complication: Definition

Due to its high surface tension, SO does not usually enter the subretinal space; rather it prevents the entry of fluid into the subretinal space. If the surface tension decreases, the SO globule begins to emulsify. The term "emulsification" is used to describe the dispersion of tiny intraocular droplets of SO from the main globule of SO (see also Chapter 19E). It has been reported in as few as 0.7%[21] and in as many as 56% of[22–25] oil-filled eyes. On the other hand,[22] anterior chamber oil emulsification occurs frequently (83%) despite inferior peripheral iridectomy in aphakic or pseudophakic eyes and the use of highly purified, higher viscosity SO. Heidenkummer[23] concluded that the lower the viscosity of the SO the higher the emulsification rate even if Scott et al.[26] in a comparative study after retinal detachment repair using 1,000- versus 5,000-cSt SO found similar rates of SO emulsification in the two groups.

Risk Factors

Individual patient factors may contribute to SO emulsification (see also Chapter 19E).

A variety of publications attempted to describe the causes for SO emulsification and/or the mechanisms influencing emulsification.[27–35] The main causes discussed have been blood constituents,[27] oligosiloxanes, 5 OH-endgroups,[27] lipoproteins and/or phospholipids,[27,28] metal ions left as remnants from catalysts,[27] viscosity,[28–31] and interfacial tension.[27,31]

Bambas[36] reported that there is a suggestion that individual patient factors may contribute to SO emulsification or even environmental poisons like polybiphenyls and dichlor-diphenyl-trichloroethane, which are present in body fat. The latter substances can be more or less dissolved in SO but attack the surface of the SO droplet. In addition, the presence of fibrin or serum may also facilitate the emulsification process.[12] Emulsification is also intensified in eyes with intraocular inflammation.

The pro-emulsifying potential of substances and blood components that may have access to the vitreous cavity was analyzed in an in vitro model for quantitative analysis of SO emulsification. In this model, red blood cell ghosts had the highest emulsifying effect; plasma and lymphocytes also had a significant emulsifying effect. Phospholipids in membranes and other soluble blood components may play important roles in this process. These results suggest the importance of avoiding and removing hemorrhage and avoiding inflammation when SO is used in vitreoretinal surgery.[37]

Pathogenesis: Why Does It Occur

The decrease in surface tension may be due to the release of inflammatory agents and blood. Despite routine cleaning and sterilization of vitreoretinal instruments and accessories, remnants of SO and detergents can remain and act as surfactant agents lowering the interfacial tension between SO and an aqueous phase leading to emulsification of SO that comes into contact with these contaminated devices during instillation of the endotamponade.

Other possible contaminants of SO are substances that are used intraoperatively such as PFCL which have to be removed at the end of surgery. Removal is performed either by direct exchange to SO or indirectly, with a previous air/fluid exchange.

Pearls on How to Prevent It

♦ A reduction of the risk of emulsification can be achieved by using a disposable device for SO injection, thus reducing the content of impurities in the SO to the lowest possible level. Contact with substances used as ocular endotamponades like PFCL should be reduced to the utmost extent. From a chemical point of view, a direct PFCL–SO exchange should be avoided as a complete removal of PFCL would be advisable before SO is injected to reduce the chance for SO emulsification to occur. In contrast, many vitreoretinal surgeons are accustomed to the direct PFCL–SO exchange technique, which can be performed easily. The additional step of PFCL–air exchange prior to insertion of SO enhances the risk of retinal slippage (see Chapter 17) in certain clinical conditions such as giant retinal tears.

◆ Our approach for removing oil is as follows: We first remove emulsified SO from the anterior chamber, before we commence the removal of SO from the vitreous cavity via the pars plana approach, in phakic or pseudophakic eyes. A superior anterior chamber paracentesis is performed with a 15-degree knife and it is kept open by pushing on the posterior lip with the knife thus allowing the SO droplets to come out of the eye; we rinse the anterior chamber with BSS or sodium hyaluronate till the anterior chamber is clean. It is also possible, if small droplets of emulsify oil persist, to aspire them with a 27G Rycroft cannula or if we have to deal with a huge amount of emulsified SO we use the irrigating–aspiring system. Once removal of emulsified SO is completed from the anterior chamber, SO and emulsified SO is removed from the vitreous cavity; the removal of emulsified oil in the vitreous cavity is best achieved by performing several fluid–air exchanges. The latter move the droplets which can then be aspirated using a flute needle or with the vitrectomy probe at the level of the fluid/air interfaces. We have to continue until all the droplets that may be trapped under iris or the ciliary processes are washed away. In aphakic patients, we remove anterior chamber emulsification via pars plana with the posterior irrigation.

◆ Another important problem is adherent SO on IOL following surgery: It induces large and irregular refractive errors and multiple images, and gives rise to glare, distorted, and often poor vision.[38] The adherence is particularly tenacious to silicone lenses, but SO has been shown also to adhere to lenses made from other materials including Polymethyl methacrylate (PMMA) and hydrophobic acrylic lenses.[39,40] It usually comes into contact with the IOL when there is a breach in the posterior capsule. The adherence of the SO may, however, not be obvious until after oil removal.[41] The oil droplets on the lenses have large contact angles, and they are dome shaped, thus changing the refractive properties of the lenses.

Several methods have been advocated for dealing with adherent SO droplets; in many cases, the method of last resort has been the explantation of the IOL.[42,43] Rinsing the IOL with sodium hyaluronate 1% Healon[43] and mechanical wiping with intraocular instruments[44] have also been advised. Dealing with acrylic IOLs we usually use a flute needle to clean the anterior and posterior side of the lens by using an anterior paracentesis and a pars plana approach respectively. A novel approach is to use solvents like SFAs and their oligomers.[45,46] SFAs are heavier-than-water transparent liquids that are tolerated by the retina.[46,47] SFAs dissolve in SO, and therefore this solubility can be used for the removal of SO. So far, F6H8 is the only certified agent for removal of SO adherent to silicone IOLs[48] requiring mechanical forces even for partial removal of the SO remnants. The search for a biocompatible substance to achieve a better and easier SO removal led to the production of F4H5, an SFA that had demonstrated excellent in vivo tolerance.[49] Experimental data showed that F4H5 is a more effective solvent than F6H8. Indeed a smaller volume of F4H5 than F6H8 is able to completely remove SO 1,000 or 5,000 from silicone lenses in vitro and also in vivo.[49]

⬖ Expected Outcomes: What Is the Worst-case Scenario

Glaucoma is a frequent and often a refractory complication related to the use of SO and has a multifactorial etiology in which emulsification plays a fundamental role[22,25,50–52] (see also Chapter 19B). Aggressive sequential therapeutic measures include medical therapy to temporize an acute elevation of intraocular pressure (IOP) and surgical management with SO removal, trabeculectomy with mitomycin C, and glaucoma shunts procedures. Cyclodestructive procedures may be reserved for refractory cases and for eyes with poor visual potential.[25,53,54]

SUBRETINAL SILICONE OIL

The Complication: Definition

Silicone oil migration into the subretinal space following vitreoretinal surgery may occur in complex cases of retinal detachment with proliferative vitreoretinopathy (PVR) and seems to relate to the presence of unrelieved retinal traction around retinal breaks. It can also occur as an intraoperative complication due to an accidental injection into the subretinal/suprachoroidal space, or if the stiffness of the retina overcomes the interface tension of the oil bubble.[54]

Displacement of SO under the retina prevents achievement of the primary goal (i.e., to attach the retina) and fails to provide the internal tamponade, leading to a permanent decrease in visual acuity. Successful and complete removal of the subretinal oil is a challenge. Internal drainage as described earlier in the literature advocates a large relaxing retinotomy.[55]

Risk Factors

Severe retinal detachment with retinal contraction, traumatic tractional retinal detachment, and/or large retinal tears with intraoperative persistence or postoperative formation of vitreoretinal proliferation, or choroidal coloboma[56] may favor this complication.

Pathogenesis: Why Does It Occur

Subretinal migration of SO is the consequence of insufficiently released or newly developed tractions in the proximity of retinal tears/holes. SO may migrate under the retina intraoperatively during its instillation at the end of surgery due to insufficient release of retinal traction or, postoperatively, if extensive contraction of the retina occurs following the developing or worsening of pre-existing proliferative vitreoretinopathy. As the retina is under tension due to the epiretinal or subretinal proliferation, eventual retinal tears reopen and enlarge, thus causing subretinal migration of the oil.

Pearls on How to Prevent It

◆ The key point is to make sure that the retina is mobile and there is no unrelieved traction around retinal tears/holes at the time of SO insertion. The use of vital staining helps in removing epiretinal membranes as much as possible. If subretinal proliferation is detected, a small central retinotomy can be performed to remove solitary and clearly visible strands; a large limbus parallel retinotomy may be necessary in order to inspect the outer side of the retina and remove multiple network and sheets of subretinal proliferation. The injection of SO after a fluid–air exchange helps in flattening the retina. However, the surface tension of air is greater than the interfacial tension between oil and water. Sometimes the retina could be flattened by air, thus masking the presence of residual tractions and causing the migration under the retina of the oil during the injection. A careful removal of traction and membranes is, thus, essential prior to the insertion of SO.

Pearls on How to Solve It

Oil evacuation can be performed by using different techniques depending on its amount and location.

◆ Subretinal SO may float up over the retina when the large bubble of SO present in the vitreous cavity is removed and, thus, subretinal SO can be removed with no major difficulty. This occurs nearly always when the SO has gone under the retina through a large retinal tear that remained under traction intraoperatively and opened or if PVR developed around a large tear soon postoperatively.

◆ In the presence of a small amount of SO, PFCL can be injected over the disk and the SO removed with a flute needle through an open tear or a small drainage retinotomy: In this case an air filling can be still indicated.

◆ Removal of larger amounts of subretinal SO represents a challenge. We usually prefer to remove first the SO tamponade and to operate with eye filled with BSS. In this manner the oil will occupy the uppermost position: Therefore the oil is often located anterior to the break unless the break is at the ora serrata. SO does not flow easily through a small retinotomy and employing active suction for removal of subretinal SO through a small retinotomy is potentially dangerous, especially in cases of emulsified oil. Therefore, a large peripheral retinotomy is often required to float the subretinal oil into the vitreous cavity and aid its removal.[55,56]

◆ If a large amount of SO is present under the retina, a persistent retinal detachment is evident often prior to and after the removal of the main bubble of oil present in the vitreous cavity. It may be useful to evacuate the subretinal SO only until after all retinal traction has been removed, as remaining epiretinal membranes are easier to remove with the retina stretched by the underlying SO bubble.[57] Once the surgeon has ensured that the retina is no longer withheld, he/she can then perform a long peripheral retinotomy, if the SO does not float up by itself through a retinal break, and inject PFCL on the disk so that the trapped SO will escape from the back to the vitreous cavity. Then the SO can be removed, endolaser can be applied, a PFCL/air exchange can be done and the surgery can be completed by a new SO filling.

◆ SO can also be removed transclerally. Eyes with subretinal SO often show complex PVR requiring a retinotomy for reattachment of the retina that may be also used for the removal of the oil. However, creating a large peripheral retinotomy in the initial stages of the surgery to remove subretinal oil is likely to make the retina mobile, complicating subsequent removal of the preretinal membranes; attempting to remove the membranes prior to the retinotomy for oil removal is made difficult by the buoyant subretinal oil that makes the retina bullous. Incomplete removal in such circumstances usually leads to recurrent retinal detachment with recurrent subretinal oil.[56] Transscleral removal of the oil has been advocated in cases where PVR is limited and a retinotomy may be necessary only for removal of the SO, as it avoids creating a retinotomy, thereby limiting the complexity of the surgery and also subsequent risk of PVR. Transscleral removal of SO has also been suggested for the treatment of suprachoroidal oil: In a serous choroidal detachment, suprachoroidal fluid can be drained through regular sclerotomies because the fluid can cleave through the suprachoroidal space due to its low surface tension and viscosity. Unfortunately, suprachoroidal oil may not flow as easily due to its high surface tension and viscosity. Therefore, an additional sclerostomy overlying the oil to drain it has been suggested.[58] Rarely, the pocket of suprachoroidal oil may be located far from the regular sclerotomies; in these cases a separate sclerostomy overlying the oil will be necessary. The technique reported is similar to that of subretinal fluid drainage during scleral buckling surgery. Insertion of an infusion cannula prior to the removal aids an increase in the intravitreal pressure that helps egress of the oil. The sclerostomy is placed just posterior to the ora serrata because the subretinal SO floats beneath the anterior retina. The SO usually egresses in toto with this technique due to the high surface tension of the oil and the lack of fluid currents in the subretinal space to break the flow of oil. The authors reported that emulsified subretinal oil may not flow out completely with this technique. Rotating the eye so that the sclerostomy remains superior and retaining this position until all oil flows out as indicated by flow of fluid also aids complete removal.

REFERENCES

1. McCuen BW 2nd, de Juan E Jr, Landers MB 3rd, et al. Silicone oil in vitreoretinal surgery. Part 2: results and complications. *Retina.* 1985;5:198–205.
2. Wolf S, Schön V, Meier P, et al. Silicone oil-RMN3 mixture ("heavy silicone oil") as internal tamponade for complicated retinal detachment. *Retina.* 2003;23(3):335–342.
3. Stappler T, Williams R, Gibran SK, et al. A guide to the removal of heavy silicone oil. *Br J Ophthalmol.* 2008;92(6):844–847. Epub 2008 May 6.
4. Romano MR, Groenwald C, Das R, et al. Removal of Densiron-68 with a 23-gauge transconjunctival vitrectomy system. *Eye (Lond).* 2009;23(3):715–717. Epub 2009 Jan 16.
5. Veckeneer MA, de Voogd S, Lindstedt EW, et al. An epidemic of sticky silicone oil at the Rotterdam Eye Hospital. Patient review and chemical analyses. *Graefes Arch Clin Exp Ophthalmol.* 2008;246:917–922.
6. Van Meurs J, Veckeneer M, de Voogd S, et al. An "epidemic" of sticky silicone oil at the Rotterdam Eye Hospital. Book of abstracts: first meeting on heavy tamponades in vitreo-retinal surgery (HEA-TAM1). Telfs, Austria; 2003.
7. Dresp JH, Menz DH. The phenomenon of "sticky" silicone oil. *Graefe's Arch Clin Exp Ophthalmol.* 2007;245:863–868.
8. Winter M, Winter C, Wiechens B. Quantification of intraocular retained perfluorodecalin after macroscopic complete removal. *Graefes Arch Clin Exp Ophthalmol.* 1999;237(2):153–156.
9. Wong D, Williams RL, German MJ. Exchange of perfluorodecalin for gas or oil: A model for avoiding slippage. *Graefes Arch Clin Exp Ophthalmol.* 1998;236(3):234–237.
10. Wong D, Van Meurs JC, Stappler T, et al. A pilot study on the use of a perfluorohexyloctane/silicone oil solution as a heavier than water internal tamponade agent. *Br J Ophthalmol.* 2005;89(6):662–665.
11. Rizzo S, Genovesi-Ebert F, Vento A, et al. A new heavy silicone oil (HWS 46-3000) used as a prolonged internal tamponade agent in complicated vitreoretinal surgery: A pilot study. *Retina.* 2007;27(5):613–620.
12. Sparrow JR, Ortiz R, MacLeish PR, et al. Fibroblast behavior at aqueous interfaces with perfluorocarbon, silicone, and fluorosilicone liquids. *Investig Ophthalmol Vis Sci.* 1990;31:638–646.
13. Prather TL, Grande J, Keese CR, et al. An agglutination assay using emulsified oils. *J Immunol Methods.* 1986;87:211–215.
14. Dresp JH, Menz DH. Interaction of different ocular endotamponades as a risk for silicone oil emulsification. *Retina.* 2005;25:902–910.
15. Rizzo S, Genovesi-Ebert F, Hagedorn N, et al. Coloring Of PFCL Facilitates Safe And Efficient Removal Of Temporary Tamponades ARVO Meeting Abstracts April 22, 2011;52:552.
16. Joussen AM, Wong D. The concept of heavy tamponades—chances and limitations. *Graefes Arch Clin Exp Ophthalmol.* 2008;246:1217–1224.
17. Joussen AM, Gardner TW, Kirchhof B. Vitrectomy in retinal vascular disease: Surgical principles. *Springer.* 2007;263.

18. Wolf S. Results of high-density silicone oil as a tamponade agent in macular hole retinal detachment in patients with high myopia. *Br J Ophthalmol.* 2007;91(6): 706–707.

19. Hoerauf H, Roider J, Kobuch K, et al. Perfluorohexylethan (O62) as ocular endotamponade in complex vitreoretinal surgery. *Retina.* 2005;25(4):479–488.

20. Stappler T, Williams R, Gibran SK, et al. *Br J Ophthalmol.* 2008;92:844–847.

21. Leaver PK, Grey RH, Garner A. Silicone oil injection in the treatment of massive preretinal retraction. II. Late complications in 93 eyes. *Br J Ophthalmol.* 1979;63: 361–367.

22. Valone J Jr, McCarthy M. Emulsified anterior chamber silicone oil and glaucoma. *Ophthalmology.* 1994;101:1908–1912.

23. Heidenkummer HP, Kampik A, Thierfelder S. Emulsification of Silicone with specific physicochemical characteristic. *Graefes Arch Clin Exp Ophthalmol.* 1991;229:88–94.

24. Dresp JH, Menz D-H. Interaction of different ocular endotamponades as a risk factor for silicone oil emulsification. *Retina.* 2005;25:902–910.

25. Honavar SD, Goyal M, Majji AB, et al. Glaucoma after pars plana vitrectomy and silicone oil injection for complicated retinal detachments. *Ophthalmology.* 1999;106: 169–177.

26. Scott IU, Flynn HW Jr, Murray TG, et al. Outcomes of complex retinal detachment repair using 1000- vs 5000-centistoke silicone oil. *Arch Ophthalmol.* 2005;123(4): 473–478.

27. Gabel VP. Polydimethylsiloxane and the factors influencing its intraocular biocompatibility. In: Heimann K, Wiedemann P, eds. *International Symposium on Proliferative Vitreoretinopathy,* Heidelberg, Kaden Verlag; 1989;156–162.

28. Heidenkummer HP, Kampik A, Thierfelder S. Experimentelle Untersuchungen zum sogenannten Emulsifikationsverhalten von Silikonöl: Einflu. der Viskosität. *Fortschr Ophthalmol.* 1990;87:226–228.

29. Heidenkummer HP, Kampik A, Thierfelder S. Experimental evaluation of in vitro stability of purified polydimethylsiloxanes (silicone oil) in viscosity ranges from 1000 to 5000 centistokes. *Retina.* 1992;12:S28–S32.

30. Crisp A, De Juan E, Tiedemann J. Effect of silicone oil viscosity on emulsification. *Arch Ophthalmol.* 1987;105:546–550.

31. Nakamura K, Refojo MF, Crabtree DV. Factors contributing to the emulsification of intraocular silicone and fluorosilicone oils. *Invest Ophthalmol Vis Sci.* 1990;31: 647–656.

32. Eckardt C, Nicolai U, Czank M, et al. Identification of silicone oil in the retina after intravitreal injection. *Retina.* 1992;12:S17–S22.

33. Eckardt C, Nicolai U, Czank M, et al. Okulare Gewebe nach intravitrealer Silikonölinjektion. *Ophthalmologe.* 1993;90:250–257.

34. Ni C, Wang WJ, Albert DM, et al. Intravitreous silicone injection. Histopathologic findings in a human eye after 12 years. *Arch Ophthalmol.* 1983;101:1399–1401.

35. Heidenkummer HP, Kampik A, Thierfelder S. Emulsification of silicone oils with specific physicochemical characteristics. *Graefes Arch Clin Exp Ophthalmol.* 1991;229: 88–94.

36. Bambas B, Eckardt C, Vowinkel E, et al. Toxische Substanzen im Silikonöl nach intraokularer Injektion. *Ophthalmologe.* 1995;92:663–667.

37. Bartov E, Pennarola F, Savion N, et al. A quantitative in vitro model for silicone oil emulsification. Role of blood constituents. *Retina.* 1992;12(3 Suppl):S23–S27.

38. Arthur SN, Peng Q, Escobar-Gomez M, et al. Silicone oil adherence to silicone intraocular lenses. *Int Ophthalmol Clin.* 2001;41:33–45.

39. Batterbury M, Wong D, Williams R, et al. The adherence of silicone oil to standard and heparin-coated PMMA intraocular lenses. *Eye.* 1994;8:547–549.

40. Wong D, Williams R, Batterbury M. Adherence of silicone oil to intraocular lenses. *Eye.* 1995;9:539.

41. Kusaka S, Kodama T, Ohashi Y. Condensation of silicone oil on the posterior surface of a silicone intraocular lens during vitrectomy. *Am J Ophthalmol.* 1996;121: 574–575.

42. Stolba U, Binder S, Velikay M, et al. Intraocular silicone lenses in silicone oil: An experimental study. *Graefes Arch Clin Exp Ophthalmol.* 1996;234:55–57.

43. Apple DJ, Federman JL, Krolicki TJ, et al. Irreversible silicone oil adhesion to silicone intraocular lenses. A clinicopathologic analysis. *Ophthalmology.* 1996;103: 1555–1561.

44. Kageyama T, Yaguchi S. Removing silicone oil droplets from the posterior surface of silicone intraocular lenses. *J Cataract Refract Surg.* 2000;26:957–959.

45. Meinert H. Patent: semifluorinated alkanes and their application. *PCT/EP96/03542.* 9 1996.

46. Roider J, Hoerauf H, Kobuch K, et al. Clinical findings on the use of long-term heavy tamponades (semifluorinated alkanes and their oligomers) in complicated retinal detachment surgery. *Graefes Arch Clin Exp Ophthalmol.* 2002;240:965–971.

47. Kirchhof B, Wong D, Van Meurs J, et al. Use of perfluorohexyloctane as a long-term internal tamponade agent in complicated retinal detachment surgery. *Am J Ophthalmol.* 2002;133:95–101.

48. Liang Y, Kociok N, Leszczuk M, et al. A cleaning solution for silicone intraocular lenses: "sticky silicone oil." *Br J Ophthalmol.* 2008;92:1522–1527.

49. Stappler T, Williams R, Wong D. F4H5: A novel substance for the removal of silicone oil from intraocular lenses. *Br J Ophthalmol.* 2010;94:364–367.

50. Genovesi-Ebert F, Rizzo S, Chiellini S, et al. Ultrasound biomicroscopy in the assessment of secondary glaucoma after vitreoretinal surgery and silicone oil injection. *Ophthalmologica.* 1998;212 (Suppl 1):4–5.

51. Avitabile T, Bonfiglio V, Cicero A, et al. Correlation between quantity of silicone oil emulsified in the anterior chamber and high pressure in vitrectomized eyes. *Retina.* 2002;22(4):443–448.

52. Nguyen QH, Lloyd MA, Heuer DK, et al. Incidence and management of glaucoma after intravitreal silicone oil injection for complicated retinal detachments. *Ophthalmology.* 1992;99:1520–1526.

53. Moisseiev J, Barak A, Manaim T, et al. Removal of silicone oil in the management of glaucoma in eyes with emulsified silicone. *Retina.* 1993;13:290–295.

54. de Juan E Jr, McCuen B, Tiedeman J. Intraocular tamponade and surface tension. *Surv Ophthalmol.* 1985;30:47–51.

55. Chitolina J, Bacin F. Treatment of a subretinal silicone oil bubble [article in French]. *J Fr Ophtalmol.* 2006;29:409–412.

56. Dithmar S, Schuett F, Voelcker HE, et al. Delayed sequential occurrence of perfluorodecalin and silicone oil in the subretinal space following retinal detachment surgery in the presence of an optic disc pit. *Arch Ophthalmol.* 2004;122:409–411.

57. Zivojnovic R. Chapter 6. *Silicone oil in Vitreoretinal Surgery.* Martinus Nyjhoff/Dr W. Junk publishers, Kluwer Academic Publisher Group, Dordrecht/Boston/Lancaster; 1987:120–124.

58. Shanmugam MP, Ramanjulu R, Kumar RM, et al. Transscleral drainage of subretinal/ suprachoroidal silicone oil. *Ophthalmic Surg Lasers Imaging.* 2012;43(1):69–71.

14 SUBRETINAL DISPLACEMENT of DYES

ARND GANDORFER

Peeling of epiretinal membranes (ERMs) and the internal limiting membrane (ILM) is a frequently performed procedure by vitreoretinal surgeons. In recent years, visualization of the membranes has been made easier by staining them with different dyes, such as indocyanine green (ICG), trypan blue, brilliant blue, and others.[1] Since their introduction, there has been some debate on whether or not these dyes are toxic to the macula, with regards to both inner and outer retinal damage.[2,3] Whereas in ERM patients, potential toxicity is primarily focused on inner retinal layers, macular hole cases are at higher risk of outer retinal damage, because the dye can directly access the subretinal space, potentially causing additional harm to the retinal pigment epithelium and photoreceptors. This complication is discussed herein, summarizing the current literature on this topic.

✥ The Complication: Definition

ICG was the first dye used to stain the ILM during macular hole surgery.[4] Two years after its introduction, Engelbrecht and coworkers[3] reported on retinal pigment epithelial changes after macular hole surgery with ICG-assisted ILM peel. In their retrospective series of 22 eyes, 10 eyes had unusual atrophic changes in the retinal pigment epithelium at the site of the previous macular hole, or in the area where the ICG solution (0.1%) had direct access to the bare retinal pigment epithelial cells. The best corrected visual acuity dropped from 20/200 preoperatively to 20/400 postoperatively, although 86% of macular holes were closed.

Arevalo and Garcia[5] report on a massive accidental subretinal ICG injection in a macular hole case. 0.3 mL of 0.5% ICG was applied to stain the ILM. The assistant pushed the syringe with too much force, and a relatively high volume of ICG entered the subretinal space, creating an iatrogenic retinal tear in the papillomacular bundle. After ILM peel and macular hole closure, retinal pigment epithelial and choriocapillaris atrophy was present. Subretinal ICG was still detectable 7 months after surgery.[5]

More recently, Ghosh and coworkers[6] published a case series of subretinal migration of trypan blue during macular hole and ERM peel. 0.3 mL of 0.15% trypan blue was used under air, and entered the subretinal space through the macular hole in two patients. Retinal pigment epithelial changes and chorioretinal atrophy corresponding to the area of dye migration was noted 1 week after surgery. In one patient with an ERM peel, the jet of dye caused an immediate subretinal bluish hue along the inferior temporal vascular arcade. On the first postoperative day subretinal dye was documented, followed by an atrophic area with pigment epithelial changes in the area where the dye had migrated.[6]

Previously, Uno and coworkers[7] also reported on subretinal migration of trypan blue during ERM peel. In a patient with idiopathic ERM, 0.3 mL of 0.15% trypan blue was administered onto the posterior pole under air. As soon as the dye was removed from the vitreous cavity, a subretinal trypan blue collection of three-disk diameters was detected inferior to the optic disk. There was no internal drainage of the subretinal trypan blue because no subretinal dye collection was present at the macula, as the authors state.[7] Four weeks after surgery, retinal pigment epithelium changes were seen in the area inferior to the optic disk, corresponding to the previous subretinal dye deposit, and a window defect was seen on fluorescein angiography. The authors assume that trypan blue "probably reached the subretinal space through a tiny retinal hole induced by the dye jet when the dye was injected into the vitreous cavity."[7]

Pathogenesis

The pathogenesis of dye toxicity is poorly understood. In theory, damage can directly occur due to the injection of dye into the subretinal space, causing retinal detachment and photoreceptor and/or retinal pigment epithelium damage, in the sense of a jet-related mechanical trauma. Chemical damage may occur due to the toxicity of trypan blue or the osmolarity of the solution. In addition, a photodynamic effect of trypan blue was proposed in combination with endoillumination.[7] There is one study investigating the effect of different dyes and osmolarities injected subretinally.

In this experimental study, 20 Dutch-belted rabbits underwent vitrectomy with subretinal injection of ICG, trypan blue, glucose, and balanced salt solution (BSS) at different concentrations equivalent to those used in human macular surgery.[8] The dye was left in the subretinal space, and the blebs that had been created were flat after 24 hours. Fluorescein angiography showed window defects after ICG and trypan blue injection. Subretinal application of 0.05% ICG resulted in more substantial retinal damage than 0.15% trypan blue injection.[8] In addition, hypo-osmolar solutions of ICG and trypan blue showed a more severe damage than iso-osmolar solutions.[8] Histologic evaluation 6, 12, and 24 hours and 14 days after surgery revealed damage to the photoreceptor outer and inner segments, to the outer nuclear layer, and to the retinal pigment epithelium.[8] Functional studies were not performed in this series.

All the above clinical and experimental reports have in common that (1) the dye directly entered the subretinal space, or (2) was iatrogenically displaced subretinally by a forceful injection. It is obvious that a dye administered to the posterior pole will get access to the subretinal space in case of a macular hole. In ERM patients, however, the way how the dye enters the subretinal space is not clear. If the retina is attached to the retinal pigment epithelium, both a retinal defect and a jet must be present for subretinal dye displacement. In these cases, a forceful injection seems to contribute to the subretinal displacement of dye. Theoretically, the dye could also migrate through the intact retina but there is no data supporting this mechanism.

Pearls on How to Prevent It

◆ In general, administration of the dye under air results in a higher concentration of dye at the retina compared with that done under fluid. This is due to the higher concentration of dye as there is a smaller distribution volume under air where the dye can only settle on the retina without dilution in BSS. In addition, in the case of a macular hole, the dye will migrate into the subretinal space promoted by gravity. As the dye cannot diffuse away from the subretinal space compared to a fluid-filled vitreous cavity, a high concentration of dye will be in direct contact with the retinal pigment epithelium and the photoreceptors of the elevated macular hole rim. Therefore, any dye injection under air should be avoided, as should be the use of ICG, given its narrow safety margins and the potential toxicity compared to other dyes, especially brilliant blue.[9,10] One advantage of brilliant blue is the fact that it can be applied into the fluid-filled eye with good staining properties of the ILM.

◆ Forceful injection should also be prevented by using suitable instruments. An easy-to-handle syringe reduces the risk of creating a pressure gradient before the dye can leave the cannula. Also, some drops of dye should be applied outside the eye to ensure that no pressure is needed for injection. We use a 23G flute needle connected to a tuberculin syringe, and administer only a few drops of heavy brilliant blue (Brilliant Peel, Fluoron GmbH, Neu Ulm, Germany) to the posterior pole.[11] Care should be taken not to inject directly into a macular hole.

◆ Any jet of dye is unnecessary for staining and can harm the retina either by pressure or by forcing the dye to enter the subretinal space. As toxicity is also dependent on the volume applied, as less dye as possible should be applied.

◆ In addition, several alternatives have been proposed to prevent direct retinal damage due to dye injection, such as the use of perfluorocarbon liquid and viscoelastic over the area of the macular hole.[12,13] There are also reports on a small number of patients using subretinal trypan blue for break identification in retinal detachment surgery with successful outcome (see Chapter 16).[14] This indicates that retinal pigment epithelial damage due to dyes is a combination of several factors, such as dye toxicity, volume applied, mechanical stress due to a jet, and possibly light toxicity. Any dye administered should be left in contact with the retina as shortly as possible. Ideally, the dye should be gently injected and washed out immediately, as described before regarding brilliant blue G.

◆ Do not inject the dye under air.

◆ Do not create any jet.

◆ Apply only a few drops of dye gently onto the posterior pole.

◆ Do not point toward the macular hole.

◆ Do not use a hard-to-control syringe.

◆ Do not apply more than 0.1 mL.

◆ Do not use ICG.

◆ Use brilliant blue G.

◆ Pearls on How to Solve It

◆ If the dye had entered the subretinal space, it should be washed out. This is not as easy to do as it sounds, because ICG and trypan blue seem to have some binding affinity to the retinal pigment epithelium and every washing maneuver itself is prone to harm the retinal pigment epithelium. A gentle flow created by a flute needle may help to carefully wash the dye out of the subretinal space, at least in macular hole cases. In ERM cases, the flute needle can be used to detect the retinal hole where the dye had entered the subretinal space. Creating a small retinotomy to get access to the subretinal dye deposit can be another rationale to remove the dye if no such tiny retinal defect is found.

◆ What Is the Worst-case Scenario

The case reports shown above demonstrate that any dye injection into the subretinal space can be a severe complication of vitreoretinal surgery associated with a potentially guarded visual prognosis. Especially in macular hole eyes, closure of the hole is worthless in functional terms if the retinal pigment epithelium is damaged by subretinal dye toxicity. The same applies for ERM cases if the dye had caused damage in the foveal area. Given today's high expectations after surgery in terms of visual quality, dye-related complications should be avoided by using the least toxic dye available, at the shortest application time, which currently is heavy brilliant blue G.[11]

REFERENCES

1. Haritoglou C, Schuttauf F, Gandorfer A, et al. An experimental approach towards novel dyes for intraocular surgery. *Dev Ophthalmol.* 2008;42:141–152.

2. Gandorfer A, Haritoglou C, Gass CA, et al. Indocyanine green-assisted peeling of the internal limiting membrane may cause retinal damage. *Am J Ophthalmol.* 2001; 132(3):431–433.

3. Engelbrecht NE, Freeman J, Sternberg P Jr, et al. Retinal pigment epithelial changes after macular hole surgery with -assisted internal limiting membrane peeling. *Am J Ophthalmol.* 2002;133(1):89–94.

4. Kadonosono K, Itoh N, Uchio E, et al. Staining of internal limiting membrane in macular hole surgery. *Arch Ophthalmol.* 2000;118(8):1116–1118.

5. Arevalo JF, Garcia RA. Macular hole surgery complicated by accidental massive subretinal indocyanine green, and retinal tear. *Graefes Arch Clin Exp Ophthalmol.* 2007; 245(5):751–753.

6. Ghosh S, Issa S, El Ghrably I, et al. Subretinal migration of trypan blue during macular hole and epiretinal membrane peel: An observational case series. Is there a safer method?. *Eye (Lond).* 2010;24(11):1724–1727.

7. Uno F, Malerbi F, Maia M, et al. Subretinal trypan blue migration during epiretinal membrane peeling. *Retina.* 2006;26(2):237–239.

8. Penha FM, Maia M, Eid Farah M, et al. Effects of subretinal injections of indocyanine green, trypan blue, and glucose in rabbit eyes. *Ophthalmology.* 2007;114(5):899–908.

9. Enaida H, Hisatomi T, Hata Y, et al. Brilliant blue G selectively stains the internal limiting membrane/brilliant blue G-assisted membrane peeling. *Retina.* 2006; 26(6):631–636.

10. Gandorfer A, Haritoglou C, Kampik A. Toxicity of indocyanine green in vitreoretinal surgery. *Dev Ophthalmol.* 2008;42:69–81.

11. Haritoglou C, Schumann RG, Kampik A, et al. Heavy brilliant blue G for internal limiting membrane staining. *Retina.* 31(2):405–407.

12. Scupola A, Giammaria D, Tiberti AC, et al. Use of perfluorocarbon liquid to prevent contact between indocyanine green and retinal pigment epithelium during surgery for idiopathic macular hole. *Retina.* 2006;26(2):236–237.

13. Kusaka S, Oshita T, Ohji M, et al. Reduction of the toxic effect of indocyanine green on retinal pigment epithelium during macular hole surgery. *Retina.* 2003;23(5): 733–734.

14. Jackson TL, Kwan AS, Laidlaw AH, et al. Identification of retinal breaks using subretinal trypan blue injection. *Ophthalmology.* 2007;114(3):587–590.

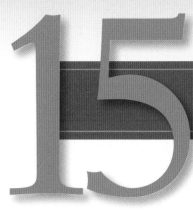

15 IATROGENIC RETINAL TEARS

Jan Van Meurs and Paul Sullivan

15A Breaks Due to Vitreous Traction (Indirect Trauma)

Most iatrogenic breaks occur due to vitreous traction, that is, the instrument does not come into direct contact with the retina but pulls in the vitreous. As the vitreous is very adherent to the retina at the vitreous base this causes breaks on the posterior border of the vitreous base.

ENTRY SITE BREAKS

These are breaks within 1 clock hour of the entry sites. They rarely occur near the infusion port. They develop due to vitreous traction associated with instrument insertion and withdrawal with associated vitreous incarceration and traction (see **Fig. 15A-1**).

◆ Pearls on How to Prevent It

- ◆ Minimize the number of instrument changes.
- ◆ Minimize aspiration during instrument movements: That is, when using the vitreous cutter, use suction only for specific intentional goals (induction of PVD).

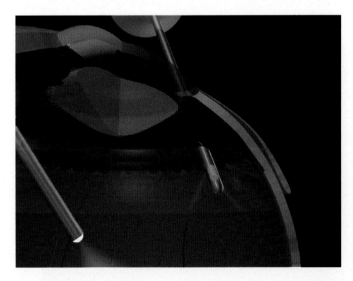

Figure 15A-1 Entry site break due to vitreous traction while withdrawing instrument.

When using a passive extrusion system (such as the Charles flute), ensure the port is covered when you do not wish to aspirate.

◆ Avoid high IOP during instrument changes.

◆ In bullous retinal detachments, reducing the height of the detachment by cutting over the break seems to reduce the risk of vitreous incarceration.

◆ Entry site breaks appear to be significantly less frequent with trocar-based systems (23G and 25G systems).[1,2]

◆ Routine retinopexy of entry site breaks has been advocated[3] but is not generally practiced because of possible complications[4] and because enhanced intraoperative inspection seems to be highly effective in preventing postoperative retinal detachment.[5]

◆ In a bullous retinal detachment vitreous incarceration is indicated by retinal folds radiating from the incarceration point. Attempts to release the incarcerated vitreous with the cutter are futile. Lowering of the infusion pressure may help release the vitreous/retinal incarceration. Re-attachment of the retina using air or perfluorocarbon liquid (PFCL) displaces the vitreous posteriorly and usually frees the incarceration. Instillation of PFCL through the port with incarceration is not advisable; this should be done through another port or even using a sharp injection needle through the infusion tubing. In case of a recalcitrant incarceration the retina or vitreous may be grasped and freed with forceps or as a last resort by creating a local retinectomy.

 ## Pearls on How to Treat It

◆ Entry site breaks detected intraoperatively and treated with retinopexy and internal tamponade rarely cause postoperative retinal detachment. It is therefore very important to examine the peripheral retina around the sclerotomies at the end of every case. Fortunately, wide-angle viewing systems have made this easier.[5]

PEROPERATIVE TRACTIONAL BREAKS DISTANT FROM THE ENTRY SITE

Risk Factors

Peripheral breaks may occur while a posterior vitreous detachment is being induced **(Fig. 15A-2)** (Chung et al., 2009, #68585). They are not adjacent to entry sites and

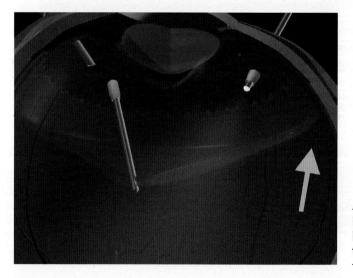

Figure 15A-2 Peripheral break (*arrow*) due to vitreous traction while inducing PVD.

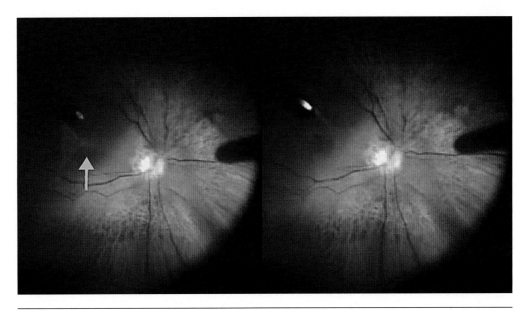

Figure 15A-3 Iatrogenic macular hole during separation of vitreous. Note the macular tissue under stress appears stretched (*arrow*) in the left panel immediately prior to the break in the right panel.

indeed often occur inferiorly.[6] They may also occur during vitrectomy in eyes with a posterior vitreous detachment if there is poor control of the aspiration and cutting rate.

Macular breaks can result from excessive traction in eyes with vitreomacular traction syndrome **(Fig. 15A-3)**.

◆ Pathogenesis

Very high vacuum is required to engage and initiate detachment of the posterior hyaloid from the retina. Continued aspiration and traction after the hyaloid starts to detach (e.g., if detachment of the hyaloid is not recognized) causes traction at the vitreous base which can cause retinal tears.

◆ Pearls on How to Prevent It

◆ While detaching the posterior hyaloid look out for signs of vitreous separation (elevating Weiss ring, vitreous tissue in the mouth of the cutter, an expanding dark ring around the optic disc) and move from aspiration to cut mode as soon as these are observed. Once signs of posterior detachment of the hyaloid are observed, further separation generally occurs by the aspiration coupled to the cutting mode and by spending some time cutting the vitreous. In some patients with more centrally adherent vitreous as in some myopes, extending the hyaloidal detachment may need more active suction, certainly at the risk of causing retinal tears. Particularly, in the presence of a retinal detachment, for instance in young patients with vitreoretinopathies, this situation ranks among the most demanding of vitreoretinal maneuvers (see also Chapter 12). The goal would be to relieve any vitreoretinal traction present around the break(s) causing the retinal detachment by trimming the posterior hyaloid around this break(s). Sometimes it helps to weigh down the detached central retina; sometimes a hydraulic jet reflux stream by the flute needle in one hand and the vitreous cutter in suction mode in the other may help to separate the hyaloid from the detached retina.

Pearls on How to Treat It

◆ Examine the whole peripheral retina (not just around the entry sites) in eyes in which a PVD has been induced.[6] Once a tear is observed, it should be surrounded by laser coagulation or cryo after relieving traction by trimming the posterior hyaloid around the break or tear. We would favor to use a gas tamponade, even when there is no associated retinal detachment.

EXCESSIVE VITREOUS TRACTION DURING VITRECTOMY IN EYES WITH A PVD

Poor control of vitrectomy fluidics and movement of instruments with vitreous incarcerated in their tips may produce peripheral distant tractional retinal breaks. Dense vitreous hemorrhage seems to be a risk factor for these breaks,[7] possibly due to the greater mass and (therefore inertia) of the vitreous in these cases.

 ## Pearls on How to Prevent It

◆ Minimization of vitreous traction during vitrectomy requires an excellent understanding of fluidic concepts like vacuum, cut rate, and duty cycle. In general the highest possible cut rate and the lowest possible vacuum minimize vitreous traction.

◆ Vitreoretinal traction during vitrectomy is a function of distance from the retina, so the aspiration should be reduced when operating close to the retina.

POSTOPERATIVE RETINAL BREAKS DUE TO TRACTION

Late tears may occur due to contraction of incarcerated vitreous base.[8] Giant retinal tears may develop following incomplete vitrectomy.[9]

 ## Pearls on How to Prevent It

◆ Wherever possible perform a complete vitrectomy, including the removal of the posterior hyaloid membrane up to the vitreous base.

The authors have the clinical impression that the combinations of extensive or circumferential laser and a remaining vitreous skirt may lead to vitreous base contraction; the risk for this event to happen may be reduced by trimming the posterior hyaloid up to the vitreous base.

REFERENCES

1. Chung SE, Kim KH, Kang SW. Retinal breaks associated with the induction of posterior vitreous detachment. *Am J Ophthalmol.* 2009; 147:1012–1016.
2. Gosse E, Newsom R, Lochhead J. The incidence and distribution of iatrogenic retinal tears in 20-gauge and 23-gauge vitrectomy. *Eye (Lond).* 2012;26:140–143.
3. Issa SA, Connor A, Habib M, et al. Comparison of retinal breaks observed during 23 gauge transconjunctival vitrectomy versus conventional 20 gauge surgery for proliferative diabetic retinopathy. *Clin Ophthalmol.* 2011;5:109–114.
4. Kim CS, Kim KN, Kim WJ, et al. Intraoperative endolaser retinopexy around the sclerotomy site for prevention of retinal detachment after pars plana vitrectomy. *Retina.* 2011;31:1772–1776.
5. Wimpissinger B, Binder S. Entry-site-related retinal detachment after pars plana vitrectomy. *Acta Ophthalmol Scand.* 2007;85:782–785.
6. Tan HS, Lesnik Oberstein SY, Mura M, et al. Enhanced internal search for iatrogenic retinal breaks in 20-gauge macular surgery. *Br J Ophthalmol.* 2010;94:1490–1492.

7. Sjaarda RN, Glaser BM, Thompson JT, et al. Distribution of iatrogenic retinal breaks in macular hole surgery. *Ophthalmology*. 1995;102:1387–1392.

8. Ritland JS, Syrdalen P, Eide N, et al. Outcome of vitrectomy in patients with Terson syndrome. *Acta Ophthalmol Scand*. 2002;80:172–175.

9. Krieger AE. The pars plana incision: Experimental studies, pathologic observations, and clinical experience. *Trans Am Ophthalmol Soc*. 1991;89:549–621.

10. McLeod D. Giant retinal tears after central vitrectomy. *Br J Ophthalmol*. 1985;69:96–98.

15B   Retinal Breaks Due to Direct Retinal Trauma

RETINAL BREAKS DURING CORE VITRECTOMY

Stereoacuity during vitrectomy surgery is limited and experienced surgeons depend on tacit awareness of subtle monocular clues to orientate their instruments in relation to the retina. For example, if the tip of the light pipe cannot be seen in the field, but a diffuse and even illumination of the retina is noted, this would indicate that the light pipe is distant from the retina. The location and distance from the retina of the tips of other instruments used during the surgery are indicated by the distance from their shadows **(Fig. 15B-1)**.

Inexperienced surgeons may lose their orientation and cause retinal trauma during core vitrectomy. This is most common when the field of view is limited (e.g., small pupil) and when the view is poor (e.g., media opacity). It may also occur due to sudden movement of the patient or uncontrolled movements of the surgeon (e.g., looking to the side causes torsional movements of the upper body which are transmitted to the instruments).

 ## Pearls on How to Prevent It

- ◆ This is primarily a training issue. Simulators for vitreoretinal surgery such as the Eyesi simulator and model eyes for wet lab use faithfully replicate the illumination features that allow orientation of instruments explained above.

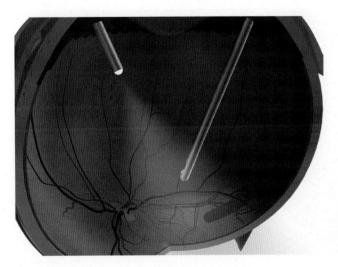

Figure 15B-1 Shadows are used to assess the distance of instrument tips from the retina.

Pearls on How to Treat It

◆ Retinal impact sites outside the vitreous base rarely cause retinal detachment and, thus, may be managed conservatively (no treatment is necessary).

BREAKS DURING SURGERY FOR SIMPLE EPIRETINAL MEMBRANES (MACULAR PUCKER)

The instruments used to peel epiretinal membranes are in contact with the neurosensory retina. Small movements of either the instruments or the patient have the potential for serious retinal trauma.

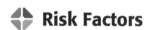 **Risk Factors**

◆ Sudden movement of the patient (e.g., due to unanticipated discomfort or misjudged level of sedation) or operating table **(Fig. 15B-2)**.

◆ Movements of distant parts of the surgeon may be transmitted via the upper body to the instruments. We have seen this occur during adjustment of the foot pedal to refocus and while looking away from the microscope to address other members of staff.

◆ Typically a surgeon would be switching from a wide-angle lens to one with greater Z-axis resolution at this stage (e.g., a plano-concave contact lens or a specialized noncontact lens). These lenses have a narrower field of view which may make the appreciation of the distance of the instrument tip from its shadow more difficult **(Fig. 15B-3)** and, inadvertently, may then touch the retina.

◆ There is a tendency to focus one's attention on the point at which the epiretinal tissue is separating from the retina—if an extensive large sheet of tissue is being peeled the tip of the forceps becomes progressively further from this point as the peel progresses and may even move out of the field of view (at which point the tip could be gouging the retina) **(Fig. 15B-4)**. Repeated regrasping of the epiretinal tissue as it delaminates avoids this as the separation point and the tip of the instrument can be viewed simultaneously.

◆ Trainee surgeons tend to extrapolate their experience of capsulorrhexis when learning epiretinal membrane peeling. During capsulorrhexis it is very important to keep the tangent of tearing flat as any elevation will cause the rhexis to

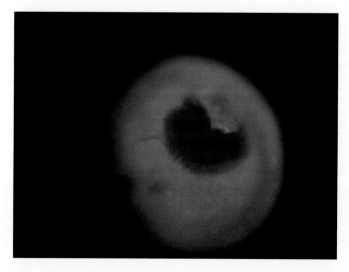

Figure 15B-2 Retinal gouging following sudden unanticipated movement of a patient.

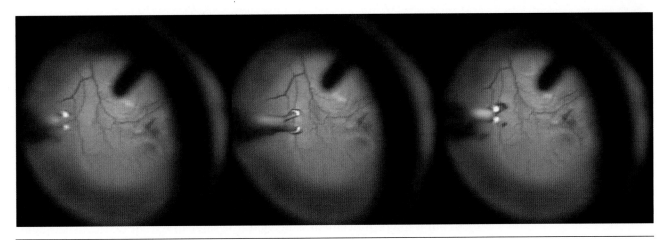

Figure 15B-3 Retinal perforation during epiretinal membrane peeling. The forceps are at the edge of the operative field where anterior capsule opacification makes the distance from the retina difficult to assess.

run out. The retina has a convex contour, however, and if the same principle is observed the instrument will gouge the retina.

Pearls on How to Prevent It

◆ Conscious patients should be comfortable at the start of the operation—for example, a pillow under the knees often prevents low back pain due to prolonged recumbent extension of the lumbar region.

◆ Patients should be made aware of the need for their full cooperation in lying still before peeling is commenced.

◆ All members of the operating room (OR) team need to be aware that a delicate maneuver is about to take place and avoid unnecessary distraction of the surgeon—a video display of the surgery is helpful in raising the level of situational awareness in the OR.

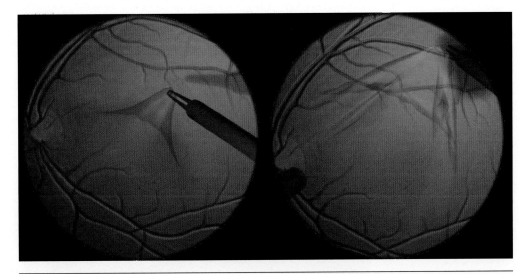

Figure 15B-4 Retinal gouging during macular surgery. The forceps are at the edge of the operative field where lack of a visible shadow and failing to adjust the angle of pulling results in retinal injury.

◆ All members of the OR team need to be made aware of the importance of avoiding sudden movements of the operating table and the need to inform the surgeon if any adjustments have to be made (e.g., for anesthetic reasons).

◆ Surgeons whose previous experience has been confined to wide-angle viewing systems need to be aware of the very different 'gestalt' of macular viewing systems and the need to be conscious of the position of the tip of the instrument.

◆ When peeling extensive membranes regrasp frequently.

◆ The desired tangent of peeling is not completely flat (as in capsulorrhexis) but about 30 degrees from the tangent to the retina.

◆ While operating near the retina surgeons should withdraw their instruments slightly before making any minor movement with any part of their body (e.g., to refocus). If a major movement is needed it is safer to withdraw the instruments from the eye altogether.

◈ Pearls on How to Treat It

Extensive damage to the nerve fiber layer causes large corresponding arcuate scotomas.

As a general rule retinal breaks in the posterior pole, in the absence of very significant traction, do not cause retinal detachment and do not require treatment. This is particularly true of lesions near the fovea where retinopexy is not only unnecessary but harmful as it increases the area of the scotoma.

RETINAL BREAKS DURING DIABETIC VITRECTOMY

Advanced diabetic eye disease is characterized by the presence of limited vitreous separation and numerous fibrovascular complexes (or pegs) that tether the posterior hyaloid to the retinal veins. These adhesions are so strong that traction on them will frequently produce a retinal break before it will shear the peg (particularly if the retina is atrophic as in long standing tractional detachment) **(Fig. 15B-5)**. Vitrectomy for advanced diabetic eye disease carries a high risk of retinal breaks because of the need to sever all of these pegs to allow removal of all the epiretinal tissue and vitreous. The risk is proportional to the degree of retinal detachment, vitreoretinal adhesion, and perfusion on fibrovascular pegs.

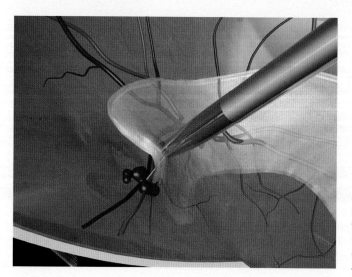

Figure 15B-5 Traction on a fibrovascular complex causing hemorrhage and a retinal break.

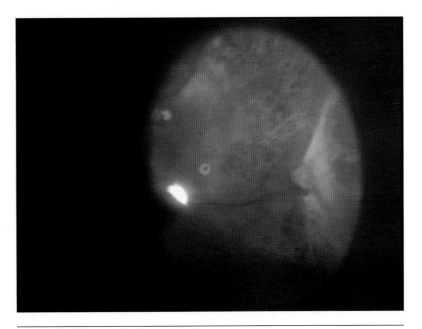

Figure 15B-6 Peripheral and posterior retinal breaks (marked by diathermy) following diabetic delamination surgery.

Peripheral retinal breaks due to traction at the vitreous base are also common in diabetic eye surgeries **(Fig. 15B-6)**. They occur due to the need to introduce large irregular-shaped instruments such as delamination scissors through the vitreous base.

Posterior breaks usually arise indirectly through excessive traction on vitreo-retinal adhesions. They may also arise if the retina is perforated with the tips of delamination scissors, typically if the retina is convoluted (by focal traction) or if the plane of dissection is incorrect **(Fig. 15B-7)**. Difficulty in identifying the correct plane of dissection is exacerbated by the presence of hemorrhage from severed

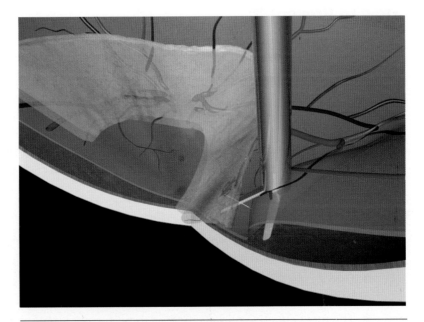

Figure 15B-7 The blade of delamination scissors passed through a retinal fold during delamination.

pegs—the bleeding seems to be worse if the pegs are ripped off (which avulses the side wall of a major retinal vessel) than if they are cleanly transected.

✛ Pearls on How to Prevent It

◆ Limiting intraoperative hemorrhage makes it easier to stay in the correct surgical plane which avoids the formation of retinal breaks. Preoperative reduction in the perfusion of fibrovascular pegs helps to achieve this. This can be obtained by preoperative pan retinal photocoagulation or by intravitreal injection of a vascular endothelial growth factor (VEGF) inhibitor 5 to 7 days preoperatively. Intraoperative bleeding can be also minimized/prevented by elevating the infusion pressure, by mechanical pressure with an instrument, such as a blunt-tipped forceps, diathermy, and laser of bleeding points (see also Chapter 26B).

◆ There are many surgical approaches to advanced diabetic eye disease. Whichever technique is used the risk of retinal breaks is reduced by limiting the amount of pulling on the membrane. In practice a little traction is often required to separate nonvascularized epiretinal membranes around the pegs, identify the correct surgical plane, and identify the exact location of individual pegs but it should be used as little as possible.

✛ Pearls on How to Treat It

◆ The key to management of posterior breaks is removal of all surrounding epiretinal tissue to prevent traction which would keep the break open. This is followed by fluid/air and air/gas exchange and laser retinopexy. Gas tamponade is usually preferable to silicone oil because of the risk of perisilicone proliferation. An adjuvant scleral buckle is not required.

BREAKS DURING PROLIFERATIVE VITREORETINOPATHY (PVR) SURGERY

Breaks may occur when peeling star folds from mobile retina.

✛ Pearls on How to Prevent It

◆ The retina is thinner and weaker peripherally than centrally. Star folds should, whenever possible, be peeled centrifugally rather than centripetally.

◆ Ensure that forceps do not pinch a fold of retina along with the star fold. If there is suspicion that this is the case rotate the instrument tip slightly to allow oblique inspection of the tissue in the tip—if only epiretinal tissue has been grasped there will be a translucent zone between the forceps and the retina.

◆ While peeling be alert for signs of mechanical stress in the surrounding retina. An area of progressively increasing retinal translucency may indicate an incipient retinal break **(Fig. 15B-8)**.

✛ Pearls on How to Treat It

◆ Management of iatrogenic breaks in star folds is quite problematic as attempts at further peeling tend to enlarge the break further.

◆ Use of episcleral explants to create high broad indents over the breaks often fails to relieve sufficient traction.

◆ The most effective management is to perform a large relieving retinectomy.

Large retinectomies are very effective at relieving traction. However, they also cause peripheral scotomas and may increase the risk of persistent postoperative hypotony by increasing uveoscleral outflow.

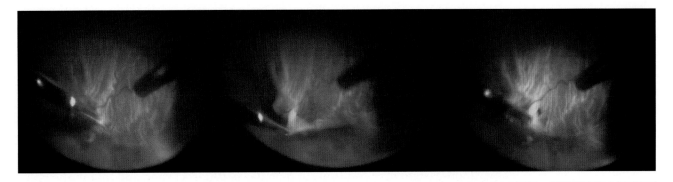

Figure 15B-8 Retinal break while peeling a star fold. Note the area of retinal translucency preceding the break.

INCARCERATION OF MOBILE RETINA

Mobile retina may be aspirated into the tip of the cutter—once partially occluded a large amount of tissue may become incarcerated very quickly indeed **(Fig. 15B-9)** resulting in very large retinal breaks.

Risk Factors

◆ Bullous retinal detachments.

◆ Use of inappropriately low cut rates or high aspiration vacuum.

Pearls on How to Prevent It

◆ Aspirate fluid through the break to reduce the height of the detachment and create space in the preretinal compartment for the cutter to operate safely.

◆ Avoid use of low cut rates and high aspiration over mobile retina.

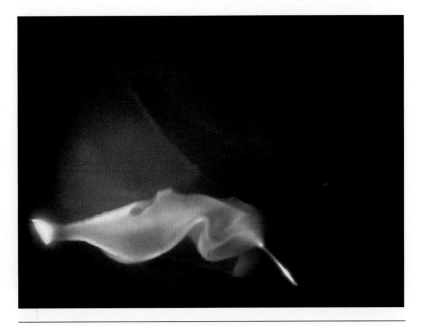

Figure 15B-9 Mobile retina may get incarcerated in the cutter, particularly in bullous retinal detachment with inappropriately low cutting rates or high aspiration vacuum.

◆ Surgeons need a full understanding of the fluidic parameters of their machine to understand how they can control these intraoperatively.

◆ Modern vitrectomy systems have many enhancements, including the potential to cut at very high rates and control the proportion of time that the port is open (the "duty cycle"), that reduce the likelihood of this. Using these systems it is possible to safely remove vitreous in cases with very mobile detachments.

◆ Perfluorocarbon liquid (PFCLs) may be used to stabilize the retina in very bullous retinal detachments and reduce the risk of incarceration but do have a number of disadvantages such as their cost, the risk that manipulation of retina under perfluorocarbon may result in submacular perfluorocarbon and that in the presence of small breaks an anterior doughnut of subretinal fluid may be created.

◆ Pearls on How to Treat It

◆ If the retina is incarcerated in the cutter use the foot pedal-controlled reflux button to free it—alternatively ask the assistant to pinch the cutter aspiration line.

◆ Inadvertent retinotomies should be treated like any other retinal break (i.e., retinopexy and tamponade).

RETINAL BREAKS RELATED TO RETINOPEXY

Intraoperative retinal breaks may occur due to excessively heavy photocoagulation in areas with shallow subretinal fluid. These are rarely of any consequence as they tend to be surrounded by photocoagulation scars.

Postoperatively large retinal breaks can occasionally develop following vitrectomy with cryotherapy.[1] These breaks are characterized by the appearance of an area of retinal necrosis corresponding to the area of the underlying chorioretinal cryopexy changes ("cryonecrosis") **(Fig. 15B-10)**.

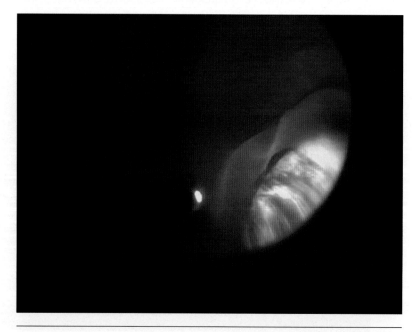

Figure 15B-10 Re-operation for retinal break due to cryonecrosis. Note the pigment loss and choroidal hemorrhages indicating very cryotherapy or multiple freeze/thaw cycles.

Pearls on How to Prevent It

The cause of this very rare phenomenon is poorly understood and it is therefore difficult to give firm guidelines to prevent it. It is well known, however, that multiple cycle freezes (i.e., retreatment of the same area) are particularly destructive to all tissues in other settings.[2] Laser retinopexy may be preferable to cryotherapy for large retinal breaks not least because the immediately visible tissue reaction reduces the risk of retreatment.

REFERENCES

1. Bowman RJ, Hodgkins PR, Soliman MM, et al. Retinal necrosis as a complication of cryotherapy. *Eye (Lond).* 1994;8:600–601.
2. Goldbaum MH, Fletcher RC, Jampol LM, et al. Cryotherapy of proliferative sickle retinopathy, II: Triple freeze-thaw cycle. *Br J Ophthalmol.* 1979;63:97–101.

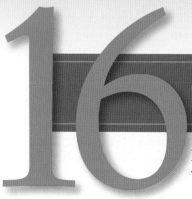

The "MISSING" BREAK

ROGER WONG AND ALISTAIR LAIDLAW

 ## The Complication: Definition

A "missing" break occurs when the clinician is not able to identify the hole or tear which is responsible for the rhegmatogenous retinal detachment. Despite meticulous indentation and indirect biomicroscopy, some breaks remain hidden. Unidentified breaks is one of the most common causes of failed retinal detachment surgery.[1] As many as 6% of cases have been found to have no break despite pars plana vitrectomy and internal search.[2] Various factors can hinder identification, but the knowledge of why these holes/tears are difficult to identify will help plan surgery and improve the rate of success.

 ## Risk Factors and Pathogenesis

Eye Factors

Media Opacity

◆ Pupil: Poorly dilating pupil (due to diabetes, previous ocular surgery, trauma, previous inflammatory eye disease).

◆ Anterior segment: Corneal pathology, lenticular opacities, intraocular lens, capsular remnants.

◆ Vitreous opacity: Tobacco dust, vitreous hemorrhage, asteroid hyalosis.

Not all retinal detachments are identifiable by biomicroscopy. Media opacities can not only obstruct views of the breaks, but also of the retinal detachment. When there is an obstruction of the fundus view, ultrasound B scan may be required for diagnosis. Surgical intervention of anterior segment disease due to factors such as corneal pathology, poorly dilating pupil, and lens opacification can be performed to improve the view of the fundus. If vitreous hemorrhage or debris is the cause of a hazy view, pars plana vitrectomy rather than an external buckling procedure may be a better approach to identify and treat retinal breaks. The surgeon opting for an external approach could elect to wait for the hemorrhage to clear before booking surgery. However, one must not wait too long to promote proliferative vitreoretinopathy (PVR) development and consequently decrease the chance of surgical success. If signs of progression are detected on serial ultrasound scanning, then surgical intervention should be contemplated sooner rather than later.

Peripheral Retinal/RPE/Choroid

In patients with a pale fundus, previous retinopexy, trauma, or peripheral retinal pigment changes, identification of breaks may be difficult due to the nonconfluent background of the choroid and retinal pigment epithelium (RPE).

Proliferative Vitreoretinopathy (PVR)

Retinal detachments with fixed folds, anterior loop traction, and funnel configuration can hide breaks from view.

Unusual Site

◆ Coloboma, macular hole.

In some rare cases such as coloboma or macular hole-associated retinal detachments, the break may not be obvious in the usual methods of peripheral indentation and search.

Patient Factors

Poor Cooperation

Patients who cannot posture supine to allow 360-degree indentation or patients who are not cooperative will make preoperative assessment difficult and therefore result in incomplete examination.

Clinician Factors

Poor Technique

◆ Pearls on How to Prevent It

◆ Meticulous preoperative indentation + indirect biomicroscopy.

◆ Identification of signs/clues to predict type/site of break (e.g., posterior vitreous detachment (PVD) usually causes horse-shoe tear; myopic chronic inferior detachments with no PVD are usually due to round holes).

◆ Understanding of Lincoff's rules (see also Chapter 4).[3]

◆ Pearls on How to Solve It

◆ Examination under general anesthesia: This eliminates the variable of patient cooperation allowing for better indentation, indirect ophthalmoscopy, and subsequent planning of surgery.

◆ Surgical removal/improvement of media opacity.

  ◆ That is, cataract extraction, corneal graft, temporary keratoprosthesis, capsulectomy, and vitrectomy.

◆ Perfluorocarbon liquid (PFCL) to push subretinal fluid (SRF) from the posterior retina to the anterior retina causing extrusion of schlieren (thick SRF) through the break and subsequent opening of the break to facilitate better identification.

◆ Bimanual shaving of vitreous base to prevent vitreous skirt obscuring break.

◆ Manual lifting of vitreous skirt with vitrector or light pipe to show underlying break.

◆ DE-Tech (Dye Extrusion Technique): Using a posterior retinotomy or direct injection into the subretinal space with a 41G cannula, trypan blue is injected into the subretinal space. PFCL is then injected to cover the retinotomy forcing the SRF and dye to migrate anteriorly. The dye and SRF extrude out of the occult break when the PFCL is injected or when the surgeon performs a search with

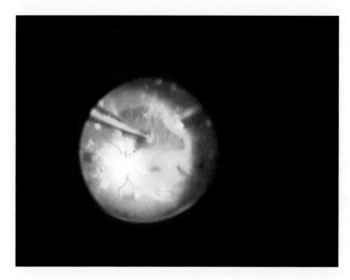

Figure 16-1 DE-Tech: Injection of trypan blue into the subretinal space through retinotomy.

external indentation. Once the occult break is identified, the area can be treated with retinopexy **(Figs. 16-1 and 16-2)**.[4]

The use of an infusion of low molecular weight silicone oil (5 millipascal seconds) as a preoperative tool to facilitate vitreous base shaving and break localization has been proposed recently.[5] Once PFCL has been injected to stabilize the posterior retina, the infusion of balance salt solution is stopped and, instead, low molecular weight silicone oil is infused. As both, PFCL and low molecular weight silicone oil are hydrophobic, when in contact with one another they join to produce a heavier-than-water bubble, displacing the vitreous base anteriorly. Although PFCL, itself, helps during vitreous shaving by stabilizing the retina, the low molecular weight silicone oil, in addition, facilitates the view of the vitreous base, given the differences in refractive index between silicone oil (1.40) and vitreous (1.34). As the view of the vitreous base is enhanced, shaving of the vitreous base can be done easily without risking iatrogenic breaks. Infusion of low molecular weight silicone oil also improves visualization of retinal breaks by reflecting anteriorly the vitreous and the operculum of U tears. It also helps on localizing the posterior border of the vitreous base, which can be seen inside the silicone oil infusion as the refractive index of the latter is 1.40 and that of vitreous, perfluorodecalin, and n-octane is 1.34, 1.31, and 1.29, respectively.

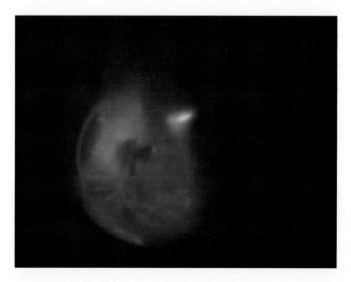

Figure 16-2 Extrusion of subretinal trypan blue found occult retinal break.

◆ If no break is found

　◆ Encirclement buckle:

　　◆ Circumferential encirclement buckling is thought to help decrease both vitreous traction and also transretinal traction (Hook's law).[6] These changes in tractional forces shift the equilibrium toward retinal reattachment. Bernoulli's principle states that as speed of fluid increases, the pressure within the fluid decreases. Due to this, a buckle can further facilitate reattachment. Some surgeons recommend this approach in high myopes, aphakic eyes, and also eyes with no PVD. However, there are certain associated complications with encirclement buckles such as changes in refractive error, motility problems, and anterior ischemia. Therefore, if the break *can* be found, a localized buckle should be applied.

　　◆ Speculative segmental buckling (i.e., buckling only the area that is detached) can reduce the complications associated with circumferential encirclement by limiting the area in which the retina is treated, but still allowing an adequate change in forces to facilitate reattachment.

　◆ 360-degree retinopexy.

In the case of vitrectomy, by performing two rows of 360-degree laser retinopexy confined to the posterior border of the vitreous base, this can potentially cause inadvertent treatment of the break or isolation of retinal detachment to a section peripheral to the retinopexy. However, a circumferential ring detachment anterior to the retinopexy may occur. To prevent this, one can extend the laser up to the ora in sections to isolate the detachment if it occurs. In conventional sclera buckling, laser retinopexy could be applied once the retina flattens and the SRF absorbs. A 360-degree cryotherapy is not necessary at the time of surgery in these cases and could promote unnecessary PVR progression if applied.

◆ Expected Outcomes

Identification of Break

◆ The identification of retinal breaks will allow targeted and localized treatment of the break preventing more invasive maneuvers such as encirclement buckling.

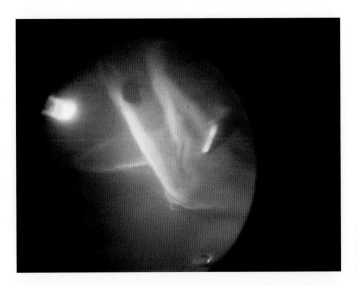

Figure 16-3 Retinal break identified on indentation.

Persistent Missed Break

◆ A missed break will progress to re-detachment of the retina.

REFERENCES

1. Norton EW. Retinal detachment in aphakia. *Am J Ophthalmol.* 1964;58:111–124.
2. Salicone A, Smiddy WE, Venkatraman A, et al. Management of retinal detachment when no break is found. *Ophthalmology.* 2006;113:398–403.
3. Lincoff H, Gieser R. Finding the retinal hole. *Arch Ophthalmol.* 1971;85:565–569.
4. Wong R, Gupta B, Aylward GW, et al. Dye extrusion technique (DE-TECH): Occult retinal break detection with subretinal dye extrusion during vitrectomy retinal detachment repair. *Retina.* 2009;29:492–496.
5. Wong D, Lai W, Yusof W. The use of continuous silicone oil infusion as a preoperative tool to facilitate break localisation, vitreous base dissection and drainage of subretinal fluid. *Ophthalmologica.* 2011;226 (suppl 1):53–57.
6. Thompson J. The effects and action of scleral buckles in the treatment of retinal detachment. In: Wilkinson CP, ed. *Retina.* vol III, 4th ed. Philadelphia, PA: Elsevier Inc; 2006:2021–2034.

17

RETINAL SLIPPAGE

Ian Y. Wong and David Wong

The Complication: Definition

Retinal slippage is the posterior displacement of subretinal fluid by an incoming bubble of tamponade, usually air, resulting in retinal folds with or without exposure of the underlying retinal pigment epithelium (RPE). It is not an uncommon problem encountered during surgery for the repair of giant retinal tears (GRTs), and cases where relaxing retinotomies were done. There have been no reports on the incidence of retinal slippage or retinal folds following slippage. In a recent report where the incidence of GRT was found to be 0.094 cases per 100,000 population in a nation-wide survey,[1] the incidence of relaxing retinotomies is yet to be documented. Hence, the occurrence of slippage may be far under-reported.[2]

Mechanism: Why Does It Occur

◆ *Presence of a GRT:* A GRT is defined as a full-thickness retinal break extending circumferentially for ≥3 hours (90 degrees) in the presence of a posteriorly detached vitreous.[3,4] The lack of vitreous attachment to the posterior flap means that it can be freely and independently mobile and thus prone to sagging posteriorly. GRT includes giant retinotomies but of course not giant dialyses, where the vitreous remains attached to the posterior edge (of the dialyses). In a GRT, the cord length is shorter than the arc length. This causes relative redundancy and a natural tendency to sag posteriorly **(Fig. 17-1)**.

◆ *Incomplete drainage of subretinal fluid:* Another important element is the presence of residual subretinal fluid, during air–fluid exchange.[5,6] This residual fluid will be displaced posteriorly toward the disc and macula by the surface tension of the incoming air bubble.[6] A perfluorocarbon liquid (PFCL) bubble in an eye filled with balanced salt solution (BSS) will assume a convex upper surface. The edge of the GRT follows this contour. During air–PFCL exchange, a "wedge" of aqueous is trapped between the air bubble above and the PFCL bubble below. This wedge is peripheral and frequently inaccessible. As the exchange progresses, this wedge of aqueous together with the edge of the GRT can be pushed by the high surface tension of the air bubble posteriorly. This results in both an exposed area of bare RPE and the formation of a curvilinear fold of retina **(Fig. 17-2)**.

◆ The mechanism of slippage in cases of retinotomies is the same as that seen in GRT.

◆ The traditional advice to prevent slippage includes the complete drying of the edge of the GRT during the exchange of PFCL and air. This is the counsel of perfection. In reality, complete evacuation of fluid is very difficult to do, partly because of problems with visualization and partly because of difficulty with access. The upper surface of the PFCL is convex. There is therefore a "wedge"

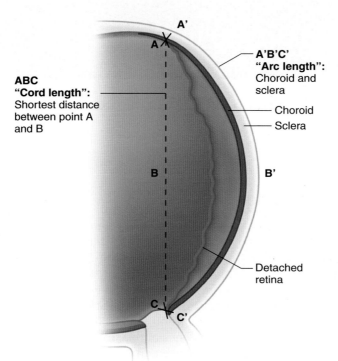

ABC
"Cord length":
Shortest distance
between point A
and B

A'B'C'
"Arc length":
Choroid and
sclera

Choroid

Sclera

B'

Detached
retina

Figure 17-1 Relative redundancy of the retina is caused by a difference in distance between the cord and arc in a giant retinal tear. This difference causes the posterior sagging of the tear when no vitreous is adhering to the posterior flap.

of aqueous between the PFCL and the eye wall. What we have been asked to do is to remove the aqueous under the air bubble before removing the PFCL. Inside the eye, there are multiple reflective and refractive interfaces (between the back of the lens/IOL and incoming air bubble, between the air and aqueous, between air and PFCL, etc.). The difference in refractive indices between air and aqueous or lens is large, whilst between PFCL and aqueous is small. To remove aqueous without unintentional removing of PFCL is not easy. The location of the aqueous also makes visualization challenging. The "wedge" of aqueous is in the far periphery. Wide-angle optics is required; there are many optical aberrations. Rotating the eye does not help. If the eye was rotated superotemporally in order to see the edge of a GRT, the aqueous would be displaced by the PFCL to

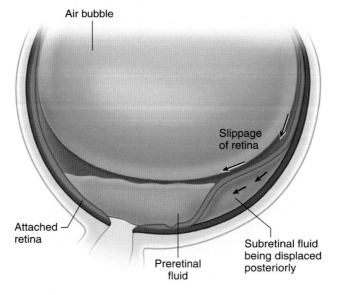

Air bubble

Slippage
of retina

Attached
retina

Preretinal
fluid

Subretinal fluid
being displaced
posteriorly

Figure 17-2 Incomplete drainage of subretinal fluid and relative redundancy of the retina cause slippage to occur when the vitreous cavity is being filled by an air bubble. The posterior displacement of subretinal fluid carries the overlying detached retina toward the macular, and causes the observable slippage.

the inferonasal quadrant. This may be fine if the retina was not totally detached. If it was, any aqueous could be loculated subretinally. If PFCL were drained before all aqueous was evacuated, then the "wedge" would simply be displaced posteriorly (to cause slippage). Another problem is the difficulty of access. The edge of the GRTs is often anterior. Unless the eye is pseudophakic, a draining needle could cause lens touch and cause lens opacity.

Risk Factors

♦ Direct fluid–air exchange is more likely to cause slippage (see above).

♦ Extent of retinal tear: GRTs greater than 180 degrees have a greater tendency to slippage using silicone oil tamponade without PFCL. Prior to the introduction of PFCL, air was used to unfold GRT in a prone patient strapped to a rotating Stryker table with the surgeon operating literally underneath the patient. If PFCL is not used, one is reliant on the surface tension of silicone oil going out to length. However, if the tear is greater than 180 degrees, the cord length separating the two horns of the giant tear will be smaller than the diameter of the eye at the ora serrata leading to retinal redundancy and more chance for retinal slippage (see **Fig. 17-3**).

♦ Location of the tear: Tears located superiorly have a higher tendency to cause postoperative retinal folds than tears situated inferiorly.[7–9] The reason for this might be due to the fact that patients adopt an erect posture soon after surgery in the presence of subretinal fluid.

♦ The use of encircling buckle, in conjunction with internal tamponade, may also predispose to slippage.[7–9] Encirclement will reduce the circumference of the eye, and give rise to circumferential redundancy and radial retinal folds.

♦ Phakic eyes: During the process of PFCL/air exchange it is necessary to drain the subretinal fluid at the posterior edge of the GRT. GRTs often occur relatively

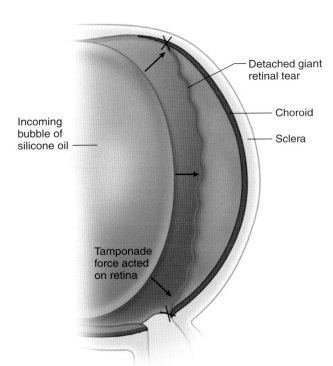

Incoming bubble of silicone oil

Detached giant retinal tear

Choroid

Sclera

Tamponade force acted on retina

Figure 17-3 If a giant retinal tear was less than 180 degrees, then the cord length between the two ends of the tear is less than the diameter of the globe. Injection of a tamponade agent such as silicone oil will separate the two ends, thus lifting any sagging of the posterior edge. If the giant retinal tear were greater than 180 degrees, then the same "pulling up" of the sagging posterior edge would not occur.

anteriorly, almost at the ora serrata. It is difficult to visualize and apply the drainage needle that far anteriorly without engendering high risk of lens touch. Failure to evacuate all subretinal or preretinal aqueous fluid before air infusion would result in slippage.

Pearls on How to Prevent It

◆ **Direct PFCL/oil exchange:** Both oil and PFCL are hydrophobic. Once in contact with one another, the two liquids will form a single bubble and displace any aqueous from the interface. Naturally if there were any residual subretinal or preretinal fluid, this would be displaced laterally and superiorly. It is necessary to explain why water, which is heavier than silicone oil, would be displaced superiorly. The reason is the oil and PFCL formed together a single bubble. In the early phase of the exchange, the combined bubble is made up of mostly PFCL and therefore heavier than water. During the latter phase of the exchange, the combined bubble is made up of mostly oil. Even then, although the water is heavier than oil, it does not quickly work its way below the silicone oil. The reason is the interfacial tension of oil tends to keep the oil as a spherical bubble. For the water to "fall" below the bubble, it needs to overcome the interfacial tension. The difference in the specific gravities between water and oil is only small. The aqueous therefore remains loculated anteriorly when the patient is supine. By definition, slippage is the posterior displacement of aqueous. If they are loculated anteriorly slippage cannot possibly occur.

An important tip: As silicone oil is injected, the drainage needle should be passed from the oil into the PFCL bubble several times. This maneuver encourages the two liquids to come into contact with one another to form a single bubble. Passing the needle through the two liquids once or twice would suffice; surface energy would do the rest.

◆ **Overfill method:** This is by far the easiest technique to adopt. However, it should only be applied if there was complete removal of traction from the retina such that there would be no risk of subretinal PFCL when it is filled beyond the anterior edge of the tear. Essentially the method requires PFCL to be filled to overfill, that is, all aqueous should be displaced out of the eye including space of the infusion tubing up to and including the three-way tap. This is done with the BSS disconnected. The intraocular pressure is maintained by a steady injection of the PFCL. Once the fill is to the three-way tap, then air or oil infusion could commence. Since the vitreous cavity now contains only PFCL and no aqueous, therefore almost by definition slippage cannot occur. We have verified this in a series of close to 100 cases of patients undergoing 360 retinotomies for macular rotation.[10] It also means that it would be perfectly safe to carry out a direct air/ PFCL or with a silicone oil/PFCL exchange.

◆ **More tips:** With 20G surgery over-fill of PFCL would expel any aqueous in the vitreous cavity provided that one of the sclerotomies is opened and the eye rotated with that sclerotomy uppermost. With smaller-gauge surgery and the use of cannulae, it may be necessary to rotate the eye/cannula to ensure that aqueous can escape from the eye during the PFCL over-filling.

Pearls on How to Solve It

◆ If slippage is minor, for example, if there was a slight circumferential fold near the edge of the tear, the following method can be used. A diamond-dusted membrane scraper (DDMS) or a soft-tipped needle can be used to engage the edge of the flap to bring the edge anteriorly. Gentle strokes should be used, otherwise tearing the retina and trauma to the underlying RPE would occur.

◆ If the slippage is more severe and the eye is filled with air, we advocate refilling the eye with saline, then PFCL.

◆ If the slippage was significant and there is already oil in situ, then great care should be taken. The removal of silicone oil has to be done under direct visualization of the retinal edge at all time. Because of the high suction pressure used, it is possible to remove the oil and inadvertently aspirate the retina into the usually wide-bore cannula used for the removal of oil.

What Is the Worst-case Scenario

Slippage of the retina may cause various complications such as retinal folds,[2] hypotony,[11] and may promote proliferative vitreoretinopathy (PVR).[2] Slippage is most likely to occur during the process of air–fluid exchange.[5,6] Historically, strategies included rapid head movements to unfold the tear,[12] performing fluid–air exchange with the patient in the prone position,[13–17] manipulation of the retinal flap under silicone oil,[3,18–20] fixating the flap by microincarceration,[21,22] intraoperative adhesives,[23] retinal tacks,[24–26] and sutures.[27] These methods have been traumatic and were of limited success.

REFERENCES

1. Ang GS, Townend J, Lois N. Epidemiology of giant retinal tears in the United Kingdom: The British Giant Retinal Tear Epidemiology Eye Study (BGEES). *Invest Ophthalmol Vis Sci. Sep.* 2010;51(9):4781–4787.
2. Heimann H, Bopp S. Retinal folds following retinal detachment surgery. *Ophthalmologica.* 2011;226(Suppl 1):18–26.
3. Scott JD. Giant tear of the retina. *Trans Ophthalmol Soc U K.* 1975;95(1):142–144.
4. Kanski JJ. Giant retinal tears. *Am J Ophthalmol.* 1975;79(5):846–852.
5. Mathis A, Pagot V, Gazagne C, et al. Giant retinal tears. Surgical techniques and results using perfluorodecalin and silicone oil tamponade. *Retina.* 1992;12(3 Suppl): S7–S10.
6. Wong D, Williams RL, German MJ. Exchange of perfluorodecalin for gas or oil: A model for avoiding slippage. *Graefes Arch Clin Exp Ophthalmol.* 1998;236(3): 234–237.
7. Lewen RM, Lyon CE, Diamond JG. Scleral buckling with intraocular air injection complicated by arcuate retinal folds. *Arch Ophthalmol.* 1987;105(9):1212–1214.
8. Pavan PR. Retinal fold in macula following intraocular gas. An avoidable complication of retinal detachment surgery. *Arch Ophthalmol.* 1984;102(1):83–84.
9. van Meurs JC, Humalda D, Mertens DA, et al. Retinal folds through the macula. *Doc Ophthalmol.* 1991;78(3–4):335–340.
10. Li KK, Wong D. Avoiding retinal slippage during macular translocation surgery with 360 retinotomy. *Graefes Arch Clin Exp Ophthalmol.* 2008;246(5):649–651.
11. Machemer R. Retinotomy. *Am J Ophthalmo.* 1981;92(6):768–774.
12. Freeman HM. Current management of giant retinal breaks with an inverted retinal flap. In: Kanski JJ, Morse PH, eds. *Disorders of the Vitreous, Retina and Choroid.* Boston, MA: Butterworths; 1983:210–217.
13. Norton EW, Aaberg T, Fung W, et al. Giant retinal tears. I. Clinical management with intravitreal air. *Am J Ophthalmo.* 1969;68(6):1011–1021.
14. Machemer R, Allen AW. Retinal tears 180 degrees and greater. Management with vitrectomy and intravitreal gas. *Arch Ophthalmol.* 1976;94(8):1340–1346.

15. Lincoff H. A small bubble technique for manipulating giant retinal tears. *Ann Ophthalmol.* 1981;13(2):241–243.

16. Freeman HM, Castillejos ME. Current management of giant retinal breaks: Results with vitrectomy and total air fluid exchange in 95 cases. *Trans Am Ophthalmol Soc.* 1981;79:89–102.

17. Vidaurri-Leal J, de Bustros S, Michels RG. Surgical treatment of giant retinal tears with inverted posterior retinal flaps. *Am J Ophthalmol.* 1984;98(4):463–466.

18. Leaver PK, Lean JS. Management of giant retinal tears using vitrectomy and silicone oil/fluid exchange. A preliminary report. *Trans Ophthalmol Soc U K.* 1981;101(1): 189–191.

19. Leaver PK, Cooling RJ, Feretis EB, et al. Vitrectomy and fluid/silicone-oil exchange for giant retinal tears: Results at six months. *Br J Ophthalmol.* 1984;68(6):432–438.

20. Glaser BM. Treatment of giant retinal tears combined with proliferative vitreoretinopathy. *Ophthalmology.* 1986;93(9):1193–1197.

21. Schepens CL, Freeman HM. Current management of giant retinal breaks. *Trans Am Acad Ophthalmol Otolaryngol.* 1967;71(3):474–487.

22. Peyman GA, Rednam KR, Seetner AA. Retinal microincarceration with penetrating diathermy in the management of giant retinal tears. *Arch Ophthalmol.* 1984; 102(4):562–565.

23. Faulborn J. Treatment of giant retinal tears after perforating injuries with vitrectomy and a cyanocrylate tissue adhesive. *Adv Ophthalmol.* 1976;33:204–207.

24. Ando F, Kondo J. A plastic tack for the treatment of retinal detachment with giant tear. *Am J Ophthalmol.* 1983;95(2):260–261.

25. de Juan E Jr, McCuen BW 2nd, Machemer R. The use of retinal tacks in the repair of complicated retinal detachments. *Am J Ophthalmol.* 1986;102(1):20–24.

26. Abrams GW, Williams GA, Neuwirth J, et al. Clinical results of titanium retinal tacks with pneumatic insertion. *Am J Ophthalmol.* 1986;102(1):13–19.

27. Federman JL, Shakin JL, Lanning RC. The microsurgical management of giant retinal tears with trans-scleral retinal sutures. *Ophthalmology.* 1982;89(7):832–839.

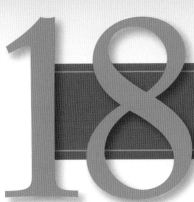

COMPLICATIONS in RELATION to the VITREORETINAL SURGICAL SYSTEMS USED

STEVE CHARLES

The Complication: Why Does It Happen and How to Prevent It

(See specific chapters with regards to how to treat it once it occurs.)

Infusion Fluidics and Intraoperative Low Intraocular Pressure

Since the inception of pars plana vitrectomy, surgeons have occasionally experienced excessively low intraocular pressure (IOP) during vitreoretinal surgery. New techniques and technologies have greatly improved surgical outcomes but created special challenges with respect to the infusion system. Gravity-fed infusion systems were simplistic and could only cause low IOP if the bottle was too low or the infusion fluid was depleted. Sutured 20G vitrectomy resulted in low intraoperative IOP if the cannula was initially placed or displaced into the suprachoroidal space and not detected. Digital display of infusion pressure associated with vented gas forced infusion created the false impression that IOP was controlled when, in fact, as much as 25 mm Hg of difference existed between infusion pressure and IOP because of pressure drop in the infusion cannula and tubing. These large pressure gradients are inherent with typical flow rates during vitreous removal, especially fragmenter use. This was the first instance of low intraoperative IOP being wrongly blamed on the machine when, in fact, surgeons were using too low infusion pressure (15–20 mm Hg). There are many causes of excessively low IOP during vitrectomy; each of these will be discussed in this section.

Inadvertent suprachoroidal infusion is a relatively common cause of low pressure as well as other more serious complications during vitrectomy with 20G, 23G, and 25G surgeries. Sutureless 25G vitrectomy initially utilized straight-in trocar–cannula trajectories to produce sclerotomies perpendicular to the sclera. When 23G sutureless surgery was introduced subsequently, oblique trocar–cannula entry was utilized in order to construct a scleral tunnel to reduce wound leakage. Initially, surgeons used a two-plane approach; the initial trocar–cannula insertion segment was approximately 30 degrees relative to the sclera and the second segment trajectory perpendicular to the sclera. Some surgeons even incorrectly believed that a biplanar incision was constructed although this is not true because the scleral tunnel was created before changing the trajectory. More recently, most surgeons using both 23G and 25G systems have switched to oblique entry in order to create a long scleral tunnel, often with very steep angles (5–10 degrees). This method is often incorrectly referred to as beveled wound construction. Although near tangential entry creates a long scleral tunnel, it increases the chances of infusing into the suprachoroidal or subretinal space. If the cannula is in the suprachoroidal space, early in the case the choroid elastically expands allowing infusion without hypotony; later the choroid can no longer expand and infusion becomes limited alerting the surgeon to the problem. Unfortunately, some surgeons incorrectly conclude that the hypotony was the primary problem which subsequently caused a choroidal effusion. A single-plane, 30-degree trajectory produces a scleral tunnel with the highest resistance to leakage (Ray Iezzi, Vail, unpublished data, 2010).

I have always advised inspecting the infusion cannula with the operating microscope or indirect ophthalmoscope after insertion and before initiating infusion to assure it is inside the vitreous cavity. Unfortunately, many surgeons have discontinued this practice since we began using 23G/25G sutureless vitrectomy; clearly we must not omit the crucial step of observing the tip of the infusion cannula. Since it is the best practice to insert the infusion port in the cannula with the infusion pressurized to prevent bubbles, it is necessary to immediately inspect the tip on the infusion port to avoid suprachoroidal infusion. The naked eye and endoilluminator provide insufficient magnification to make the determination that the cannula has penetrated the choroid and nonpigmented pars plana epithelium; microscope visualization is essential.

Adhesively fastening the infusion cannula tubing and associated stopcock(s) and connectors to the drape is imperative to prevent traction on the infusion cannula and the eye. Inadvertent and unrecognized pulling on the tubing by the assistant or surgeon can easily cause the cannula to pull partially out causing a suprachoroidal infusion later in the case. Adhesively fastening the infusion cannula tubing to the drape with the eye in the primary position with a short tubing loop can result in a suprachoroidal infusion when the eye is rotated to view the periphery creating tension on the cannula.

Scleral depression, while valuable to examine peripheral vitreoretinal traction, is another opportunity to cause inadvertent suprachoroidal infusion by causing pressure on the cannula as the eye is rotated by the depressor. In addition, scleral depression can force blood clots, dense scar tissue, peripheral vitreous, or silicone oil into the infusion cannula and tubing, effectively plugging it giving the false impression of machine failure.

Placing the infusion cannula too close to the lower lid rather than just inferior to the horizontal meridian is a common cause of suprachoroidal infusion created when the eye is rotated down to visualize the inferior periphery and the cannula is rotated into the suprachoroidal space.

Kinking of the more flexible silicone tubing terminal segment of the infusion cannula can be caused by the surgeon or assistant accidentally pulling on the tubing. This problem is exacerbated by using excessively low infusion pressure settings (10–25 mm Hg) insufficient to straighten out the tubing kink. The author has always used 45 mm Hg except when operating on small children or patients with very low systemic blood pressure, typically under general anesthesia.

Frictional losses in the infusion line are often underestimated by the surgeon. There are significant frictional losses in the infusion system with typical flow rates, typically 10 to 20 mm Hg. Although the Alcon Constellation Vision System has an IOP Compensation System, this technology cannot always overcome frictional losses in the line when excessively low pressure settings (10–25 mm Hg) are combined with high outflow rates. Kinking as well as multiple bubbles in the infusion line increase resistance to flow and cause pressure drop ultimately resulting in excessively low IOP. The IOP Compensation System is most effective when used to slow the rate of IOP drop when using 23G or especially 25G infusion, and a 20G fragmenter to remove dense lens fragments. Occlusion break will result in ocular collapse if the surgeon does not respond quickly enough; the IOP Compensation System gives the surgeon more time to reduce vacuum when an occlusion break is recognized. The IOP Compensation System utilizes an ultrasonic flow sensor; when the flow rate rapidly increases the infusion pressure is automatically increased in an attempt to maintain the selected IOP.

✚ Aspiration Fluidics and Intraoperative Retinal Breaks

Retinal breaks are less common than in the early days of vitrectomy but are still a highly significant issue. There are many causes of preventable retinal breaks (see also Chapter 15) but the focus of this chapter is on machine parameters and technical choices.

The highest possible cutting rate should be used for all tasks and all cases in order to minimize pulsatile vitreoretinal traction and collagen fiber travel before shearing. Higher cutting rates confine pulsatile flow to the region near the port thereby reducing remote effects. It is a common misconception that lower cutting rates, 3D mode, or dual linear mode should be used for so-called "core vitrectomy" to increase flow rates. Optimal phaco technique requires mobilizing lens material away from the capsule; the tissue to be removed is moved to the port. In sharp contrast, the vitrectomy cutter port should be brought to the vitreous to be removed rather than using excessive flow rates to pull vitreous to the port. Withdrawing the cutter while cutting and aspirating is another common mistake during vitrectomy; continuous engage and advance is least likely to produce iatrogenic retinal breaks.

A common cause of iatrogenic retinal breaks during vitrectomy is aggressive creation of a posterior vitreous detachment (PVD) in macular hole surgery (see also Chapter 12). The cutter in suction-only mode should be positioned at the nasal, superior, and inferior borders of the optic nerve head and pulled straight anteriorly without lateral motion to prevent shear forces on the vitreous base to create a PVD. The author never uses pics, diamond-dusted membrane scrapers, or forceps designed to place one blade under the epiretinal membrane (ERM). Epimacular membranes (EMMs), ERM in proliferative vitreoretinopathy (PVR) cases, and internal limiting membrane (ILM) in all macular hole and EMM cases are managed using disposable end-gripping Alcon DSP ILM forceps which have 120 μm deep gripping surface so-called pinch peeling. With this method, both forceps and blades are always on the anterior surface of the ERM or ILM, never in contact with the retina. Forceps with deeper gripping surfaces, especially if reusable, are unable to sustain apposition of the gripping surface at the tip.

The ERM in diabetic traction retinal detachment cases is usually highly adherent to retina therefore peeling results in retinal breaks (see also Chapter 15). The ERMs should be managed with:

1. Conformal cutter delamination: Feeding, not sucking, rigid ERM into the port while adjusting the angle of attack to rotate the port away from the retina, thereby reducing the chances of retina entering the port; conformal emphasizes the need to modify the angle of attack to conform to changes in retinal contour (**Fig. 18-1**).

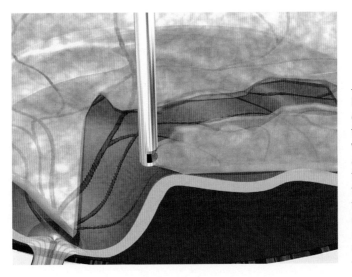

Figure 18-1 Conformal cutter delamination: Rigid ERM is fed, not sucked, into the port while adjusting the angle of attack to rotate the port away from the retina, thus reducing the chances of retina entering the port. "Conformal" emphasizes the need to modify the angle of attack to conform to changes in retinal contour.

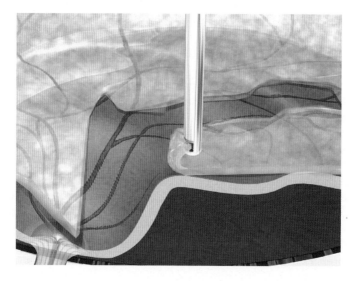

Figure 18-2 Foldback delamination: Positioning of the cutter on the anterior surface of the flexible ERM behind the leading edge allowing the ERM to fold back into the port. This technique, although less likely to create iatrogenic retinal breaks than conformal cutter delamination, is only for rather flexible ERM.

2. Foldback delamination: Placing the cutter on the anterior surface of flexible ERM behind the leading edge allowing the ERM to fold back into the port **(Fig. 18-2)**. This technique, although less likely to create iatrogenic retinal breaks than conformal cutter delamination, is only for rather flexible ERM.

3. Inside-out scissors delamination with the Alcon 25G curved DSP scissors **(Fig. 18-3)**: Curved scissors are better than vertical scissors for access segmentation because blade width is greater than blade thickness. Forcing a wide vertical scissors blade between the ERM and the retina causes retinal breaks. Rotation of the curved scissors after access segmentation produces the correct blade orientation for scissors delamination. Curved scissors are better for delamination than horizontal scissors because they conform to the curvature of the retina **(Figs. 18-3 and 18-4)**.

✦ Intraoperative Hemostasis and Machine Issues

Bleeding is often caused by excessively low IOP (see also Chapter 26); as stated above, the author always uses 45 mm Hg IOP settings except for children and the rare adult with very low perfusion pressure. The Alcon Accurus and Constellation

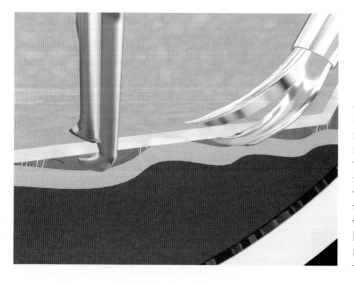

Figure 18-3 Inside-out scissors delamination: Curved scissors are better than vertical scissors for access segmentation because blade width is greater than blade thickness. Forcing a wide vertical scissors blade between the ERM and the retina causes retinal breaks.

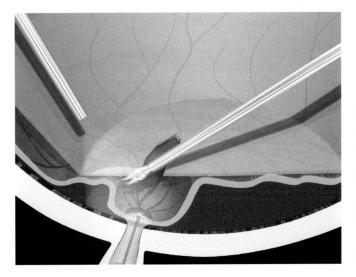

Figure 18-4 Curved scissors: Curved scissors are advantageous for delamination because they conform to the curvature of the retina. Rotation of the curved scissors after access segmentation produces the correct blade orientation for scissors delamination.

systems have a secondary infusion setting selectable by foot pedal, console graphical user interface, or remote control to raise the IOP and control bleeding or prevent bleeding when working on highly vascular tissues. Retinal surface bleeding is better controlled by endophotocoagulation than by using the bipolar diathermy because the energy and necrosis is more spatially confined thereby eliminating late atrophic retinal holes.

Air, Air–gas Mixture, or Silicone Oil in the Anterior Chamber

Visualization is impaired at times preventing drainage of subretinal fluid or retinopexy when air, air–gas mixtures, or silicone oil enter the anterior chamber in phakic or pseudophakic eyes. This problem can be reduced by taking care that the infusion cannula tip does not rotate anteriorly when the fluid–air exchange is initiated and the eye is momentarily soft. This problem as well as silicone oil in the anterior chamber is best managed by making a 20G incision at the limbus, like a phaco sideport, and injecting viscoelastic in the anterior chamber thereby expressing the air, gas, or oil out of the anterior chamber around the viscocannula. The viscoelastic is usually left in place and pharmacologic methods used to control IOP.

Venting air from an open superonasal cannula during air–silicone exchange is essential; the infusion pressure can be left at 45 mm Hg with this method. Aspiration of air with a soft-tip cannula during slow, manual syringe-based infusion of an isoexpansive air–gas mixture facilitates a normotensive exchange process.

Intraocular Lens Fogging

It is a common misconception that intraocular lens (IOL) fogging occurs solely with silicone IOLs. Silicone IOLs have much higher posterior chamber opacification (PCO) rates than acrylic IOLS and greater thermal mass, but fogging can occur with polymethylmethacrylate (PMMA) and acrylic IOLs as well. The reason why PCO is a factor in creating lens fogging is because it results in neodymium-doped yttrium aluminium garnet (YAG) laser capsulotomy being done more frequently allowing the water vapor saturated air bubble to condense on the colder IOL. If a YAG laser capsulotomy is present the anterior vitreous cortex should not be removed to prevent air bubble contact with the IOL. Viscoelastic materials cannot be placed on the IOL surface in 23/25 cases to manage the fogging. It is better to attach the retina with perfluorocarbon liquid (PFCL) under BSS, laser all retinal breaks, and then exchange the PFCL for an air–gas mixture with the soft-tip cannula in the optic cup.

Miosis and Infusion Fluidics

Miosis is best prevented by initiating infusion before making second and third sclerotomies and never turning off the infusion; first in, last out strategy. The author uses 45 mm Hg as discussed above to avoid intraoperative low IOP and secondary miosis. Iris instrument contact will result in miosis as well. The vast majority of miosis situations can be managed by using contact-based wide-angle visualization (Volk or Panoramic Viewing System from Advanced Visual Instruments (AVI)); iris hooks should be used only if wide-angle viewing is ineffective.

Cataract and Infusion Fluids

Intraoperative cataract is almost always caused by using substandard infusion fluids, additives to the infusion fluid, or excessive fluid volumes. Balanced Salt Solution (BSS) Plus is the ideal infusion fluid. There is simply no rationale for adding dextrose in diabetic cases since intraoperative serum glucose monitoring became available and the patients are maintained in a euglycemic state. Preservatives and stabilizers in epinephrine are potentially toxic to the lens and corneal endothelium. It is unnecessary to add antibiotics to the fluid. Subconjunctival antibiotics should be used in every case however. BSS Plus requires no additional buffer.

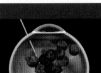

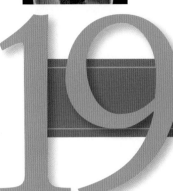

COMPLICATIONS RELATED to the TAMPONADE AGENT

19A   Anterior Displacement of the Tamponade Agent (Subconjunctivally and to the Anterior and Posterior Chambers)

SOFIA ANDROUDI, CHRYSANTHOS SYMEONIDIS, AND PERIKLIS BRAZITIKOS

◆ The Complication: Definition

Anterior displacement of the tamponade is defined as the postoperative migration of the internal tamponade (air, gas, perfluorocarbon liquid, silicone oil), either under the conjunctiva or in the anterior or posterior chambers.

◆ Risk Factors

Subconjunctival Migration

Conventional 20G pars plana vitrectomy (PPV), which involves suturing of the scleral incisions, rarely causes subconjunctival tamponade migration. This problem is more frequently encountered postoperatively with sutureless surgical techniques (Fig. 19A-1). This can be commonly observed following trocar removal and can be solved either by applying light pressure or massaging the sclerotomies or (in cases with persistent leakage) with suture placement. Less commonly, subconjunctival SO migration in the form of small bubbles may occur postoperatively (Fig. 19A-2). A recent study reported an SO leakage rate of 9.7% in a series of 23G PPVs.[1] In our experience, subconjunctival migration occurs more frequently with silicone oil (SO) of 1,000 centistokes (cs) when compared with 5,000 cs and also following heavy silicone oil (HSO) injection, due to the lower viscosity of 1,000 cs SO.

Small-bore 25G transconjunctival sclerotomies do not usually require suturing because of their small diameter.[2] The classic technique for the cannula placement includes the insertion of the trocar–microcannula directly, pointing to the center of the vitreal cavity. On extraction of the cannula, the wound usually closes by a

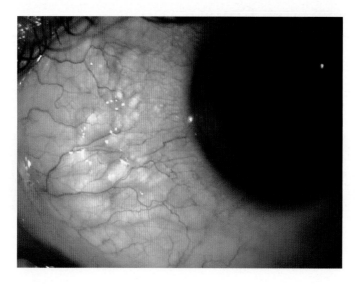

Figure 19A-1 Subconjunctival migration of silicone oil under the conjunctiva, after 25G PPV (1st postoperative day).

self-sealing mechanism, but formation of a growing conjunctival bleb, resulting from incomplete wound closure, has been described.[3] Recent studies on 25G wound closure have shown that oblique 25G sclerotomies may prevent wound leakage.[4,5] In contrast, Singh and Stewart[6] showed that oblique incisions may not be secure in the immediate postoperative period. It has been postulated that oblique sclerotomies may become lax and deformed because of pivoting motions of the instruments during peripheral vitrectomy.[7] The degree of scleral rigidity also plays a role, because the more flexible sclera in younger patients may be a risk factor for incomplete closure of the sclerotomy sites (see also Chapter 9). Trocar wound construction may be important for avoiding gas leakage in some cases. Another possible mechanism for 25G wound closure is the plug created by vitreous incarceration into the scleral wound.[2] In most retinal detachment, meticulous anterior vitreous removal is necessary. Therefore, a well-constructed oblique sclerotomy may leak because of vitreous absence.

Anterior or Posterior Chamber Migration of the Tamponade Agent

Tamponade migration in the anterior chamber (AC) is more frequently encountered with air than with liquid tamponades. Zonulysis is the pathologic change that allows migration of the tamponade agent from the vitreous cavity into the posterior

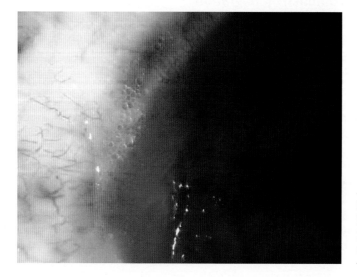

Figure 19A-2 Small perilimbal silicone oil bubbles after 25G PPV for complicated retinal detachment surgery.

chamber and then into the AC. Such changes are usually observed after trauma, previous vitrectomy with shaving of vitreous base, and possible zonular trauma or in cases of weak zonules such as pseudoexfoliation or high myopia. Another mechanism may be the intraoperative anterior misdirection of the infusion cannula toward the anterior segment that may cause zonular trauma and influx directly to the AC. Finally, sclerotomies placed anteriorly (less than 3 mm) may also cause zonular trauma and subsequent anterior tamponade migration.

In eyes filled with SO, SO can migrate into the AC during phacoemulsification if the pressure in the AC drops intraoperatively. This can occur also postoperatively subsequently to a leaking corneal wound. Maintaining a positive pressure in the AC during phacoemulsification and suturing the corneal wound at the end of the procedure at the end of the procedure are necessary to avoid SO migration to the AC.

Pathogenesis: Why Does It Occur

Over-fill of the eye with air tamponade or SO, a breach in the posterior capsule, or loose/defects in the zonules are risk factors for migration of the tamponade into the posterior and the anterior chamber.

SO has a tendency for emulsification and droplet formation.[8] Varying degrees of SO emulsification have been described with an incidence between 56% and 100% of cases, months to years from SO injection.[9,10] These droplets may potentially leak through surgical incisions or areas of compromised anatomy such as areas of zonular dehiscence.[10]

Emulsified droplet migration has been observed in phakic, pseudophakic, and aphakic eyes. Several factors may play a role in the process of emulsification: Hemorrhage, use of low viscosity silicone oil,[8] or residual fluid in the vitreous cavity[11,12] (see Chapter 19E).

Pearls on How to Prevent It

Subconjunctival Migration

◆ In the case of 20G PPVs, tight suturing of the sclerotomies is imperative.

◆ In small-gauge vitrectomy, modification of the oblique sutureless technique with selective sclerotomy suturing may be important in achieving better wound closure and avoiding possible postoperative complications. In the case of 23G to 25G PPVs, an oblique one- or two-step tight trocar incision that will self-seal at the end of the surgical procedure is advocated. In the later case, an incision of approximately 20 to 30 degrees through the sclera in addition to slight rotation of the trocars during insertion will facilitate the creation of a tight incision and reduce scleral stretching.

◆ Throughout the surgical procedure, it is advisable to minimize lateral movements of the instruments (in case of 20G PPVs) or the instruments in addition to the trocars (in case of 23–25G PPVs) as well as the abrupt movement of the instruments toward the centre of the globe. These manipulations may not result in visible complications intraoperatively but may well facilitate scleral stretching. Gentle rotation of the instruments during surgery around the axis of the microcannulae has proven to be an efficient technique for the prevention of intraoperative scleral stretching.

◆ Massaging or applying light pressure sclerotomies at the end of surgery with a cotton tip.

◆ Avoid tamponade over-fill (air, SO).

◆ Sclerotomy suturing is advisable if leakage still persists despite all of the above.

Anterior and Posterior Chamber migration

◆ Considerable emphasis must be given to correct posturing of the patient post-operatively. It is essential that a face-down head position must be maintained in order to prevent forward lens–iris movement caused by anterior pressure of the gas bubble,[13] especially in cases of floppy or atrophic iris. Otherwise, migration of gas tamponade into the AC can displace the iris diaphragm anteriorly, resulting in pupillary block. For patients recovering from general anesthesia, appropriate (face-down) posturing is not always feasible to adopt immediately postoperatively. In these cases, side posturing according to the location of retinal break may be an alternative option for the immediate postoperative recovery.

◆ The prevention of SO migration in the AC can decrease significantly the risk of corneal damage and elevated intraocular pressure (IOP).[14] An effective prophylactic measure is the creation of an inferior peripheral iridotomy located at the 6 o'clock position during SO injection in aphakic eyes. Physiologic aqueous flow from the posterior to the anterior chamber is facilitated by the considerable buoyancy of the SO combined with the inferior location of the iridotomy. In this way, in aphakic eyes, pupillary block may be prevented while SO migration in the AC may be considerably limited.[15]

◆ In pseudophakic eyes, a central capsulotomy in silicone-filled eyes may increase the risk of silicone entry into the AC.

◆ In pseudophakic eyes with AC intraocular lenses (IOLs), migration of SO is more common despite intraoperative measures such as AC filling with air, viscoelastic, or intraoperative miosis. When using viscoelastic, the viscoelastic is left in the AC at the end of the procedure with careful monitoring of the IOP in the postoperative period and treatment if necessary. In some cases, AC IOL removal may be the only strategy for effectively preventing SO migration into the AC.

◆ In pseudophakic eyes with posterior chamber IOLs, SO migration is more common in cases with posterior capsule rupture and sulcus-fixated IOLs. In these circumstances, filling of AC with air and pupillary miosis may decrease the risk of SO migration into the AC. Still, in some cases, IOL removal is required.

◆ In pseudophakic eyes, as well as in phakic eyes, SO may still migrate in the AC if zonules are weak. In addition, over-filling with SO may result in zonular damage and displacement of SO in the AC.

◆ In all cases, it is important to have a tight AC prior to the injection of SO. It is better to avoid any limbal incision when SO injection is planned. When limbal incisions must be performed, (i.e., combined surgical approaches), the latter must always be sutured prior to SO injection since migration of SO into the AC may be massive when AC collapses following accidental air, aqueous, or balanced salt solution loss through limbal incisions.

Pearls on How to Solve It

Subconjunctival Migration

◆ Subconjunctival air migration postoperatively, is rarely a problem by itself. In all cases, the air mixture is absorbed. Intense lubrication may be needed to avoid dellen formation, in cases of severe conjunctival chemosis.

◆ Generally, a small subconjunctival SO bubble is well tolerated in the majority of cases and requires no immediate management. In rare occasions, a significantly increased bubble volume that impedes eyelid closure may require bubble removal.

Anterior and Posterior Chamber migration

Silicone Oil

◆ As the presence of SO has been associated with corneal endothelial damage, band keratopathy, secondary glaucoma, and cataract progression, its removal not only decreases the risk of the above complications,[16] but may also improve visual acuity. The duration required to keep the SO tamponade varies with each case but is definitely longer for more complicated ones (e.g., involving PVR grade C); this has an impact on the occurrence of emulsification. Newer, heavy tamponade agents are characterized by increased viscosity and improved tolerance. This can be demonstrated by a longer time window for removal: From 108 days up to 4 months with Densiron 68,[17] from 88 days up to 4 months with Oxane HD,[18,19] and up to 3 months with HWS 46-3000.[20] SO removal can therefore be carried out within that time frame provided that complications such as recurrence are not imminent.

◆ SO migration to the posterior chamber can result in adhesion of SO droplets to the crystalline lens or implanted silicone IOLs **(Fig. 19A-3)**. The latter can cause significant visual disturbances. Although aspiration with a soft-tipped extrusion needle or viscoelastic agent has been used to remove small oil droplets, it is difficult to remove them from the IOL surface.[21-23] The way to remove the SO droplets from the surface of the IOL is by placing an infusion cannula to irrigate the vitreous cavity and AC with balanced salt solution. A cutter is inserted through the limbal incision at the 10 o'clock position to aspirate discrete oil bubbles. A lens hook is inserted through the sclerotomy at the 2 o'clock position and is quickly moved from side to side, parallel to the IOL surface, to scrape away the oil droplets.[24] In severe cases, the IOL must be removed and replaced.[25] Others advocate the use of F4H5, PFCL, or sponge with methycellulose to remove the SO droplets.

◆ When removing SO from the AC, the goal is to remove the oil bubble and also prevent subsequent migration. Pupillary miosis and viscoelastic injection may decrease subsequent SO migration and confine the AC SO bubble toward the limbal incision. SO bubble can then be removed with aspiration or passively with pressure on the corneal incision while injecting the viscoelastic agent.

◆ Emulsified SO or HSO that adheres to the iris surface can be removed using a soft-tip cannula and gentle aspiration or by gentle scrubbing of the iris surface with a soft-tip needle.

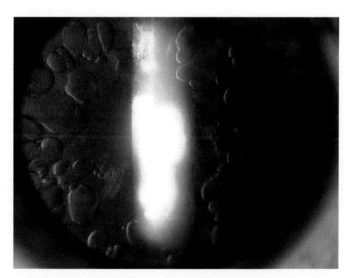

Figure 19A-3 Heavy silicone oil bubbles in the posterior chamber of a phakic patient after 25G PPV.

PFCL

◆ PFCL in AC usually migrates from the vitreous cavity due to incomplete aspiration during PFCL/air exchange. Small quantities of PFCL are usually well tolerated and inert. For larger quantities or symptomatic patients, the residual AC PFCL can be aspirated through a limbal incision with a 25G soft-tip needle.

Air Tamponades

◆ A permanent iridocorneal apposition may occur if there is no early recognition and intervention. A Nd:YAG laser iridotomy at 6 o'clock is sufficient to treat the pupillary block. An early Nd:YAG laser iridotomy is a suitable way to reduce IOP in similar cases.

◆ With regard to elevated IOP, aqueous suppressants can be used in order to achieve pressure reduction. If IOP is still very elevated, and especially if IOP level obstructs perfusion, partial gas aspiration may be advisable.

◈ Expected Outcomes: What Is the Worst-case Scenario

Subconjunctival Migration

Massive subconjunctival migration may result in hypotony. Lai and Von Fricken[26,27] reported occurrences of postoperative choroidal hemorrhage in sutureless 25G RD repair. Acar and associates[28] reported postoperative hypotony in 9% of the eyes that had undergone oblique 25G sclerotomies after RD repair. In another series, with selected sclerotomy suturing, the authors did not observe postoperative hypotony or choroidal hemorrhage.[29]

Anterior or Posterior Chamber Migration

Silicone Oil

In this case, a number of complications may occur: Postoperative patient discomfort decreased the SO endotamponade effect and potentially glaucoma requiring surgery. Complications from the anterior segment that have been linked to SO use involve elevated IOP,[30] cataract development or progression in case of existing cataractous changes,[16] and corneal pathologic changes.[31] SO has been shown to be toxic to the cornea: Endothelial cell structural damage, decreased cell density, and eventually cell damage that may lead to endothelial cell necrosis, edema, and/or band keratopathy were observed histopathologically following long-term use of SO.[32] Incidence of keratopathy following SO injection has been reported to vary between 4.5% and 63%.[33]

Incidence of IOP increase following SO injection has been reported to vary between 5.9% and 56% of eyes[13,34–36] (see also Chapter 19B). The advent of higher viscosity SOs has been associated with a lower quantity of silicone droplets in the AC as well as a lower risk of glaucoma.[37] Previous diagnosis of glaucoma,[38–40] aphakia,[38] as well as diabetes mellitus[38,39,41] have been identified as risk factors for IOP elevation secondary to SO injection.

Air Tamponades

In case of pure (100%) SF_6 use, the incidence of IOP increase has been reported to be significantly higher and a considerable percentage of patients (11%) develop central retinal artery occlusion.[42] On the other hand, IOP increase secondary to intravitreal injection of an SF_6 mixture has been reported to have an incidence between 6.1% and 67%.[42,43] According to the Silicone Study Group, an IOP higher than 30 mm Hg following 20% SF_6 use was observed in only 6.1% of the patients[43] while a comparable IOP was observed in 18% of the patients following 14% C_3F_8 use.[44] A greater risk of elevated IOP was reported in eyes with fibrinous AC exudates as usually observed in diabetic eyes.[42]

PFCL

Residual PFCL droplets may pass through inferior iridectomies and the pupil of aphakic eyes. In such cases, PFCL material deposition can be observed in the inferior angle which may lead to moderate or severe AC reaction (cells+/flare+). Regarding potential complications, corneal toxicity has been previously observed in cases of perfluorooctane, perfluoropolyether, and perfluoro-phenanthrene use.[45,46] Perfluorodecalin may also contribute to a number of pathologic changes, such as corneal edema and deep corneal vascularization in the area of contact with the endothelium. Direct endothelium contact with perfluorodecalin may result in corneal toxicity in a relatively short period of 1 to 2 months. It is assumed that perfluorodecalin presence may have a negative effect on cell density and induce morphologic changes. Pathologic changes have been reported to be reversible in case of immediate perfluorodecalin aspiration.[46]

REFERENCES

1. Siqueira RC, Gil AD, Jorge R. Retinal detachment surgery with silicone oil injection in transconjunctival sutureless 23-gauge vitrectomy. *Arq Bras Oftalmol.* 2007;70: 905–909.
2. Fujii GY, De Juan E Jr, Humayun MS, et al. Initial experience using the transconjunctival sutureless vitrectomy system for vitreoretinal surgery. *Ophthalmology.* 2002; 109:1814–1820.
3. Lakhanpal RR, Humayun MS, de Juan E Jr, et al. Outcomes of 140 consecutive cases of 25-gauge transconjunctival surgery for posterior segment disease. *Ophthalmology.* 2005;112:817–824.
4. López-Guajardo L, Pareja-Esteban J, Teus-Guezala MA. Oblique sclerotomy technique for prevention of incompetent wound closure in transconjunctival 25-gauge vitrectomy. *Am J Ophthalmol.* 2006;141:1154–1156.
5. Rizzo S, Genovesi-Ebert F, Vento A, et al. Modified incision in 25-gauge vitrectomy in the creation of a tunneled airtight sclerotomy: An ultrabiomicroscopic study. *Graefes Arch Clin Exp Ophthalmol.* 2007;245:1281–1288.
6. Singh A, Stewart JM. 25-gauge sutureless vitrectomy: variations in incision architecture. *Retina.* 2009;29:451–455.
7. Byeon SH, Chu YK, Lee SC, et al. Problems associated with the 25-gauge transconjunctival sutureless vitrectomy system during and after surgery. *Ophthalmologica.* 2006;220:259–265.
8. Nakamura K, Refojo MF, Crabtree DV. Factors contributing to the emulsification of intraocular silicone and fluorosilicone oils. *Invest Ophthalmol Vis Sci.* 1990;31: 647–656.
9. Federman JL, Schubert HD. Complications associated with the use of silicone oil in 150 eyes after retina-vitreous surgery. *Ophthalmology.* 1988;95:870–876.
10. Donahue SP, Friberg TR, Johnson BL. Intraconjunctival cavitary inclusions of silicone oil complicating retinal detachment repair. *Am J Ophthalmol.* 1992;114: 639–640.
11. Bartov E, Pennarola F, Savion N, et al. A quantitative in vitro model for silicone oil emulsification. Role of blood constituents. *Retina.* 1992;12:S23–S27.
12. Heidenkummer HP, Kampik A, Thierfelder S. Emulsification of silicone oils with specific physicochemical characteristics. *Graefes Arch Clin Exp Ohthalmol.* 1991; 229:88–94.
13. Gedde SJ. Management of glaucoma after retinal detachment surgery. *Curr Opin Ophthalmol.* 2002;13:103–109.

14. Friberg TR, Guibord NM. Corneal endothelial cell loss after multiple vitreoretinal procedures and the use of silicone oil. *Ophthalmic Surg Lasers.* 1990;30: 528–534.

15. Madreperla SA, McCuen MW 2nd. Inferior peripheral iridectomy in patients receiving silicone oil. Rates of postoperative closure and effect on oil position. *Retina.* 1995;15:87–90.

16. Hutton WL, Azen SP, Blumenkranz MS, et al. The effects of silicone oil removal. Silicone Study Report 6. *Arch Ophthalmol.* 1994;112:778–785.

17. Wong D, Van Meurs JC, Stappler T, et al. A pilot study on the use of a perfluorohexyloctane/silicone oil solution as a heavier than water internal tamponade agent. *Br J Ophthalmol.* 2005;89(6):662–665.

18. Rizzo S, Genovesi-Ebert F, Belting C, et al. A pilot study on the use of silicone oil-RMN3 as heavier-than- water endotamponade agent. *Graefes Arch Clin Exp Ophthalmol.* 2005;243(11):1153–1157.

19. Cheung BT, Lai TY, Yuen CY, et al. Results of high-density silicone oil as a tamponade agent in macular hole retinal detachment in patients with high myopia. *Br J Ophthalmol.* 2007;91(6):719–721.

20. Rizzo S, Genovesi-Ebert F, Vento A, et al. A new heavy silicone oil (HWS 46-3000) used as a prolonged internal tamponade agent in complicated vitreoretinal surgery: A pilot study. *Retina.* 2007;27:613–620.

21. Mein CE. Posterior surface condensation on silicone IOLs. *Ophthalmology.* 1995;102: 1412–1413.

22. Robertson JE Jr. The formation of moisture droplets on the posterior surface of intraocular lenses during fluid/gas exchange procedures. *Arch Ophthalmol.* 1992; 110:168.

23. Horgan SE, Cooling RJ. Irreversible silicone oil adhesion. *Ophthalmology* 1997;104: 898–900.

24. Kageyama T, Yaguchi S. Removing silicone oil droplets from the posterior surface of silicone intraocular lenses. *J Cataract Refract Surg.* 2000;26:957–959.

25. Apple DJ, Federman JL, Krolicki TJ, et al. Irreversible silicone oil adhesion to silicone intraocular lenses. A clinicopathologic analysis. *Ophthalmology.* 1996;103: 1555–1562.

26. Lai MM, Ruby AJ, Sarrafizadeh R, et al. Repair of primary rhegmatogenous retinal detachment using 25-gauge transconjunctival sutureless vitrectomy. *Retina.* 2008; 28:729–734.

27. Von Fricken MA, Kunjukunju N, Weber C, et al. 25-Gauge sutureless vitrectomy versus 20-gauge vitrectomy for the repair of primary rhegmatogenous retinal detachment. *Retina.* 2009;29:444–450.

28. Acar N, Kapran Z, Altan T, et al. Primary 25-gauge sutureless vitrectomy with oblique sclerotomies in pseudophakic retinal detachment. *Retina.* 2008;28:1068–1074.

29. Bourla DH, Bor E, Axer-Siegel R, et al. Outcomes and complications of rhegmatogenous retinal detachment repair with selective sutureless 25-gauge pars plana vitrectomy. *Am J Ophthalmol.* 2010;149:630–634.

30. Barr CC, Lai MY, Lean JS, et al. Postoperative intraocular pressure abnormalities in the Silicone Study. Silicone Study Report 4. *Ophthalmology.* 1993;100: 1629–1635.

31. Abrams GW, Azen SP, Barr CC, et al. The incidence of corneal abnormalities in the Silicone Study. Silicone Study Report 7. *Arch Ophthalmol.* 1995;13:764–769.

32. Gao RL, Neubauer L, Tang S, et al. Silicone oil in the anterior chamber. *Graefes Arch Clin Exp Ophthalmol.* 1989;227(2):106–109.

33. Falkner CI, Binder S, Kruger A. Outcome after silicone oil removal. *Br J Ophthalmol.* 2001;85:1324–1327.

34. Burk LL, Shields MB, Proia AD, et al. Intraocular pressure following intravitreal silicone oil injection. *Ophthalmic Surg.* 1988;19:565–569.

35. Riedel KG, Gabel VP, Neubauer L, et al. Intravitreal silicone oil injection: Complications and treatment of 415 consecutive patients. *Graefes Arch Clin Exp Ophthalmol.* 1990;228:19–23.

36. Henderer JD, Budenz DL, Flynn HW Jr, et al. Elevated intraocular pressure and hypotony following silicone oil retinal tamponade for complex retinal detachment: Incidence and risk factors. *Arch Ophthalmol.* 1999;117:189–195.

37. Petersen J, Ritzau-Tondrow U. Chronic glaucoma following silicone oil implantation: A comparison of 2 oils of differing viscosity. *Fortschr Ophthalmol.* 1988;85:632–634.

38. Honavar SG, Goyal M, Majji AB, et al. Glaucoma after pars plana vitrectomy and silicone oil injection for complicated retinal detachments. *Ophthalmology.* 1999;106:169–176.

39. Henderer JD, Budenz DL, Flynn HW, et al. Elevated intraocular pressure and hypotony following silicone oil retinal tamponade for complex retinal detachment: Incidence and risk factors. *Arch Ophthalmol.* 1999;117:189–195.

40. Nguyen QH, Lloyd MA, Heuer DK, et al. Incidence and management of glaucoma after intravitreal silicone oil injection for complicated retinal detachments. *Ophthalmology.* 1992;99:1520–1526.

41. Ando F. Usefulness and limit of silicone oil in management of complicated retinal detachment. *Jpn J Ophthalmol.* 1987;31:138–146.

42. Abrams GW, Swanson DE, Sabates WI. The results of sulfur hexafluoride gas in vitreous surgery. *Am J Ophthalmol.* 1982; 94:165–171.

43. The Silicone Study Group. Vitrectomy with silicone oil or sulfur hexafluoride gas in eyes with severe proliferative vitreoretinopathy: Results of a randomized clinical trial. Silicone Study Report 1. *Arch Ophthalmol.* 1992; 110:770–779.

44. Silicone Study Group. Vitrectomy with silicone oil or perfluoropropane gas in eyes with severe proliferative vitreoretinopathy: Results of a randomized clinical trial. Silicone Study Report 2. *Arch Ophthalmol.* 1992;110:780–792.

45. Moreira H, de Queiroz JM Jr, Liggett PE, et al. Corneal toxicity study of two perfluorocarbon liquids in rabbit eyes. *Cornea.* 1992;11:376–379.

46. Willbanks GA, Apel AJ, Jolly SS, et al. Perfluorodecalin corneal toxicity: Five case reports. *Cornea.* 1996;15:329–334.

19B Glaucoma Following Vitreoretinal Surgery

EOIN GUERIN AND ANTHONY J. KING

✦ The Complication

In the setting of vitreoretinal surgery this can best be described as a postoperative acute or chronic increase in intraocular pressure (IOP) that would be sufficient to cause optic neuropathy if left untreated.

One of the problems with reported glaucoma following vitreoretinal surgery is that often no distinction is made between an isolated elevation of IOP (ocular hypertension) and an elevation of IOP resulting in optic disc damage and visual field loss (glaucoma). This may reflect the difficulty in undertaking visual field assessment on many of these patients. However, it is an important distinction in determining the visual prognosis and need for treatment in this group of patients.

In addition, an elevation of IOP is defined in different ways and at different time points in different studies (as indicated in Table 19B-1 using the * markers) making direct comparisons difficult (Table 19B-1).

Table 19B-1 • Published Literature Reporting on Raised Intraocular Pressure after Vitreoretinal Surgery

Author	Early IOP Elevation	Late IOP Elevation	Type of Surgical Intervention	Risk Factors for IOP Elevation
Han et al.[51]	36%		Miscellaneous VR (vitreoretina)	Buckle, endolaser, lensectomy, fibrinous reaction
Tranos et al.[97]		4.8%[a]		
Al-Jazzaf et al.[98]		11%[b]	Oil for complex detachment	
Nguyen et al.[8]		48%	Oil for complex detachment	
Burk et al.[6]	43%	7%	Oil for complex detachment	Preoperative status, oil AC
Leaver et al.[9]		15%	Oil	Traction detachment, oil in AC, preoperative glaucoma
Honavar et al.[12]	33%	40%[c]	Oil for PVR, diabetic retinopathy, and rhegmatogenous detachment	Rubeosis, oil in AC, diabetes, aphakia
Riedel et al.[11]		6%	Oil for PVR, diabetic retinopathy, and rhegmatogenous detachment	Oil
Henderer et al.[13]	48.5%	29.5%	Oil for complex detachment	Pre-existing glaucoma, diabetes
Barr et al.[19]		5%	Oil and gas (C_3F_8) for PVR	Gas use
Chen PP[11]	38%		C_3F_8 and SF_6 all VR surgery	Expansile gas concentrations, C_3F_8, circumferential buckles
Mittra RA[12]	55%		C_3F_8 and SF_6 all VR surgery	
Abrams et al.[4]	45%		SF_6 and vitrectomy	Fibrinous AC reaction
Smith et al.[40]	4%	0%	Buckling	Buckle nil else. Shallow AC
Oshima Y[15]	0%	0%	Retinal detachment repair (gases and buckle used)	
Scott IU[16]	38%	3%	Perfluoron heavy liquid	Perfluoron used per op Buckle and various tamponades in situ post op
Hussain RN[17]		50%	Densiron 68 heavy liquid for inferior retinal detachment	
Chen[96]	52%	7.5%	Macular hole C_3F_8	

[a]Consistently elevated IOP was defined as any postoperative IOP of at least 25 mm Hg in three or more consecutive follow up visits requiring long-term use of antiglaucoma treatment.

[b]Elevation of IOP > 21 mm Hg sustained for greater than 6 weeks.

[c]IOP > 24 mm Hg and >10 mm Hg above preoperative IOP for longer than 6 weeks.

◆ Risk Factors

Surgical Risk Factors

Vitrectomy

Vitrectomy alone has been shown to increase the IOP to 30 mm Hg or greater in 40% of those operated.[1]

Use of Intraocular Tamponade Agents

◆ **Gas:** The reported incidence of IOP elevation with the use of intraocular gas ranges from 6.1% to 100% depending on the gas used and its concentration. The maximum expansion of gas is in the first 24 to 72 hours and therefore this is exclusively a complication of the early postoperative period.[2–5] A fibrinous postoperative anterior chamber exudate seems to increase the risk of a gas-related IOP elevation.[4]

◆ **Silicone Oil:** Intravitreal silicone oil is associated with both short- and long-term IOP elevation.[6–8] The reported incidence of IOP elevation after use of silicone oil ranges from 2.2% to 56%.[6,8–21] There is good evidence that postoperative IOP elevation is associated with emulsified oil droplets in the anterior chamber **(Fig. 19B-1)**.[11,17,18,22–24] Higher viscosity silicone oil is less likely to emulsify and thus carries a lower risk of glaucoma.[25,26] There is weaker evidence that preexisting glaucoma, diabetes mellitus, proliferative diabetic retinopathy, aphakia, and the duration that silicone remains in the eye increase the risk of silicone oil-related IOP rise.[8,12,13,26–31] Over-filling the eye with silicone oil may also produce secondary glaucoma.[31,32]

◆ **Heavy Liquid:** A rise in IOP has been reported with Oxane HD and Densiron. Rates for Oxane HD range from 14% to 42%[33–35] and from 19% to 40% for Densiron 6.[36,37] For both agents the complication is more common early rather than late after liquid removal.

Scleral Buckling

The risk of angle-closure glaucoma after scleral buckling is estimated to be between 1.4% and 4.4%[38–42] and is associated with pre-existing narrow angles,[39,41] use of an

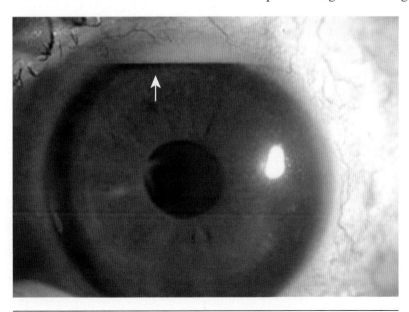

Figure 19B-1 Emulsified oil in the anterior chamber (*arrow showing oil aqueous interface*).

encircling band,[42,43] placement of band anterior to the equator[39] and high myopia,[41] older patient age,[41] and postoperative ciliochoroidal detachment.[39]

Retinal Photocoagulation

The incidence of transient early glaucoma from performing Pan retinal photocoagulation (PRP) alone is reported to be as high 22%.[44]

Preoperative Pathology

Prior Glaucoma

Retinal detachment has been reported to be 4 to 12 times more common in patients with glaucoma than in the general population.[38,45] This may be a consequence of myopia being a common risk factor for both disorders,[46] an increased risk of retinal holes in pigment dispersion syndrome,[47] or an association of retinal detachment with the use of miotics for glaucoma treatment.[48,49]

Vitreous Hemorrhage

This can induce ghost cell glaucoma and may be secondary to retinal vascular disease such as diabetes mellitus, retinal vein occlusion, and macular degeneration.[50–52]

Postoperative Complications

Failed Retinal Detachment Repair

Retinal detachment is known to induce both uveitic and rubeotic glaucoma.[53,54] The neovascularization is associated with anterior retinal detachment or residual anterior retina after retinectomy.[55–57] The role played by anterior proliferative vitreoretinopathy is less clear.[56,57]

Pathogenesis: Why Does It Occur

Several distinct mechanisms have been postulated to account for elevated IOP following vitreoretinal surgery (Table 19B-2). These mechanisms may coexist.

Table 19B-2 • Mechanisms Underlying Intraocular Pressure Elevation Following Vitreoretinal Surgery	
Open Angle	
Steroid response	
Ghost cell	
Emulsified silicone oil	
Inflammation/uveitis	
Closed Angle	
Pupil block (aphakic eyes)	Silicone oil
	Gas tamponade
Anterior displacement of lens–iris diaphragm	Gas/liquid tamponade
	Overtight scleral buckle
	Ciliary body edema
	Retinal photocoagulation
Iris neovascularization	

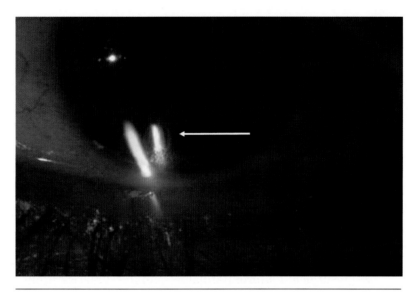

Figure 19B-2 Heavy liquid droplets in the anterior chamber (*arrow*).

Mechanisms of Secondary Open-angle Glaucoma

Ghost Cell Glaucoma: Ghost cell glaucoma is a rare complication of vitrectomy.[58] It occurs when red blood cells associated with a vitreous hemorrhage degenerate and pass into the anterior chamber. The degenerated and poorly deformable red blood cells become lodged in the trabecular meshwork.[59,60] Depending upon the volume of ghost cells in the trabecular meshwork, mild to severe elevations of IOP may occur and may last for months. Khaki-colored ghost cells may be seen within the anterior chamber as a layer of cells in the inferior angle on gonioscopy.[61] The eye will not normally appear inflamed.

Steroid Induced Glaucoma: Steroid-induced IOP rise affects up to 5% of the general population[62,63]; however, this may be higher in those undergoing vitreoretinal procedures.[64] Increased IOP typically occurs 2 to 6 weeks following initiation of treatment. The magnitude of this elevation depends upon many factors including potency, frequency, route of administration, and duration of treatment.

Silicone Oil: Intravitreal silicone oil is associated with both short- and long-term IOP elevation caused by both nonemulsified oil and emulsified oil droplets.[8,9,12–14,16,17,65–67] Mechanisms of open-angle glaucoma with silicone oil use include inflammation, migration of emulsified and nonemulsified silicone oil into the anterior chamber, infiltration of the trabecular meshwork by silicone bubbles, and idiopathic open-angle glaucoma.[6,8–18,23,24,65–71] The widely believed hypothesis that emulsified oil droplets mechanically obstruct the trabecular meshwork has not been unequivocally proven, though fibrotic changes to the trabecular meshwork that could affect outflow have been documented in eyes with a silicone oil fill.[72]

Heavy Liquid: Emulsified heavy liquid in the anterior chamber has been noted with Densiron 68 and Oxane HD, though a statistically significant association with raised IOP has not been demonstrated **(Fig. 19B-2)**.[36,73–75]

Mechanisms of Secondary Angle-closure Glaucoma

Buckle/Encirclement: Blood flow from the ciliary body into the vortex veins can be obstructed by the scleral buckle leading to congestion and swelling of the ciliary body which consequently rotates anteriorly and pushes the lens–iris diaphragm forward generating angle-closure glaucoma.[76,77]

Silicone Oil: Mechanisms of angle-closure glaucoma with silicone oil use include pupillary block, inflammation, angle closure, and rubeosis iridis.[6,8–18,23,24,65–71] Pupil block promotes the development of secondary angle-closure glaucoma[6,9–14,65,68–71] which may lead to synechial angle closure.[9,13,65] Pupil block occurs infrequently in phakic and pseudophakic eyes unless zonular defects allow silicone oil migration and the development of pupillary block.[69–71]

Intravitreal Gas Tamponade Expansion: The expansion of the commonly used gases SF6, C2F6, and C3F8 may result in forward displacement of the lens–iris diaphragm producing either a pupil block or non-pupil block form of angle-closure glaucoma early in the postoperative period.[32]

Heavy Liquid: Acute pupillary block type of elevation of the IOP has been noted with Densiron 68.[78,79]

Retinal Photocoagulation: Glaucoma following panretinal photocoagulation is produced by angle closure.[44] A postulated explanation is choroidal vascular occlusion resulting in choroidal and ciliary body swelling and anterior rotation of the ciliary body with resultant forward shifting in the lens–iris diaphragm.[80]

Surgical Failure: Retinal ischemia or anterior proliferative vitreoretinopathy associated with persistent peripheral retinal detachment probably is the source of an angiogenic/inflammatory stimulus that leads to rubeosis iridis and/or uveitis with secondary glaucoma (that may be open if purely uveitic as opposed to rubeotic).[53,54]

Iris Neovascularization: There is equivocal evidence associating iris neovascularization with the use of silicone oil but strong evidence associating such neovascularization with retinectomy (most probably secondary to a residual anterior ischemic retinal frill).[6,12,14,16,81]

Pearls on How to Prevent It

Intraocular Tamponade Agents

Gas

- Slow and reduce gas expansion by use of concentrations diluted with air (20% SF6 and 14% C3F8 should be nonexpansile depending on atmospheric pressure).

- Ensure by digital compression that the globe is not tense at the end of surgery.

- Routine use of postoperative oral acetazolamide for 48 hours.

- Head-down posture following surgery.

- Avoid reduced atmospheric pressure (e.g., flying).

Silicone Oil

- Use high viscosity (5,000 centistokes) and high purity oil as this is less likely to emulsify[25] or induce inflammation.

- Early removal may reduce risk.[21]

- Inferior peripheral iridotomy (PI) to prevent pupillary block: It should be performed in aphakic patients routinely[82] and considered in pseudophakic and phakic patients particularly if zonular defects are suspected.

- An iridotomy should be at least 150 to 200 μm in diameter but too large an iridotomy may allow forward migration of the oil **(Fig. 19B-3)**.[83–85]

- In aphakic patients remove all capsular remnants to minimize risk of PI occlusion.

- Control inflammation to reduce risk of inflammatory membrane occluding inferior PI.

- Avoid over-fill.[32]

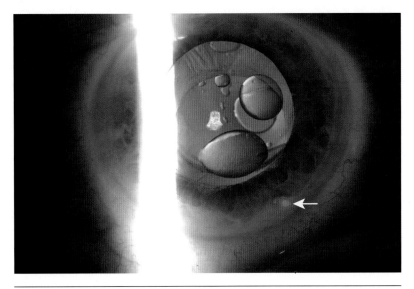

Figure 19B-3 Silicone oil in the anterior chamber. Note inferior peripheral iridotomy (*arrow*).

Heavy Liquid

◆ Superior PI when heavy liquid is used for tamponade for the same reasons as inferior PI is performed for silicone oil.[21]

◆ Avoid over-fill.[86]

Encirclement/Buckling

◆ Avoid placement of encirclements too anteriorly to prevent anterior segment ischemia that can induce neovascularization.

◆ Perform anterior chamber paracentesis preoperatively if the central retinal artery is not perfused after applying the explant. It is mandatory to ensure perfusion at the end of surgery.

Ghost Cell Glaucoma

◆ To prevent neovascularization treat retinal ischemia secondary to vascular disease with PRP.

◆ Ensure posterior segment hemostasis before the end of surgery by transiently raising IOP (fluid infusion pressure) or using endodiathermy preoperatively.

◆ Ensure complete removal of any vitreous containing hemorrhage with attention to the inferior vitreous base where blood gravitates.

Retinectomy

◆ Ensure that any significant anterior frill of retina that is not likely to achieve apposition to the retinal pigment epithelium (RPE) is removed to prevent ischemia and inflammation.

◆ Pearls on How to Solve It

Specific Measures to Address Causative Mechanisms

Ciliary Body Swelling Causing Angle-closure Glaucoma

◆ This normally settles over a few days to weeks as the swelling reduces and so no treatment is required unless IOP is significantly elevated.

◆ Cycloplegics shift the lens–iris diaphragm posteriorly and open the angle.

◆ Topical steroids will reduce swelling within the ciliary body and Peripheral anterior synechiae (PAS) formation.

◆ Avoid miotics as they may worsen inflammation by affecting blood–iris barrier and may shift the lens–iris diaphragm forward.

◆ Iridotomy is not useful[32] as pupil block is not the underlying mechanism.

◆ Laser iridoplasty may be helpful in opening up the angle.[87]

Intravitreal Gas Tamponade Expansion

◆ Head-down position to reverse pupil block.

◆ Cycloplegics shift the lens–iris diaphragm posteriorly and open the angle.

◆ Iridotomy may be useful if pupil block is the underlying mechanism.[32]

◆ Release of gas if necessary by needle aspiration through the pars plana.

Silicone Oil

◆ Despite occasional reported success with oil removal it does not seem that this procedure is sufficient to control the pressure.[12,14,23,30–32,65,88–90]

◆ Face-down positioning may reverse pupillary block in some cases.[90]

Ghost Cell Glaucoma

◆ Medical treatment with aqueous suppression is often sufficient to control IOP until all the ghost cells have dissipated.

◆ An anterior chamber washout to remove residual ghost cells or a more extensive vitrectomy where there are concerns about residual vitreous hemorrhage producing ghost cells.

Steroid-induced Glaucoma

◆ The use of a steroid such as loteprednol with a lower ocular hypertensive effect or the use of less frequent applications of lower strength may be helpful.

◆ A nonsteroidal anti-inflammatory may be substituted for the steroid in cases where anti-inflammatories cannot be withdrawn.

Medical Management

Topical ocular hypotensive medications: As the mechanism of secondary glaucoma following vitreoretinal surgery is often related to outflow obstruction, the use of medications which reduce the production of aqueous as their primary effect (β-blockers, carbonic anhydrase inhibitors) are often the most useful.

IV mannitol or acetazolamide: These may reduce IOP quickly when it has become excessively elevated or does not respond to topical treatment.

Surgical Management

Retinal Reattachment: Patients with rubeosis iridis associated with peripheral retinal detachment, may respond favorably to surgical removal or reattachment of peripheral detached retina.[54]

Cyclodestruction: Cyclodestructive approaches to controlling IOP have been described with success reported between 44% to 100%.[91–93] Trans-scleral application of diode laser (cyclodiode) is the usual method though an intraocular approach has also been described.[94] Cryodestruction has largely been abandoned due to a higher complication rate.[95]

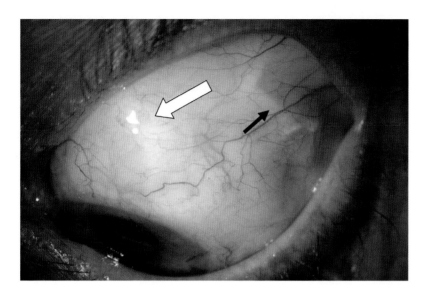

Figure 19B-4 Trabeculectomy bleb (*white arrow*) in an eye with a segmental scleral buckle (*black arrow*). Conjunctiva remained mobile following VR surgery.

Incisional Glaucoma Surgery: In patients in whom postoperative IOP elevation persists despite conservative medical management and addressing the underlying mechanism, surgical intervention is likely to be necessary. Factors that influence the choice of intervention are:

◆ **Extent of conjunctival scarring and mobility:** Many patients have considerable conjunctival scarring following vitreoretinal intervention. This limits the ability to use some incisional surgical approaches. Consequently, cyclodestructive treatment and insertion of glaucoma drainage devices (GDD) are commonly used when medical interventions have failed. When mobile conjunctiva is present successful outcomes to control IOP may be achieved with augmented trabeculectomy **(Fig. 19B-4)**.

◆ **Extent and position of any scleral buckles:** Ideally glaucoma surgery is best undertaken in positions where there are no underlying scleral buckles. This is likely to be an area of least conjunctival disturbance and scarring which allows for easier dissection either for an augmented trabeculectomy or placement of a GDD **(Fig. 19B-4)**. In addition, placement of a GDD is much easier in areas where there is no encircling band.

◆ **Areas of scleral thinning:** Scleral thinning affects the ability to fashion a scleral flap for trabeculectomy or provide adequate tissue to anchor the plates of GDD. In such instances it may be necessary to first repair the scleral thinning with a scleral patch before undertaking GDD implantation. In addition, it is best to avoid areas of scleral thinning when undertaking cyclodiode treatment as there is an increased risk of scleral perforation.

◆ **Presence of silicone oil:** Silicone oil within the eye prevents superior drainage operations and effectively excludes trabeculectomy. Inferiorly placed GDD devices have been used to overcome the floating silicone oil. Any leakage of silicone oil produces a severe conjunctival inflammatory response with scarring.

◆ **Presence of peripheral anterior synechiae:** Small areas of synechiae should be avoided and this will dictate the position of the tube, but wide bands of synechiae may make implantation in the anterior chamber difficult. Disinsertion of the iris root or iris damage may generate a hyphema, and excessive anterior placement of a tube may lead to later corneal problems. It may be possible in such cases to place the tube in the ciliary sulcus or pars plana of pseudophakic eyes. (See **Figs. 19B-5** and **19B-6** for a summary systematic approach to treatment.)

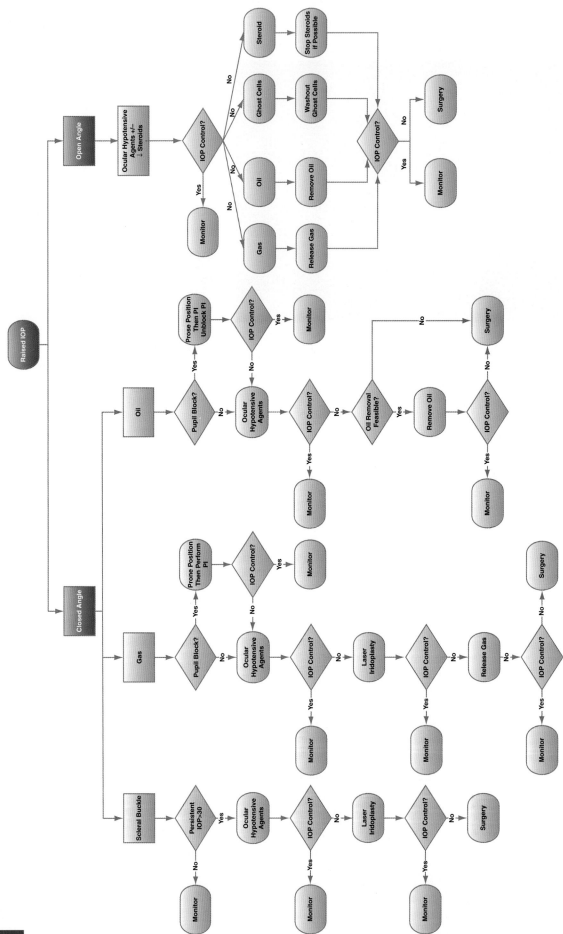

Figure 19B-5 Algorithm for management of glaucoma post vitreoretinal surgery.

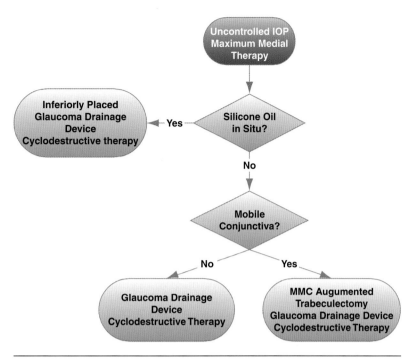

Figure 19B-6 Algorithm for surgical management of glaucoma post vitreoretinal surgery.

✦ Expected Outcomes: What Is the Worst-case Scenario

In the majority of cases, postsurgical IOP elevation is a transient self-limiting complication requiring no treatment.[96] In those requiring treatment, the use of antihypotensive medications is usually sufficient.[12,96–98] In addition to medical treatment, some cases may require adjustment to the original procedure to reverse the mechanism underlying the glaucoma.[12] A minority of patients (17–39%)[12,97,98] require glaucoma surgery. This is generally successful[65] but may result in chronic hypotony in some.[65]

REFERENCES

1. Desai UR, Alhalel AA, Schiffman RM, et al. Intraocular pressure elevation after simple pars plana vitrectomy. *Ophthalmology*. 1997;104(5):781–786.
2. Vitrectomy with silicone oil or perfluoropropane gas in eyes with severe proliferative vitreoretinopathy: Results of a randomized clinical trial. Silicone Study Report 2. *Arch Ophthalmol*. 1992;110(6):780–792.
3. Vitrectomy with silicone oil or sulfur hexafluoride gas in eyes with severe proliferative vitreoretinopathy: Results of a randomized clinical trial. Silicone Study Report 1. *Arch Ophthalmol*. 1992;110(6):770–779.
4. Abrams GW, Swanson DE, Sabates WI, et al. The results of sulfur hexafluoride gas in vitreous surgery. *Am J Ophthalmol*. 1982;94(2):165–171.
5. Chang S, Lincoff HA, Coleman DJ, et al. Perfluorocarbon gases in vitreous surgery. *Ophthalmology*. 1985;92(5):651–656.
6. Burk LL, Shields MB, Proia AD, et al. Intraocular pressure following intravitreal silicone oil injection. *Ophthalmic Surg*. 1988;19(8):565–569.
7. Lucke KH, Foerster MH, Laqua H. Long-term results of vitrectomy and silicone oil in 500 cases of complicated retinal detachments. *Am J Ophthalmol*. 1987;104(6):624–633.
8. Nguyen QH, Lloyd MA, Heuer DK, et al. Incidence and management of glaucoma after intravitreal silicone oil injection for complicated retinal detachments. *Ophthalmology*. 1992;99(10):1520–1526.

9. Leaver PK, Grey RH, Garner A. Silicone oil injection in the treatment of massive preretinal retraction. II. Late complications in 93 eyes. *Br J Ophthalmol.* 1979;63(5):361–367.

10. Federman JL, Schubert HD. Complications associated with the use of silicone oil in 150 eyes after retina-vitreous surgery. *Ophthalmology.* 1988;95(7):870–876.

11. Chen PP, Thompson JT. Risk factors for elevated intraocular pressure after the use of intraocular gases in vitreoretinal surgery. *Ophthalmic Surg Lasers.* 1997;28(1):37–42.

12. Mittra RA, Pollack JS, Dev S, et al. The use of topical aqueous suppressants in the prevention of postoperative intraocular pressure elevation after pars plana vitrectomy with long-acting gas tamponade. *Ophthalmology.* 2000;107(3):588–592.

13. Henderer JD, Budenz DL, Flynn HW Jr, et al. Elevated intraocular pressure and hypotony following silicone oil retinal tamponade for complex retinal detachment: Incidence and risk factors. *Arch Ophthalmol.* 1999;117(2):189–195.

14. Jonas JB, Knorr HL, Rank RM, et al. Intraocular pressure and silicone oil endotamponade. *J Glaucoma.* 2001;10(2):102–108.

15. Oshima Y, Yamanishi S, Sawa M, et al. Two-year follow-up study comparing primary vitrectomy with scleral buckling for macula-off rhegmatogenous retinal detachment. *Jpn J Ophthalmol.* 2000;44(5):538–549.

16. Scott IU, Murray TG, Flynn HW Jr, et al. Perfluoron Study Group. Outcomes and complications associated with giant retinal tear management using perfluoro-n-octane. *Ophthalmology.* 2002;109(10):1828–1833.

17. Hussain RN, Banerjee S. Densiron 68 as an intraocular tamponade for complex inferior retinal detachments. *Clin Ophthalmol.* 2011;5:603–607.

18. La Heij EC, Hendrikse F, Kessels AG. Results and complications of temporary silicone oil tamponade in patients with complicated retinal detachments. *Retina.* 2001;21(2):107–114.

19. Barr CC, Lai MY, Lean JS, et al. Postoperative intraocular pressure abnormalities in the Silicone Study. Silicone Study Report 4. *Ophthalmology.* 1993;100(11):1629–1635.

20. Flaxel CJ, Mitchell SM, Aylward GW. Visual outcome after silicone oil removal and recurrent retinal detachment repair. *Eye (Lond).* 2000;14(Pt 6):834–838.

21. Ichhpujani P, Jindal A, Jay Katz L. Silicone oil induced glaucoma: A review. *Graefes Arch Clin Exp Ophthalmol.* 2009;247(12):1585–1593.

22. Ni C, Wang WJ, Albert DM, et al. Intravitreous silicone injection. Histopathologic findings in a human eye after 12 years. *Arch Ophthalmol.* 1983;101(9):1399–1401.

23. Moisseiev J, Barak A, Manaim T, et al. Removal of silicone oil in the management of glaucoma in eyes with emulsified silicone. *Retina.* 1993;13(4):290–295.

24. Valone J Jr, McCarthy M. Emulsified anterior chamber silicone oil and glaucoma. *Ophthalmology.* 1994;101(12):1908–1912.

25. Petersen J, Ritzau-Tondrow U. [Chronic glaucoma following silicone oil implantation: A comparison of 2 oils of differing viscosity]. *Fortschr Ophthalmol.* 1988;85(6):632–634.

26. Gonvers M, Andenmatten R. Temporary silicone oil tamponade and intraocular pressure: An 11-year retrospective study. *Eur J Ophthalmol.* 1996;6(1):74–80.

27. Alexandridis E, Daniel H. Results of silicone oil injection into the vitreous. *Dev Ophthalmol.* 1981;2:24–27.

28. Billington BM, Leaver PK. Vitrectomy and fluid/silicone-oil exchange for giant retinal tears: Results at 18 months. *Graefes Arch Clin Exp Ophthalmol.* 1986;224(1):7–10.

29. Gonvers M. Temporary use of intraocular silicone oil in the treatment of detachment with massive periretinal proliferation. Preliminary report. *Ophthalmologica.* 1982;184(4):210–218.

30. Leaver PK, Cooling RJ, Feretis EB, et al. Vitrectomy and fluid/silicone-oil exchange for giant retinal tears: Results at six months. *Br J Ophthalmol.* 1984;68(6):432–438.

31. Ando F. Usefulness and limit of silicone in management of complicated retinal detachment. *Jpn J Ophthalmol.* 1987;31(1):138–146.

32. Gedde SJ. Management of glaucoma after retinal detachment surgery. *Curr Opin Ophthalmol.* 2002;13(2):103–109.

33. Wolf S, Schon V, Meier P, et al. Silicone oil-RMN3 mixture ("heavy silicone oil") as internal tamponade for complicated retinal detachment. *Retina.* 2003;23(3):335–342.

34. Rizzo S, Genovesi-Ebert F, Belting C, et al. A pilot study on the use of silicone oil-RMN3 as heavier-than-water endotamponade agent. *Graefes Arch Clin Exp Ophthalmol.* 2005;243(11):1153–1157.

35. Cheung BT, Lai TY, Yuen CY, et al. Results of high-density silicone oil as a tamponade agent in macular hole retinal detachment in patients with high myopia. *Br J Ophthalmol*. 2007;91(6):719–721.

36. Sandner D, Engelmann K. First experiences with high-density silicone oil (Densiron) as an intraocular tamponade in complex retinal detachment. *Graefes Arch Clin Exp Ophthalmol*. 2006;244(5):609–619.

37. Wong D, Van Meurs JC, Stappler T, et al. A pilot study on the use of a perfluorohexyloctane/silicone oil solution as a heavier than water internal tamponade agent. *Br J Ophthalmol*. 2005;89(6):662–665.

38. Becker B. Discussion of Smith JL: Retinal detachment and glaucoma. *Trans Am Acad Ophthalmol Otolaryngol*. 1963;67:726–732.

39. Sebestyen J, Schepens C, Rosenthal M. Retinal detachments and glaucoma I, Tonometric and gonioscopic study of 160 cases. *Arch Ophthalmol*. 1962;67:736–745.

40. Smith T. Acute glaucoma developing after scleral buckling procedures. *Am J Ophthalmol*. 1967;63:1807–1808.

41. Kreiger AE, Hodgkinson BJ, Frederick AR Jr, et al. The results of retinal detachment surgery. Analysis of 268 operations with a broad scleral buckle. *Arch Ophthalmol*. 1971;86(4):385–394.

42. Perez RN, Phelps CD, Burton TC. Angel-closure glaucoma following scleral buckling operations. *Trans Sect Ophthalmol Am Acad Ophthalmol Otolaryngol*. 1976;81(2):247–252.

43. Hartley RE, Marsh RJ. Anterior chamber depth changes after retinal detachment. *Br J Ophthalmol*. 1973;57(8):546–550.

44. Huamonte FU, Peyman GA, Goldberg MF, et al. Immediate fundus complications after retinal scatter photocoagulation. I. Clinical picture and pathogenesis. *Ophthalmic Surg*. 1976;7(1):88–99.

45. Phelps CD, Burton TC. Glaucoma and retinal detachment. *Arch Ophthalmol*. 1977;95(3):418–422.

46. Podos SM, Becker B, Morton WR. High myopia and primary open-angle glaucoma. *Am J Ophthalmol*. 1966;62(6):1038–1043.

47. Scheie HG, Cameron JD. Pigment dispersion syndrome: A clinical study. *Br J Ophthalmol*. 1981;65(4):264–269.

48. Beasley H, Fraunfelder FT. Retinal detachments and topical ocular miotics. *Ophthalmology*. 1979;86(1):95–98.

49. Pape LG, Forbes M. Retinal detachment and miotic therapy. *Am J Ophthalmol*. 1978;85(4):558–566.

50. Singh H, Grand MG. Treatment of blood-induced glaucoma by trans pars plana vitrectomy. *Retina*. 1981;1(3):255–257.

51. Han DP, Murphy ML, Mieler WF, et al. Outpatient fluid-air exchange for severe postvitrectomy diabetic vitreous hemorrhage. Long-term results and complications. *Retina*. 1991;11(3):309–314.

52. Rodriguez FJ, Foos RY, Lewis H. Age-related macular degeneration and ghost cell glaucoma. *Arch Ophthalmol*. 1991;109(9):1304–1305.

53. Schwartz A. Chronic open-angle glaucoma secondary to rhegmatogenous retinal detachment. *Trans Am Ophthalmol Soc*. 1972;70:178–189.

54. Barile GR, Chang S, Horowitz JD, et al. Neovascular complications associated with rubeosis iridis and peripheral retinal detachment after retinal detachment surgery. *Am J Ophthalmol*. 1998;126(3):379–389.

55. Comaratta MR, Chang S, Sparrow J. Iris neovascularization in proliferative vitreoretinopathy. *Ophthalmology*. 1992;99(6):898–905.

56. Bourke RD, Cooling RJ. Vascular consequences of retinectomy. *Arch Ophthalmol*. 1996;114(2):155–160.

57. van Meurs JC, Bolt BJ, Mertens DA, et al. Rubeosis of the iris in proliferative vitreoretinopathy. *Retina*. 1996;16(4):292–295.

58. Campbell DG, Simmons RJ, Tolentino FI, et al. Glaucoma occurring after closed vitrectomy. *Am J Ophthalmol*. 1977;83(1):63–69.

59. Campbell DG, Simmons RJ, Grant WM. Ghost cells as a cause of glaucoma. *Am J Ophthalmol*. 1976;81(4):441–450. PubMed PMID: 1266922.

60. Campbell DG, Simmons RJ, Grant WM. Ghost cells as a cause of glaucoma. *Am J Ophthalmol.* 1976;81(4):441–450.

61. Campbell D, Schertzer R. Ghost cell glaucoma. In: Ritch R, Shields M, Krupin T, eds. *The Glaucomas.* 2nd ed. St Louis, MO: Mosby; 1996:1277–1285.

62. Armaly MF. Effect of corticosteroids on intraocular pressure and fluid dynamics. I. The effect of dexamethasone in the normal eye. *Arch Ophthalmol.* 1963;70:482–491.

63. Becker B. Intraocular pressure response to topical corticosteroids. *Invest Ophthalmol.* 1965;4:198–205.

64. Shammas HF, Halasa AH, Faris BM. Intraocular pressure, cup-disc ratio, and steroid responsiveness in retinal detachment. *Arch Ophthalmol.* 1976;94(7):1108–1109.

65. Budenz DL, Taba KE, Feuer WJ, et al. Surgical management of secondary glaucoma after pars plana vitrectomy and silicone oil injection for complex retinal detachment. *Ophthalmology.* 2001;108(9):1628–1632.

66. Chan C, Okun E. The question of ocular tolerance to intravitreal liquid silicone. A long-term analysis. *Ophthalmology.* 1986;93(5):651–660.

67. Yeo JH, Glaser BM, Michels RG. Silicone oil in the treatment of complicated retinal detachments. *Ophthalmology.* 1987;94(9):1109–1113.

68. McCuen BW 2nd, de Juan E Jr, Landers MB 3rd, et al. Silicone oil in vitreoretinal surgery. Part 2: Results and complications. *Retina.* 1985;5(4):198–205.

69. Zborowski-Gutman L, Treister G, Naveh N, et al. Acute glaucoma following vitrectomy and silicone oil injection. *Br J Ophthalmol.* 1987;71(12):903–906.

70. Ardjomand N, El-Shabrawi Y. Pupillary block after silicone oil implantation in a phakic eye. *Eye (Lond).* 2001;15(Pt 3):331.

71. Jackson TL, Thiagarajan M, Murthy R, et al. Pupil block glaucoma in phakic and pseudophakic patients after vitrectomy with silicone oil injection. *Am J Ophthalmol.* 2001;132(3):414–416.

72. Cvenkel B, Zupan M, Hvala A. Transmission electron microscopic analysis of trabecular meshwork in secondary glaucoma after intravitreal silicone oil injection. *Int Ophthalmol.* 1996;20(1–3):43–47.

73. Wong D, Kumar I, Quah SA, et al. Comparison of postoperative intraocular pressure in patients with Densiron-68 vs conventional silicone oil: A case-control study. *Eye (Lond).* 2009;23(1):190–194.

74. Stappler T, Heimann H, Wong D, et al. Heavy tamponade 2 Densiron 68 in routine clinical practice: Anatomical and functional outcomes of a consecutive case series. *Eye (Lond).* 2008;22(10):1360–1365.

75. Theelen T, Tilanus MA, Klevering BJ. Intraocular inflammation following endotamponade with high-density silicone oil. *Graefes Arch Clin Exp Ophthalmol.* 2004;242(7):617–620.

76. Hayreh SS, Baines JA. Occlusion of the vortex veins. An experimental study. *Br J Ophthalmol.* 1973;57(4):217–238.

77. Diddie KR, Ernest JT. Uveal blood flow after 360 degrees constriction in the rabbit. *Arch Ophthalmol.* 1980;98(4):729–730.

78. Pavlidis M, Scharioth G, de Ortueta D, et al. Iridolenticular block in heavy silicone oil tamponade. *Retina.* 2010;30(3):516–520.

79. Li W, Zheng J, Zheng Q, et al. Clinical complications of Densiron 68 intraocular tamponade for complicated retinal detachment. *Eye (Lond).* 2010;24(1):21–28.

80. Mensher JH. Anterior chamber depth alteration after retinal photocoagulation. *Arch Ophthalmol.* 1977;95(1):113–116.

81. Bourke RD, Cooling RJ. Vascular consequences of retinectomy. *Arch Ophthalmol.* 1996;114(2):155–160.

82. Grey RH, Leaver PK. Results of silicone oil injection in massive preretinal retraction. *Trans Ophthalmol Soc U K.* 1977;97(2):238–241.

83. Bartov E, Huna R, Ashkenazi I, et al. Identification, prevention, and treatment of silicone oil pupillary block after an inferior iridectomy. *Am J Ophthalmol.* 1991;111(4): 501–504.

84. Fleck BW. How large must an iridotomy be? *Br J Ophthalmol.* 1990;74(10): 583–588.

85. Reddy MA, Aylward GW. The efficacy of neodymium: YAG laser iridotomy in the treatment of closed peripheral iridotomies in silicone-oil-filled aphakic eyes. *Eye (Lond)*. 1995;9(Pt 6):757–759.

86. Tognetto D, Minutola D, Sanguinetti G, et al. Anatomical and functional outcomes after heavy silicone oil tamponade in vitreoretinal surgery for complicated retinal detachment: A pilot study. *Ophthalmology*. 2005;112(9):1574.

87. Burton TC, Folk JC. Laser iris retraction for angle-closure glaucoma after retinal detachment surgery. *Ophthalmology*. 1988;95(6):742–748.

88. Ober RR, Blanks JC, Ogden TE, et al. Experimental retinal tolerance to liquid silicone. *Retina*. 1983;3(2):77–85.

89. Cairns JD, Anand N. Combined vitrectomy, intraocular microsurgery and liquid silicone in the treatment of proliferative vitreoretinopathy. *Aust J Ophthalmol*. 1984; 12(2):133–138.

90. Leaver PK, Grey RH, Garner A. Complications following silicone-oil injection. *Mod Probl Ophthalmol*. 1979;20:290–294.

91. Han SK, Park KH, Kim DM, et al. Effect of diode laser trans-scleral cyclophotocoagulation in the management of glaucoma after intravitreal silicone oil injection for complicated retinal detachments. *Br J Ophthalmol*. 1999;83(6):713–717.

92. Ghazi-Nouri SM, Vakalis AN, Bloom PA, et al. Long-term results of the management of silicone oil-induced raised intraocular pressure by diode laser cycloablation. *Eye (Lond)*. 2005;19(7):765–769.

93. Sivagnanavel V, Ortiz-Hurtado A, Williamson TH. Diode laser trans-scleral cyclophotocoagulation in the management of glaucoma in patients with long-term intravitreal silicone oil. *Eye (Lond)*. 2005;19(3):253–257.

94. Murthy GJ, Murthy PR, Murthy KR, et al. A study of the efficacy of endoscopic cyclophotocoagulation for the treatment of refractory glaucomas. *Indian J Ophthalmol*. 2009;57(2):127–132.

95. Goldenberg-Cohen N, Bahar I, Ostashinski M, et al. Cyclocryotherapy versus transscleral diode laser cyclophotocoagulation for uncontrolled intraocular pressure. *Ophthalmic Surg Lasers Imaging*. 2005;36(4):272–279.

96. Chen CJ. Glaucoma after macular hole surgery. *Ophthalmology*. 1998;105(1):94–99; discussion 99–100.

97. Tranos P, Asaria R, Aylward W, et al. Long term outcome of secondary glaucoma following vitreoretinal surgery. *Br J Ophthalmol*. 2004;88(3):341–343.

98. Al-Jazzaf AM, Netland PA, Charles S. Incidence and management of elevated intraocular pressure after silicone oil injection. *J Glaucoma*. 2005;14(1):40–46.

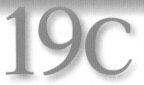

Subfoveal Displacement of the Tamponade Agent

MARTA S. FIGUEROA AND INÉS CONTRERAS

SUBRETINAL DISPLACEMENT OF PERFLUOROCARBON LIQUIDS

 ## The Complication: Definition

Perfluorocarbon liquids (PFCL), due to their physical properties, are employed during retinal detachment surgery to flatten the detached retina and displace the subretinal fluid anteriorly. They also stabilize the retina during the surgical maneuvers. They must be removed completely during fluid–air exchange. However, occasionally, PFCLs slide under the detached retina and are trapped subretinally after retinal re-attachment.

Retained intraocular PFCL has been shown to elicit a prominent macrophage reaction. This response may lead to a secondary cellular reaction that, in severe cases, results in subretinal, epiretinal, or retrocorneal membrane formation.[1] PFCL has toxic effects when it remains in contact with the retina for more than 48 hours.[2–4] In addition to interrupting the physical contact with the retinal pigment epithelium (RPE) that the retinal photoreceptors require for metabolic nourishment and trophic factor support, subretinal PFCL interferes with the physiologic electrolytic balance of the retina.

Several authors have reported poor visual outcomes after delayed removal of subfoveal PFCL, probably due to the permanent damage it inflicts on photoreceptors and the RPE.[5,6] Long-standing subretinal PFCL has been reported to lead to retinal hole formation.[7]

When compared with other available perfluorocarbons, perfluoro-*n*-octane (PFO) has the most visible interface, which aids complete intraoperative removal. PFO also has the lowest viscosity of the PFCL, offering less resistance to injection and aspiration through microsurgical instruments, and it has the highest vapor pressure, allowing for more complete evaporation of residual PFO from the retinal surface after fluid–air exchange. Despite these characteristics (which have led to PFO being the most commonly used PFCL by retinal surgeons), inadvertent postoperative retention of PFO occurs in approximately 1% to 7.5% of eyes.[8,9]

In a case series, Tewari et al.[10] presented four cases in which retained subretinal PFCL was associated with changes in retinal sensitivity as determined with scanning laser ophthalmoscope microperimetry. In one case, movement of the droplet during the postoperative period was associated with a relative scotoma in the area where the droplet was originally located and an absolute scotoma at the new site. This suggests that at least partial recovery of function is possible if the PFCL is removed. However, there was significant RPE atrophy throughout the area vacated by the migrating droplet. Hence, subretinal PFCL beneath the fovea or at risk for migration beneath the fovea may be associated with a poor visual outcome, and surgical removal of PFCL should be considered in such cases.

Characteristics on OCT

Optical coherence tomography can provide the diagnosis of retained PFCL and facilitate the differential diagnosis with persistence of subretinal fluid. It is essential to distinguish retained subretinal PFCL from residual subretinal fluid since the implications of each situation are completely different.

PFCL remnants show the following tomographic characteristics:

A. Retinal contour in the shape of the Greek letter Ω.
   We have observed that the retina adapts itself to the shape of the PFCL droplet, which has more surface tension than subretinal fluid. Thus, the angle between the RPE and the neurosensory retina at the base of the PFCL droplet is always acute (Fig. 19C-1A). On the other hand, persistent subretinal fluid leads to a retinal contour resembling a hat, with an obtuse angle between the RPE and the neurosensory retina at its base (Fig. 19C-1B).

B. Undefined retinal layers.[5–7,11–13]
   The retinal layers above the subretinal PFCL droplets cannot be identified as if the whole retina were being squeezed by the force generated by PFCL (Fig. 19C-2A). If there is persistent subretinal fluid, the retinal layers are clearly visible above the fluid (Fig. 19C-2B). When the PFCL droplet is removed, the retina regains a recognizable structure (Fig. 19C-3).

C. Elevation of the RPE hyper-reflective band.
   The RPE hyper-reflective band is elevated at the level of the PFCL/RPE interface when compared to the course of the RPE adjacent to the droplet (Figs. 19C-1A,

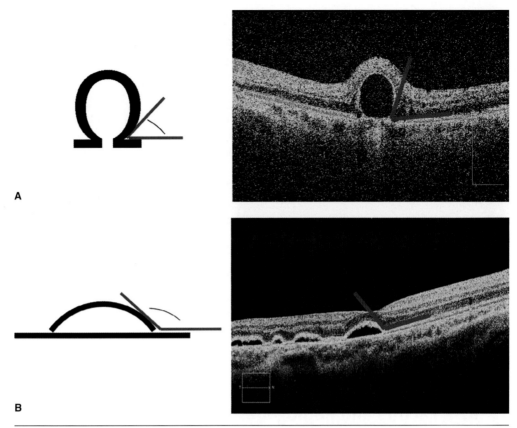

Figure 19C-1 **A:** Retained subretinal PFO droplet: The retina adapts to the shape of the PFO resembling a Greek letter Ω. Thus, the angle formed between the RPE and the neurosensory retina at the base of the PFO is acute. **B:** Persistent subretinal fluid leads to a retinal contour resembling a hat, with an obtuse angle between the RPE and the neurosensory retina at its base.

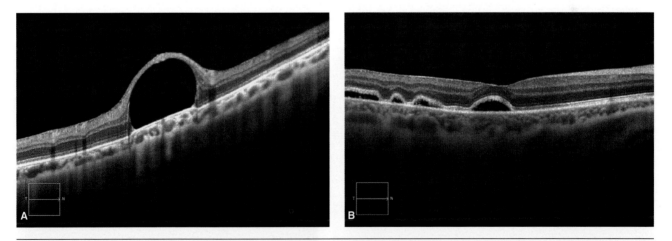

Figure 19C-2 **A:** Retained subretinal PFO. The retinal layers cannot be identified above the PFO drop, as if the whole retina were being squeezed by the PFO. **B:** Persistent subretinal fluid: The retinal layers above the fluid are easily identified.

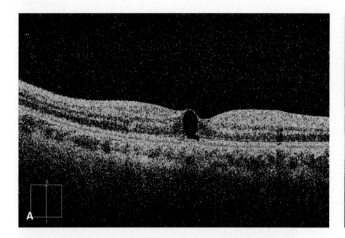
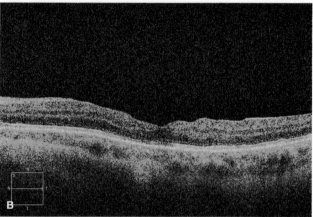

Figure 19C-3 **A:** The retinal layers cannot be identified above the subretinal perfluoro-*n*-octane droplet. **B:** When the droplet is removed, the retina regains a recognizable structure.

19C-2A, 19C-3A, 19C-4A, and 19C-5A). The band is not elevated in the presence of persistent subretinal fluid **(Fig. 19C-4B)**.

D. Hyper-reflective shadow at the choroid in high-definition OCT.

In some of our cases the remnants of subretinal PFCL produce a hyper-reflective shadow obscuring the choroid **(Fig. 19C-4 and 19C-5)**.

Risk Factors and Pathogenesis

During membrane peeling under PFCL, the traction exerted on the retina creates a suctional force that may draw the PFCL into the subretinal space. PFCL may also gain access to the subretinal space through the retinal break during fluid–air exchange. This can be avoid by careful aspiration of the fluid at the breakwhile the PFCL leve descends. However, in most cases, PFCL probably reaches the subretinal space during the initial postoperative period. PFCL droplets retained preretinally may migrate under the retina during changes in the patient's head position before a stable retina–RPE adhesion forms at the edge of the retinal breaks.[11] Unrelieved traction at the edge of the breaks may facilitate this migration.

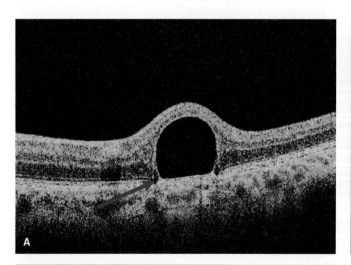
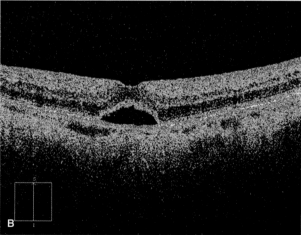

Figure 19C-4 **A:** Retained subretinal PFO. Elevation of the RPE hyper-reflective band at the level of the PFCL/RPE interface when compared to the course of the RPE adjacent to the droplet (*arrow*). **B:** The band is not elevated in the presence of persistent subretinal fluid.

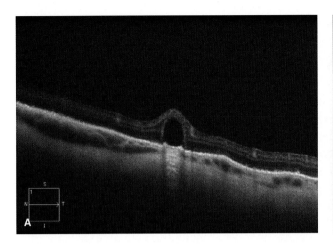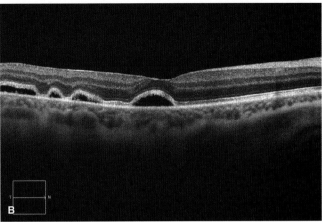

Figure 19C-5 Retained PFO produces a hyper-reflective shadow at the choroid **(A)** that is absent if there is persistent subretinal fluid **(B)**.

In an extensive retrospective study, García-Valenzuela et al.[8] found retained subretinal PFCLs in 8 of 72 eyes (11.1%). All cases of subretinal PFCL had a peripheral retinotomy of 120 degrees or larger. Subretinal PFCL was found in 40% of eyes with a 360-degree retinotomy. Another surgical procedure that significantly correlated with subretinal PFCL was lack of a saline rinse after fluid–air exchange. Only one of the eyes that were rinsed had subretinal PFCL, although many had large retinotomies. Among 10 eyes with a 360-degree peripheral retinotomy, 7 were not rinsed after removal of PFCL; 6 of these 7 eyes retained subretinal PFCL postoperatively. All eyes that had retained subretinal PFCL were filled with silicone oil. However, the authors did not believe that the use of silicone oil was an independent risk factor, since eyes that had large retinotomies were preferentially tamponaded with silicone oil.[8] Other reports also suggest an increased risk of subretinal displacement of the tamponade agent after large retinotomies combined with silicone oil.[5,6,11]

PFCL could be also injected accidentally by the surgeon into the subretinal space at the time of fluid–air exchange if PFCL and subretinal fluid are drained with the same flute needle. After removing PFCL, if the surgeon goes back to the tear/hole to remove further subretinal fluid, PFCL remnants inside the flute can be flushed accidentally into the subretinal space.

In our experience, in the treatment of primary retinal detachment with 23G vitrectomy without buckling, retained subretinal PFCL was found in 5% of eyes (6/119). This represents an unexpectedly high rate, since only 5 out of 119 eyes had giant tears (and in fact none of these had retained PFCL) and no retinectomies were performed. Several factors may contribute to this increased rate. Fluid–air exchange with 23G is slower than with 20G, increasing the possibility of PFCL slipping under the retina if the surgeon is not especially careful. Also, the scleral cannulas may hinder the release of evaporated PFCL through the sclerotomies during fluid–air exchange.

Pearls on How to Prevent It

◆ Complete release of retinal traction at the edge of the retinal breaks. Avoid injecting PFCL to a level close to that of the edge of retinal tears or retinectomy in which traction is still present. All traction should be relieved before raising the level of PFCL higher.

◆ Avoid emulsification of PFCL, which occurs when the infusion fluid impacts on the surface of PFCL. This happens more often during indentation maneuvers for peripheral laser applications and when checking the sclerotomies. In order to prevent emulsification, indentation should be performed gently and with low infusion pressures.

◆ Any emulsified droplets of PFCL should be thoroughly removed before fluid–air exchange.

◆ Careful aspiration of PFCL should be performed at the retinotomy edge or at the retinal breaks during fluid–air exchange as the liquid level descends below this point. This maneuver is slower with small-gauge vitrectomy.

◆ The surface of the retina should be rinsed with clean irrigating solution after fluid–air exchange in order to eliminate any residual PFCL. A silicone-tipped cannula connected to a syringe can be used for manual injection of a few droplets of irrigating solution on the retinal surface, avoiding the tears, holes, or retinotomies. This fluid can be aspirated manually with the same syringe and cannula, passively with a flute needle or mechanically through an extrusion line.

◆ After extraction of the rinsing solution with a soft-tipped cannula, the cannula should be placed in the centre of the vitreous cavity and used to aspirate some air, allowing evaporated PFO to exit the eye.

◆ Early postoperative face-down or prone positioning, so that any PCFL droplets that may have migrated beneath the retina will accumulate away from the sub-macular space.[11]

⬥ Pearls on How to Solve It

◆ Direct subretinal PFCL suction through a cannula inserted into the subretinal space with a pars plana vitrectomy approach has been reported to improve visual function.[12,14] However, most authors have reported poor visual results in most cases. It is unclear whether this was due to delayed extraction of the PFCL or to damage inflicted on the retina or the RPE during the procedure.[5,6,13] In our experience, the 41G/23G cannulas employed for macular translocation allow for proper removal of the droplets with minimal RPE alteration. The 41G retinotomy is performed over the PFCL or right next to it, depending on the location and the size of the subretinal droplet. The most complicated step is the penetration of the retina detached by the PFCL droplets. This requires a controlled pressure to avoid damaging the RPE and the underlying choroid. Although passive or active aspiration can be used in this maneuver, we prefer active aspiration by a trained assistant because passive aspiration with a Charles flute increases the risk of accidental re-injection of PFCL into the subretinal space.

◆ An alternative technique is to create a retinal detachment at the posterior pole and the middle inferior periphery by slowly injecting saline solution through a retinal puncture near the superotemporal arcade using a 41G flexible cannula connected to the silicone injection line of the vitrectomy machine at an injection pressure enough to generate a constant flow of fluid. Fluid–air exchange is then performed, and the patient must keep an upright head positioning during the immediate postoperative period to force the subretinal PFCL toward the inferior peripheral area.[11] Visual improvement has been reported after this technique, with postoperative visual acuities as high as 20/32.[11] However, the subretinal injection of fluid may lead to the production of a macular hole in eyes that have sustained damage to the retina either by the retained PFCL or the original surgical procedure.

⬥ Expected Outcomes

Although one case report described no deterioration in visual acuity after 10 years of retained PFCL,[15] subfoveal PFCL should be removed promptly since in most case reports, delayed extraction of the PFCL leads to poor visual outcomes.[5,6,13] In order to remove the PFCL, pars plana vitrectomy must be performed. Visual improvement may be modest if the retained droplet has already produced RPE damage.

SUBRETINAL DISPLACEMENT OF SILICONE OIL AND HEAVY SILICONE OILS

The Complication: Definition

Silicone oil and heavy silicone oil are used as endotamponades following intraoperative retinal reattachment in complicated retinal detachment cases with proliferative vitreoretinopathy (PVR). The new generation of heavy silicone oils (Oxane HD, Densiron 68, and HWS 46-3000) seems to be comparable to conventional silicone oil tamponades, while providing better support for the inferior retina. They can be instilled in the vitreous cavity either with the vitreous cavity filled with PFCL (PFCL–silicone exchange) or with air (after PFCL–air exchange). Subretinal displacement of these endotamponades can occur either intraoperatively or postoperatively.

Risk Factors

- Persistence of retinal traction at the edges of a tear or a retinectomy in RD cases with severe PVR during endotamponade instillation.

- Postoperative re-detachment due to new postoperative breaks.

- Postoperative re-detachment due to the reopening of old breaks.

- Postoperative re-detachment due to elevated edges of the retinectomy.

Pathogenesis: Why Does It Occur

The endotamponade can gain access to the subretinal space through breaks and retinectomies with elevated edges due to the persistence or development of retinal traction. This occurs most commonly in RD or re-detachment cases complicated by PVR.

Pearls on How to Prevent It

- It is important to confirm intraoperatively the elimination of all retinal traction under PFCL (with epiretinal membrane removal and retinectomies as necessary) prior to PCFL/endotamponade exchange or PFCL/air/endotamponade exchange. A fluid–air exchange is very useful to test whether tears/retinectomies are free of traction and the retina around them is flattened prior to endotamponade insertion.

Pearls on How to Solve It

- The presence of silicone oil or heavy silicone oil under the retina in the postoperative period means that the retinal breaks have not been correctly sealed and that the retina will eventually suffer a new detachment. There is always concern about the ease and safety of the removal of any endotamponade agent. Silicone removal can be performed via an anterior approach (through a posterior capsulotomy at the time of phacoemulsification) or via a posterior approach (through the pars plana). Removal of heavy silicone oils should always be performed via a posterior approach. Endoillumination is required for complete removal of the agent.

- Some reports have provided tips to facilitate removal of heavier-than-water endotamponades: The use of prewarmed balanced salt solution as the infusion in order to reduce viscosity and allow for easier aspiration; aspiration of heavy silicone oil through a 20G intravenous plastic cannula cut obliquely to maximize the surface area for aspiration;[16] or aspiration through a 20G cannula, shortened to 7.5 mm, but with no other modifications of the cannula tip.[17]

Expected Outcomes

The presence of subretinal silicone oil/oxane/Densiron under the fovea can lead to retinal degeneration and poor visual outcomes. The surgical removal of subretinal silicone oil or heavy silicone oil remnnats, elimination of retinal traction, and retinal re-attachment may be followed only in certain cases by visual acuity improvement, since both the original condition that led to the use of these tamponade agents and the damage they produce to the retina usually produce permanent visual loss. Case reports are scarce; in one case of retinal detachment associated with an optic disc pit, removal of subretinal silicone oil improved visual acuity only to 20/100.[18] However, in another case series, removal of subretinal silicone oil led to an improvement of visual acuity in all five eyes.[19] Thus we believe that removal of these substances should be attempted unless there is clear evidence of irreversible retinal damage.

REFERENCES

1. Elsing SH, Fekrat S, Green WR, et al. Clinicopathologic findings in eyes with retained perfluoro-n-octane liquid. *Ophthalmology*. 2001;108:45–48.
2. Chang S, Sparrow JR, Iwamoto T, et al. Experimental studies of tolerance to intravitreal perfluoro-n-octane liquid. *Retina*. 1991;11:367–374.
3. Eckardt C, Nicolai U, Winter M, et al. Experimental intraocular tolerance to liquid perfluorooctane and perfluoropolyether. *Retina*. 1991;11:375–384.
4. Winter M, Eberhardt W, Scholz C, et al. Failure of potassium siphoning by Muller cells: A new hypothesis of perfluorocarbon liquid-induced retinopathy. *Invest Ophthalmol Vis Sci*. 2000;41:256–261.
5. Joondeph BC, Nguyen H. Ocular coherence tomography findings with retained submacular perfluoron. *Clin Experiment Ophthalmol*. 2006;34:85–66.
6. Lesnoni G, Rossi T, Gelso A. Subfoveal liquid perfluorocarbon. *Retina*. 2004;24:172–176.
7. Cohen SY, Dubois L, Elmaleh C. Retinal hole as a complication of long-standing subretinal perfluorocarbon liquid. *Retina*. 2006;26:843–844.
8. Garcia-Valenzuela E, Ito Y, Abrams GW. Risk factors for retention of subretinal perfluorocarbon liquid in vitreoretinal surgery. *Retina*. 2004;24:746–752.
9. Scott IU, Murray TG, Flynn HW Jr, et al. Outcomes and complications associated with perfluoro-n-octane and perfluoroperhydrophenanthrene in complex retinal detachment repair. *Ophthalmology*. 2000;107:860–865.
10. Tewari A, Eliott D, Singh CN, et al. Changes in retinal sensitivity from retained subretinal perfluorocarbon liquid. *Retina*. 2009;29:248–250.
11. Le Tien V, Pierre-Kahn V, Azan F, et al. Displacement of retained subfoveal perfluorocarbon liquid after vitreoretinal surgery. *Arch Ophthalmol*. 2008;126:98–101.
12. Lai JC, Postel EA, McCuen BW. Recovery of visual function after removal of chronic subfoveal perfluorocarbon liquid. *Retina*. 2003;23:868–870.
13. Soheilian M, Nourinia R, Shoeibi N, et al. Three-Dimensional OCT Features of Perfluorocarbon Liquid Trapped Under the Fovea. *Ophthalmic Surg Lasers Imaging*. 2010;1–4.
14. Roth DB, Sears JE, Lewis H. Removal of retained subfoveal perfluoro-n-octane liquid. *Am J Ophthalmol*. 2004;138:287–289.
15. Nowilaty SR. Ten-year follow-up of retained subfoveal perfluoro-N-octane liquid. *Retinal Cases & Brief Reports*. 2007;1:41–43..
16. Ang GS, Murphy AL, Ng WS, et al. Oxane HD and retinal detachment surgery in routine clinical practice. *Ophthalmologica*. 2010;224:347–353.

17. Stappler T, Williams R, Gibran SK, et al. A guide to the removal of heavy silicone oil. *Br J Ophthalmol.* 2008;92:844–847.

18. Dithmar S, Schuett F, Voelcker HE, et al. Delayed sequential occurrence of per-fluorodecalin and silicone oil in the subretinal space following retinal detachment surgery in the presence of an optic disc pit. *Arch Ophthalmol.* 2004;122(3):409–411.

19. Chitolina J, Bacin F. Traitement du passage de l'huile de silicone sous la rétine. *J Fr Ophtalmol.* 2006;29(4):409–412.

19D   Silicone Oil Associated Visual Acuity Loss

Morten la Cour and Ulrik Correll Christensen

The Complication: Definition

Silicone oil associated visual acuity loss is an unexpected loss in best corrected visual acuity (BCVA) that occurs in eyes where silicone oils are used as intravitreal tampon-ade. This complication was first described by Newsom et al.[1] The degree of visual loss in the reported cases varies from relatively mild to severe losses in acuity, equivalent to 80 Early Treatment Diabetic Retinopathy Study (ETDRS) letters or more.[2]

Patients usually report a gray or dark area in the central visual field, and in cases where formal visual field testing was performed, a central scotoma was found without overt evidence of glaucomatous damage.[1–3]

The key to the diagnosis is that the visual loss in *unexpected*. It occurs typically in eyes operated for rhegmatogenous retinal detachment (RRD) where the macula has never been detached, and where the BCVA has been good shortly after the retina was reattached under silicone oil.

Risk Factors

The risk factors for silicone oil associated visual acuity loss are vitrectomy with the use of silicone oil, and good preoperative BCVA.[1,2,4–8] Almost all described cases have occurred in eyes with RRD, but the condition has also been described in an eye operated with silicone oil for a full thickness macular hole.[7]

In the first case series the silicone oil associated visual acuity loss occurred in conjunction with silicone oil removal, and in these reports the preoperative BCVA was not reported.[1,3,4,7] Recent reports have shown that the silicone oil associated visual acuity loss frequently occurs while the oil is still in the eye.[2,6,9] **Figure 19D-1** shows the changes in BCVA in nine cases of macula-on RRD operated with sili-cone oil. In all cases with severe visual loss, the major part of the visual acuity loss occurred while oil was in the eye.

The risk of silicone oil associated visual acuity loss in eyes with good visual potential is difficult to assess without a prospective study. However, such a study is less likely to be forthcoming, as the use of silicone oil in such eyes is rather rare, and interpretation of the results will be hampered by the many causes of poor outcome in complicated RRD cases. Nevertheless, some indication of the frequency of this complication might be inferred from the published case series. In the initial report of seven cases from the Moorfields group, it was stated that these represented only

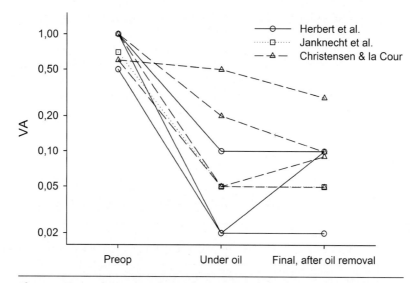

Figure 19D-1 Nine cases of macula-on RRD, and preoperative BCVA ≥0.5, operated with silicone oil, anatomical success after a single procedure, and subsequent BCVA loss equivalent to 15 ETDRS letters or more. The BCVA are the preoperative measurement (preop), the measurement just prior to oil removal (under oil), and the final recorded BCVA after oil removal (final, after oil removal). The cases are 1, 3, 4, and 5, as from Herbert et al.,[2] as their case 2 did not have BCVA loss. There is a case from Janknecht et al.,[6] and four cases fulfilling the above criteria from Christensen and la Cour.[5]

around 1% of oil removal procedures performed in the "study period."[1] Later, Herbert et al.[10] reported that the increased awareness of the condition resulted in more frequent identification of unexplained visual loss accompanying the use of silicone oil. They identified this complication in 12 cases out of 118 oil removal procedures, corresponding to a risk of 10%. The denominator in these estimates is the total number of oil cases during a certain period. However, silicone oil associated visual acuity loss is more likely to manifest itself in eyes with good visual potential, and such cases probably constitute a very small part of the total number of oil cases. The condition might therefore be much more common in such eyes. To address this, we performed a chart review of 162 consecutive patients operated for primary RRD with silicone oil in our institution in 2004 and 2005.[5] We identified, eyes where the RRD was documented macula-on, the preoperative visual acuity was 0.5 or better; first surgery anatomical success had been obtained, and the macula thus never detached, silicone oil had been removed, cataract surgery had been performed if the eye was phakic, and retina was completely attached at last follow-up. Nine eyes in nine individuals fulfilled these criteria, and were examined. **Figure 19D-2** shows the visual acuities of these eyes 4 to 5 years after the primary surgery. Only four eyes (44%) had retained a visual acuity of 0.5 (Snellen equivalent 6/12) or better at follow-up; in three eyes (33%) the visual acuity had dropped below 0.1 (Snellen equivalent 6/60). Five eyes (56%) had suffered a visual loss corresponding to 15 ETDRS letters or more. We compared this with seven similar eyes operated with gas, of which none had suffered significant visual loss.[5] Our study confirmed that even in an institution where a relatively high proportion of primary RRD cases were operated with silicone oil (approximately 35%, la Cour, unpublished), this tamponade was only used in few cases with excellent visual potential during the study period. On the other hand, among those few cases the risk of silicone oil associated visual loss was unexpectedly, and alarmingly, high.

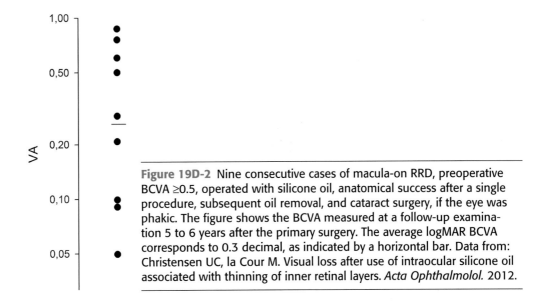

Figure 19D-2 Nine consecutive cases of macula-on RRD, preoperative BCVA ≥0.5, operated with silicone oil, anatomical success after a single procedure, subsequent oil removal, and cataract surgery, if the eye was phakic. The figure shows the BCVA measured at a follow-up examination 5 to 6 years after the primary surgery. The average logMAR BCVA corresponds to 0.3 decimal, as indicated by a horizontal bar. Data from: Christensen UC, la Cour M. Visual loss after use of intraocular silicone oil associated with thinning of inner retinal layers. *Acta Ophthalmolol.* 2012.

Pathogenesis: Why Does It Occur

The pathogenesis of silicone oil associated visual acuity loss is currently unknown. Electrophysiologic investigations after silicone oil removal have shown compromised central retinal function as evidenced by reduced amplitudes in central multifocal electroretinography (ERG) amplitudes, and reduced pattern ERG amplitudes, indicating a retinal cause for the visual loss.[1,3,4]

In almost all reported cases, optical coherence tomography (OCT) of the macular region was performed, and did not show fibrosis, edema, or other findings that readily could explain the visual loss.[1-4,9] We performed follow-up high definition OCT scanning of 16 cases of primary macula-on RRD operated with vitrectomy and single operation successfully: Nine oil cases and seven gas cases (**Figs. 19D-3A** and **C**). We found that the inner retinal layers in oil eyes were highly significantly thinned when compared to the gas cases, and the degree of thinning was correlated with the degree of visual loss.[5]

Both in experimental animals and in enucleated human eyes, intravitreal tamponade with silicone oil has resulted in oil droplets being identified in both epiretinal membranes, retina, and retrolaminar optic nerve.[11-15] Intraretinal vacuoles have been reported histopathologically as early as 2 months after oil instillation.[14] Intraretinal emulsified silicone oil could cause neuronal damage, and functional loss. However, Chung and Spaide[16] performed OCT on an eye operated for a full thickness macular hole, with the use of silicone oil tamponade for a duration of only 2 months. They did find vacuoles in the retina suggestive of migration of emulsified silicone oil into the retina, but despite this a relatively good visual acuity of 20/60.[16] We also found two eyes in our series with such vacuoles on OCT (**Fig. 19D-3B**). As in the case by Chung and Spaide[16] these eyes did not have silicone oil associated visual loss. Nevertheless, intraretinal oil droplets, or mechanical displacement of them during the turbulence involved in silicone oil removal, might theoretically result in neuronal damage.

Recently, a number of case reports have appeared where intravitreal silicone seemingly have migrated along the optic nerve to the cerebral ventricles.[8,17,18] However, this complication is not common, as we found no evidence of it in a consecutive series of 19 patients who were examined by magnetic resonance imaging with sequences specific for silicone oil.[19] Thus, while silicone oil droplets in the optic nerve or central visual pathways can occur, it is an unlikely explanation for silicone oil associated visual acuity loss.

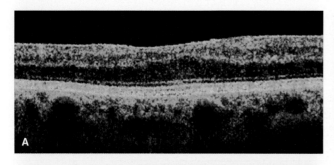
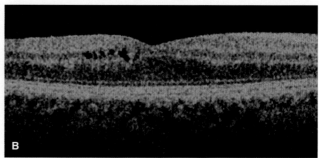
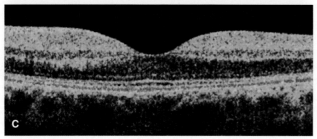

Figure 19D-3 Macular OCT scans of three eyes that underwent anatomical successful vitrectomy for macula-on RRD. **Panel A:** Shows an eye with preoperative BCVA of 1, operated with silicone oil that was subsequently removed. BCVA at the time of the scan was 0.1. OCT shows thinning of the inner retinal layers. **Panel B:** Oil case with a preoperative BCVA of 0.5. After silicone oil removal, at the time where the scan was obtained, the BCVA was 0.76. OCT shows small vacuoles seen in the inner plexiform layer, but otherwise the inner retina is quite normal. **Panel C:** Case operated successfully with vitrectomy and gas. BCVA preoperatively 0.6, improved to 1.15 at the time the scan was obtained. OCT shows a normal inner retina. Data from: Christensen UC, la Cour M. Visual loss after use of intraocular silicone oil associated with thinning of inner retinal layers. *Acta Ophthalmol.* 2011.

Light toxicity during the oil removal procedure, local changes in the concentration of potassium, Ca++, Mg++, or changes in the levels of various cytokines in front of the retina are likely to be implicated in the inner retinal damage seen in silicone oil associated visual acuity loss.[1,5]

Animal experiments suggest a possible optic nerve or retinal ganglion cell involvement in silicone oil associated visual acuity loss.[20]

Pearls on How to Prevent It

◆ Be aware that the risk of silicone oil associated visual acuity loss might be considerable in eyes with good visual potential, and avoid the use of silicone oil in such eyes, whenever possible. Remember that the silicone study included eyes with severe proliferative vitreoretinopathy (PVR), and got the same anatomical results with C3F8 gas as with silicone oil.[21,22]

◆ Acquire the skills to make a vitrectomy thorough enough that you will be successful by using gas as intravitreal tamponade. If the vitrectomy is thorough enough, it is possible to obtain excellent anatomical success in non-PVR RRD cases with only air tamponade, or even without any nonaqueous tamponade. This has been shown also for cases with inferior breaks and unseen breaks.[23–25]

◆ Remove silicone oil as soon as possible.

Pearls on How to Solve It

◆ Once silicone oil associated visual acuity loss has occurred, no treatment has been shown to be helpful.

◆ Be aware of other, treatable, causes of visual acuity loss, such as epiretinal membranes, shallow redetachment, macular holes, cystoid macular edema, and so on.

◈ Expected Outcomes: What Is the Worst-case Scenario

The final outcome of silicone associated visual acuity loss is variable (Figs. 19D-1 and 19D-2). In some cases, a slight improvement over time has been observed, particularly in cases without severe visual loss (a loss of 30 ETDRS letters or more).[2]

The worst-case scenario could be a patient with a macula-on, superior RRD with multiple breaks, and BCVA of 1 (Snellen equivalent 6/6). The surgeon feels that vitrectomy is necessary because some of the breaks are quite posterior. He also feels that gas tamponade will be sufficient, but opts for oil because of convenience such as patients' preference for air travel over surface transportation. If the surgery is anatomically successful, but the patient suffers silicone oil associated visual acuity loss to hand motions vision, the outcome will not be conceived as optimal by neither the patient nor the surgeon.

REFERENCES

1. Newsom RS, Johnston R, Sullivan PM, et al. Sudden visual loss after removal of silicone oil. *Retina.* 2004;24:871–877.
2. Herbert EN, Habib M, Steel D, et al. Central scotoma associated with intraocular silicone oil tamponade develops before oil removal *Graefes. Arch Clin Exp Ophthalmol.* 2006;244:248–252.
3. Michel G, Meyer L, Naoun O. Sudden visual loss following silicone oil removal: Three patients treated for giant retinal tear. *J Fr Ophtalmol.* 2009;32:104–111.
4. Cazabon S, Groenewald C, Pearce IA, et al. Visual loss following removal of intraocular silicone oil. *Br J Ophthalmol.* 2005;89:799–802.
5. Christensen UC, la Cour M. Visual loss after use of intraocular silicone oil associated with thinning of inner retinal layers. *Acta Ophthalmol.* 2012;90:733–737.
6. Janknecht P, Zdenek GJ, Park C, et al. Diagnostic and therapeutic challenges. *Retina.* 2004;24:293–296.
7. Satchi K, Bolton A, Patel CK. Loss of vision once silicone oil has been removed. *Retina.* 2005;25:807–808.
8. Williams RL, Beatty RL, Kanal E, et al. MR imaging of intraventricular silicone: Case report. *Radiology.* 1999;212:151–154.
9. Williams PD, Fuller CG, Scott IU, et al. Vision loss associated with the use and removal of intraocular silicone oil. *Clin Ophthalmol.* 2008;2:955–959.
10. Herbert EN, Liew SH, Williamson TH. Visual loss after silicone oil removal. *Br J Ophthalmol.* 2005;89:1667–1668.
11. Budde M, Cursiefen C, Holbach LM, et al. Silicone oil-associated optic nerve degeneration. *Am J Ophthalmol.* 2001;131:392–394.
12. Eckardt C, Nicolai U, Czank M, et al. Identification of silicone oil in the retina after intravitreal injection. *Retina.* 1992;12:S17–S22.
13. Kirchhof B, Tavakolian U, Paulmann H, et al. Histopathological findings in eyes after silicone oil injection. *Graefes Arch Clin Exp Ophthalmol.* 1986;224:34–37.
14. Knorr HL, Seltsam A, Holbach L, et al. [Intraocular silicone oil tamponade. A clinico-pathologic study of 36 enucleated eyes]. *Ophthalmologe.* 1996;93:130–138.
15. Wickham LJ, Asaria RH, Alexander R, et al. Immunopathology of intraocular silicone oil: Retina and epiretinal membranes. *Br J Ophthalmol.* 2007;91:258–262.
16. Chung J, Spaide R. Intraretinal silicone oil vacuoles after macular hole surgery with internal limiting membrane peeling. *Am J Ophthalmol.* 2003;136:766–767.
17. Eller AW, Friberg TR, Mah F. Migration of silicone oil into the brain: A complication of intraocular silicone oil for retinal tamponade. *Am J Ophthalmol.* 2000;129:685–688.

18. Fangtian D, Rongping D, Lin Z, et al. Migration of intraocular silicone into the cerebral ventricles. *Am J Ophthalmol.* 2005;140:156–158.

19. Kiilgaard JF, Milea D, Logager V, et al. Cerebral migration of intraocular silicone oil: An MRI study. *Acta Ophthalmol.* 2011;89:522–525.

20. Papp A, Kiss EB, Timar O, et al. Long-term exposure of the rabbit eye to silicone oil causes optic nerve atrophy. *Brain Res Bull.* 2007;74:130–133.

21. Silicone study group. Vitrectomy with silicone oil or perfluoropropane gas in eyes with severe proliferative vitreoretinopathy: Results of a randomized clinical trial. Silicone Study Report 2. *Arch Ophthalmol.* 1992;110:780–792.

22. Abrams GW, Azen SP, McCuen BW 2nd, et al. Vitrectomy with silicone oil or long-acting gas in eyes with severe proliferative vitreoretinopathy: Results of additional and long-term follow-up. Silicone Study report 11. *Arch Ophthalmol.* 1997;115:335–344.

23. Martinez-Castillo V, Boixadera A, Verdugo A, et al. Pars plana vitrectomy alone for the management of inferior breaks in pseudophakic retinal detachment without facedown position. *Ophthalmology.* 2005;112:1222–1226.

24. Martinez-Castillo V, Zapata MA, Boixadera A, et al. Pars plana vitrectomy, laser retinopexy, and aqueous tamponade for pseudophakic rhegmatogenous retinal detachment. *Ophthalmology.* 2007;114:297–302.

25. Martinez-Castillo V, Boixadera A, Garcia-Arumi J. Pars plana vitrectomy alone with diffuse illumination and vitreous dissection to manage primary retinal detachment with unseen breaks. *Arch Ophthalmol.* 2009;127:1297–1304.

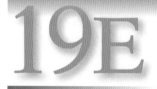

19E Emulsification of Tamponade Agents

Rachel Williams and Theodor Stappler

 ## The Complication: Definition

Emulsification can be defined as the process of dispersing one liquid in a second immiscible liquid. Emulsification occurs when shear forces are exerted at the interface of two immiscible liquids. This results in one fluid being extended into the other and at a particular shear stress, large enough to overcome the cohesive forces in the liquid and the interfacial tension, the pull-out ligament will fracture (**Fig. 19E-1**). The bulk liquid will retract and the fractured droplet becomes separated. The emulsified droplets will only be stabilized if there are surfactants present, otherwise they will coalesce into the bulk liquid.

Risk Factors

Viscosity is defined as the property of a fluid to resist the force tending to cause the fluid to flow. Shear viscosity is the property of a fluid to resist shear forces and extensional viscosity is the property to resist extensional forces and is highly dependent on the molecular weight of the fluid. For tamponade agents the viscosity parameters are generally shear viscosity and these values for a range of commonly used tamponades agents are presented in Table 19E-1. A tamponade agent has recently been developed with a modified extensional viscosity.[1] This was achieved

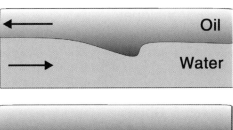

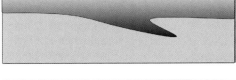

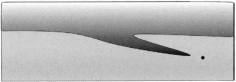

Figure 19E-1 Diagrammatic representation of ligament "pull out" under shear at the oil/water interface.

by modifying the molecular weight distribution in the silicone oil, specifically by adding 5% of a high molecular weight additive to a lower molecular weight bulk oil. The high molecular weight additive increases the shear viscosity of the bulk oil at low shear rates due to the entanglement of the large molecules; however, at higher shear rates the large molecules tend to become aligned to the direction of the shear forces and thus the shear viscosity is decreased **(Fig. 19E-2)**. This has the potential to increase the ease of injection of the tamponade agent.[2] At low shear rates the entangled molecules will have little resistance of extensional forces; however, as the shear rate increases the elongation of the large molecules in the direction of the shear forces has the potential to resist break-up of the bulk oil. When break-up does occur the small droplets are less likely to form and, thus, less emulsification would be expected **(Fig. 19E-3)**.

Table 19E-1 • Viscosities of Commonly Used Tamponade Agents	
Tamponade Agent	**Viscosity**
Siluron 5000	5,000 mPas
Siluron 2000	2,000 mPas
Siluron 1000	1,000 mPas
Densiron 68	1,400 mPas
Oxane HD	3,300 mPas
Oxane 1300	1,000 mPas
Oxane 5700	5,000 mPas
F6H8	2.5 mPas
F-Octane	2.5 mPas
F-decalin	3.7 mPas

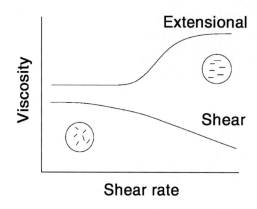

Figure 19E-2 Diagram to demonstrate the influence of a high molecular weight additive on the shear and extensional viscosity.

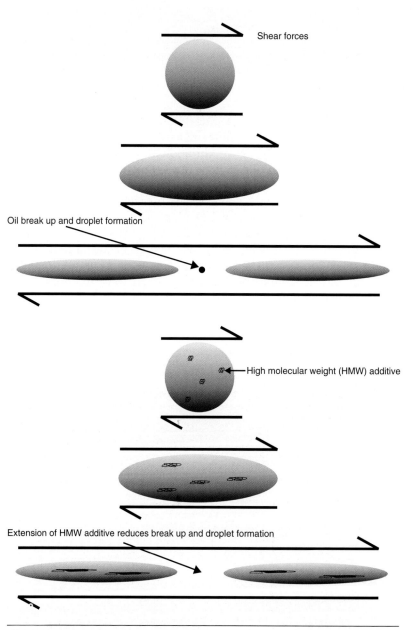

Figure 19E-3 Diagram to demonstrate how the high molecular weight additive could reduce droplet formation.

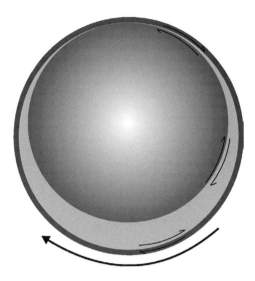

Figure 19E-4 Diagram of the potential shear forces in the vitreous cavity at the tamponade/aqueous/retina interface.

Shear Forces

The shear forces that have the potential to cause emulsification of tamponade agents are complex. At the top of the vitreous cavity the oil will be in contact with the retina (although there may be an ultrathin layer of fluid between the retina and the oil). Thus as the eye moves shear forces will be generated between the retina and the oil (Fig. 19E-4). As it is very difficult to completely fill the vitreous cavity with oil and as the oil has a tendency to float, it is likely that there would be a small amount of fluid in the lower part of the vitreous cavity. There will be shear forces generated at the interface retina/aqueous fluid and at the interface oil/aqueous fluid. The shear forces generated at the oil/retina and oil/aqueous interfaces will have the potential to cause emulsification of the oil.

Surfactants

A surfactant is a surface active agent that tends to reduce the surface tension. They generally have a hydrophilic head and a hydrophobic tail; thus, in a water/oil mixture the hydrophobic tail becomes embedded in the oil phase and the hydrophilic head makes contact with the water phase. By congregating at the oil/water interface it tends to stabilize it and thus will allow emulsified oil droplets to remain dispersed in the aqueous phase (Fig. 19E-5). Proteins in the remaining aqueous are the most likely molecules to act as surfactants at the oil/aqueous interface. Analysis of aqueous fluid collected from around silicone oil tamponades[3] has demonstrated raised levels of basic fibroblast growth factor (bFGF), interleukin-6 (IL-6), and total protein levels in comparison to normal vitreous or aqueous fluid collected at the time of revision vitrectomy. The presence of growth factors and cytokines in the vitreous cavity are capable of inducing the production of extracellular proteins from the cells present and may be a contributing factor in the development of proliferative vitreoretinopathy (PVR) in these cases.[4] It is also reported that, should the blood–retinal barrier be broken, plasma lipoproteins, apolipoproteins, and red blood cell membrane fragments could support silicone oil emulsification.[5] Thus there is evidence of protein and lipoprotein substances in the vitreous cavity postretinal detachment that could act as surfactants to stabilize oil droplets. The different levels present in different eyes may account for the variations observed in amount of emulsification observed for the same oil in different patients. When a silicone oil tamponade is present the relatively small amount of aqueous around the oil will have a concentrating effect on these soluble protein components.

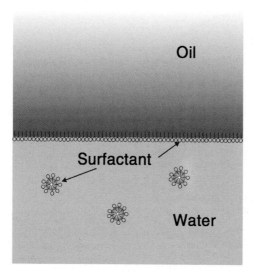

Figure 19E-5 Diagram to demonstrate the surfactant interactions at the oil/aqueous interface.

 Pathogenesis

In Vivo Emulsified Silicone Oil

Emulsification of silicone oil-based tamponades has been observed (**Fig. 19E-6**). It is generally believed that emulsified droplets are always there to some extent, particularly after the tamponade agent has been left in the eye for a long period but often they are difficult to see as they tend to accumulate in the anterior chamber angle. Gonioscopy, rarely performed during routine vitreoretinal examination, would be required to detect it. The number of patients in which emulsification was observed and reported by Scott et al.,[6] however, was very low (4% for 1,000 cS oil and 2% for 5,000 cS oil). In this study, emulsification was determined by the presence of oil droplets visible on clinical examination. Furthermore, histopathology studies of enucleated eyes following the use of silicone oil to treat complicated retinal detachments found the presence of silicone oil in many tissues of the eye, including iris, ciliary body, retina, trabecular meshwork, and epiretinal membranes.[7,8] In general the silicone oil observed in these tissues was associated with local inflammation mediated by macrophages and this is observed even after the silicone oil has been removed.

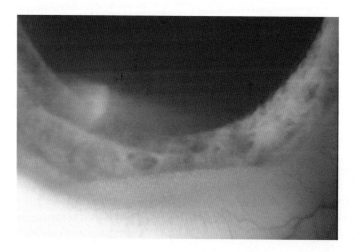

Figure 19E-6 Emulsified heavy tamponade agent in the anterior chamber.

Since kinetic energy needs to be supplied to the aqueous/oil interface to produce emulsification, it has been reported that nystagmus may increase the risk of emulsified droplet formation and the consequent clinical complications.[9] It was suggested that silicone oil emulsification may occur earlier in these patients and therefore silicone oil removal should not be delayed. In cases complicated by PVR, increased emulsification may be observed due to previous surgeries involving the use of silicone oil or perfluorocarbon liquid (PFCL), each of which can increase emulsification on its own. Furthermore, in PVR cases, the vitreoretinal surgeon may opt for leaving the silicone oil for a more extensive period of time which will increase the risk of emulsification. A further complicating factor that may influence the risk of emulsification is the possible contamination of the silicone oil from the intraoperative use of PFCL and semifluorinated alkanes (SFAs). Analysis of emulsified oil removed from eyes in which PFCL had been used, even with an indirect exchange of the PFCL for the silicone oil, has shown the silicone oil to be contaminated with the PFCL.[10] PFCL has the ability to reduce the interfacial tension of the silicone oil and, thus, increases the risk of emulsified droplets forming. SFAs are soluble in silicone oil to a certain amount and high levels have been measured in retrieved emulsified oil. Following on from this discussion the specific injection of silicone oil and PFCLs or SFAs as separate tamponade agents into the vitreous cavity to create a heavy tamponade in situ would be expected to lead to significant problems and thus would seem unwise.

Characterizing and quantifying silicone oil droplets produced in vivo is not a trivial task. When examining the emulsion clinically it is likely that only the larger droplets will be observed, for example, with slit lamp examination. Retrieval of the droplets at silicone oil removal is also complicated by the fact that the oil droplets will float and therefore are often lost during initial breach of the globe. Collection of the silicone oil and the washing balanced saline solution (BSS) should allow retrieval of the remaining droplets that are free within the vitreous cavity, that is, those not already attached or incorporated within the tissues. In the collected solution there is now a need to separate the bulk oil from the BSS wash taking care to leave the emulsified droplets undisturbed remembering that they will be present at the interface of the bulk oil and the BSS. Once separated there is a need to characterize the droplets in the BSS in terms of the total number of droplets and the size of the droplets. The most appropriate way to quantify the total number of droplets is probably by using a coulter counter or particle size analyzer. These techniques should give a total droplet count and a size distribution. Preliminary data (Wong D. Unpublished communication) using a coulter counter suggests that the majority of the droplets are less than 5 μm and many of the droplets are around 1 μm in diameter.

Clinical Significance

Secondary glaucoma has been reported associated with the use of silicone oil. A recent review[11] suggests that there are four different mechanisms by which the silicone oil can influence the development of glaucoma (see also Chapter 19B). One of these mechanisms relates to the formation of emulsified droplets of silicone oil and their migration into the trabecular meshwork. Migration of silicone oil droplets into the anterior chamber may cause a mechanical barrier to filtration, whereas migration of droplets into the trabecular meshwork may result in inflammation that causes resistance to aqueous outflow. More recently, several studies have reported case studies showing evidence of silicone oil migration and accumulation intracranially using CT and MRI.[12-15] In particular silicone oil droplets have been identified in the subarachnoid and intraventricular space and in the lateral ventricles. However, a prospective neuroimaging study[16] involving 19 patients found no evidence of silicone oil migration into the visual pathways or intracranially and concluded that the incidence of silicone oil migration into the brain is probably very rare.

In Vitro Emulsified Silicone Oil

Several studies have generated silicone oil emulsions in vitro as a way of studying how the properties of the oil, the properties of the aqueous or emulsifier, or the amount of mechanical energy imparted to the interface influences the characteristics of the emulsified droplets and the biologic significance of the droplets.

In the eye, emulsification is formed without an air interface and it is important when modeling this process in vitro that the air interface is excluded. Closed chambers[1,17] are therefore preferable to open test tube type systems. Some studies use an extrusion method in which the oil is injected through a membrane with particular pore sizes.[18,19] This approach can be useful to produce a significant volume of droplets, for example, as used in these studies, to evaluate the cellular response to the droplets. Several different methods are used to quantify the emulsion formed in terms of the total amount of droplets and the size of the droplets. In some cases the volume of the emulsified layer is measured.[20–22] Care must be taken in this approach to ensure that the emulsion is oil-in-water as in vivo not water-in-oil. Other studies evaluate emulsification microscopically.[17–19,23] This approach is particularly useful to evaluate the droplet size distribution but it is more difficult to quantify total amount of emulsified droplets. The means of producing the kinetic energy also varies considerably between studies, including high speed vortexing, sonication,[20] shaking,[17,22] and ultrasound using a phacofragmentation handpiece.[23] Studies using a range of different surfactants or emulsion stabilizers are available including various blood components,[20] whole serum and individual proteins,[22] and chemical silicone oil surfactants (Pluronics).[1,18]

All these studies add to our understanding of the potential emulsification of silicone oil tamponades. In particular, how the properties of the oils, the properties of the aqueous environment and the kinetic energy influence the amount and character of the emulsions. This understanding could help us to develop strategies to reduce the detrimental clinical significance of this behavior.

⬥ Pearls on How to Prevent It

The controlling factors for silicone oil emulsification are the viscosity of the oil, the shear forces at the interface and the presence of surfactants.

◆ There is little that can be done about the surfactants although removal of the oil earlier may be warranted in cases of pre-existing glaucoma.[11] However, knowing that lipoproteins and other components from blood[5] can cause emulsification, there may be a case to minimize bleeding intraoperatively and postoperatively and to ensure that any blood that has got into the vitreous cavity is removed as far as possible prior to injection of the oil. Furthermore, since raised levels of inflammatory mediators[3] such as bFGF and IL-6 have been found in the aqueous fluid surrounding silicone oil tamponades and that these can induce the production of extracellular proteins[4] there may be a case to attempt to control inflammation to reduce the concentration of these surfactants. One way to achieve this might be to use the silicone oil as a reservoir to release anti-inflammatory agents in a controlled and sustained manner to ensure that they are presented at a therapeutic level, are bioactive, and are not cytotoxic. Any PFCL or SFA left in the vitreous cavity prior to injection of the silicone oil should be minimized also to reduce their influence on increasing the risk of emulsification.

◆ It is also difficult to do anything about the shear forces in terms of controlling eye movement. However, ensuring maximum removal of vitreous will allow the best possible silicone oil fill and therefore may minimize the influence of shear forces at the interface and it has been suggested that using an encircling band to cause an indent can reduce the movement between the oil and the vitreous cavity and thus reduce emulsification.[17]

◆ Clearly the higher the viscosity of the oil the greater the kinetic energy required to break off oil droplets. Increasing the shear viscosity will increase resistance to emulsification but will also increase resistance to injection. Modifying the molecular composition of the poly(dimethylsiloxane) by adding a small proportion of very high molecular weight material or adding a proportion of poly(dimethylsiloxane) with a branched molecular structure may modify the extensional viscosity thus enhancing emulsification resistance without making the shear viscosity so high as to be detrimental to the clinical use in terms of injection and removal.

✦ Pearls on How to Solve It

Once silicone oil emulsification has occurred then there is a need to try to remove as much of the droplets at possible.

◆ Some advocate consecutive fluid/air exchanges to try and bring the droplets to the air/fluid interface and thus make it easier to remove them. However, this is not universally advocated and some people question its effectiveness.

◆ SFAs such as F4H5 are used to dissolve silicone oil from intraocular lens.[24] Could this be used to dissolve and thus remove silicone oil droplets stuck to the retina? Could other SFAs such as F6H8 be used? Are there surfactants that would be safe to use in the vitreous cavity that would preferentially attach to silicone oil droplets thus reducing their attachment to the retina and allowing the droplets to be washed out more easily? Future studies may help to answer these questions.

REFERENCES

1. Williams RL, Day M, Garvey MJ, et al. Increasing the extensional viscosity of silicone oil reduces the tendency for emulsification. *Retina.* 2010;30(2):300–304.
2. Williams RL, Day MJ, Garvey MJ, et al. Injectability of silicone oil-based tamponade agents. *Br J Ophthalmol.* 2011;95(2):273–276.
3. Asaria RH, Kon CH, Bunce C, et al. Silicone oil concentrates fibrogenic growth factors in the retro-oil fluid. *Br J Ophthalmol.* 2004;88(11):1439–1442.
4. Pennock S, Rheaume MA, Mukai S, et al. A novel strategy to develop therapeutic approaches to prevent proliferative vitreoretinopathy. *Am J Pathol.* 2011;179(6): 2931–2940.
5. Savion N, Alhalel A, Treister G, et al. Role of blood components in ocular silicone oil emulsification. Studies on an in vitro model. *Invest Ophthalmol Vis Sci.* 1996; 37(13):2694–2699.
6. Scott IU, Flynn HW Jr, Murray TG, et al. Outcomes of complex retinal detachment repair using 1000- vs 5000-centistoke silicone oil. *Arch of Ophthalmol.* 2005;123(4): 473–478.
7. Wickham L, Asaria RH, Alexander R, et al. Immunopathology of intraocular silicone oil: Enucleated eyes. *Br J Ophthalmol.* 2007;91(2):253–257.
8. Wickham LJ, Asaria RH, Alexander R, et al. Immunopathology of intraocular silicone oil: Retina and epiretinal membranes. *Br J Ophthalmol.* 2007;91(2):258–262.
9. Yilmaz T, Güler M. The role of nystagmus in silicone oil emulsification after pars plana vitrectomy and silicone oil injection for complex retinal detachment. *Eur J Ophthalmol.* 2008;18(1):150–154.
10. Dresp JH, Menz DH. Interaction of different ocular endotamponades as a risk factor for silicone oil emulsification. *Retina.* 2005;25(7):902–910.

11. Ichhpujani P, Jindal A, Jay Katz L. Silicone oil induced glaucoma: A review. *Graefes Arch Clin Exp Ophthalmol.* 2009;247(12):1585–1593.

12. Fangtian D, Rongping D, Lin Z, et al. Migration of intraocular silicone into the cerebral ventricles. *Am J Ophthalmol.* 2005;140(1):156–158.

13. Eller AW, Friberg TR, Mah F. Migration of silicone oil into the brain: A complication of intraocular silicone oil for retinal tamponade. *Am J Ophthalmol.* 2000;129(5): 685–688.

14. Jabbour P, Hanna A, Rosenwasser R. Migration of silicone oil in the cerebral intraventricular system. *Neurologist,* 2011;17(2):109–110.

15. Tatewaki Y, Kurihara N, Sato A, et al. Silicone oil migrating from intraocular tamponade into the ventricles: Case report with magnetic resonance image findings. *J Comput Assist Tomogr.* 2011;35(1):43–45.

16. Kiilgaard JF, Milea D, Logager V, et al. Cerebral migration of intraocular silicone oil: An MRI study. *Acta Ophthalmol.* 2011;89(6):522–525.

17. de Silva DJ, Lim KS, Schulenburg WE. An experimental study on the effect of encircling band procedure on silicone oil emulsification. *Br J Ophthalmol.* 2005; 89(10):1348–1350.

18. Kociok N, Gavranic C, Kirchhof B, et al. Influence on membrane-mediated cell activation by vesicles of silicone oil or perfluorohexyloctane. *Graefes Arch Clin Exp Ophthalmol.* 2005;243(4):345–358.

19. Ma LN, Hui YN, Wang YS, et al. Inhibition of migration but stimulation of proliferation of human retinal pigment epithelial cells cultured with uniform vesicles of silicone oil. *Graefes Arch Clin Exp Ophthalmol.* 2010;248(4):503–510.

20. Caramoy A, Schroder S, Fauser S, et al. In vitro emulsification assessment of new silicone oils. *Br J Ophthalmol.* 2010;94(4):509–512.

21. Caramoy A, Hagedorn N, Fauser S, et al. Development of emulsification-resistant silicone oils: Can we go beyond 2000 mPas silicone oil? *Invest Ophthalmol Vis Sci.* 2011;52(8):5432–5436.

22. Heidenkummer HP, Kampik A, Thierfelder S. Emulsification of silicone oils with specific physiochemical characteristics. *Graefes Arch Clin Exp Ophthalmol.* 1991; 229(1):88–94.

23. Francis JH, Latkany PA, Rosenthal JL. Mechanical energy from intraocular instruments cause emulsification of silicone oil. *Br J Ophthalmol.* 2007;91(6):818–821.

24. Stappler T, Williams R, Wong D. F4H5: A novel substance for the removal of silicone oil from intraocular lenses. *Br J Ophthalmol.* 2010;94(3):364–367.

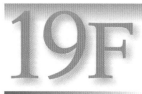

Retinal Redetachment Following Removal of the Tamponade Agent

ADRIANA RAMIREZ, VALENTINA FRANCO-CARDENAS, AND STEVEN D. SCHWARTZ

The Complication: Definition

Retinal Redetachment after Silicone Oil Removal

In order to reduce the incidence of postoperative complications in silicone oil filled eyes, many authors recommend silicone oil removal as soon as a stable retinal situation is achieved. Others feel that if a silicone oil filled eye is stable after multiple surgeries and has moderate to low visual potential even post-oil removal, a reasonable strategy is to observe with oil in. In other words, if silicone oil removal is not likely to change the visual acuity (i.e., fellow eye is healthy) or quality of life, observation is a reasonable strategy simply given the risk of a recurrent retinal detachment (RD).[1]

Indications for the removal of silicone oil include:

◆ Attached retina with stable retinal examination for at least 3 months.

◆ Possibility of visual acuity improvement, complications such as ocular hypertension, band keratopathy, oil-corneal touch, or silicone emulsification.[2,3] Increased intraocular pressure (IOP) may not improve following oil removal though.

In special circumstances, it is reasonable to consider long-term silicone oil tamponade. Eyes with recurrent proliferative vitreoretinopathy (PVR), hypotony, and repeated vitreous hemorrhage often become silicone oil dependent eyes.[4]

The Silicone Study has provided useful information on the advisability of removing silicone oil from eyes after surgery complicated by PVR. As reported in the Silicone Study (1994), eyes with Grade C PVR or worse that undergo oil removal are at an increased risk for recurrent retinal detachment (odds ratio 2.1). Visual improvement occurred in 29% of the oil-removed eyes compared to 2% of eyes with retained oil.[5] Incidence rates of band keratopathy and hypotony were lower in oil-removed eyes, although not statistically significantly. Limitations of the Silicone Study include the fact that this study was conducted many years ago and the impact of new surgical strategies could have potentially changed current outcomes and the fact that only 45% of all the eyes with silicone oil underwent oil removal. It is important to keep in mind that selection for silicone oil tamponade in the Silicone Study was likely biased to the most complicated retinal detachments.

In a case series of complicated retinal detachments, Goezinne et al.[6] described time to redetach after silicone oil removal. 19% of eyes redetached after silicone oil removal. Of those eyes, 26/38 eyes (68%) redetached after 3 months and 33/38 eyes (87%) at 6 months. After 1 year, an additional 3/38 eyes (8%) developed redetachment. The majority of eyes that developed a redetachment within 3 months were due to reopening of old retinal tears or formation of new defects attributable to PVR. In general, the literature suggests that retinal detachment recurrence rates are approximately 6% to 28%[5–13] (Table 19F-1). In contrast, the success rate using SF-6

Table 19F-1 • Redetachment Rate after Silicone Oil Removal		
	Redetachment Rate	**Number of Eyes/Year**
Zilis JD	With PVR 9%	55 eyes/1989
Lesloni	PVR grade C 6%	83 eyes/2000
Jiang, F	20%	94 eyes/2002
Goezinne	Complicated retinal detachment 19%	287 eyes/2007
Silicone Study	20%	99 eyes/1994
Soheilian	28%	82 eyes/2006
Lam RF	19%	147 eyes/2008
Jonas JB	25.3%	225 eyes/2001
Pavlovic	Mix of attached and detached eyes, 12%. For completely attached, 8%. In detached eyes, 34%	324 eyes/1995

in complicated retinal detachment surgery was 26% to 54%.[14] Retinal redetachment after silicone oil removal occurred an average of 3.4 weeks after initial surgery,[14] but can occur intraoperatively or years later.

The Heavy Silicone Oil Study compared heavy silicone oil versus standard silicone oil in a randomized, prospective clinical trial. There was no significant difference between both groups regarding anatomic success.[15] The removal of heavy silicone oil may be challenging; however, this may also be the case in some cases in which conventional silicone oil is inserted (see Chapter 13C). Use of perfluorocarbon liquid (PFCL) can aid in the removal of conventional and heavy silicone oil under these circumstances (see Chapter 13C).

◈ Risk Factors

The literature suggests important risk factors for redetachment following silicone oil removal including the number of previous surgeries[3,9,11,12] and long axial length.[11] Patients requiring further retinal reattachment surgery after their first oil removal procedure are at two-fold risk of redetachment after oil removal.[16] Pathology involving giant retinal tears as well as less than ambulatory vision can lead to anatomic failure.[9] Absence of scleral buckle[3] and an incomplete removal of the vitreous base and lack of an encircling element in eyes with PVR in the absence of inferior retinectomy are factors that can lead to a higher incidence of redetachment.[12,17]

Other complications related to removal of silicone oil (besides retinal redetachment following oil removal) include:

a. Poor visual outcome

Visual outcome following retinal detachment repair is an enormous topic beyond the scope if this chapter. Suffice to say that anatomic success is necessary to achieve a meaningful visual outcome. Further, even poor vision can be very important to patients during the course of their lifetime as the risk of vision-threatening events in the fellow eye for patients with PVR is 50% over 10 years.[18] Risk factors for poor visual outcome include male sex, preoperative visual activity (VA) of less than 20/200, proliferative diabetic retinopathy, performance of three or more surgeries, retinectomy, postoperative hypotony, and partial detachment at time of tamponade removal.[6]

b. Hypotony

Transient hypotony has been reported in 39.3% of eyes after silicone oil removal. Most eyes (94%) recovered within 1 week. The only risk factor found to be associated with transient hypotony was long axial length. A number of surgical procedures and severity of PVR were not correlated with transient hypotony.[19] Long-term hypotony is a complex condition and can be due to ciliary body detachment, atrophy, or traction. Rarely, silicone oil removal leads to chronic hypotony with an attached retina. For details on this topic, see Chapter 23.

c. Unexplained loss of vision

Unexplained, profound, and permanent visual acuity loss has been reported after silicone oil removal (see Chapter 19D).[20] This loss of vision was not associated with presence of cystoid macular edema (CME), epiretinal membrane (ERM), or redetachment. In these cases, opticall coherence tomography (OCT) and fluorescein angiography (FA) remained normal, but multifocal electroretinogram (ERG) showed severe macular dysfunction.[20,21] ERG alterations suggested specific damage to the middle and outer layers of the retina in the central macula. The cause of vision loss after silicone oil removal remains unknown. Potential explanations include a release of harmful soluble growth factors and free radicals, as well as alterations to blood perfusion after silicone oil removal.[21]

d. Retention of silicone oil causing floaters

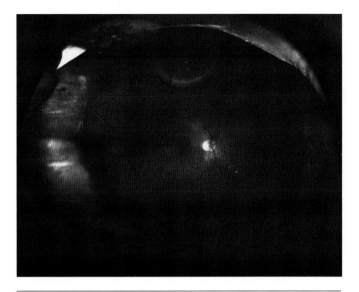

Figure 19F-1 Color fundus photograph of right eye with residual silicone oil.

Silicone oil removal can be associated with floaters due to residual oil droplets in up to 73% of patients[22] **(Fig. 19F-1)** (see also Chapter 13C). There is no significant difference in the incidence of floaters after silicone oil removal with passive drainage compared to passive drainage with air–fluid exchange.[22] In vitro experiments have showed that the amount of residual nonemulsified silicone oil left in the eye after removal is 0.0037% to 0.0179%.[23] In emulsified silicone oil, this residual oil percentage may be higher.[23]

Pathogenesis

Retinal redetachment after removal of silicone oil can occur as a result of:

◆ PVR
Retinal detachment after silicone oil removal is often associated with residual or secondary PVR.[24] In a case series by Lewis et al.,[25] perisilicone PVR developed in 61% of eyes and led to recurrent retinal detachments in 49% of eyes. It occurred at an average of 5 weeks after oil removal. Microscopic examination revealed droplets of silicone oil and necrotic cells on the PVR membranes. Silicone oil was present in these membranes months after silicone oil removal.

◆ Formation of new holes or tears
Tangential vitreoretinal traction from new PVR or residual vitreous gel may lead to new holes or tears after silicone oil removal.

◆ Previous tears or holes not/inadequately treated
Silicone oil's high surface tension can overcome the tractional forces from residual gel and can seal occult breaks that may lead to redetachment after its removal.

Pearls on How to Prevent It

◆ "Get it right the first time"
Doing things right the first time the patient is taken to the operating room (complete vitreous removal, encircling band when indicated, membrane removal in PVR) **(Fig. 19F-2)** is critical in achieving the best anatomic and visual outcome.

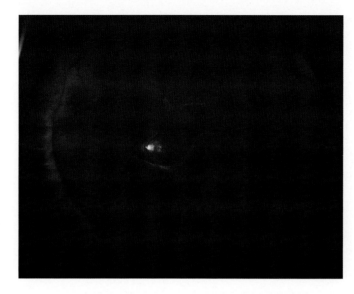

Figure 19F-2 Color fundus photograph of left eye. Patient status—postscleral buckle for primary retinal detachment with subsequent formation of proliferative vitreous membranes causing traction.

◆ Laser before oil removal

In a study by Tufail et al.,[26] application of prophylactic argon laser retinopexy with two rows of laser throughout 360 degrees 3 to 6 weeks before removal of silicone oil appeared to reduce retinal detachment rate from 25% to 6.7%. A 360-degree prophylactic laser retinopexy, either at the time of the final retinal detachment procedure or as a separate supplementary procedure, was associated with a reduction from 26% to 14% in the incidence of redetachment after removal of silicone oil.[16] Retinopexy prior to oil removal can help detect subclinical fluid and close occult breaks before changing the surface tension relationships of the oil–retina interface.

◆ Look for holes, tears, or subclinical retinal detachment meticulously prior to silicone oil removal; consider using a contact lens for this purpose.

◆ Consider use of an encircling band at the time of repair in complex retinal detachments. Scleral buckle encirclement seems to improve anatomic success after silicone oil removal.[3,12]

◆ Perform complete removal of the vitreous base.[12]

◆ Look for holes, tears, or subclinical retinal detachment intraoperatively immediately after silicone oil removal. Treatment of this pathology may prevent redetachment after silicone oil removal.[27]

Pearls on How to Solve It

◆ Retinal detachment after silicone oil removal is often associated with residual or secondary PVR.[24] Tangential vitreoretinal traction from new PVR or residual vitreous gel may lead to new holes or tears after silicone oil removal; thus, removal of all remaining vitreous and peeling of membrane would be advisable. In selected cases, retinectomies may be needed.

◆ Scleral buckle encirclement: Scleral buckle encirclement seems to improve anatomic success after silicone oil removal.[3,12]

◆ Careful internal search to find and treat any retinal tears/holes or suspicious lesions.

◆ 360-degree prophylactic laser retinopexy, either at the time of the retinal rede-tachment procedure or as a separate supplementary procedure, was associated with a reduction from 26% to 14% in the incidence of redetachment after removal of silicone oil and, thus, is recommended.[16]

◆ Consider performing retinectomies in cases of retinal redetachments complicated with PVR if remaining traction is still present following removal of residual vitreous and PVR membranes.[28]

◆ For most cases, tamponade with silicone oil would be recommended in cases of retinal redetachment after silicone oil removal. Consider keeping the silicone oil tamponade for longer than 6 months in these cases.[29]

Expected Outcomes: What Is the Worst-case Scenario

◆ Set visual expectations appropriately; explain to the patient that the primary goal is to save the eye and that this may require several surgeries including long-term silicone oil tamponade.

◆ Loss of only eye or loss of fellow eye due to missed pathology.

◆ Hypotony long term: Hypotony is a complex condition and can be due to ciliary body detachment, atrophy, or traction. Rarely, silicone oil removal leads to chronic hypotony with an attached retina. An estimated 10% to 16% of patients can experience hypotony after oil removal.[30,31]

◆ Phthisis

◆ Blind, painful eye

◆ Cosmetic disfigurement associated with enophthalmos

REFERENCES

1. Schwartz SD, Kreiger AE. Proliferative vitreoretinopathy: A natural history of the fellow eye. *Ophthalmology.* 1998;105(5):785–788.
2. Zhang MN, Li XY. [Long-term follow-up and prognostic analysis on the silicone oil-dependent eyes]. *Zhonghua Yan Ke Za Zhi.* 2008;44(12):1108–1111.
3. La Heij EC, Hendrikse F, Kessels AG. Results and complications of temporary silicone oil tamponade in patients with complicated retinal detachments. *Retina.* 2001;21(2):107–114.
4. Dong FT, Dai RP, Jia Y. [Clinical features of silicone oil dependent eyes]. *Zhonghua Yan Ke Za Zhi.* 2008;44(11):998–1001.
5. Hutton WL, Azen SP, Blumenkranz MS, et al. The effects of silicone oil removal. Silicone Study Report 6. *Arch Ophthalmol.* 1994;112(6):778–785.
6. Goezinne F, La Heij EC, Berendschot TT, et al. Risk factors for redetachment and worse visual outcome after silicone oil removal in eyes with complicated retinal detachment. *Eur J Ophthalmol.* 2007;17(4):627–637.
7. Zilis JD, McCuen BW 2nd, de Juan E Jr, et al. Results of silicone oil removal in advanced proliferative vitreoretinopathy. *Am J Ophthalmol.* 1989;108(1):15–21.
8. Lesnoni G, Rossi T, Nistri A, et al. Long-term prognosis after removal of silicone oil. *Eur J Ophthalmol.* 2000;10(1):60–65.
9. Jiang F, Krause M, Ruprecht KW, et al. Risk factors for anatomical success and visual outcome in patients undergoing silicone oil removal. *Eur J Ophthalmol.* 2002; 12(4):293–298.
10. Soheilian M, Mazareei M, Mohammadpour M, et al. Comparison of silicon oil removal with various viscosities after complex retinal detachment surgery. *BMC Ophthalmol.* 2006;6:21.

11. Lam RF, Cheung BT, Yuen CY, et al. Retinal redetachment after silicone oil removal in proliferative vitreoretinopathy: A prognostic factor analysis. *Am J Ophthalmol.* 2008;145(3):527–533.

12. Jonas JB, Knorr HL, Rank RM, et al. Retinal redetachment after removal of intraocular silicone oil tamponade. *Br J Ophthalmol.* 2001;85(10):1203–1207.

13. Pavlovic S, Dick B, Schmidt KG, et al. [Long-term outcome after silicone oil removal]. *Ophthalmologe.* 1995;92(5):672–676.

14. Hoing C, Kampik A, Heidenkummer HP. [Results of pars plana vitrectomy with intraocular SF-6 gas tamponade in complicated retinal detachment]. *Der Ophthalmologe: Zeitschrift der Deutschen Ophthalmologischen Gesellschaft.* 1994;91(3):312–318.

15. Joussen AM, Rizzo S, Kirchhof B, et al. Heavy silicone oil versus standard silicone oil in as vitreous tamponade in inferior PVR (HSO Study): Interim analysis. *Acta Ophthalmol.* 2011;89(6):e483–e489.

16. Laidlaw DA, Karia N, Bunce C, et al. Is prophylactic 360-degree laser retinopexy protective? Risk factors for retinal redetachment after removal of silicone oil. *Ophthalmology.* 2002;109(1):153–158.

17. Quiram PA, Gonzales CR, Hu W, et al. Outcomes of vitrectomy with inferior retinectomy in patients with recurrent rhegmatogenous retinal detachments and proliferative vitreoretinopathy. *Ophthalmology.* 2006;113(11):2041–2047.

18. Gonzales CR, Gupta A, Schwartz SD, et al. The fellow eye of patients with rhegmatogenous retinal detachment. *Ophthalmology.* 2004;111(3):518–521.

19. Kim SW, Oh J, Yang KS, et al. Risk factors for the development of transient hypotony after silicone oil removal. *Retina.* 2010;30(8):1228–1236.

20. Newsom RS, Johnston R, Sullivan PM, et al. Sudden visual loss after removal of silicone oil. *Retina.* 2004;24(6):871–877.

21. Cazabon S, Groenewald C, Pearce IA, et al. Visual loss following removal of intraocular silicone oil. *Br J Ophthalmol.* 2005;89(7):799–802.

22. Dabil H, Akduman L, Olk RJ, et al. Comparison of silicone oil removal with passive drainage alone versus passive drainage combined with air-fluid exchange. *Retina.* 2002;22(5):597–601.

23. Scholda CD, Egger SF, Lakits A, et al. In vitro effectiveness of silicone oil removal. *Acta Ophthalmol Scand.* 1998;76(2):192–195.

24. Halberstadt M, Domig D, Kodjikian L, et al. PVR recurrence and the timing of silicon oil removal. *Klin Monbl Augenheilkd.* 2006;223(5):361–366.

25. Lewis H, Burke JM, Abrams GW, et al. Perisilicone proliferation after vitrectomy for proliferative vitreoretinopathy. *Ophthalmology.* 1988;95(5):583–591.

26. Tufail A, Schwartz SD, Gregor ZJ. Prophylactic argon laser retinopexy prior to removal of silicone oil: A pilot study. *Eye (Lond).* 1997;11(pt 3):328–330.

27. Herbert EN, Williamson TH. Combined removal of silicone oil plus internal search (ROSO-plus) following retinal detachment surgery. *Eye (Lond).* 2007;21(7):925–929.

28. Tsui I, Schubert HD. Retinotomy and silicone oil for detachments complicated by anterior inferior proliferative vitreoretinopathy. *Br J Ophthalmol.* 2009;93(9):1228–1233.

29. Hoing C, Kampik A, Heidenkummer HP. [Possibilities of silicone oil removal after complex vitreoretinal surgery]. *Fortschr Ophthalmol.* 1991;88(6):593–597.

30. Casswell AG, Gregor ZJ. Silicone oil removal. II. Operative and postoperative complications. *Br J Ophthalmol.* 1987;71(12):898–902.

31. Wesolek-Czernik A. [The influence of silicone oil removal on intraocular pressure]. *Klin Oczna.* 2002;104(3–4):219–221.

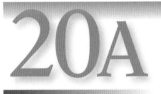

COMPLICATIONS FOLLOWING PHACO-VITRECTOMY

20A Posterior Capsule Opacification Following Phaco-Vitrectomy

KAZUAKI KADONOSONO

⬥ The Complication: Definition

Performance of vitrectomy in combination with cataract surgery has been recently come to be widely accepted because it has the advantages of avoiding nuclear cataract formation as a postoperative complication, enables a clear view of the fundus during vitrectomy, has an economical benefit for patients and may be more convenient for them, and, finally, reduces surgical costs.[1] Posterior capsule opacification (PCO) is a major complication after phacoemulsification and implantation of an intraocular lens (IOL).[2,3] The incidence of PCO after cataract surgery is reported to be approximately 11% at 1 year, and increase to 30% by 5 years.[3,4] Since postoperative inflammation may be more severe after phaco-vitrectomy than after cataract surgery alone, the incidence and severity of PCO may be greater in eyes on which simultaneous surgery has been performed[5,6]; PCO is a still major problem after vitrectomy combined with cataract surgery as well as after cataract surgery alone.[5]

PCO after phaco-vitrectomy has two major disadvantages.[2,3] The first major disadvantage is the visual impairment caused by PCO. PCO can impair vision significantly, not only by causing a marked decrease in visual acuity, but also by impairing contrast sensitivity, glare disability, and monocular diplopia. PCO is the most common long-term complication of phaco-vitrectomy. The second major disadvantage of PCO after phaco-vitrectomy is that it reduces the visibility of the fundus. PCO may prevent physicians from being able to examine the macula as well as the peripheral retina. Since it is important to maintain clear visualization of the fundus in patients with vitreoretinal diseases, PCO is sometimes a more serious complication after vitrectomy combined with cataract surgery than after cataract surgery alone.

⬥ Risk Factors

Diabetes. PCO following phaco-vitrectomy is associated with postoperative inflammation. Diabetic patients have more extensive PCO after vitrectomy combined with cataract surgery than nondiabetic patients.[6] Some reports have shown a significantly higher incidence of PCO in diabetic patients at 3, 6, and 12 months postoperatively than in nondiabetic patients, and diabetic patients should be carefully monitored for the development of postoperative PCO.[6,7] Patients with proliferative diabetic retinopathy (PDR) often have cataracts, which are strongly associated with their diabetes mellitus, and vitrectomy combined with cataract surgery may be performed in these patients. Since diabetic PDR patients have an associated breakdown of the blood–aqueous barrier and blood–retinal barrier, severe postoperative inflammation is observed in them after phaco-vitrectomy, which is often seen as fibrin formation.[7] On the other hand, when panretinal photocoagulation has been performed in diabetic patients, there appears to be less inflammation after surgery than in diabetic patients in whom photocoagulation has not been performed.[3] The hemoglobin A1c in diabetic patients is also associated with the progression of PCO.[7] Patients with extremely high serum HbA1c values, above 10%, may develop severe postoperative inflammation that causes PCO.

Proliferative vitreoretinopathy (PVR). Patients with PVR may develop severe postoperative PCO. Since some may have further increased preoperative inflammation due to the presence of choroidal detachment, combined surgery may have an impact on increasing inflammation further.

Type of surgery performed. Microincision 23G, 25G, and 27G vitrectomy have become popular recently, and have the advantage of causing less postoperative inflammation.[8,9] An experimental study showed that the postoperative inflammation is less in 25G vitrectomy than 20G vitrectomy, and a meta-analysis showed that small-gauge vitrectomy has the benefits of more rapid healing, less discomfort, and milder ocular inflammation.[10] Since the incidence of PCO can be caused by ocular inflammation,[2,3] it is postulated that the incidence of PCO is lower after microincision vitrectomy surgery.

Posturing following the vitreoretinal procedure. Face-down positioning is very often prescribed after vitreoretinal surgery. The duration of face-down positioning may have an impact on the incidence of PCO. Many factors, including cytokine IL-2, inflammatory cells, that is, macrophages, are able to come into contact with the lens capsule while the patient's head is in the face-down position which may facilitate the development of PCO.

Other factors. The incidence of postoperative PCO is higher in eyes with pre-existing inflammation, for example, in eyes with uveitis, eyes that have been subjected to trauma, and eyes with atopic dermatitis.[3,4]

✤ Pathogenesis

The pathogenesis of PCO after phaco-vitrectomy is likely to be similar to that following cataract surgery. In the latter, lens epithelial cells (LECs) left behind in the capsular bag following lens extraction are mainly responsible for the development of PCO. PCO is thought to represent a wound-healing response to the opening of the capsular bag and removal of the lens fibers. Factors involved in the development of PCO include proliferation, migration, and epithelial-to-mesenchymal transition of LEC, collagen deposition, and lens fiber regenerations.[3] There are two types of PCO, a fibrosis type and a pearl type **(Fig. 20A-1)**. The fibrosis type causes severe visual impairment; in this LECs undergo an epithelial-to-mesenchymal transition to create fibrous metaplasia. The clinical findings are a whitened appearance and formation of folds and wrinkles in the posterior capsule. Pearl-type PCO is caused by LECs located in the equatorial lens region causing regeneration of crystalline-expressing lenticular fibers and forming Elschnig pearls and Soemmering's ring, thereby causing, if affecting the visual axis, severer visual loss than the fibrosis type.

After phaco-vitrectomy it is postulated that, in addition, cytokines and growth factors as well as astrocytes/fibroblasts/myofibroblasts present in the posterior segment and related to the vitreoretinal condition and/or elicited by the posterior segment surgery itself may migrate anteriorly and increase the incidence of PCO.[3] Cytokines and growth factors include transforming growth factor β, fibroblast growth factor 2 (FGF-2), hepatocyte growth factor, interleukins 1 and 6 (IL-1 and IL-6), and epithelial growth factor among others. Transforming growth factor β seems to play an important role in the pathogenesis of PCO.[11] FGF-2 has an important role in the

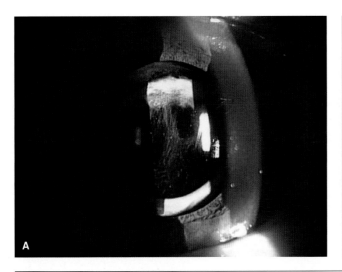
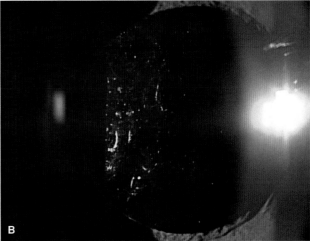

Figure 20A-1 The picture of posterior capsular opacification types. This is a picture of fibrous type **(A)** of PCOs after vitrectomy combined with cataract surgery for the eye with PDR. This type is more popular in PCO after phaco-vitrectomy, which often also have anterior capsular opacification, than pearl type **(B)** of PCO.

proliferation, migration, and fiber differentiation of normal LECs, which contribute to the development of PCOs. Matrix metalloproteinases are a group of proteolytic enzymes that are essential for cell migration and cell-mediated contraction during wound healing, and the changes in lens capsule structure during PCO development may include remodeling of the extracellular matrix by matrix metalloproteinases.

 Pearls on How to Prevent It

PCO after Phaco-vitrectomy

Surgical Technique

◆ Primary posterior capsulotomy with a 25G vitreous cutter is a useful and simple surgical technique when vitrectomy is combined with cataract surgery[12] **(Fig. 20A-2)**. It is advisable to undertake primary posterior capsulotomy at the end of the vitrectomy rather than at the beginning of it, because the posterior capsule should be preserved to keep the IOL well positioned during the surgery.

◆ Our usual procedure is described as follows. After the vitrectomy is completed but before implantation of the IOL, an ophthalmic viscosurgical device (OVD, viscoelastic, Healon) is inserted into the anterior chamber and capsular bag, and a foldable acrylic IOL having a 6-mm-round optic is implanted in the capsular bag. The posterior capsule is then removed from the center toward the periphery with a 25G vitreous cutter. A pars plana approach makes it possible to remove a well-centered posterior capsule having a diameter of approximately 5 mm.

◆ Finally, the OVD is gently removed with irrigation/aspiration. This surgical technique is an easy technique to afford the stabilization of vision after surgery, and to allow better visualization of the retinal fundus during examinations. This planned posterior capsulotomy can be performed in any eye undergoing phaco-vitrectomy. In gas-filled eyes tilt or dislocation of IOL is rarely seen postoperatively after complete disappearance of intraocular gas.

IOL Materials and Designs

◆ There are strong associations between IOL designs and the incidence of PCO. There have been many advances in IOL design, and they have reduced the inci-

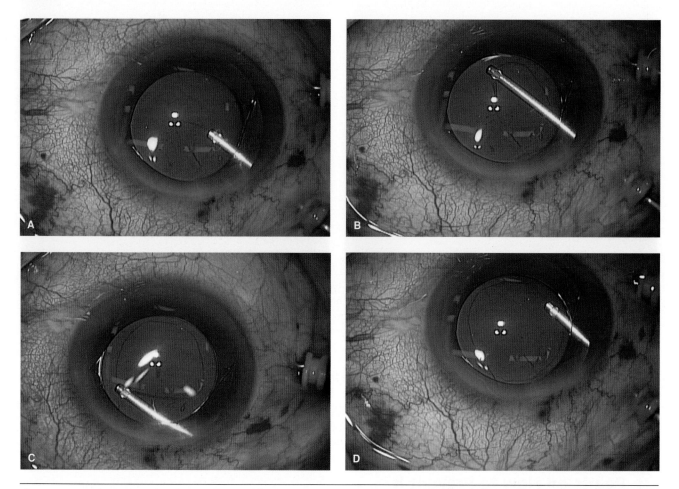

Figure 20A-2 The technique of posterior capsular membranectomy. This is a procedure of posterior capsulotomy during vitrectomy. After vitrectomy and the intraocular lens implantation performed, 25-gauge cutter is inserted into the vitreous cavity to cut the posterior capsular membrane (**20A-2A**), and the posterior capsular membrane is removed along the edge of IOL (**20A-2B and 20A-2C**). Finally IOL is tightly positioned without posterior capsular membrane in its optic area (**20A-2D**).

dence of PCO. A greater preventive effect against PCO has been observed with IOLs that provide a mechanical barrier effect on the posterior lens capsule. The sharp-edge optic IOL and the formation of a capsular bend are highly effective in reducing PCO.[13,14] Adhesion of the IOL material to the lens capsule also plays a role in preventing PCO by creating a sharp capsular bend, which inhibits LEC migration onto the posterior capsule. Contact inhibition of migrating LECs is induced at the capsular bend, which leads to PCO prevention.

◆ The material of which the IOL is made may have an effect on PCO development. IOLs are made of two types of material: Acrylic and silicone. Since IOLs made of silicone have moist drops during fluid–gas exchange, and the drops impair visibility of the fundus, IOLs made of acrylic materials are most suitable for the phaco-vitrectomy. Although hydrophilic acrylic materials are more biocompatible, IOLs made of hydrophilic acrylic material have been shown to promote LEC adhesion, migration, and proliferation. Modification of the IOL surface is also an effective method of preventing PCO.

◆ In a recent systematic review of the literature, Findl et al.[15] found a statistically significant lower PCO score and YAG rates in sharp-edged compared with round-edged IOLs, but no statistically significant differences between one-piece and three-piece IOLs. There was no statistically significant difference in PCO development among the different IOL materials (Polymethylmethacrylate (PMMA), hydrogel, hydrophobic acrylic, silicone), although hydrogel IOLs tended to have higher PCO scores and silicone IOLs lower PCO scores than the other materials, or among different types of intraoperative/postoperative anti-inflammatory treatments with the exception of treatment with an immunotoxin which led to a statistically significantly lower rate of PCO.[15]

◆ It has been suggested that the IOL size may be important in the development of PCO. IOLs having a large optic size of 7 mm have some advantages in eyes undergoing phaco-vitrectomy **(Fig. 20A-3)** (see also Chapter 20B). There is a

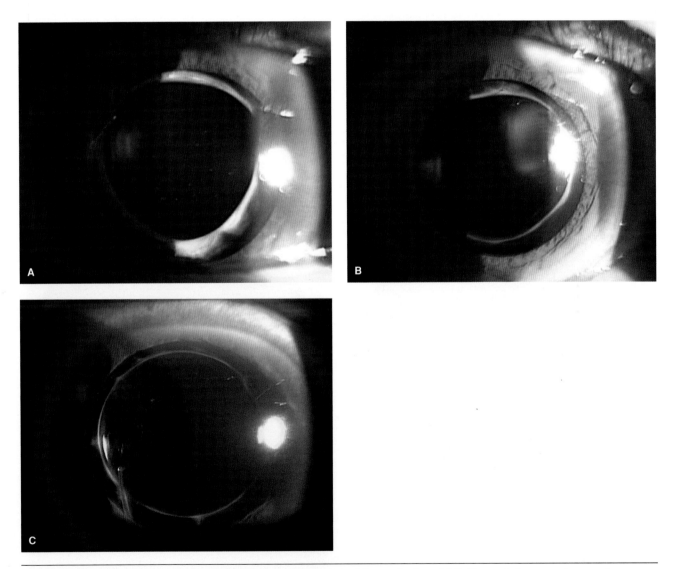

Figure 20A-3 The anterior capsular membrane opacification and the optic size of IOL. The anterior capsular membrane opacification due to fibrosis is associated with the IOL optic size. The smallest optic size IOL (5.5 mm, **A**) has the largest anterior capsular fibrosis, while the middle size IOL (6 mm, **B**) has the moderate fibrosis and the largest optic size IOL (7 mm, **C**) has the least anterior capsular fibrosis.

lower incidence of decentered IOLs which may occur as a result of the presence of a tamponade agent and head posturing following implantation of IOLs having a larger optic size than IOL with a smaller optic size.[16] A larger IOL will allow a larger capsulorrhexis to be made still maintaining the optic of the IOL under the anterior capsule; this may reduce PCO and, additionally, may reduce also the area of anterior capsule opacification which, on its turn, will allow better visualization of the fundus postoperatively **(Fig. 20A-4)**.

⬥ Pearls on How to Solve It

Nd:YAG Laser

◆ The neodymium-doped yttrium aluminum garnet (Nd:YAG) laser is the only effective treatment for PCO and involves clearing the visual axis by creating a central opening in the opacified posterior capsule. This procedure may lead to complications, including retinal detachment, damage to the IOL, cystoid macular edema, an increase in intraocular pressure, iris hemorrhage, and floaters. It is not clear whether the complications observed following Nd:YAG laser in nonvitrectomized eyes may also occur in eyes that had previously undergone vitrectomy surgery. The vitreous traction is likely to occur in some eyes with YAG laser, and then may be a main cause of post-YAG laser complications as described earlier.[17]

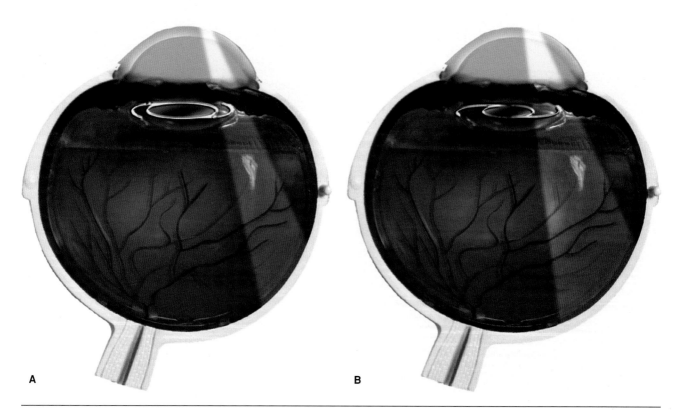

A   B

Figure 20A-4 The size of IOL optic and the fundus visibility. Since the light passing through the optic edge has a different reflection from the optics of IOL, the images obtained during vitrectomy in the area outside the optics are damaged. This obscured image is less in the large optic size IOL **(A)** than in the small optic size IOL **(B)**. The large optic size IOL has the less obscured visibility caused by the IOL edge than the small optic size IOL.

◆ Some patients who have undergone phaco-vitrectomy for PDR or PVR may have such a tough posterior capsular membrane that the YAG laser is ineffective. In such cases, primary posterior capsule membranectomy is very helpful in order to avoid the complications caused by the high-power YAG laser. For eyes with thickened posterior capsule membrane, posterior capsule membranectomy can be achieved using the vitreous cutter, using lower cutting rates and high vacuum. If this technique does not allow to create an adequate opening in the posterior capsule then vitrectomy scissors may be used for this purpose.

✛ Expected Outcomes

PCO after phaco-vitrectomy can be successfully managed, in most cases, by using the methods described above. If untreated, PCO following phaco-vitrectomy may thicken severely the posterior capsule leading to patient's impaired visual function and a poor view of the posterior segment structures.

REFERENCES

1. Chang MA, Parides MK, Chang S, et al. Outcome of phacoemulsificaiton after pars plana vitrectomy. *Ophthalmology.* 2002;109:948–954.
2. Apple DJ, Solomon KD, Tetz MR, et al. Posterior capsule opacification. *Surv Ophthalmol.* 1992;37:73–116.
3. Awasthi N, Guo S, Wagner BJ. Posterior capsular opacification. *Arch Ophthalmol.* 2009;127:555–562.
4. Schaumberg DA, Dana MR, Christen WG, et al. A systematic overview of the incidence of posterior capsule opacification. *Ophthalmology.* 1998;105:1213–1221.
5. Roh JH, Sohn HJ, Lee DY, et al. Comparison of posterior capsular opacification between a combined procedure and a sequential procedure of pars plana vitrectomy and cataract surgery. *Ophthalmologica.* 2010;224:42–46.
6. Toda J, Kato S, Oshika T, et al. Posterior capsule opacification after combined cataract surgery and vitrectomy. *J Cataract Refract Surg.* 2007;33:104–107.
7. Ebihara Y, Kato S, Oshika T, et al. Posterior capsule opacification after cataract surgery in patients with diabetic mellitus. *J Cataract Refract Surg.* 2006;32:1184–1187.
8. Recchia FM, Scott IU, Brown GC, et al. Small-gauge pars plana vitrectomy: A report by the American Academy of Ophthalmology. *Ophthalmology.* 2010;117:1851–1857.
9. Oshima Y, Wakabayashi T, Sato T. A 27-gauge instrument system for transconjunctival sutureless microincision vitrectomy surgery. *Ophthalmology.* 2010;117:93–102.
10. Inoue Y, Kadonosono K, Yamakawa T, et al. Surgically-induced inflammation with 20-, 23-, and 25-gauge vitrectomy systems: An experimental study. *Retina.* 2009;29:477–478.
11. Kurosaka D, Nagamoto T. Inhibitory effect of TGF-beta 2 in human aqueous humor on bovine lens epithelial cell proliferation. *Invest Ophthalmol Vis Sci.* 1994;35:3408–3412.
12. Sato S, Inoue M, Kobayashi S, et al. Primary posterior capsulotomy using a 25-gauge vitreous cutter in vitrectomy combined with cataract surgery. *J Caratact Refract Surg.* 2010;36:2–5.
13. Sugita M, Kato S, Sugita G, et al. Migration of lens epithelial cells through haptic root of single-piece acrylic-foldable intraocular lens. *Am J Ophthalml.* 2004;137:377–379.
14. Menapace R. Posterior capsulorhexis combined with optic buttonholing: An alternative to standard in-the-bag implantation of sharp-edged intraocular lenses? A critical analysis of 1000 consecutive cases. *Graefes Arch Clin Exp Ophthalmol.* 2008;246:787–801.

15. Findl O, Buehl W, Bauer P, et al. Interventions for preventing posterior capsule opacification. *Cochrane Database Syst Rev.* 2010;(2):CD003738.

16. McDonnell PJ, Spalton DJ, Falcon MG. Decentration of the posterior chamber lens implant: The effect of optic size on the incidence of visual aberrations. *Eye (Lond).* 1990;4:132–137.

17. Georgalas I, Petrou P, Kalantzis G, et al. Nd: YAG capsulotomy for posterior capsule opacification after combined clear corneal phacoemulsification and vitrectomy. *Ther Clin Risk Manag.* 2009;5(1):133–137.

20B Intraocular Lens Decentration/Luxation/Subluxation

WENSHENG LI, PEI JIAN MIAO, AND QINXIANG ZHENG

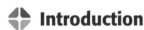

Introduction

The practice of combining phacoemulsification and intraocular lens (IOL) implantation with pars plana vitrectomy (PPV) in eyes with signification cataract and coexisting vitreoretinal diseases is becoming increasingly common. There have been some reports supporting combined vitreoretinal surgery and phacoemulsification with foldable IOL implantation as a safe and effective method of treating vitreoretinal abnormalities coexisting with cataract.[1–3] The key issue of providing sufficient IOL stability in the capsular bag appears to be of outstanding importance when cataract surgery is combined with PPV. IOL decentration or dislocation may appear intraoperatively as a result of the additional surgical stress on the capsular bag and zonular fibers during vitrectomy, or postoperatively, as a result of the increased inflammation and zonular stress from the additional vitrectomy procedure.[4,5] The first case of spontaneous in-the-bag IOL dislocation was reported by Yasuda et al.,[6] following a triple procedure of vitrectomy, phacoemulsification, and IOL implantation. Decentration/luxation/subluxation of posterior chamber (PC) IOL can occur after combined phacoemulsification and vitrectomy surgery; the approximate incidence ranges between 1.3% and 6.3%,[2,4] but the exact incidence of this complication is not known.

The Complication: Definition

IOL malpositions range from simple IOL decentration to luxation into the posterior segment. Decentration of an IOL may be the result of the original surgical placement of the lens, or it may develop in the postoperative period because of external (e.g., trauma, eye rubbing) or internal forces (e.g., scarring, peripheral anterior synechiae, capsular contraction, Soemmering's ring formation, size disparity). The design of the lens optic also influences the risk of visually significant decentration. An increase in the optical diameter of an implant from 6 to 7 mm will increase the surface area by more than 36%. Lenses are available with positioning holes outside the optical area to increase the effective optical zone further. In one group of pseudophakic patients, dialing holes were seen in the scotopic pupil in 37% of patients with a 6-mm lens optic and in 3% with a 7-mm optic[7] **(Fig. 20B-1).** Subluxated IOLs

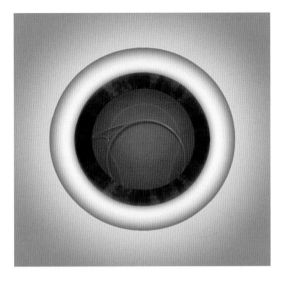

Figure 20B-1 Decentration of an IOL.

involve such extreme decentration that the IOL optic covers only a small fraction of the pupillary space **(Fig. 20B-2)**. Luxation involves total dislocation of the IOL into the posterior segment or anterior segment too **(Fig. 20B-3)**. Posterior dislocation of an IOL is an uncommon complication of combining phacoemulsification and IOL implantation with PPV.

Symptoms

The most commonly presenting complaint of a decentered IOL is unwanted optical images caused by the edge of the optic within the pupil.

- ◆ Patients may complain of decreased vision, edge glare, diplopia, streaks of light, haloes, photosensitivity, and ghost images.

- ◆ A sudden loss of vision due to uncorrected aphakia, retinal detachment, cystoid macular edema, or vitreous hemorrhage occurs with a dislocated IOL. If the IOL is mobile in the vitreous cavity, the patient may complain of unusual floaters or optical effects.

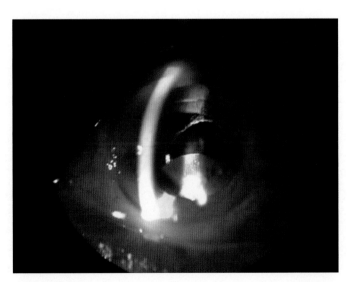

Figure 20B-2 Subluxation of an IOL.

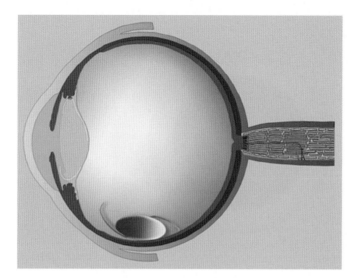

Figure 20B-3 Luxation of an IOL.

Signs

◆ Visual acuity can be compromised by optical aberrations and refractive changes. Slit lamp examination usually does not reveal evidence of inflammation unless contact of a portion of the IOL with the cornea or vitreous prolapse is present.

◆ Corneal edema from IOL or vitreous touch can be found. In these cases, cystoid macular edema (CME) may be a complication.

◆ Vitreous traction can increase the risk of a retinal detachment, while vitreous to the wound can be implicated in endophthalmitis.

◆ The posterior capsule usually has an obvious defect.

◆ Zonulodialysis may be present.

◆ The IOL may be freely mobile in the vitreous cavity; it may be in apparent contact with the retina or it may have one haptic attached to the posterior capsule, iris, or ciliary body.

Risk Factors

The pathogenesis of IOL malposition may be related to a variety of locations of haptic fixation, to the forces of capsular contraction, or to a combined mechanism.[8]

◆ Asymmetric haptic placement: Before the development of capsulorrhexis, it was common for the surgeon to place the inferior IOL haptic within the capsule, while releasing the superior haptic into the ciliary sulcus producing asymmetric haptic fixation.

◆ Inadequate zonular or capsular support: This can be due to posterior capsular rupture or zonular dialysis both of which are more prevalent in patients with pseudoexfoliation.

◆ Capsular contraction syndrome: Capsulorrhexis is a major surgical advance that contributes to long-term IOL stability and centration. Despite an intact capsulorrhexis, IOL decentration may still occur due to capsular contraction syndrome.

◆ Capsular fusion: An eccentric capsulorrhexis may allow one of its edges to be more peripheral than the optic in one area, with fusion developing, producing decentration away from the area of contact. A large symmetric, round, central capsulorrhexis is recommended to reduce significant decentration (see also pearls on how to prevent it later).

♦ Postoperative trauma: In general, the main cause of dislocation is lack of capsular support for the IOL. This may be caused by any of the following:

♦ Unrecognized posterior capsule rupture

♦ Progressive zonular dehiscence: Patients with pseudoexfoliation syndrome are at risk of developing zonular dehiscence.

◈ Pathogenesis: Why Does It Occur

IOL dislocation can be subdivided into early and late dislocation. Early dislocation refers to dislocation occurring within 3 months of combined surgery, whereas late dislocation occurs more than 3 months after combined surgery.

Posterior dislocation of an IOL may occur during or shortly after combined surgery. In these cases, posterior capsular rupture or zonular dialysis usually is present. It occurs because of improper fixation within the capsular bag and instability of the IOL–capsular bag complex.[9] The implementation of a continuous curvilinear capsulorrhexis (CCC) during phacoemulsification has decreased the rate of early IOL dislocation. CCC gives support to the IOL optic for 360 degrees and permits excellent IOL fixation. Prior to CCC, most IOL dislocation occurred secondary to asymmetric IOL fixation or IOL malposition within the capsular bag. Rarely, it may occur following neodymium-doped yttrium aluminum garnet (Nd:YAG) capsulotomy or beyond the immediate postoperative period. Trauma may be a precipitant in these cases.

Late IOL dislocation has been noted to occur more frequently than previously thought.[10] Late IOL dislocation results from zonular weakness since the IOL is adequately fixed within the capsular bag. Several risk factors, including pseudoexfoliation syndrome, trauma, prior vitreoretinal surgery, and connective tissue disorders, have been associated with zonular weakness. In a retrospective case series of 86 late IOL dislocations, the IOL dislocated on average 8.5 years after phacoemulsification and IOL implantation. These same authors reported that patients with any type of IOL were at risk for late in-the-bag IOL dislocation.[11]

The IOL rarely dislocates completely onto the retinal surface. It usually lies meshed into the anterior vitreous with one haptic still adherent to the capsule or iris. It may cause a vitreous hemorrhage by mechanical contact with ciliary body vessels. The dislocated IOL may lead to retinal detachment or cystoid macular edema secondary to vitreous changes and may cause pupillary block or corneal contact with secondary corneal edema. On many occasions, it does not cause any complications and may be left alone if the patient is able to use aphakic spectacles or contact lenses.

After a thorough vitrectomy with sclera depression, however, there may be nothing left to support the IOL in the capsular bag, except some of the zonules, because of damage to the anterior hyaloid membrane and the posterior zonules. Also, chronic centripetal traction caused by capsular contraction may trigger dialysis of the remaining zonules. Grusha et al.[12] reported cases of weakness or dialysis of the zonules during phacoemulsification and IOL implantation after vitrectomy. In addition, pathophysiologic effects of vitrectomy on the capsule and zonules may exist, as well as possible pathology in the zonules, in patients with diabetes mellitus. We recognize that the anterior hyaloid membrane and posterior zonules are important to maintain the long-term stability of the IOL; however, the anterior hyaloid may serve also as scaffold for the development of anterior proliferative vitreoretinopathy. Therefore, the anterior hyaloid membrane should be left in place in patients at low risk for the development of postoperative anterior proliferation. Introduction of trocars through the overlying sclera and pars plana likely traumatizes zonules at their insertion. Port manipulation throughout the vitreoretinal procedure likely continues the mechanical trauma initiated by the introduction of trocars. Because of the geometry of the zonular apparatus, focal surgical disruption of zonules unevenly distributes the increased stress on the remaining intact zonules. Other factors such as the energy of the vitrector delivered indirectly to the zonules, intraoperative and postoperative pressure changes within the globe, and postoperative inflammation also may contribute to the zonular insufficiency.

◆ Pearls on How to Prevent It

The recognition of predisposing factors for this complication suggests a modified approach in cases at risk. Several measures to prevent bag dislocation have been suggested.[13]

◆ The CCC diameter should be smaller than the optic,[14] but a particularly small opening should be avoided.[11,15]

◆ During surgery, particular attention should be paid to preserving the integrity of zonules and capsule bag. This may be technically difficult in eyes with pseudo-exfoliation due to the small pupil, poor resistance by the zonules, and possible lens subluxation. Once the CCC is not intact and has extended, but when the PC remains intact and then when the IOL is placed, one haptic comes out of the bag while the other remains in the bag, if the capsule tear is less than half of the whole capsule, we can implant the IOL in the capsular bag by rotating the other loop; conversely, if the capsule tear is more than half or even three-quarters of the whole capsule, we can implant the IOL in the ciliary sulcus by rotating the other loop.

◆ IOL material and design may affect capsule contraction and IOL dislocation. Single-piece poly (methyl methacrylate) (PMMA) IOLs may counteract capsule shrinkage better than three-piece PMMA IOLs.[16,17] It has also been suggested that a three-piece hydrophobic acrylic IOL may reduce CCC contraction through a combination of decreased anterior capsule fibrosis and greater haptic rigidity.[15,18] Several recent reports support that one-piece acrylic IOLs may induce more capsule contraction or offer less haptic resistance to contraction than three-piece acrylic lenses.[19,20] It is clear that plate-haptic silicone IOLs induce the most capsulorrhexis contracture, suggesting they may be contraindicated in high-risk cases.[18]

◆ Subluxation can also occur as a result of the use of wrong type of IOL, for example, the one-piece acrylic lenses are meant for placement in the bag. When surgeons encounter complications, they sometimes continue to use these lenses because they are foldable. Their overall diameter is such that they are not stable in the sulcus and sublux inferiorly. Under this situation, a wrong IOL must be exchanged. The wrong IOL may be removed through the pars plana or through a limbal incision at the surgeon's discretion. But pars plana removal increases the risk of retinal detachment and severe choroidal bleeding.

◆ Capsular tension rings (CTRs) are indicated in cases in which there is zonular rupture or dehiscence after blunt or surgical trauma or in cases of inherently weak zonules, as in pseudoexfoliation.[21–23] Eyes with zonular dehiscence or weakness are at greater risk for developing asymmetrical capsule shrinkage and dislocation because the remaining zonules cannot resist the centripetal forces exerted by the anterior capsule rim.[24] However, in cases in which the extent of zonular dehiscence is limited (≤1/3 or 1/4), phacoemulsification with CTR insertion followed by PPV and gas tamponade may provide an alternative surgical option. This approach has the advantage of preserving the zonular and capsular complex for endocapsular phacoemulsification and implantation of the IOL within the capsular bag. CTR also strengthened the zonular and capsular complex for intravitreal gas tamponade during and after

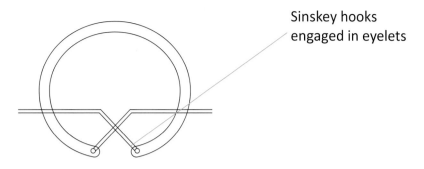

Sinskey hooks
engaged in eyelets

Figure 20B-4 CTR being "tire-ironed" into the capsular bag.

surgery. The presence of a CTR inside the capsular bag may help to redistribute the prevailing forces so that it becomes more difficult for air or gas to escape from the vitreous cavity into the anterior chamber (AC). Our experiences showed that combined phacoemulsification with CTR insertion followed by PPV with or without gas tamponade is a feasible surgical option for managing patients with limited zonular dehiscence who require combined cataract and vitreoretinal surgery.

There are CTRs with loops and hooks that can be used to suture the IOL back to its proper position. The CTR can be inserted through tunnel or paracentesis with forceps or by injectors. A CTR inserter consists of a spring-loaded plunger assembly with a hook at its distal end. The easiest way to manipulate a CTR is by using MacPherson forceps or a Sinskey hook. In profound zonular weakness, a CTR should not be dialed into the capsular bag. In such cases, the leading fixation hole is positioned at its desired location and then "tire-ironed" **(Fig. 20B-4)** into the capsular bag. For localized zonular dehiscence, a CTR should be positioned so that the body of the ring is coincident with the weakened zonular fibers. In profound zonular weakness, the modified ring by Cionni can be sutured to the scleral wall. Preplaced 10-0 prolene suture is taken through the eyelet. Each of the two needles is then placed through the incision and diverted over the area of maximum zonular dialysis to exit through the ciliary sulcus and scleral wall, once corresponding sclera flaps have been prepared. The ring is then inserted in the capsular bag and the fixating element captures itself anterior to the residual anterior capsular rim **(Fig. 20B-5)**.

◆ Alternative IOL fixation sites have also been proposed as a preventive measure to IOL dislocation in patients with pseudoexfoliation. Implantation of the IOL in

10-0 prolene taken through eyelets

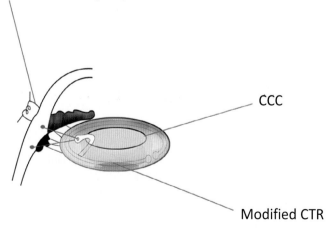

CCC

Modified CTR

Figure 20B-5 Modified CTR by Cionni sutured to the sclera wall.

the ciliary sulcus, transscleral fixation, and primary implantation of an AC-IOL have been advocated.[25,26] Alternative implantation sites should be considered in patients who have compromised zonules at the time of surgery. Finally, to avoid dislocation of the IOL into the vitreous after PPV, the preservation of the anterior hyaloid membrane has been advocated.[6]

Pearls on How to Solve It

Selection of treatment in the case of a decentered IOL should be based on the patient's symptoms, needs, and expectations.

Observe

In the absence of symptoms and no evidence of inflammatory sequelae observation is an option. In the case of an IOL associated with a peaked or oval pupil, careful observation is warranted if there are no signs or symptoms of intraocular inflammation.

Observation may be recommended in dislocated IOLs if the following conditions are met:

◆ The IOL is not mobile.

◆ There are no retinal complications.

◆ The patient is satisfied with aphakic spectacle correction or contact lenses.

Medical Treatment

If symptoms from a decentered PC-IOL are infrequent and limited to evening, due to a dilated pupil, these patients may be treated conservatively by using a topical miotic such as pilocarpine 0.5% to 1%. A trial of miotic agents may be warranted before removing or repositioning an implant.

Surgical treatment

When more severe and disabling symptoms are present or if inflammation occurs with the potential for further complications in the future, treatment should include either repositioning, explanting, or exchanging the decentered IOL. Selection of treatment is based on the patient's symptoms, visual needs, and expectations, and an assessment of which option is likely to provide the best long-term benefit with the least risk.

IOL reposition

An IOL may become decentered due to either insufficient zonular support or irregular fibrosis of the posterior capsule or Soemmering's ring formation. In the case of inadequate support, early in the postoperative period the surgeon may attempt to rotate the IOL surgically where there is clinical evidence of sufficient capsule and zonules to support the implant.

IOL explantation

Certain circumstances warrant removal of an IOL without secondary IOL implantation. This is determined on an individual basis and by taking into account the patient's expectations.

IOL exchange

The most common indications for removal or exchange of a modern PC-IOL are wrong IOL power and malposition. Deformation of the implant due to irregular capsular fibrosis may make simple rotation insufficient to properly center the IOL. The IOL may be exchanged for an AC-IOL, a sulcus-fixated IOL with or without McCannel sutures, a transsclerally sutured PC-IOL, or an iris-claw IOL.

Under certain situations, an IOL must be exchanged. For instance, if the dislocated IOL is damaged (i.e., broken haptic), it must be removed. The damaged IOL may be removed through the pars plana or through a limbal incision at the surgeon's discretion. Pars plana removal increases the risk of retinal detachment and severe choroidal bleeding. The surgeon has the choice of suturing a posterior IOL or inserting an AC-IOL[27] or an iris-claw IOL? Modern flexible open-loop AC-IOLs do not appear to result in the complications seen with older types (i.e., corneal decompensation, uveitis–glaucoma–hyphema syndrome). Another option is to manipulate the dislocated IOL into the AC and leave it there. Potential drawbacks of this option are endothelial cell and trabecular meshwork damage. This technique works well with three-piece PMMA IOLS but requires a peripheral iridectomy to prevent pupillary block. Perfluorocarbon liquids are very useful if a retinal detachment is also present.[28] The perfluorocarbon liquid bubble displaces the subretinal fluid through the retinal breaks reattaching the retina and, at the same time, serves as a cushion between the IOL and the retina. Thus, the retina is protected from potential damage from IOL impact during surgical manipulation.

Expected Outcomes: What Is the Worst-case Scenario

Complications from a decentered IOL

Complications associated with AC-IOL, iris-fixated IOLs, and older PC-IOLs are much more severe than those encountered with modern PC-IOL decentration. Corneal edema and inflammatory consequences such as uveitis–glaucoma–hyphema syndrome and chronic CME were common reasons for explantation in the above cases.

Complications from a dislocated IOL

◆ Vitreous hemorrhage

◆ Retinal detachment has been estimated to occur in at least 2% of cases. It is frequently caused by attempts at relocation by the cataract surgeon or as a complication of vitreoretinal surgery.

◆ Cystoid macular edema

◆ Uncorrected aphakia, glare, or distortion

Complications from transscleral suture fixation

◆ Late endophthalmitis through the suture track has been reported.

◆ IOL torque may occur. In addition, to place the IOL truly in the sulcus, the suture must be placed about 1 mm posterior to the limbus in the vertical meridian and about 0.5 mm in the horizontal meridian. The effective lens power is probably less than the desired one.

◆ Vitreous hemorrhage may occur if the major arterial circle of the iris is pierced inadvertently during the maneuvers required to suture the IOL. In addition, these maneuvers also may raise the risk of a postoperative retinal detachment.

REFERENCES

1. Treumer F, Bunse A, Rudolf M, et al. Pars plana vitrectomy, phacoemulsification and intraocular lens implantation. Comparison of clinical complications in a combined versus two-step surgical approach. *Graefes Arch Clin Exp Ophthalmol.* 2006;244(7):808–815.
2. Li W, Sun G, Wu R, et al. Longterm results after phacovitrectomy and foldable intraocular lens implantation. *Acta Ophthalmol.* 2009;87:896–900.
3. Wensheng L, Wu R, Wang X, et al. Clinical complications of combined phacoemulsification and vitrectomy for eyes with co-existing cataract and vitreoretinal diseases. *Eur J Ophthalmol.* 2009;19:37–45.
4. Mingels A, Koch J, Lommatzsch A, et al. Comparison of two acrylic intraocular lenses with different haptic designs in patients with combined phacoemulsification and pars plana vitrectomy. *Eye (Lond).* 2007;21:1379–1383.

5. Ohara K, Kato S, Hori S, et al. Tilt and decentration of the intraocular lens following combined vitrectomy and pars plana lensectomy. *Acta Ophthalmol Scand.* 2006;84:388–389.

6. Yasuda A, Ohkoshi K, Orihara Y, et al. Spontaneous luxation of encapsulated intraocular lens onto the retina after a triple procedure of vitrectomy, phacoemulsification, and intraocular lens implantation. *Am J Ophthalmol.* 2000;130:836–837.

7. McDonnell PJ, Spalton DJ, Falcon MG. Decentration of the posterior chamber lens implant: The effect of optic size on the incidence of visual aberrations. *Eye (Lond).* 1990;4:132–137.

8. Tappin MJ, Larkin DF. Factors leading to lens implant decentration and exchange. *Eye (Lond).* 2000;14:773–776.

9. Gross JG, Kokame GT, Weinberg DV, et al. In-the-bag intraocular lens dislocation. *Am J Ophthalmol.* 2004;137:630–635.

10. Gimbel HV, Condon GP, Kohnen T, et al. Late in-the-bag intraocular lens dislocation: Incidence, prevention, and management. *J Cataract Refract Surg.* 2005;31:2193–2204.

11. Davis D, Brubaker J, Espandar L, et al. Late in-the-bag spontaneous intraocular lens dislocation: Evaluation of 86 consecutive cases. *Ophthalmology.* 2009;116:664–670.

12. Grusha YO, Masket S, Miller KM. Phacoemulsification and lens implantation after pars plana vitrectomy. *Ophthalmology.* 1998;105:287–294.

13. Lindstrom RL, Samuelson TW, Anderson NJ. Cataract surgical problem. *J Cataract Refract Surg.* 2002;28:580.

14. Olson RJ, Mamalis N, Werner L, et al. Cataract treatment in the beginning of the 21st century [perspective]. *Am J Ophthalmol.* 2003;136:146–154.

15. Chang DF. Prevention of bag-fixated IOL dislocation in pseudoexfoliation [letter]. *Ophthalmology.* 2002;109:1951–1952.

16. Shigeeda T, Nagahara M, Kato S, et al. Spontaneous posterior dislocation of intraocular lenses fixated in the capsular bag. *J Cataract Refract Surg.* 2002;28:1689–1693.

17. Gross JG, Kokame GT, Weinberg DV, et al. In-the-bag intraocular lens dislocation. *Am J Ophthalmol.* 2004;137:630–635.

18. Werner L, Pandey SK, Escobar-Gomez M, et al. Anterior capsule opacification: A histopathological study comparing different IOL styles. *Ophthalmology.* 2000;107:463–471.

19. Izak AM, Werner L, Pandey SK, et al. Single-piece hydrophobic acrylic intraocular lens explanted within the capsular bag: Case report with clinicopathological correlation. *J Cataract Refract Surg.* 2004;30:1356–1361.

20. Titiyal JS, Sinha R, Verma K. Bent haptic of a single-piece AcrySof intraocular lens implantation from capsular contraction [letter]. *J Cataract Refract Surg.* 2004;30:1812–1813.

21. Sun R, Gimbel HV. In vivo evaluation of the efficacy of the capsular tension ring for managing zonular dialysis in cataract surgery. *Ophthalmic Surg Lasers.* 1998;29:502–505.

22. Menapace R, Findl O, Georgopoulos M, et al. The capsular tension ring: Designs, applications, and techniques. *J Cataract Refract Surg.* 2000;26:898–912.

23. Jacob S, Agarwal A, Agarwal A, et al. Efficacy of a capsule tension ring for phacoemulsification in eyes with zonular dialysis. *J Cataract Refract Surg.* 2003;29:315–321.

24. Smiddy WE, Ibanez GV, Alfonso E, et al. Surgical management of dislocated intraocular lenses. *J Cataract Refract Surg.* 1995;21:64–69.

25. Jehan FS, Mamalis N, Crandall AS. Spontaneous late dislocation of intraocular lens within the capsular bag in pseudoexfoliation patients. *Ophthalmology.* 2001;108:1727–1731.

26. Auffarth GU, Tsao K, Wesendahl TA, et al. Centration and fixation of posterior chamber intraocular lenses in eyes with pseudoexfoliation syndrome. An analysis of explanted autopsy eyes. *Acta Ophthalmol Scand.* 1996;74:463–467.

27. Kazemi S, Wirostko WJ, Sinha S, et al. Combined pars plana lensectomy-vitrectomy with open-loop flexible anterior chamber intraocular lens (AC IOL) implantation for subluxated lenses. *Trans Am Ophthalmol Soc.* 2000;98:247–251.

28. Yoshida K, Kiryu J, Kita M, et al. Phacoemulsification of dislocated lens and suture fixation of intraocular lens using a perfluorocarbon liquid. *Jpn J Ophthalmol.* 1998;42:471–475.

20C

Synechiae

KUHL HUH

The Complication: Definition

Posterior iris synechiae arise when the pupillary margin and/or back surface of the iris bind to the front surface of the lens. Posterior iris synechiae result from postoperative hyperplasia and myofibroblastic metaplasia of lens epithelial, iris epithelial, or iris stromal cells, and adhesion of the posterior iris to the anterior lens capsule. Posterior iris synechiae are found more frequently in cases of iris trauma or inflammation and are a common complication after phacovitrectomy.[1-6] The frequency of posterior iris synechiae formation after phacovitrectomy has been reported to range from 7% to 30%.[1,2,4-7] In a univariate analysis, the rates of posterior iris synechiae depended on the indication for surgery. Rates were higher following retinal detachment or complicated diabetic retinopathy surgery compared with simple epiretinal membrane peeling or macular hole surgery.[1,8]

Risk Factors

Known risk factors for posterior iris synechiae include preoperative posterior iris synechiae, history of uveitis, underlying proliferative diabetic retinopathy (PDR), vitreous tamponade with C3F8 gas or silicone oil, excessive panretinal photocoagulation (PRP), single-piece acrylic intraocular lens (IOL) implantation, postoperative anterior chamber (AC) fibrin deposition, postoperative inflammation, and postoperative use of long-acting mydriatics.[1,2,8,9] Uncontrolled diabetes or systemic inflammatory disease may also be risk factors for posterior iris synechiae after phacovitrectomy.

Preoperative Posterior Iris Synechiae

Damage to the posterior surface of the iris or pupillary margin during synechiolysis and postoperative inflammation are thought to increase the risk of postoperative posterior iris synechiae formation.

Vitreous Tamponade with C3F8 Gas or Silicone Oil

In eyes injected with an expandable gas, tighter apposition of the IOL to the posterior iris surface may lead to a higher incidence of posterior iris synechiae. In particular, if a patient cannot maintain a prone position after gas or oil tamponade, the buoyancy of the expanding gas or oil may lead to the IOL protruding anteriorly. Hanemoto et al.[10] demonstrated the effect of gas tamponade on eyes that had scleral-fixated IOL implantation after combined pars plana lensectomy and vitrectomy. IOLs were sutured horizontally, obliquely, or vertically. In eyes in which the IOL was horizontally fixated, the upper part of the IOL tilted anteriorly, causing peripheral anterior iris synechiae due to the enhanced effect of the gas bubble on the upper vitreous cavity. This outcome might have been avoided through the use of vertical or oblique suturing. The accumulation of growth factors in the anterior segment due to the patient's prone position after tamponade may also contribute to synechiae formation.[11] Silicone oil may be associated with increased inflammation, fibrin formation, and posterior synechiae, particularly when compared to expanding gas tamponade.[12,13]

Excessive PRP

PRP for PDR can induce a breakdown of the blood–aqueous barrier, leading to increases in protein and cells in the AC and increased rates of posterior synechiae.[14]

Single-piece Acrylic IOL Implantation

The three-piece acrylic IOL has haptics of polymethylmethacrylate, which are angulated by 10 degrees. In contrast, the single-piece acrylic IOL has supporting haptics of the same soft acrylic material as the optic but without haptic angulation (0 degrees). Due to the softness of the optic–haptic junction, the single-piece acrylic IOL has a reduced ability to resist the effect of the vitreous replacement tamponade and thus tends to protrude anteriorly, shifting the anterior capsule forward toward the iris. Since the IOL optic is not sufficiently held in place, a horizontal optic–haptic junction positions the optic relatively anteriorly. Therefore, single-piece acrylic IOL implantation could be a risk factor for posterior iris synechiae.[1]

In one case of C3F8 gas tamponade, the image of a single-piece IOL on POD 7 was captured on the UBM (Optikon 2000 International SpA, Rome, Italy), showing that the optic–haptic junction was bent outward, causing the IOL optic (arrow head) to move forward and attach to the iris (large arrows). The IOL haptic (small arrows) remained in its original position **(Figure 20C-1)**.

Iwase and Sugiyama[11] compared degrees of IOL movement among eyes that received a single-piece acrylic IOL after phacovitrectomy. The AC depth in eyes with gas tamponade increased with time, coinciding with gas dissipation from the vitreous cavity.

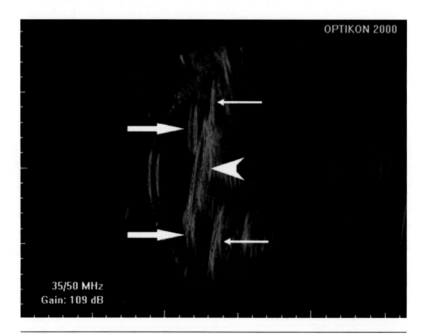

Figure 20C-1 Ultrasound biomicroscopic photograph of a single-piece IOL at 1 week after combined surgery with a C3F8 gas tamponade. The vertical view shows that the optic of the IOL (*arrow head*) has protruded anteriorly due to buoyancy of the expanding C3F8 gas and has contacted the iris margin (*large arrows*). The two haptics (*small arrows*) of the IOL were located posteriorly when the patient was positioned supine for this examination.

Postoperative AC Fibrin Deposition

The phacovitrectomy must result in an increased liberation of inflammatory cytokines. If fibrin is postoperatively deposited in the AC, the patient is six times more likely to develop posterior iris synechiae.[1]

Postoperative Use of Long-acting Mydriatics

Maintaining mydriasis with long-acting mydriatics can increase the contact duration between the iris and the lens capsule epithelium and therefore increases the risk of posterior iris synechiae. In contrast, the repeated use of short-acting mydriatics appears to reduce the risk of posterior iris synechiae.[9]

Pathogenesis: Why Does It Occur

Posterior iris synechiae are the result of inflammation within the AC. The synechiae site is between the iris and the peripheral capsule that remains after continuous curvilinear capsulorrhexis or between the iris and an inflammatory membrane that may form and cover the anterior surface of the IOL. Adhesions do not form between the iris and the IOL itself.[4,15,16] Posterior iris synechiae are formed when iritis, which may occur during the early postoperative period, causes the remaining lens epithelium or iris stroma to undergo hyperplasia and myofibroblastic metaplasia.[17–19] Lens epithelial cells present in the inner aspect of the anterior lens capsule and at the bow of the lens proliferate in response to "wounding" such as capsulorrhexis or factors present in the aqueous fluid.[20] Fibrous metaplasia in the anterior segment may not only originate from lens cells, but may also arise from inflamed or traumatized iris tissue.[17–19] Iritis or iris trauma with iris cell release contributes to posterior iris synechiae formation. Cells of iris origin in association with lens epithelial cells play an important role in the formation of posterior iris synechiae. Therefore, minimization of iris manipulation and trauma during surgery may be important in preventing posterior iris synechiae. A relevant question is whether the IOL itself may directly trigger some of the processes involved in posterior iris synechiae formation. Macrophages are deposited on the surface of most IOLs soon after implantation as part of the foreign body reaction.[21–23] These cells can subsequently undergo metaplasia to fibroblast-like cells[22] and may contribute to synechiae formation at the IOL edges, particularly in the presence of iris trauma or inflammation. While macrophages may play some role, iris and lens epithelial cell myofibroblastic metaplasia seems to play a more important causative role in posterior iris synechiae. Posterior synechiae form less commonly between the iris and inflammatory membranes that cover the anterior surface of the IOL optic. Posterior synechiae also occur in patients with iritis alone who have never experienced any cataract surgery or iris trauma, which implies that adhesions from fibrinous exudates also play an important role in this process.

Pearls on How to Prevent It

To prevent postoperative posterior iris synechiae:

◆ Minimize iris trauma at the time of the surgery.

◆ Use larger continuous curvilinear capsulorrhexis of a slightly smaller size (0.5 mm) than the optic diameter to assure complete circumferential overlap of the IOL edge[24] (e.g., 5 ~ 5.5 mm diameter).

◆ Use angled three-piece acrylic IOL rather than single-piece acrylic IOL. (If you do not favor a three-piece acrylic IOL due to difficulty of insertion and management of IOL in the capsular bag, a single-piece hydrophobic acrylic four haptic IOL can be used instead).

◆ Minimize intraoperative photocoagulation for PDR using short-acting mydriatics after surgery (e.g., the mixture of 0.5% phenylephrine and 0.5% tropicamide three times with a 10-minute interval only in the morning for 2 weeks).

◆ Adequately control postoperative inflammation (e.g., 1% prednisolone acetate eye drops every 2 hours daily starting the day after the operation. The application frequency and duration of the eye drops could be adjusted according to the inflammatory state in the AC).

Consider the use of pre- and postoperative systemic steroids in high-risk patients with uveitis or systemic inflammatory disease (e.g., oral prednisolone [1 mg/kg/day] can be given each morning for 2 days before surgery. Then, postoperatively, doses of systemic prednisolone therapy can be tapered depending on the amount of inflammation and discontinued when postoperative inflammation has resolved).

◆ Keep the patient in a prone position to avoid anterior protrusion of the IOL due to buoyancy of the expanding gas or oil.

◈ Pearls on How to Solve It

◆ If posterior iris synechiae are noticed early in the postoperative period, short-acting topical mydriatics with topical steroid eye drops could be repetitively used in order to move the pupil and resolve the posterior synechiae.

◆ If the posterior synechiae are so severe that they increase the intraocular pressure, cover the visual axis or impair the peripheral fundus examination; surgical release with a 26G needle, microcannula, iris hook, or viscoelastic material could be performed.

◈ Expected Outcomes: What Is the Worst-case Scenario

Posterior iris synechiae create problems for both patients and ophthalmologists. They can cause impaired pupillary movement and create difficulties with peripheral retinal examination. They can also cause a fixed pupil in response to light and near objects, which may lead to photophobia and a decrease in visual quality. The most disastrous consequence of posterior iris synechiae is seclusio pupillae (100% posterior iris synechiae) or/and occlusio pupillae (small miosed pupil with a covering membrane). Seclusio pupillae can lead to the formation of iris bombe and pupillary block glaucoma.[25,26] In one study, the occurrence rate of iris bombe requiring Neodymium-Yttrium-Aluminium-Garnet (Nd:YAG) laser iridotomy was as high as 2.2% after phacovitrectomy.[26] Occlusio pupillae can severely compromise visual acuity. Though these factors sometimes limit the advisability of a combined operation, the incidence and the extent of posterior iris synechiae have decreased significantly with the advancement of surgical techniques and newly developed instruments such as phacoemulsification and the vitrectomy machine, along with improvements in postoperative management. Therefore, phacovitrectomy is still recommended if necessary, but the ophthalmologist must be aware of potential complications such as posterior iris synechiae.

REFERENCES

1. Kim SW, Oh J, Song JS, et al. Risk factors of iris posterior synechia formation after phacovitrectomy with three-piece acrylic IOL or single-piece acrylic IOL. *Ophthalmologica*. 2009;223:222–227.

2. Shinoda K, O'hira A, Ishida S, et al. Posterior synechia of the iris after combined pars plana vitrectomy, phacoemulsification, and intraocular lens implantation. *Jpn J Ophthalmol*. 2001;45:276–280.

3. Lavin M, Jagger J. Pathogenesis of pupillary capture after posterior chamber intraocular lens implantation. *Br J Ophthalmol*. 1986;70:886–889.

4. Lahey JM, Francis RR, Kearney JJ. Combining phacoemulsification with pars plana vitrectomy in patients with proliferative diabetic retinopathy: A series of 223 cases. *Ophthalmology*. 2003;110:1335–1339.

5. Heiligenhaus A, Holtkamp A, Koch J, et al. Combined phacoemulsification and pars plana vitrectomy: Clear corneal versus scleral incisions: Prospective randomized multicenter study. *J Cataract Refract Surg*. 2003;29:1106–1112.

6. Senn P, Schipper I, Perren B. Combined pars plana vitrectomy, phacoemulsification, and intraocular lens implantation in the capsular bag: A comparison to vitrectomy and subsequent cataract surgery as a two-step procedure. *Ophthalmic Surg Lasers*. 1995;26:420–428.

7. Honjo M, Ogura Y. Surgical results of pars plana vitrectomy combined with phacoemulsification and intraocular lens implantation for complications of proliferative diabetic retinopathy. *Ophthalmic Surg Lasers*. 1998;29:99–105.

8. Rudnisky CJ, Cheung J, Nanji JA. Intraocular lens capture in combined cataract extraction and pars plana vitrectomy: Comparison of 1-piece and 3-piece acrylic intraocular lenses. *J Cataract Refract Surg*. 2010;36:1645–1649.

9. Lee SB, Lee DG, Kwag JY, et al. The effect of mydriatics on posterior synechia after combined pars plana vitrectomy, phacoemulsification, and intraocular lens implantation. *Retina*. 2009;29:1150–1154.

10. Hanemoto T, Ideta H, Kawasaki T, et al. Suture fixation of an intraocular lens combined with pars plana vitrectomy and gas tamponade. *J Cataract Refract Surg*. 2003;29:2458–2460.

11. Iwase T, Sugiyama K. Investigation of the stability of one-piece acrylic intraocular lenses in cataract surgery and in combined vitrectomy surgery. *Br J Ophthalmol*. 2006;90:1519–1523.

12. Johnson RN, Flynn HW Jr, Parel JM, et al. Transient hypopyon with marked anterior chamber fibrin following pars plana vitrectomy and silicone oil injection. *Arch Ophthalmol*. 1989;107:683–686.

13. Krzystolik MG, D'Amico DJ. Complications of intraocular tamponade: Silicone oil versus intraocular gas. *Int Ophthalmol Clin*. 2000;40:187–200.

14. Larsson LI, Nuija E. Increased permeability of the blood-aqueous barrier after panretinal photocoagulation for proliferative diabetic retinopathy. *Acta Ophthalmol Scand*. 2001;79:414–416.

15. Lahey JM, Francis RR, Fong DS, et al. Combining phacoemulsification with vitrectomy for treatment of macular holes. *Br J Ophthalmol*. 2002;86:876–878.

16. Holland GN, Van Horn SD, Margolis TP. Cataract surgery with ciliary sulcus fixation of intraocular lenses in patients with uveitis. *Am J Ophthalmol*. 1999;128:21–30.

17. McDonnell PJ, Zarbin MA, Green WR. Posterior capsule opacification in pseudophakic eyes. *Ophthalmology*. 1983;90:1548–1553.

18. Yeo JH, Jakobiec FA, Pokorny K, et al. The ultrastructure of an IOL 'cocoon membrane'. *Ophthalmology*. 1983;90:410–419.

19. Odrich MG, Hall SJ, Worgul BV, et al. Posterior capsule opacification: Experimental analyses. *Ophthalmic Res*. 1985;17:75–84.

20. Weinsieder A, Reddan J, Wilson D. Aqueous humor in lens repair and cell proliferation. *Exp Eye Res*. 1976;23:355–363.

21. Wolter JR, Felt DP. Proliferation of fibroblast-like cells on failing intraocular lenses. *Ophthalmic Surg.* 1983;14:57–64.
22. Wolter JR. Cytopathology of intraocular lens implantation. *Ophthalmology.* 1985; 92:135–142.
23. Ohara K. Biomicroscopy of surface deposits resembling foreign-body giant cells on implanted intraocular lenses. *Am J Ophthalmol.* 1985;99:304–311.
24. Rahman R, Rosen PH. Pupillary capture after combined management of cataract and vitreoretinal pathology. *J Cataract Refract Surg.* 2002;28:1607–1612.
25. Makhzoum O, Crosby NJ, Hero M. Secondary angle-closure glaucoma due to posterior synechiae formation following phacovitrectomy. *Int Ophthalmol.* 2011;31:481–482.
26. Ling R, Simcock P, McCoombes J, et al. Presbyopic phacovitrectomy. *Br J Ophthalmol.* 2003;87:1333–1335.

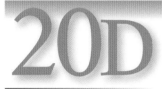

Refractive Outcome and Possible Errors Following Combined Phaco-vitrectomy

DAVID STEEL

When assessing refractive outcome after phaco-vitrectomy, the following issues need to be considered:

1. The refractive accuracy of the procedure: This can be assessed by the proportion of patients achieving a refractive outcome within 0.5 diopter (D) and 1 D of the planned refraction and/or by the mean absolute postoperative prediction error (MAE), that is, the absolute difference in diopters from the planned result.

2. The overall direction of the refractive error or refractive shift: This can be assessed by the mean postoperative prediction error (ME) after combined phaco-vitrectomy as compared to phacoemulsification alone particularly as there are several reports supporting the occurrence of a small myopic shift in refraction when vitrectomy is added to phacoemulsification.

3. The astigmatic change produced: The addition of vitrectomy to phacoemulsification may lead to an increased astigmatic change as compared to phacoemulsification alone.

The above aspects are discussed separately below.

 ## The Complication: Refractive Accuracy and Possible Errors Following Phaco-vitrectomy

Phaco-vitrectomy is often performed routinely in conditions such as macular hole and pucker and it is important to assess the refractive accuracy of this procedure in these cases.

Patel et al.[1] found an MAE of 0.83 D with 45% and 68% of patients achieving a refractive outcome within 0.5 and 1 D respectively of the planned result using A-scan ultrasound to assess axial length in a series of macular hole cases. Results are generally slightly improved using optical interferometry with the intraocular lens (IOL) master (Carl Zeiss, Germany) to assess axial length.[2] Kojima et al.[3]

reported 56% and 92% within 0.5 and 1 D of planned refraction using partial coherence interferometry (PCI) in a series of patients with a variety of macular diseases undergoing phaco-vitrectomy. Manvikar et al.[4] found an MAE of 0.39 D with 70% and 96% of patients achieving a planned refraction within 0.5 and 1 D respectively using the IOL master on patients with macular hole and pucker. Although this was significantly different to a control group of normal eyes without macular pathology undergoing uncomplicated phacoemulsification (MAE of 0.26 D and 87% and 100% within 0.5 and 1 D of planned refraction), it was very similar to the outcomes obtained in a sequential phacoemulsification control group of patients with maculopathy previously treated by vitrectomy (MAE of 0.38 D and 66% and 93% within 0.5 and 1 D of planned refraction) and close to published standards for uncomplicated phacoemulsification.[5] In conclusion, although the refractive results in patients undergoing combined phaco-vitrectomy for macular pathology such as macular hole and pucker are not as good as those undergoing solitary phacoemulsification without macular pathology, they can be as good as those undergoing sequential surgery with vitrectomy followed by phacoemulsification for the same conditions.

Risk Factors

There are several potential reasons why the refractive outcome following combined phaco-vitrectomy may be less accurate than that obtained following phacoemulsification alone. Inaccuracies mostly relate to the underlying vitreoretinal condition being treated and may occur as a result of:

1. Poor vision with unstable, inaccurate, or eccentric fixation and, hence, axial length measurement along an axis other than the optimal.

2. High myopia with the presence of posterior staphyloma.

3. The presence of uneven, elevated, or thickened retinas with variable axial length readings.

Pearls on How to Prevent It

◆ Under the above circumstances and in order to prevent inaccurate refractive results the surgeon may opt to avoid performing a combined phaco-vitrectomy, unless absolutely necessary in some of these conditions. If combined surgery is required then occasionally the fellow eye can be used to guide IOL choice; however, be warned that ~one-fourth of fellow eyes are greater than 1 mm different (= 2.5–3 D) in axial length to the operative eye. Several biometry protocols can maximize the chances of an accurate refraction. (See *Pearls on How to Prevent It: Refractive Errors Postoperatively and Optimize Refractive Accuracy following Phaco-vitrectomy* at the end of this chapter.)

The Complication: Refractive Shift Following Phaco-vitrectomy

Many authors have described a myopic shift in refraction (i.e., ME) of around 0.5 D.[6–13]

Risk Factors and Why Does It Occur

There are several possible explanations for the myopic shift observed, which include:

1. **Errors in the estimation of the axial length.**

    Ultrasound measures axial length from the anterior surface of the cornea to the anterior surface of the retina and hence it is plausible that measurement of eyes with macular pathology associated with macular thickening corrected by surgery, for example, epiretinal membranes (ERMs) and macular holes, could lead to an axial length that is longer postoperatively and hence a myopic shift in refraction postoperatively. An error of 100 μm in axial length can result in a 0.25 D error in refractive outcome.[14] In support of this, some authors have reported longer axial lengths as measured using ultrasound postoperatively secondary to resolution of retinal thickening[10] and that if an adjustment for macular thickening is made with optical coherence tomography (OCT) preoperatively then this can eliminate the myopic shift.[15,16] Others, however, have found no myopic shift using ultrasound.[1] It should also be noted that if the axial length is measured from the centre of a macular hole then the axial length could be over- rather than underestimated using ultrasound.

    Using optical interferometry with the IOL master (Carl Zeiss, Germany) axial length is measured from the anterior surface of the cornea to the retinal pigment epithelium (RPE).[17] Using this system retinal thickening should not affect axial length estimation and hence a myopic shift should not occur if this was the explanation of the effect. Indeed Manvikar et al.[4] found no myopic shift using the IOL master in a series of narrow-gauge phaco-vitrectomies for ERMs and macular holes. However, other authors have found a persistent myopic shift postoperatively using the IOL master.[11] Opacity in the neurosensory retina can lead to errors in axial length estimation in some eyes. A double peak in the IOL master scans has been recorded in ~20% of eyes undergoing vitrectomy for macular thickening or hole and can represent the two sides on the retina—the RPE surface and the anterior retinal surface in certain situations. Use of the posterior peak led to a reduction in the myopic shift seen.[3]

2. **Increased axial length.**

    An alternative explanation for the myopic shift observed postoperatively is that there is a real increase in the axial length of the eye related to stretching of the sclera at the sclerostomy sites. To go along with this, Jeoung et al.[10] reported that the myopic shift observed in a series of phaco-vitrectomies was increased in eyes with longer axial length. This phenomenon may explain at least some cases and has also been proposed as an explanation for an occasional paradoxical myopic shift seen in pseudophakic patients undergoing vitrectomy with 20 g self-sealing tunnels and scleral elongation secondary to wound stretch.[18] Despite these observations a myopic shift can be seen during phaco-vitrectomy in eyes with IOL master biometry and without an increase in axial length postoperatively,[12] meaning that axial length errors cannot explain all cases of myopic shift seen and different mechanisms must account for some cases. Alternative theories have therefore been proposed.

3. **Anterior chamber (AC) depth changes.**

    A reduction in AC depth postoperatively after phaco-vitrectomy, compared with phacoemulsification alone, associated with an anterior displacement of the IOL would result in a myopic shift in refraction and explain the phenomena. A gas-filled eye might be associated with shallowing of the AC postoperatively and in support of this theory some authors have found a correlation between gas tamponade and a myopic shift.[6,7] However, others have not found such an effect.[4,8,10] A randomized clinical trial showed, in fact, the reverse effect with lesser degrees of myopic shift in gas-filled eyes undergoing macular hole surgery than in eyes undergoing ERM peeling with no gas.[11]

    An alternative theory is that posterior capsular bag contraction occurs to a greater extent in vitrectomized eyes leading to a shallower AC. Posterior capsule opacification and anterior capsule phimosis may occur more often after combined phaco-vitrectomy when compared with vitrectomy with subsequent cataract surgery.[19] However, capsule contraction with anterior capsular phimosis has been reported to result in a more posterior position of the IOL with a hypermetropic, rather than a myopic, shift.[20] IOL tilt and decentration have not been seen, however, more frequently following combined surgery.[21,22]

IOL design may play a part in the occurrence of AC depth changes in combined surgery with potentially more myopic shift seen when using flexible one-piece IOLs with planar, as opposed to more rigid IOLs with angulated haptics. Indeed AC shallowing has been measured in the first week following combined phaco-vitrectomy surgery with one-piece IOL as compared to more rigid three-piece IOLs; this, however, corrected by 1 month postoperatively.[21]

Complications relating to the IOL may result in AC shallowing and a possible myopic shift including optic capture by the iris from posterior gas pressure, optic capture through a large rhexis, or extensive posterior synechiae formation. It should be noted that these complications have often been excluded from published series of phaco-vitrectomy and are not the cause of the myopic shift seen in uncomplicated case series.

Finally two other findings have suggested that changes in AC depth are not the cause of the myopic shift in all cases. AC depth changes have not been seen after vitrectomy in already pseudophakic eyes[18] and an randomised controlled trial (RCT) comparing combined phaco-vitrectomy with phacoemulsification alone with AC depth measurements pre- and postoperatively found no correlation of any observed AC depth changes with refractive outcome.[11]

4. Refractive effects of the vitreous.
   The refractive index of formed vitreous (1.3346) differs from that of aqueous (1.3336) which could account for as much as 0.13 D of myopic shift but not the entire amount observed in some series.

✥ The Complication: Surgically Induced Astigmatism Following Phaco-vitrectomy

Although vitrectomy can lead to short-term astigmatic changes, combined phaco-vitrectomy does not appear to induce significantly more astigmatic change than phacoemulsification alone.[23]

✥ Pearls on How to Prevent It

Refractive Errors Postoperatively and Optimize Refractive Accuracy Following Phaco-vitrectomy

◆ Develop clear quality assurance criteria to be used in the Department of biometry,[24] for example:

  ◆ Follow guidelines for formulas to be used.

  ◆ Look at inter-eye differences and ensure consistency with spectacle prescriptions. (See Knox-Cartwright NE, Johnston RL, Jaycock PD, Tole DM, and Sparrow JM. The Cataract National Dataset electronic multicentre audit of 55,567 operations: When should IOL master biometric measurements be rechecked? *Eye*. 2009:1–7, for more details.)

  ◆ Use dedicated trained biometry staff.

  ◆ Perform regular assessments of your results and adjust as needed to improve accuracy.

◆ Use of fourth generation formulas such as the Haigis or Holladay II should be considered especially in eyes with nonaverage axial lengths. Alternatively, use third generation formulas according to axial length.

The Hoffer Q for axial lengths from 20 to 20.99 mm.

The Hoffer Q or Holladay 1 for axial lengths from 21 to 21.49 mm.

The SRK/T or Holladay I for axial lengths 21.50 to 25.99 mm.

The SRK/T for axial lengths of 26 mm or longer.[25]

◆ Axial length measurement using optical interferometry with the IOL master (Carl Zeiss, Germany) gives more accurate refractive results than axial length measurement with ultrasound. Therefore, where possible, this method should be used. When using optical interferometry ideally, readings are taken undilated to maximize fixation accuracy and without corneal disruption, for example, not after contact intraocular pressure (IOP) measurements or recent contact lens wear. When measuring axial length with the IOL master, glasses can be used to maximize fixation without affecting the measurement. If fixation using the internal fixation light is impossible, a fixation light directly ahead of the fellow eye can be used to help.

◆ When measuring axial length with the IOL master in eyes with thickened maculae then inspection and editing of the graph display should be carried out if necessary. PCI uses the reflection from the RPE to assess axial length and a fixed constant is added to compensate for the normal inner retinal location. In certain situations the inner retinal reflectivity can be high (e.g., dense ERMs) and the device can inappropriately interpret this reflective peak as the RPE. In this situation the graph cursor can be adjusted to the lower RPE peak manually. Details on adjustment and other potential errors in measurement can be found in the manufacturer's device manuals and http://doctor-hill.com/iol-master/interpretation.htm, and readers are encouraged to review this.

◆ If using ultrasound axial length measurement consider using OCT measurements to correct for axial length in cases where the neurosensory retina at the foveal centre is pathologic

   ◆ For example, in ERM cases with a thick macula. In this situation assuming that the macula will assume a normal thickness of ~250 μm in due course following surgery, the axial length measurement can be adjusted.

   ◆ For example, true axial length = measured axial length (23.77 mm) + (measured central macular thickness (640 μm) – 250 μm) = 23.77 + 0.39 mm = 24.16 mm.

These calculations; however, are imprecise and a variable outcome may be expected.

◆ In general a small degree of myopic shift is rarely a clinical problem, and indeed may be an advantage. However, if it were important to avoid, then adding 0.5 D to the targeted refractive outcome should be considered in phaco-vitrectomy cases where the axial length and refractive outcome cannot be accurately predicted, for example, in macular hole cases where ultrasound axial length measurement is used.

◆ In cases of macular-off retinal detachment the important variable is to assess which peak the axial length is being measured from. In some cases ultrasound measures the axial length wrongly from the RPE, in which case 250 μm can be **added** to give the true axial length fortuitously. Sometimes the IOL Master measures an accurate RPE peak but sometimes it erroneously picks up the retinal peak. **Scan graphs need to be visually assessed to work out what is going on!** Occasionally the IOL master scan peak can be adjusted to the posterior RPE peak and an axial length surmised. Again refractive uncertainty should be explained to the patient.

◆ Maximize the chances of IOL stability, for example, by creating a rhexis with a smaller diameter than the IOL optic and ensuring AC depth stability intra- and postoperatively with a carefully constructed watertight wound with sutures if necessary. One-piece folding IOLs have been used successfully in cases where these rules are followed. Consider the use of angulated three-piece IOLs with large optic diameters however, where anterior capsulorrhexis size is larger than the optic diameter. Consider the use of a capsule tension ring if there is any doubt about zonule integrity or oil is to be used.

REFERENCES

1. Patel D, Rahman R, Kumarasamy M. Accuracy of intraocular lens power estimation in eyes having phacovitrectomy for macular holes. *J Cataract Refract Surg.* 2007; 33(10):1760–1762.
2. Lege BA, Haigis W. Laser interference biometry versus ultrasound biometry in certain clinical conditions. *Graefes Arch Clin Exp Ophthalmol.* 2004;242:8–12
3. Kojima T, Tamaoki A, Yoshida N, et al. Evaluation of axial length measurement of the eye using partial coherence interferometry and ultrasound in cases of macular disease. *Ophthalmology.* 2010;117(9):1750–1754.
4. Manvikar SR, Allen D, Steel DH. Optical biometry in combined phacovitrectomy. *J Cataract Refract Surg.* 2009;35(1):64–69.
5. Gale RP, Saldana M, Johnston RL, et al. Benchmark standards for refractive outcomes after NHS cataract surgery. *Eye (Lond).* 2009;23(1):149–152.
6. Shioya M, Ogino N, Shinjo U. Change in postoperative refractive error when vitrectomy is added to intraocular lens implantation. *J Cataract Refract Surg.* 1997;23(8):1217–1220.
7. Suzuki Y, Sakuraba T, Mizutani H, et al. Postoperative refractive error after simultaneous vitrectomy and cataract surgery. *Ophthalmic Surg Lasers.* 2000;31(4):271–275.
8. Manvikar S, Steel D, Pimenidis D. Refractive outcome of phacovitrectomy. *J Cataract Refract Surg.* 2008;34(12):2009–2010.
9. Lee DK, Lee SJ, You YS. Prediction of refractive error in combined vitrectomy and cataract surgery with one-piece acrylic intraocular lens. *Korean J Ophthalmol.* 2008;22(4):214–249.
10. Jeoung JW, Chung H, Yu HG. Factors influencing refractive outcomes after combined phacoemulsification and pars plana vitrectomy: Results of a prospective study. *J Cataract Refract Surg.* 2007;33(1):108–114.
11. Falkner-Radler CI, Benesch T, Binder S. Accuracy of preoperative biometry in vitrectomy combined with cataract surgery for patients with epiretinal membranes and macular holes: Results of a prospective controlled clinical trial. *J Cataract Refract Surg.* 2008;34(10):1754–1760.
12. Ehmann D, García R. Investigating a possible cause of the myopic shift after combined cataract extraction, intraocular lens implantation, and vitrectomy for treatment of a macular hole. *Can J Ophthalmol.* 2009;44(5):594–597.
13. Schweitzer KD, García R. Myopic shift after combined phacoemulsification and vitrectomy with gas tamponade. *Can J Ophthalmol.* 2008;43(5):581–583.
14. Olsen T, Thorwest M. Calibration of axial length measurements with the Zeiss IOL-Master. *J Cataract Refract Surg.* 2005;31:1345–1350
15. Kovács I, Ferencz M, Nemes J, et al. Intraocular lens power calculation for combined cataract surgery, vitrectomy and peeling of epiretinal membranes for macular oedema. *Acta Ophthalmol Scand.* 2007;85(1):88–91.
16. Sun HJ, Choi KS. Improving intraocular lens power prediction in combined phacoemulsification and vitrectomy in eyes with macular oedema. *Acta Ophthalmol.* 2011; 89(6):575–578.
17. Attas-Fox L, Zadok D, Gerber Y, et al. Axial length measurement in eyes with diabetic macular edema: A-scan ultrasound versus IOLMaster. *Ophthalmology.* 2007; 114(8):1499–1504.

18. Byrne S, Ng J, Hildreth A, et al. Refractive change following pseudophakic vitrectomy. *BMC Ophthalmol.* 2008;8:19.
19. Senn P, Schipper I, Perren B. Combined pars plana vitrectomy, phacoemulsification, and intraocular lens implantation in the capsular bag: A comparison to vitrectomy and subsequent cataract surgery as a two-step procedure. *Ophthalmic Surg Lasers.* 1995;26(5):420–428.
20. Nishigaki S, Inaba I, Minami H, et al. The postoperative change of depth of anterior chamber, refraction and anterior capsulorhexis size after intraocular lens implantation. *Nippon Ganka Gakkai Zasshi.* 1996;100:156–158.
21. Watanabe A, Shibata T, Ozaki M, et al. Change in anterior chamber depth following combined pars plana vitrectomy, phacoemulsification, and intraocular lens implantation using different types of intraocular lenses. *Jpn J Ophthalmol.* 2010;54(5):383–386.
22. Iwase T, Sugiyama K. Investigation of the stability of one-piece acrylic intraocular lenses in cataract surgery and in combined vitrectomy surgery. *Br J Ophthalmol.* 2006; 90:1519–1523.
23. Yuen CY, Cheung BT, Tsang CW, et al. Surgically induced astigmatism in phacoemulsification, pars plana vitrectomy, and combined phacoemulsification and vitrectomy: A comparative study. *Eye (Lond).* 2009;23(3):576–580.
24. Gale RP, Saha N, Johnston RL. National biometry audit. *Eye (Lond).* 2004;18(1): 63–66.
25. Aristodemou P, Knox Cartwright NE, Sparrow JM, et al. Formula choice: Hoffer Q, Holladay 1, or SRK/T and refractive outcomes in 8108 eyes after cataract surgery with biometry by partial coherence interferometry. *J Cataract Refract Surg.* 2011; 37(1):63–71.

20E Lack of Capsular Support

Nur Acar

Lack of Capsular Support

Combined phaco-vitrectomy surgery has recently been performed in an increased fashion. The main indications for a combined surgery are:

The patient is already in a presbyopic age with a senile cataract.

Some form of cataract may accompany the vitreoretinal (VR) pathology such as in posttraumatic cases, and no matter at what age of the patient a combined procedure is necessary/beneficial.

To be able to clean the vitreous base and to perform a more complete pars plana vitrectomy (PPV) depending on the indication of PPV such as in rhegmatogenous retinal detachment (RRD), especially more complicated forms accompanied by proliferative vitreoretinopathy (PVR) or posttraumatic RRDs, peripheric traction retinal detachments (TRD) in which peripheric maneuvers needed are more challenging to perform in a phakic eye. Near-complete vitrectomy is the preferred technique especially in eyes without buckling and combined phaco-vitrectomy allows more space and comfort for the surgeon.

The incidence of cataract development increases following PPV. Two years after vitrectomy half of the eyes require cataract extraction and the opacification progresses faster in patients older than 50 years.[1] This is the rationale behind performing combined phaco-vitrectomy in cases within the presbyopic age group without coexisting vision-threatening cataract.

Sometimes, lens touch during vitrectomy may occur as a complication, and phacoemulsification may be needed although it is unplanned.

The Complication: Definition

Lack of capsular support is the situation in which there is inadequate capsular support for implantation of an intraocular lens (IOL) even in the ciliary sulcus. Some form of defect in the iris diaphragm may coexist depending on the etiology of the ocular pathology.

Risk Factors

Cataract surgery combined with vitrectomy may be more complicated technically than cataract surgery alone as a result of different accompanying vitreoretinal and/or anterior chamber (AC) pathologies and their etiologies so that the complication of capsular rupture may result during the combined surgery.

In posttraumatic eyes, anterior and/or posterior lens capsule may already be damaged.

Zonules may be weak as a result of trauma, pseudoexfoliation, or accompanying systemic diseases such as Marfan syndrome leading to subluxation/dislocation of the lens.

Iatrogenic; the posterior or peripheric capsule or the zonules may be cut by the vitrector as a complication during PPV.

Pathogenesis: Why Does It Occur

It may occur during combined surgery as a complication as it may be more difficult to observe the fundus reflex in an eye with vitreoretinal pathology. In addition, accompanying issues such as a small pupil with synechiae, a hazy cornea due to a recent trauma, a deep anterior chamber in a highly myopic or a traumatized eye, iridodialysis, subluxation/dislocation of the lens, and so on, may coexist frequently.

In posttraumatic eyes, there may already be a rupture of the anterior and/or posterior capsule. The zonules may be disrupted or loose (Figure 20E-1). Similarly, in aged eyes with pseudoexfoliation zonules may be weak, and the capsule may be lost due to zonulodialysis if not recognized on time and managed properly.

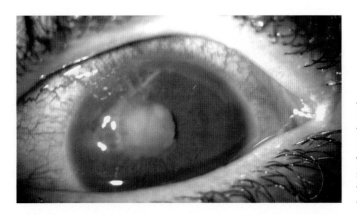

Figure 20E-1 Penetrating trauma in a 13-year-old boy. Posttraumatic cortical cataract with lens dislocation, corneal sutures, and zonulodialysis temporally

In a combined phaco-vitrectomy, some surgeons prefer to implant the IOL after PPV is completed to avoid the glare of the IOL and disturbance in visualization of the peripheral vitreous during PPV, whereas others implant the IOL first and continue with PPV. In the first scenario, the capsular bag is usually distended using viscoelastic. The implanted IOL or viscoelastic stretches the capsular bag and helps it to keep its normal anatomic position in the eye. Especially during peripheral vitrectomy with scleral indentation, the surgeon should be careful not to cut the posterior capsule or the zonules with the vitrector. Unless recognized, the defect in the capsule may enlarge and may even hinder IOL implantation. Similarly, during surgical separation of anterior hyaloid from posterior lens capsule, the posterior capsule may be caught by the vitrector, and torn or even lost almost totally. Albeit rarely seen, these complications may occur even in the second scenario with the IOL already implanted, and may lead to dislocation of the IOL into the vitreous and necessitate its extraction.

In some complicated cases such as severe PVR or trauma, the surgeon may prefer to extract the whole capsule deliberately during vitrectomy not to leave any tissue plane for reproliferation, and/or to dissect the cyclitic membranes over the pars plicata when present.

Pearls on How to Prevent It

- Surgical experience dealing with difficult cataracts is mandatory to avoid complications since phaco surgery in combined procedures may be more challenging due to the previously mentioned reasons (see above).[2,3] Keeping the cornea clear is crucial to obtain good visualization during the surgery. Synechiotomy, stable pupil dilatation using iris hooks,[4] staining the capsule with 0.06% trypan blue,[5] or performing capsulorrhexis with the help of endoillumination[6] may help to prevent the standard complications. In posttraumatic eyes in which the lens capsule is damaged, staining the capsule is helpful to localize its borders. Especially, curved VR microscissors are very helpful to transform the anterior capsule tear into a circular rhexis.

- Subluxation/dislocation of the lens and loose or disrupted zonules should be suspected especially in a traumatized eye. Preoperative diagnosis is important as the surgeon can plan the surgery with according precautions. A careful examination is valuable with special attention to phacodonesis, iridodonesis, as well as observing wrinkles while performing capsulorrhexis intraoperatively. The capsular bag can be stabilized by iris hooks or Mackool-modified capsule hooks (The Mackool Cataract Support System, FCI Ophthalmics, USA) **(Figure 20E-2)**

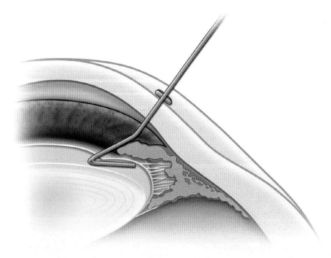

Figure 20E-2 Mackool-modified capsule hooks

Figure 20E-3 Ahmed capsule tension segment

after capsulorrhexis. A capsular tension ring (CTR) or sutured segments, which are only segments or arcs of a CTR, with a hole to be sutured to fix the localized area of capsular instability such as an Ahmed CT segment (Morcher GmbH, Stuttgart, Germany) **(Figure 20E-3)** are necessary for localized zonulodialysis, whereas sutured CTR such as a Cionni CTR (Morcher GmbH) **(Figure 20E-4)** or Malyugin-modified CTR (Morcher GmbH) **(Figure 20E-5)** is needed in eyes with extended zonule disruption.[3,7,8] These sutured CTRs are also preferred in eyes with progressive zonule weakness such as pseudoexfoliation. A controlled phaco surgery is fundamental to avoid capsule loss or other complications. **Figure 20E-6** demonstrates how the above devices can be inserted and sutured in the eye.

◆ To avoid inadvertent capsular rupture during PPV, the capsular bag should be distended either by injecting viscoelastic or implanting an IOL before vitrectomy. Despite some difficulties of visualization during PPV, the author prefers to implant the IOL before PPV, and especially in eyes in which more complete peripheric vitrectomy with scleral indentation will be performed. Three-piece IOLs with PMMA haptics are implanted as they stay more stable during surgery. If PPV is performed for a macular pathology, a single-piece IOL may also be preferred. If the surgeon does not want to implant IOL before PPV, an alternative may be an insertion of a CTR to stabilize the capsular bag to prevent capsule damage avoiding disturbed peripheral visualization during PPV, and implanting the IOL at the end of PPV.[8]

◆ Special attention should be paid not to engage the posterior capsule with the vitrector during peripheral vitrectomy with scleral indentation or during the separation of anterior hyaloid from posterior lens capsule. Recently, triamcinolone acetonide (TA)-assisted vitrectomy has been suggested by several authors as it enables the vitreous to be seen more clearly during vitrectomy.[9,10] It has been published to decrease intraoperative complications.[11] There is also FDA-approved preservative-free form available (Triesence Suspension, Alcon, USA). The author has been using peroperative TA as a routine practice and experienced that during both maneuvers

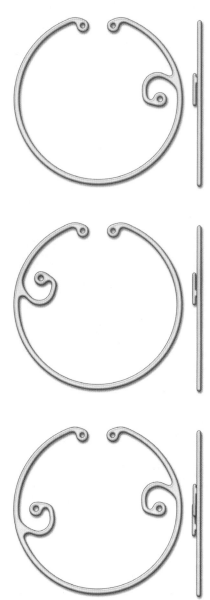

Figure 20E-4 A Cionni capsule tension ring

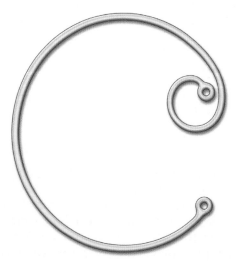

Figure 20E-5 A Malyugin-modified capsule tension ring

is a macular surgery, or a dislocated IOL, provided that the peripheral vitrectomy is done properly, the surgeon may opt to go ahead with one of the above IOL alternatives. An AC-IOL should probably be avoided if a tamponade agent is planned to be used due to the risk of corneal touch and damage. Except in eyes with ACIOLs, air or gas, however, may not be much of a problem with regards to corneal damage as they stay transiently in the eye and usually the patient can be asked to maintain a prone position postoperatively. Also if the PPV is properly performed and the iris diaphragm is preserved, with the Ando peripheral iridectomy silicone oil is avoided to fill into the anterior chamber. Sometimes, if the pupil is dilated at the end of PPV, it is advisable to constrict it with the injection of carbachol into the anterior chamber; if silicone oil is threatening to move forward into the anterior chamber at the end of PPV, air or viscoelastic could be used to fill the anterior chamber and prevent the oil to come forward. With the prone position of the patient postoperatively anterior chamber depth is usually preserved without problems.

Implanting an IOL also requires appropriate IOL measurements before the surgery. When silicone oil is used as an endotamponade silicone IOLs must be avoided. Postoperative close follow-up for any complications such as increased inflammation, pupillary membrane formation, iris capture, IOL decentralization/tilt, corneal touch of an AC-IOL, gas/silicone oil in the AC, and so on is important for timely management of these complications after combined surgery.

◆ Alternatively, the surgeon may prefer to leave the eye aphakic and plan for a secondary surgery depending on the indication of PPV, endotamponade left in the eye, the presence or absence of an intact iris diaphragm, and prognosis of vitrectomy. If the eye is to be left aphakic and silicone oil is used, an inferior iridectomy must be performed to avoid silicone oil to fill into the anterior chamber and touch the cornea. Preoperatively, endothelial cell density should be examined before secondary IOL implantation.

✦ Expected Outcomes: What Is the Worst-case Scenario

For decades, AC-IOLs and scleral-fixated PC-IOLs have been the most popular types of lenses used for secondary IOL implantation in eyes lacking capsular support. The literature supports the safe and effective use of open-loop AC, scleral-sutured PC, and iris-sutured PC-IOLs for the correction of aphakia in eyes without adequate capsular support.[12,13] However, there are both advantages and disadvantages to both, and there is no consensus regarding the indications or relative safety of either of these alternatives.[12,14–16]

1. The implantation of an AC-IOL is technically easy and takes shorter time and may be preferred in the elderly. However, angle-supported AC-IOLs are associated with short- and long-term complications such as corneal edema, hyphema, cystoid macular edema (CME), glaucoma, IOL instability, decentration, pupil distortion, and RRD; some of which are a direct consequence of the presence of haptics in the iridocorneal angle.[14,15,17] The implantation of angle-supported AC-IOL may have to be avoided in vitrectomized eyes that already have some changes in the anatomy of the AC or iridocorneal angle. Since they stay closer to the cornea they should be avoided when a gas endotamponade is left during PPV. Also, it should be avoided to overfill the eye with silicone oil and the patient should cooperate firmly with prone positioning following surgery. To implant an AC-IOL the pupil is constricted. A corneal incision of approximately 5.2 mm is performed for a rigid AC-IOL, VES is injected, and the IOL holds with a fine smooth forceps is gently placed into the AC. A lens glide may be used to protect the iris. First, the inferior and then the superior haptics are carefully placed into the inferior angle and the superior angle. Peripheric iridectomy is performed. The surgeon checks for any distortion of the pupil and decentration of the IOL. VES is aspirated, and the corneal incision is sutured. The place of the haptics may be checked by an angle lens intraoperatively.

2. Transscleral fixation of a PC-IOL (see **Figure 20E-8A–C**) is technically challenging, requiring more surgical time and the possibility of associated complications that can include ciliary choroidal body hemorrhage, RRD, giant retinal tears, vitreous hemorrhage, CME, lens tilting, decentration, late IOL dislocation due to breakage of polypropylene sutures, and conjunctival erosion by transscleral sutures with associated risk of endophthalmitis.[14,15,18,19] Ultrasound biomicroscopy showed the difficulty in reliably placing the haptics in the ciliary sulcus with this technique.[20] As a primary implantation, it lengthens the total surgical time that may be difficult for the patient to tolerate under local anesthesia. IOL should be implanted before the endotamponade is given with the sclerotomies plugged. Gas or silicone oil endotamponades can be left in the eye as PC-IOL would be an effective barrier if the iris diaphragm is intact. As a secondary implantation in a vitrectomized eye, transscleral fixation may be more difficult as a result of tight conjunctival adhesions, scarring, or conjunctival/scleral thinning frequently observed in eyes after reoperation. The association of scleral-fixated PC-IOLs with posterior segment complications such as RRD may also be a concern. In an eye with silicone oil, it may be performed after silicone oil extraction. PPV with endoscope-guided sutured PC-IOL implantation has also recently been described in an academic setting.[21] Another good alternative without the need of suturing is to fixate the haptics of a standard PC-IOL in scleral tunnels as described by Gabor S, Pavlidis MM.[22,23] The advantages of this technique is faster surgery, avoiding suture-related complications as erosion or astigmatism. As a standard technique, a single-piece PMMA-IOL or a foldable scleral-fixation IOL may be used. The foldable IOL allowing a smaller corneal incision and working in a closed chamber in these vitrectomized eyes is more frequently preferred. Pupil is fully dilated. After a localized conjunctival peritomy, two triangular scleral flaps of 3×3 mm located 180 degrees apart are prepared usually at oblique sites such as the 1- and 7-o'clock positions, or 8- and 2-o'clock positions to avoid horizontally located long posterior ciliary vessels and nerves. Vitrectomized eyes may be hypotonous and a paracentesis can be made to inject VES into the AC. As these eyes are already vitrectomized, no additional vitrectomy is needed. In the ab externo technique, from one scleral flap an insulin needle is entered about 0.75 to 1 mm away from the limbus, and advanced into the AC behind and parallel to iris. From the opposite scleral bed, a long-tipped polypropylene suture is entered 0.75 to 1 mm away from the limbus, and its end is put into the lumen of the guiding insulin needle in the middle of the anterior chamber, and this complex is pulled out of the eye. The main corneal incision is made and the suture is pulled out of the eye through this incision and cut in the middle into two. Each end of the suture is tied to each hole located in each haptic of the IOL. Then the scleral-fixation IOL is placed in the AC. Both ends of the suture are pulled from both sides so that the IOL is centered properly without tilt, and the sutures are tied to the sclera at both sides. Scleral flaps are sutured at the apex of the flap, and then the conjunctiva is sutured. The corneal incision is sutured, particularly, if large. The IOLs with two holes in each haptic may also be preferred to minimize lens tilt further.

3. Iris fixation of a foldable PC-IOL by suturing the IOL to the overlying iris in the outer periphery **(Figure 20E-8D–F)** is another method which is proven safe and effective and avoid the sight-threatening complications of AC-IOLs, although complications such as dislocation of the IOL, RRD, transient low-grade uveitis, and transient pigment dispersion have been rarely described.[13,24,25] The technique has been modified and simplified.[26] Moreover, iris-sutured PC-IOLs were found to respect the angle anatomy with no evidence of angle closure or synechia on ultrasound microscopic analysis.[27] Carefully performed pupil distortion is avoided and the dilatation remains unaffected **(Figure 20E-8G)**. There may be a transient hemorrhage and increased AC reaction during early postoperative period. The surgical technique starts with making a paracentesis and injection of viscoelastic into the AC. The three-piece IOL is placed in front of the iris through

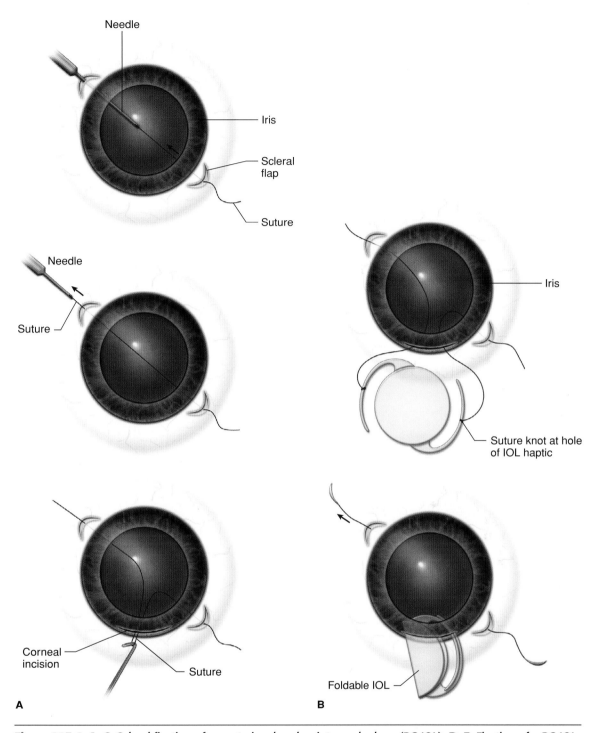

Figure 20E-8 A–C: Scleral fixation of a posterior chamber intraocular lens (PC-IOL). **D–F:** Fixation of a PC-IOL behind the iris by suturing it to the iris itself. **G:** PC-IOL sutured to the iris following 23G PPV for PC-IOL dislocation after a complicated phacoemulsification and PC-IOL implantation—early postoperative photograph. **H:** Fixation of an iris-claw IOL in the anterior surface of the iris. **I:** Anterior fixation of an iris-claw IOL in a vitrectomized eye for posttraumatic rhegmatogenous retinal detachment, after pupillary dilatation. **J:** Fixation of an iris-claw IOL in the posterior surface of the iris **K:** Secondary posterior iris surface fixation of an iris-claw IOL in a vitrectomized eye for aphakic retinal detachment.

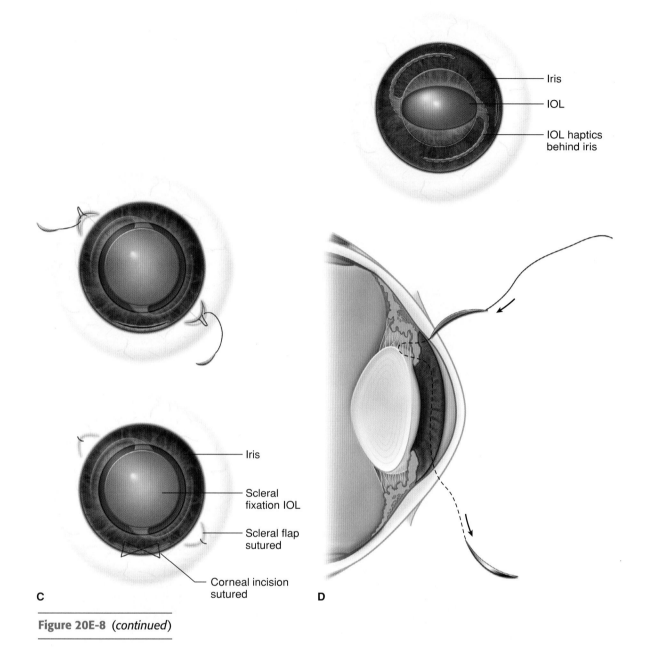

Figure 20E-8 (*continued*)

the main corneal incision. Then, the foldable optic remains in front of the iris while two haptics are placed behind the iris. Nondegradable sutures such as 10-0 or 9-0 polypropylene on a long-curved needle are then passed through the cornea, through the iris from anterior to posterior, behind the IOL haptic, through the iris from posterior to anterior and out through the cornea. The sutures are usually placed between the midperiphery of the iris and the angle to minimize the distortion of the IOL. A positioning instrument behind the IOL may be helpful to push the IOL anteriorly so that it will highlight the position of the lens haptics behind the iris as the needle passes through the iris and behind the haptics. A second paracentesis is made in peripheral cornea adjacent to the area of suture fixation. The suture ends are pulled out through this paracentesis with a hooked instrument, and tied externally. The knot is trimmed and the iris is repositioned. The same procedure is repeated for the other haptic paying attention to the centration of the IOL. Then, the optic of the IOL is repositioned posterior to the iris. The viscoelastic is aspirated and the corneal incision is closed.

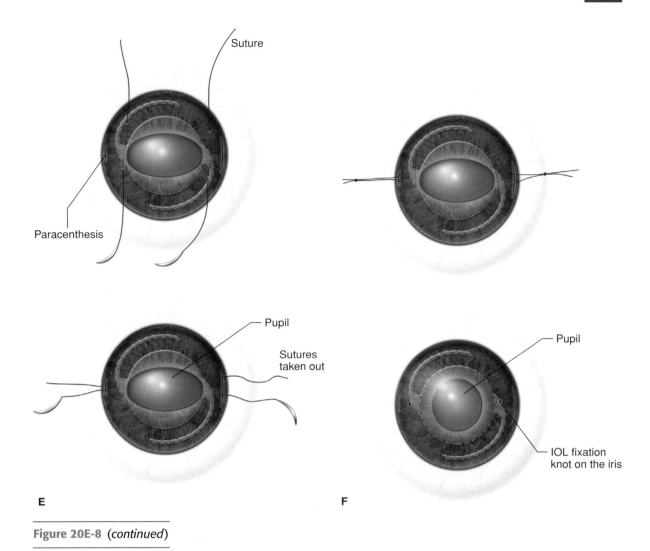

Figure 20E-8 *(continued)*

4a. Alternatively, iris-claw IOLs introduced by Worst[28,29] in the early 1980s, and improved thereafter, have been implanted successfully in aphakic eyes operated for congenital and traumatic cataracts in pediatric patients and in adults, and favorable visual outcomes and a low incidence of complications have been reported with the current model.[24,30–37] The Artisan Aphakia IOL (Ophtec BV, Groningen, The Netherlands) is one of the latest versions of the iris-fixated IOL. This single-piece polymethyl methacrylate (PMMA) IOL attaches to the anterior midperipheral iris stroma with clips on both sides of the optic. The foldable form manufactured from polysiloxane with PMMA haptics is not approved for aphakia yet. The surgical technique **(Figure 20E-8H)** starts with performing two vertical paracenteses at the 10- and 2-o'clock positions. Acetylcholine 1% is injected intracamerally followed by viscoelastic injection. A biplanar 5.2-mm posterior vascular corneal incision is made at the 12-o'clock position with a disposable slit knife. The iris-claw IOL is then inserted, rotated with Artisan lens manipulator to a horizontal position, and centered over the pupil. A special lens fixation forceps (Ophthec) is introduced through the main corneal incision. While holding the IOL with the IOL forceps, a special blunt enclavation needle (Ophthec) is introduced through the paracentesis and approximately 1 mm of iris tissue located in the middle is trapped by applying gentle pressure over it through the slotted center of the lens haptic. The same maneuver is performed for the second haptic in an effort to make the iris entrapment symmetrical to achieve ideal centration of the IOL. Special attention is paid to preventing IOL displacement, pupil ovalization, and deformation by positioning the iris claw

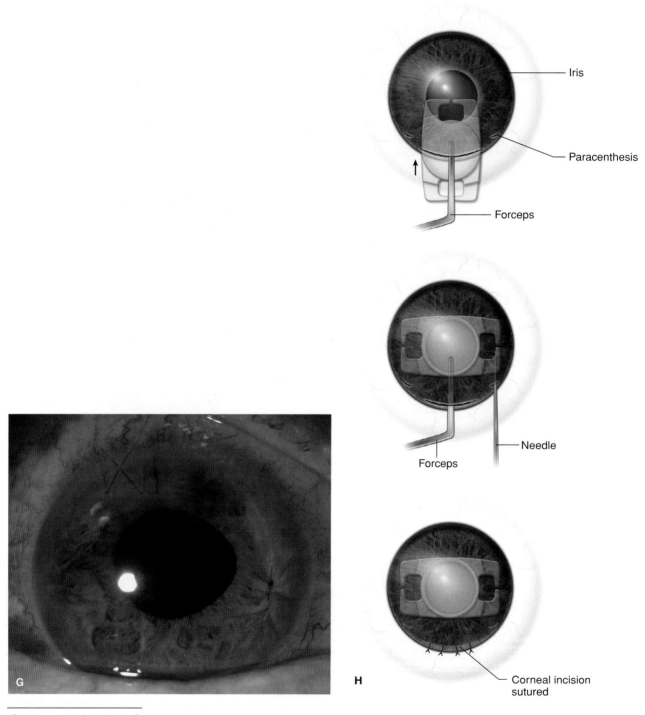

Figure 20E-8 (*continued*)

with an adequate amount of iris tissue to enable pupil movement. A peripheral slit iridotomy is performed at the 12-o'clock position if the eye had not already had a peripheral iridectomy at the 6-o'clock position. The viscoelastic is removed and the corneal incision is sutured. Alternatively, to fix the IOL to the iris a new vacuum enclavation system, the BO150 Vacufix (Ophthec, the Netherlands), is designed recently. It has two disposable handpieces, each one for the right and the left haptics. It is compatible with phaco machines, and aspirates and clips a fixed amount of iris tissue between the haptics of the IOL. Favorable outcomes were reported in 13 eyes that underwent vitrectomy for posteriorly dislocated lens fragments, and iris-claw lenses were implanted at the end.[34] However, the literature reflects limited experience with secondary Artisan iris-claw IOL implantation in aphakic eyes following PPV. Riazi et al.[36] reported that implantation of this type of IOL procedure was safe and effective in their series. We recently reported in our prospective series that secondary iris-claw IOL implantation is clinically safe and effective to correct aphakia in vitrectomized eyes without capsular support **(Figure 20E-8I)**.[37] In our series of 12 vitrectomized eyes, mean BCVA increased 10 ETDRS letters and complications were transient IOP increase, CME, and haptic dislocation replaced by surgery in one eye each. Retinas remained attached in all eyes. One concern was the mean endothelial cell density loss of 23.87% at the last visit despite no corneal decompensation.[37] Larger studies with longer follow-up are warranted with these IOLs. The Artisan IOL did not prevent pupil dilatation, and thus allowed good visualization of the peripheral retina. The lenses were stable. Besides, the reversibility of the procedure is also an advantage.

4b. Recently, we have been fixating the iris-claw IOLs onto the posterior face of iris as an alternative method in vitrectomized eyes **(Figure 20E-8J–K)**. Posterior iris surface fixation during keratoplasty was first described by Rijneveld et al.[30] in 1994, and posterior fixation through a scleral tunnel incision has also been reported.[38] Mohr et al.[39] reported favorable outcomes with retropupillary fixation in 48 aphakic eyes. Hara et al.,[40] has recently reported that retropupillary fixation of an iris-claw IOL that provides early visual recovery, has a low risk of postoperative increase in IOP, and is a time-saving method compared with transscleral suturing fixation for aphakic eyes without sufficient capsular support. However, to the best of author's knowledge the literature lacks experience with posterior iris surface fixation of iris-claw IOL implantation in aphakic eyes following PPV. According to our experience (unpublished data of the series of Z. Kapran, MD), the implantation of the iris-claw IOL behind the iris better preserves the anatomy of the anterior segment with respect to the iridocorneal angle. The technique is similar to the anterior fixation except the IOL is hold retropupillary from its optic with the forceps. The two haptics are gently introduced behind the iris, and the optic is slightly pulled forward to highlight the iris claws behind the iris. Then, 1 mm of midperipheral iris above the IOL claw is trapped through the slotted center of the lens haptic by applying gentle pressure over it and repeated on the other side. The centration of the IOL as well as pupil distortion is controlled. A small peripheric iridectomy is performed superiorly if it does not exist already. Viscoelastic is aspirated and the corneal incision is sutured. We believe that the posterior fixation of iris-claw lenses seems to have the advantages of a true PC implantation. Both the fixation techniques are easy, albeit necessitate a learning period, and especially in vitrectomized aphakic eyes one should be careful about intraoperative hypotony. The surgery is fast and reversible. The posteriorly fixated Artisan IOL does not interfere with pupil dilatation, and thus allows good visualization of the peripheral retina. Posterior fixation has the advantage to implant it with an endotamponade, and recently we have switched from our previous routine of fixating iris-claw IOLs anteriorly to posterior fixation instead. Although theoretically possible, to the best of our knowledge, there are no reports of spontaneous dislocation of the posteriorly fixated iris-claw lenses. In one study, secondary trauma resulted in dislocation of one haptic of the retroiridially placed Artisan IOLs in two out of 48 eyes, which were refixated easily by enclavation of the iris claw.[41] In a case report, subluxation of a retroiridially placed iris-claw lens from atrophic iris after an uncomplicated diode laser photocoagulation has been described.[42]

5. If there is an iridodialysis which is usually secondary to trauma, this can be repaired before or at the end of PPV before tamponade is given. When iris defects

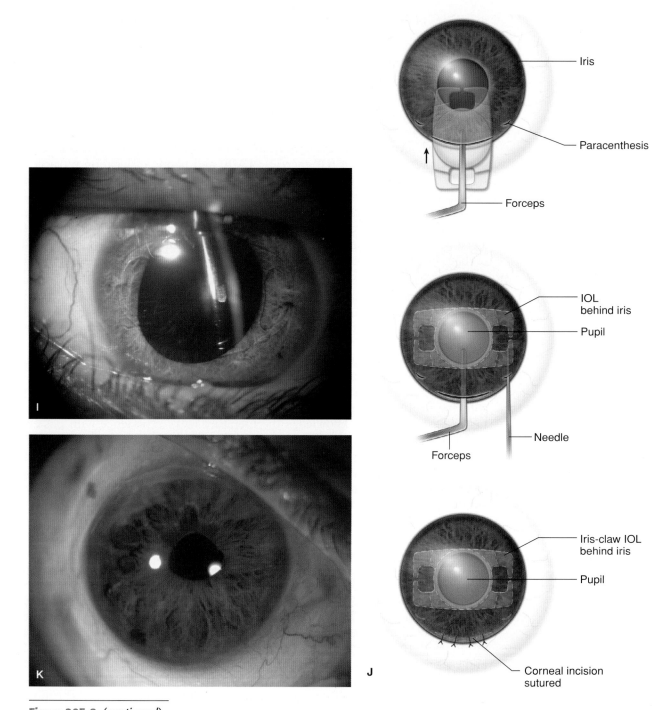

Figure 20E-8 *(continued)*

accompany aphakia following PPV, iris diaphragm IOLs, iris reconstruction implants, or aniridia IOLs, and even custom designed ones usually manufactured from PMMA and designed for scleral fixation may be preferred to avoid photophobia and glare or for cosmetic reasons. These have a fixed central transparent area through which peripheric retinal examination and laser photocoagulation can be performed with the help of contact wide-angle lenses. Dong et al.[43] reported favorable results with secondary black diaphragm IOL implantation in 15 aphakic eyes with traumatic aniridia and previous PPV. However, long-term results with larger series are warranted.

REFERENCES

1. Petermeier K, Szurman P, Bartz-Schmidt UK, et al. [Pathophysiology of cataract formation after vitrectomy]. *Klin Monbl Augenheilkd.* 2010;227:175–180. Review. German.

2. Artzén D, Lundström M, Behndig A, et al. Capsule complication during cataract surgery: Case-control study of preoperative and intraoperative risk factors: Swedish Capsule Rupture Study Group report 2. *J Cataract Refract Surg.* 2009;35:1688–1693.

3. Arbisser LB. Managing intraoperative complications in cataract surgery. *Curr Opin Ophthalmol.* 2004;15:33–39. Review.

4. Akman A, Yilmaz G, Oto S, et al. Comparison of various pupil dilatation methods for phacoemulsification in eyes with a small pupil secondary to pseudoexfoliation. *Ophthalmology.* 2004;111:1693–1698.

5. Goldman JM, Karp CL. Adjunct devices for managing challenging cases in cataract surgery: Capsular staining and ophthalmic viscosurgical devices. *Curr Opin Ophthalmol.* 2007;18:52–57. Review.

6. Nishimura A, Kobayashi A, Segawa Y, et al. Endoillumination-assisted cataract surgery in a patient with corneal opacity. *J Cataract Refract Surg.* 2003;29:2277–2280.

7. Blecher MH, Kirk MR. Surgical strategies for the management of zonular compromise. *Curr Opin Ophthalmol.* 2008;19:31–35. Review.

8. Menapace R, Findl O, Georgopoulos M, et al. The capsular tension ring: Designs, applications, and techniques. *J Cataract Refract Surg.* 2000;26:898–912. Review.

9. Yamakiri K, Sakamoto T, Noda Y, et al. One-year results of a multicenter controlled clinical trial of triamcinolone in pars plana vitrectomy. *Graefes Arch Clin Exp Ophthalmol.* 2008;246:959–966.

10. Acar N, Kapran Z, Altan T, et al. Pars plana vitrectomy with and without triamcinolone acetonide assistance in pseudophakic retinal detachment complicated with proliferative vitreoretinopathy. *Jpn J Ophthalmol.* 2010;54:331–337.

11. Yamakiri K, Sakamoto T, Noda Y, et al. Reduced incidence of intraoperative complications in a multicenter controlled clinical trial of triamcinolone in vitrectomy. *Ophthalmology.* 2007;114:289–296.

12. Wagoner MD, Cox TA, Ariyasu RG, et al; American Academy of Ophthalmology. Intraocular lens implantation in the absence of capsular support: A report by the American Academy of Ophthalmology. *Ophthalmology.* 2003;110:840–859.

13. Michaeli A, Assia EI. Scleral and iris fixation of posterior chamber lenses in the absence of capsular support. *Curr Opin Ophthalmol.* 2005;16:57–60. Review.

14. Kwong YY, Yuen HK, Lam RF, et al. Comparison of outcomes of primary scleral-fixated versus primary anterior chamber intraocular lens implantation in complicated cataract surgeries. *Ophthalmology.* 2007;114:80–85.

15. Evereklioglu C, Er H, Bekir NA, et al. Comparison of secondary implantation of flexible open-loop anterior chamber and scleral-fixated posterior chamber intraocular lenses. *J Cataract Refract Surg.* 2003;29:301–308.

16. Johnston RL, Charteris DG. Pars plana vitrectomy and sutured posterior chamber lens implantation. *Curr Opin Ophthalmol.* 2001;12:216–221. Review.

17. Rattigan SM, Ellerton CR, Chitkara DK, et al. Flexible open-loop anterior chamber intraocular lens implantation after posterior capsule complications in extracapsular cataract extraction. *J Cataract Refract Surg.* 1996;22:243–246.

18. Asadi R, Kheirkhah A. Long-term results of scleral fixation of posterior chamber intraocular lenses in children. *Ophthalmology.* 2008;115:67–72.

19. Vote BJ, Tranos P, Bunce C, et al. Long-term outcome of combined pars plana vitrectomy and scleral fixated sutured posterior chamber intraocular lens implantation. *Am J Ophthalmol.* 2006;141(2):308–312.

20. Sewelam A, Ismail AM, El Serogy H. Ultrasound biomicroscopy of haptic position after transscleral fixation of posterior chamber intraocular lenses. *J Cataract Refract Surg.* 2001;27:1418–1422.

21. Olsen TW, Pribila JT. Pars plana vitrectomy with endoscope-guided sutured posterior chamber intraocular lens implantation in children and adults. *Am J Ophthalmol.* 2011;151:287–296.

22. Gabor SG, Pavlidis MM. Sutureless intrascleral posterior chamber intraocular lens fixation. *J Cataract Refract Surg.* 2007;33:1851–1854.

23. Scharioth GB, Prasad S, Georgalas I, et al. Intermediate results of sutureless intrascleral posterior chamber intraocular lens fixation. *J Cataract Refract Surg.* 2010;36:254–259.

24. Hirashima DE, Soriano ES, Meirelles RL, et al. Outcomes of iris-claw anterior chamber versus iris-fixated foldable intraocular lens in subluxated lens secondary to Marfan syndrome. *Ophthalmology.* 2010;117:1479–1485.

25. Condon GP, Masket S, Kranemann C, et al. Small-incision iris fixation of foldable intraocular lenses in the absence of capsule support. *Ophthalmology.* 2007;114:1311–1318.

26. Condon GP. Simplified small-incision peripheral iris fixation of an AcrySof intraocular lens in the absence of capsule support. *J Cataract Refract Surg.* 2003;29:1663–1667.

27. Mura JJ, Pavlin CJ, Condon GP, et al. Ultrasound biomicroscopic analysis of iris-sutured foldable posterior chamber intraocular lenses. *Am J Ophthalmol.* 2010;149:245–252.

28. Worst JG, Massaro RG, Ludwig HH. The introduction of an artificial lens into the eye using Binkhorst's technique. *Ophthalmologica.* 1972;164:387–391.

29. Worst JG. Iris claw lens. *J Am Intraocul Implant Soc.* 1980;6:166–167.

30. Rijneveld WJ, Beekhuis WH, Hassman EF, et al. Iris claw lens: Anterior and posterior iris surface fixation in the absence of capsular support during penetrating keratoplasty. *J Refract Corneal Surg.* 1994;10:14–19.

31. Menezo JL, Martinez MC, Cisneros AL. Iris-fixated Worst claw versus sulcus-fixated posterior chamber lenses in the absence of capsular support. *J Cataract Refract Surg.* 1996;22:1476–1484.

32. Güell JL, Velasco F, Malecaze F, et al. Secondary Artisan–Verysise aphakic lens implantation. *J Cataract Refract Surg.* 2005;31:2266–2271.

33. Odenthal MT, Sminia ML, Prick LJ, et al. Long-term follow-up of the corneal endothelium after artisan lens implantation for unilateral traumatic and unilateral congenital cataract in children: Two case series. *Cornea.* 2006;25:1173–1177.

34. van der Meulen IJ, Gunning FP, Vermeulen MG, et al. Artisan lens implantation to correct aphakia after vitrectomy for retained nuclear lens fragments. *J Cataract Refract Surg.* 2004;30:2585–2589.

35. De Silva SR, Arun K, Anandan M, et al. Iris-claw intraocular lenses to correct aphakia in the absence of capsule support. *J Cataract Refract Surg.* 2011;37:1667–1672.

36. Riazi M, Moghimi S, Najmi Z, et al. Secondary Artisan–Verysise intraocular lens implantation for aphakic correction in post-traumatic vitrectomized eye. *Eye.* 2008;22:1419–1424.

37. Acar N, Kapran Z, Altan T, et al. Secondary iris claw intraocular lens implantation for the correction of aphakia after pars plana vitrectomy. *Retina.* 2010;30:131–139.

38. Baykara M, Ozcetin H, Yilmaz S, et al. Posterior iris fixation of the iris-claw intraocular lens implantation through a scleral tunnel incision. *Am J Ophthalmol.* 2007;144:586–591.

39. Mohr A, Hengerer F, Eckardt C. [Retropupillary fixation of the iris claw lens in aphakia. 1 year outcome of a new implantation techniques]. *Ophthalmologe.* 2002;99:580–583. German.

40. Hara S, Borkenstein AF, Ehmer A, et al. Retropupillary fixation of iris-claw intraocular lens versus transscleral suturing fixation for aphakic eyes without capsular support. *J Refract Surg.* 2011; 30:1–7.

41. Wolter-Roessler M, Küchle M. Correction of aphakia with retroiridally fixated IOL. *Klin Monbl Augenheilkd.* 2008;225:1041–1044.

42. Kičová N, Sekundo W, Mennel S. Subluxation of a retropupillary iris claw lens after cyclophotocoagulation. *Ophthalmologe.* 2011;108:167–169.

43. Dong X, Yu B, Xie L. Black diaphragm intraocular lens implantation in aphakic eyes with traumatic aniridia and previous pars plana vitrectomy. *J Cataract Refract Surg.* 2003;29:2168–2173.

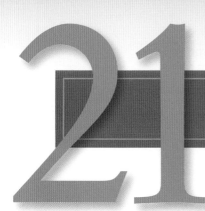

MACULAR FOLDS

RICHARD HAYNES

The Complication: Definition

Macular folds are folds of redundant retina that occur when the detached retina fails to return to the original topographical position following detachment surgery. Macular folds are effectively the result of a micro- or macroscopic (usually downward) translocation of the retina. Large folds tend to lie at the lower edge of the translocation where the redundant retina becomes rucked up. The excess of redundant retina becomes possible because retina elsewhere is stretched **(Figs. 21-1 and 21-2)**.

The clinical effect of the fold depends on the extent of the translocation and the exact location of the fold. A fold across the fovea can lead to poor acuity and severe metamorphopsia; however, a fold well below the fovea, caused by a large downward translocation of the whole macula, can result in relatively good acuity with little distortion but significant incyclotorsion or tilting of the image and resultant diplopia.

The metamorphopsia or cyclotorsion associated with macular folds can be extremely distracting, often being more problematic for the patient than reduced acuity alone. It is notable that visual acuity alone may be surprisingly well preserved, but this is in striking contrast to the dissatisfaction of the patient. This mismatch is due to the dissociating effect of the metamorphopsia and/or cyclotorsion, which make fusion of the image from the two eyes impossible (fusional range for cyclotorsion being small).

Macular folds have to be distinguished from folding of the retina caused by epiretinal membranes or proliferative vitreoretinopathy (PVR), which usually present later.

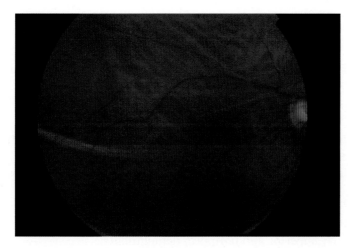

Figure 21-1 Fundus photograph of a macular fold

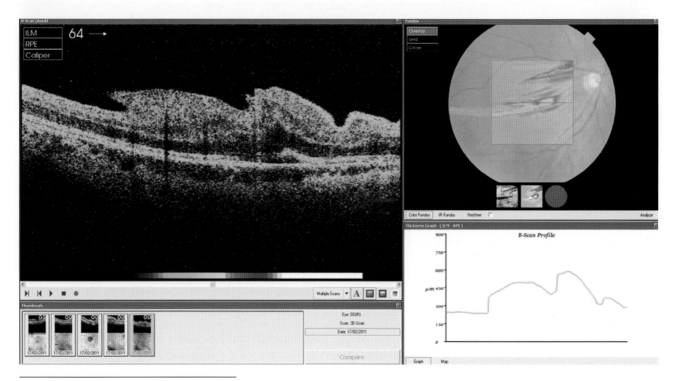

Figure 21-2 OCT image of a macular fold

◆ Risk Factors

Surgical Technique

◆ Most contemporary reports of retinal folds are associated with vitrectomy surgery, particularly where the gas bubble is large in comparison to the area of detachment and sits in front of the macula in the upright position (folds are less likely to occur with small gas bubbles).[1]

◆ The incidence of macular folds is almost certainly underestimated. Two separate recent autofluorescence imaging studies have revealed a degree of retinal translocation or macular fold formation as high as 62.8%[2] and 57.6%[3] of successful detachment operations. However, although anecdotally almost all VR surgeons will recall seeing a case with significant clinical macular folds, these cases are much less common, major units seeing perhaps one or two significant cases every few years.

◆ Folds have been reported with conventional buckling surgery when a large air bubble is injected to flatten a fish-mouthing tear.[4] The incidence of fold formation with buckling surgery has been reported as 2.8% with affected cases having large encircling elements and gas injection.[5]

◆ Incomplete drainage of subretinal fluid in the presence of a large gas/air bubble in either vitrectomy or buckling cases is a prerequisite for fold formation, particularly in a fresh detachment where subretinal fluid has low viscosity and is more mobile.[5]

Detachment Configuration

◆ Folds occur more commonly the greater the area of bullous detachment, particularly superior and temporal detachments.

◆ Macular-off or fovea splitting detachments. If the macula is detached or becomes detached during the surgery, it is easier for the macula to inadvertently translocate at a later time point. In addition, subretinal fluid gravitates more easily into the submacular space if subretinal fluid has been present in this location previously, this can occur while the patient is in the supine position at the end of the surgery.

◆ Giant retinal tears are more likely to lead to downward slippage of the retina; however, this is a well-recognized problem that is usually noted intraoperatively and effectively dealt with by direct heavy liquid to oil exchange.[6]

Immediate Postoperative Posture

◆ Upright postoperative posture or a face-down posture after even a brief period of being upright are most likely to lead to inadvertent translocation and fold formation if enough subretinal fluid is present.[7]

◆ Pathogenesis: Why Does It Occur

The above risk factors set the scene for the conditions necessary to allow inadvertent translocation of the retina and development of a retinal fold. The sequence of events that lead to a fold are as follows:

Residual subretinal fluid still present following a fluid–air exchange (almost inevitably present unless all subretinal fluid is evacuated with heavy liquid) will gravitate to the submacular space, which is the most dependent position while the patient is still lying supine at the end of the surgery. As soon as the patient adopts an upright position the denser submacular fluid will gravitate inferiorly **(Figure 21-3)**.

When it reaches the lower edge of the detachment, at the dependent border between the detached and the attached retina, the sequestered subretinal fluid will pool in this location causing the retina to bulge out like a drip of viscous paint, the mass of this bulge of subretinal fluid stretches and pulls the retina down, creating a translocation that is limited by the elasticity of the retina. This migration of subretinal fluid occurs rapidly in a completely gas-filled eye, taking at the most, minutes if not seconds. If face-down posture is adopted once this migration has occurred the macula will stick in this translocated position with fold formation at the lower border of the subretinal fluid.

(Note: This process only occurs because the premacular and submacular spaces contain substances of different density [gas and subretinal fluid respectively]. If, however, the gas bubble is small enough to not sit in front of the macula when the patient is in the upright position, then the premacular and the submacular

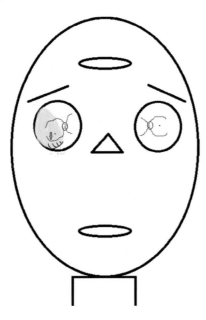

Figure 21-3 Upright posture showing submacular fluid migrating inferiorly creating fold

fluid have very similar density and there will be no relative inferior movement of submacular fluid, no translocation and no fold formation.)

✛ Pearls on How to Prevent It

◆ When we look at the risk factors listed above, the detachment configuration is out of our control; therefore, the only modifiable risk factors are the surgical technique and postoperative posturing.

◆ Regarding surgical technique:

  ◆ Small gas bubbles can be used, but many cases require large gas bubbles to provide adequate tamponade for inferior breaks.

  ◆ Heavy liquid can be used to evacuate all subretinal fluid in high risk detachments, but subretinal fluid can still sequester anteriorly at the ora serrata, reappearing later when the heavy liquid is removed.

  ◆ A posterior drainage retinotomy has been advocated to allow a more complete internal drainage of subretinal fluid,[1] but creating more holes in the retina may increase the risk of PVR.

  ◆ Large buckling elements can be avoided in high risk cases, particularly when intraocular gas is injected.

  ◆ However, given that surgical technique is not always amenable to modification (large gas bubbles and buckling elements are sometimes unavoidable and subretinal fluid is not always completely drained), the remaining risk factor that can be consistently controlled is the position of the patient in the critical minutes at the end of the operation. Unless the patient is positioned so that subretinal fluid gravitates away from the macula in a harmless direction, an inadvertent translocation and fold could develop.

◆ Whenever subretinal fluid has been under the macula or when there is any possibility that subretinal fluid could track under the macula, the following routine should help minimize the risk of a fold developing:

Position 1 = Operated side-down

  ◆ Immediately at the end of the vitrectomy, roll the patient so the operated side ear is on the pillow and their face is completely horizontal. This position is tolerated well by patients under local anesthetic, and anesthetists are generally happy to recover general anesthetic patients in this position too.

  ◆ In this position if there is any submacular fluid, it will run temporally away from the disc, but the retina will have limited possibility of moving with the fluid and will "hang" anchored to the disc, it may stretch slightly but will recoil later **(Figure 21-4)**. There will be no inferior or superior movement

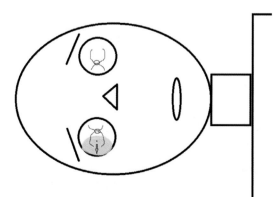

Figure 21-4 Operated side-down posture showing subretinal fluid gravitating temporally harmlessly

of the fovea. Any microscopic temporal movement of the fovea is likely to be within the horizontal fusion range.

◆ The patient should be transported to the ward *on a trolley* in this operated side-down position (with no upright period).

◆ By the time the patient arrives at the ward on the trolley (5 to 10 minutes later), the subretinal fluid will be lying temporal to the macula.

Position 2 = Face-down

◆ The patient should then roll to a face-down position for about 30 minutes *with no upright period during the transfer from operated side-down to face-down* (i.e., no upright period during the transfer from Position 1 to Position 2).

◆ The face-down position will cause the macula to "stick" with re-establishment of the macular RPE pump. The subretinal fluid will gravitate anteriorly and safely toward the ora serrata.

Position 3 = Nonoperated side-down

◆ Finally, the patient should roll on to their nonoperated side completing a 180-degree log roll.

◆ This last maneuver is probably not critical but it is a more comfortable position for the patient than remaining face-down and will usually tamponade temporal or superior breaks that led to the macular detachment.

◆ In addition, the nursing staff will become used to performing the log roll as a routine, and therefore, inappropriate posturing positions are avoided.

◆ It is best to advise the ward nursing staff that if the patient has to become upright for any reason before the above sequence has been completed (e.g., to visit the lavatory), then it is best to lie the patient supine for 10 minutes (to relocate the macula) and then repeat the sequence again from Position 1 to Position 3.

◆ In the past, posturing techniques described to move fluid away from the macula have been called "steam rolling." This is not an accurate description of the events that occur in the posturing sequence described above, as at no point is subretinal fluid "forced" into any position by a "floating" gas bubble, the subretinal fluid is simply migrating downhill in response to gravity to the most dependent position.

◆ It is to be remembered that the above posturing sequence is *not* designed to ensure adequate tamponade of retinal breaks postoperatively or successful primary repair, but is solely to prevent a macular fold developing. That is, the business of ensuring the retina remains attached in the long term is subordinate, in the first postoperative minutes, to ensuring that a macular fold does not develop. This is because a flat retina with a macular fold can be just as problematic for both the patient and the surgeon as failed primary detachment surgery.

◆ The patient can be instructed regarding the appropriate postoperative posture to ensure adequate tamponade of retinal breaks to maximize the chance of successful primary repair on day 1 post-op or at the point of discharge (if a day-case procedure), once the log roll sequence has been performed.

◆ There are those who argue that folds are such a rare event and that any attempt to prevent them is a wasted effort. However, autofluorescence studies show that small subclinical, inadvertent translocations are common, occurring in up to 62.8% of detachments with immediate upright posture (even for just a few minutes) before face-down posture.[2] In these subclinical cases, only a trivial translocation of the macula occurred (causing up to 5 degrees of torsion), presumably because the volume of subretinal fluid was low. However, this study emphasizes that the immediate upright posture position should be avoided at all costs as it clearly predisposes to downward translocation, with translocation being significantly associated with the extent of the detachment ($p = 0.019$) and the macular-off status ($p = 0.016$).[2] When a greater volume of subretinal fluid is present, a large translocation is possible with symptoms that are so intrusive that the simple measures outlined above should be taken to prevent its occurrence. The increasing trend for day-case surgery may risk an increased incidence of macular fold formation due to the reduced opportunity for performing the log roll sequence.[8] Therefore, even in the absence of a postoperative recovery ward, facilities should be available to allow the patient to remain on a trolley while the log roll sequence is performed, before being discharged home in the upright position (with instructions on how to posture when home to maximize primary success).

Pearls on How to Solve It

- Once a fold has developed, surgery may be required to correct the situation, particularly, if the patient suffers severe metamorphopsia, diplopia, or a tilted image.

- Treatment of macular folds requires surgical redetachment of the macula, which is a maneuver that can be complex and may increase the risk of PVR and late redetachment.

- The techniques for the surgical correction are borrowed from those developed for macular translocation surgery.

- There are no clear indications for the timing of corrective surgery. Animal experiments have shown apoptosis of photoreceptors and thinning of the outer nuclear layer can be detected as early as 1 week after limited macular translocation.[7] Earlier intervention therefore may enhance the restoration of normal photoreceptor–RPE anatomical relations, which are essential for photoreceptor preservation and visual function.

- Earlier intervention may also be more successful because adhesion of the inner surfaces of the fold could make unfurling progressively more difficult with time.

- Appropriate consent and setting of patient expectations, explaining that the aim is to reduce distortion, diplopia, and tilt, and that central visual acuity may not improve or could even deteriorate. It should also be pointed out that more than one operation is needed (corrective surgery plus oil removal).

- Several techniques have been described including induction of detachment with a 41-gauge needle and "ironing" out the fold with perfluorohexyloctane (F_6H_8) heavy liquid which is left in the eye with supine posture followed by removal of the heavy liquid 5 days later.[9]

- An alternative technique used by the author in a small series of cases with macular folds[10] has been adapted from a technique described by Toth et al.[11] This involves detachment of the retina with a subretinal infusion of BSS via a retinotomy and a soft silicone ball-tipped cannula, and will be described in more detail below:

  - A small superior retinotomy is made with diathermy of the edges.

  - A Duke Roundball Cannula (Alcon/Grieshaber)[11] is attached via flexible tubing to a 10-mL syringe of BSS plus (held by the assistant) for the induction of the retinal detachment. The Duke Roundball Cannula is used to simultaneously

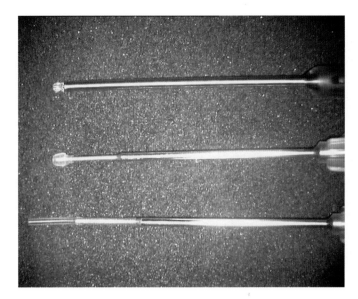

Figure 21-5 Images of the Duke Roundball Cannula (Alcon/Grieshaber)[11] (*top*), a modified 20-g Subretinal Fluid Cannula (BD Visitec) rolled back on itself to produce a bulbous end (*middle*) and an unmodified 20-g Subretinal Fluid Cannula (BD Visitec) (*bottom*).

inject BSS into the subretinal space and "plug" the retinotomy to allow enlargement of the detachment.[11] If a Duke Roundball Cannula is not available, a bulbous-ended cannula can be fashioned by folding a 20-g, soft silicone-tipped Subretinal Fluid Cannula (BD Visitec) back on itself **(Figure 21-5)**. Alternatively, a 41-gauge needle can be used to create the detachment but multiple injection sites may be needed.

◆ A 19-gauge trocar is inserted into one (enlarged 20 g) sclerostomy port to allow the escape of fluid from the vitreous cavity during induction of the detachment; if this is not done, the progress of the developing detachment may halt, due to equilibration between the pressure in the subretinal space with that in the vitreous cavity.

◆ If the retinal detachment stops progressing or does not progress as far as the fold, a fluid–air exchange will encourage the subretinal fluid to localize below the macula, agitation of the eye will then encourage further stripping off of the retina.

◆ In the air-filled eye, the detachment can be enlarged by dripping further BSS through the retinotomy into the subretinal space. Repeated aspiration of any preretinal fluid with a silicone-tipped cannula and agitation of the eye leads to complete macular detachment.

◆ Heavy liquid is then dripped on to the inferior-attached retina first (with the eye rotated downwards) to flatten the retina from below upward (attached to detached) so as to unfold the retina. The injecting cannula is attached to a modified Tano scraper to allow simultaneous injection of the heavy liquid and gentle engagement of the retina to translocate the retina back up to its correct position. When the macula is judged to be in the correct position it is held in place with the Tano scraper while heavy liquid is injected (by the assistant) to completely fill the vitreous cavity.

◆ Endolaser retinopexy is applied to all retinal breaks and silicone oil injected in a heavy liquid–oil exchange (to prevent further slippage[6]).

◆ The log roll sequence described above is performed to prevent recurrence.

◆ The silicone oil should be left in for 8 to 12 weeks before removal.

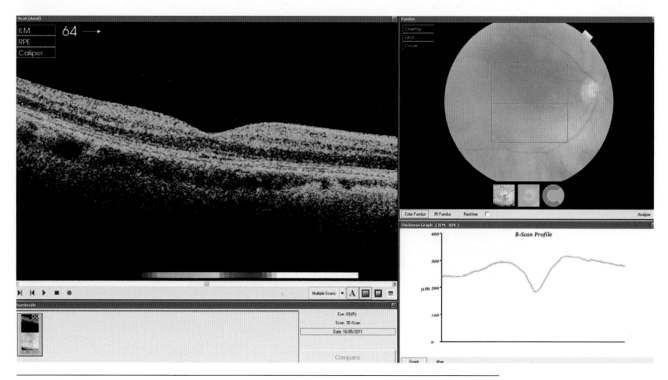

Figure 21-6 OCT scan showing the fold from Figs 21-1 and 21-2 following corrective surgery

Expected Outcomes: What Is the Worst-case Scenario

Larrison et al.[1] reported that *without* corrective surgery, one-third of macular fold cases had postoperative acuity of 6/60 or worse and only one-third managed 6/18 or better. As mentioned previously, however, poor visual acuity is only part of the spectrum of symptoms; visual acuity may be well preserved with patients still suffering severe metamorphopsia, torsion, and diplopia.

Surgery to correct a macular fold theoretically risks complications such as PVR detachment and hypotony, although reported cases have led to symptomatic improvements and can result in good visual outcomes (e.g., 6/9 in the case from **Figs. 21-1** and **21-2**) with resolution of diplopia, distortion, and restoration of the normal macular architecture on OCT **(Figure 21-6)**.

REFERENCES

1. Larrison WI, Frederick AR Jr, Peterson TJ, et al. Posterior retinal folds following vitreoretinal surgery. *Arch Ophthalmol.* 1993;111:621–625.
2. Shiragami C, Shiraga F, Yamaji H, et al. Unintentional displacement of the retina after standard vitrectomy for rhegmatogenous retinal detachment. *Ophthalmology.* 2010;117:86–92.
3. Dell'Omo R, Mura M, Lesnik Oberstein SY, et al. Early simultaneous fundus autofluorescence and optical coherence tomography features after pars plana vitrectomy for primary rhegmatogenous retinal detachment. *Retina.* 2012;32:719–728.
4. Pavan PR. Retinal fold in macula following intraocular gas. *Arch Ophthalmol.* 1984;102:83–84.
5. Van Meurs JC, Humalda D, Mertens DA, et al. Retinal folds through the macula. *Doc Ophthalmol.* 1991;78:335–340.

6. Wong D, Williams RL, German MJ. Exchange of perfluorodecalin for gas or oil: A model for avoiding slippage. *Graefes Arch Clin Exp Ophthalmol.* 1998;236:2 34–237.

7. Hayashi A, Usui S, Kawaguchi K, et al. Retinal changes after retinal translocation surgery with scleral imbrication in dog eyes. *Invest Ophthalmol Vis Sci.* 2000;41: 4288–4292.

8. Isaico R, Malvitte L, Bron AM, et al. Macular folds after retinal detachment surgery: The possible impact of outpatient surgery. *Graefes Arch Clin Exp Ophthalmol.* 2013;251(1):383–384.

9. Herbert EN, Groenewald C, Wong D. Treatment of retinal folds using a modified macula relocation technique with perfluoro-hexyloctane tamponade. *Br J Ophthalmol.* 2003; 87(7): 921–922.

10. Haynes RJ. Postoperative macular folds, their aetiology, prevention and treatment. In press.

11. Toth C, Freedman S. Macular translocation with 360-degree peripheral retinectomy: Impact of technique and surgical experience on visual outcomes. *Retina.* 2001;21(4): 293–303.

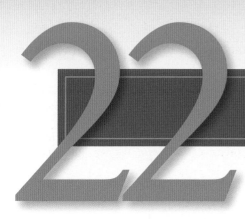

VISUAL FIELD LOSS

Silvia Bopp

 ## The Complication: Definition

Peripheral visual field defects (VFDs) are a complication that may occur following uneventful vitrectomy. Most often, these scotomas become apparent immediately after surgery or gas resorption. Typically, kinetic or static perimetry reveals dense, peripherally located scotomas without affecting the blind spot or the central visual field. Visual field loss usually remains unchanged. Despite of their presence, patients may be asymptomatic.

Postoperative peripheral visual field loss must be differentiated from **central/paracentral VFD** following vitrectomy. The latter may occur as a result of accidental, surgical, toxic, or vascular damage of the posterior retina or optic nerve head (ONH). In this context, visual loss associated with silicone oil tamponade presents with a central scotoma and shows particular features (see Chapter 19D).

Visual field loss after uncomplicated **vitrectomy with intraocular gas tamponade** has been reported sporadically since the mid-90th, in particular when macular hole surgery (MHS) emerged.[1,2] This was an incidental finding as a few patients subjectively noticed a scotoma. Systematic prospective investigations revealed that this complication was more frequent than expected. Rates up to 70% have been reported in prospective studies.[3,4] Despite of that, the findings often remained asymptomatic, because the central visual field was not affected. Most publications describe peripheral visual field loss after MHS, but few reports also showed this complication after other indications for vitrectomy, such as surgery for epiretinal membranes (ERM), optic pit maculopathy, exudative age-related macular degeneration (ARMD), and retinal detachment.[5–8]

The VFD pattern varies, but most often they appear as wedge-shaped scotomas, sometimes arcuate or altitudinal. Most frequently, the inferotemporal quadrant is affected and the scotoma extends more or less above or below the horizontal, but other sectors may also be involved **(Figure 22-1)**.[2,4,6,9–15]

Since the introduction of ICG (indocyanine green)-assisted macular surgery, **ICG-related postoperative scotomas** have been reported as well,[7,16–19] which are not necessarily associated with intravitreal gas application. Different from those mentioned above, they appear more pronounced and are predominantly located in the nasal quadrants **(Figure 22-2)**.

Clinical findings in eyes with postoperative VFD are subtle; most cases do not show any ophthalmoscopic changes **(Figure 22-3)**. Segmental optic disc pallor is the most frequent finding.[2,9–11,20] Other signs include focal narrowing of the arteriole in the corresponding retinal area[21] and regional mottling of the retinal pigment epithelium (RPE), atrophic retinal defects and epiretinal membrane formation.[20] Visible fundus changes correspond to the VFD. They become clinically visible months after surgery whereas the scotoma can be measured in the immediately postoperative period. We have observed one patient who had an inferotemporal scotoma and

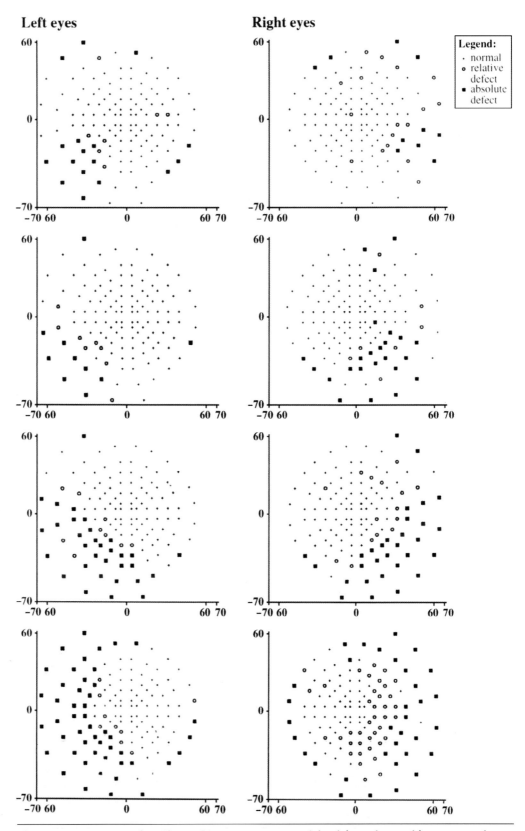

Figure 22-1 Automated perimetry (Octopus program 07) in eight patients with postoperative scotoma after MHS with gas tamponade. No ICG staining for ILM peeling was used. VFD affects the inferotemporal and temporal quadrants. The infusion port was always placed in the infero-temporal quadrant. The central visual field is not involved and all macular holes were closed. (From: Bopp S, Lucke K, Hille U. Peripheral visual field loss after vitreous surgery for macular holes. *Graefes Arch Clin Exp Ophthalmol.* 1997;235:362–371)

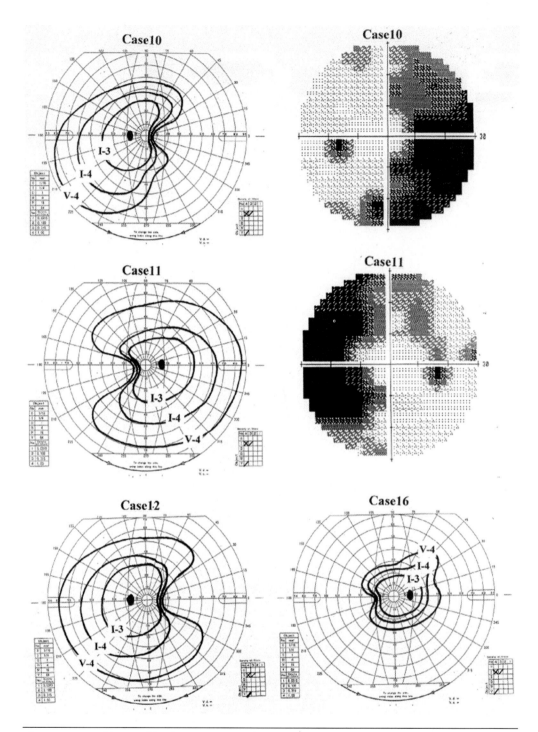

Figure 22-2 Goldmann kinetic perimetry and Humphrey central 30-degrees visual field in patients with postoperative VFD after vitrectomy with ICG-assisted ILM peeling for epiretinal membranes. The nasal half is always affected, sometimes extensive concentric constriction occurs, but the center is usually spared. (From: Uemura A, Kanda S, Sakamoto Y, et al. Visual field defects after uneventful vitrectomy for epiretinal membrane with indocyanine green-assisted internal limiting membrane peeling. *Am J Ophthalmol.* 2003;136:252–257, with permission of Elsevier, Limited).

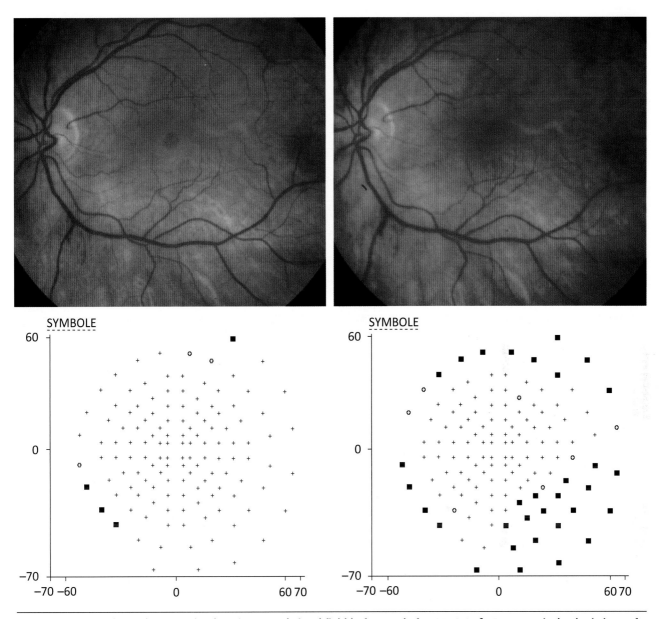

Figure 22-3 Correlation between fundus picture and visual field before and after MHS. **Left:** Preoperatively, depictions of a macular hole stage 3 based on Gass' classification and normal full visual field test. **Right:** Postoperatively the macular hole is closed, but a wedge-shaped visual field defect inferotemporal is present. Note: No optic nerve pallor is present.

showed honeycomb-like retinal changes superonasally with subsequent formation of atrophic holes at this site few months after surgery **(Figure 22-4)**.

Diagnostic tests: Except for the scotoma measured by visual field examination, the most consistent finding is thinning of the retinal nerve fiber layer (RNFL) when measuring out the peripapillary RNFL thickness.[9,10,22,23] RNFL defects, however, could not be demonstrated by red-free photography.[9,12] Fundus fluorescein angiography (FFA) and indocyanine green angiography (ICG-A) may show window defects in areas of pigment mottling and delayed choroidal filling as a hint on damage to the choriocapillaris.[11,20] Multifocal electroretinography (mERG) was found to be normal in the area of visual field loss,[22] which largely rules out a previous arterial occlusive event. Some eyes also reveal a relative afferent papillary defect (RAPD) and show more or less optic disc pallor.[2]

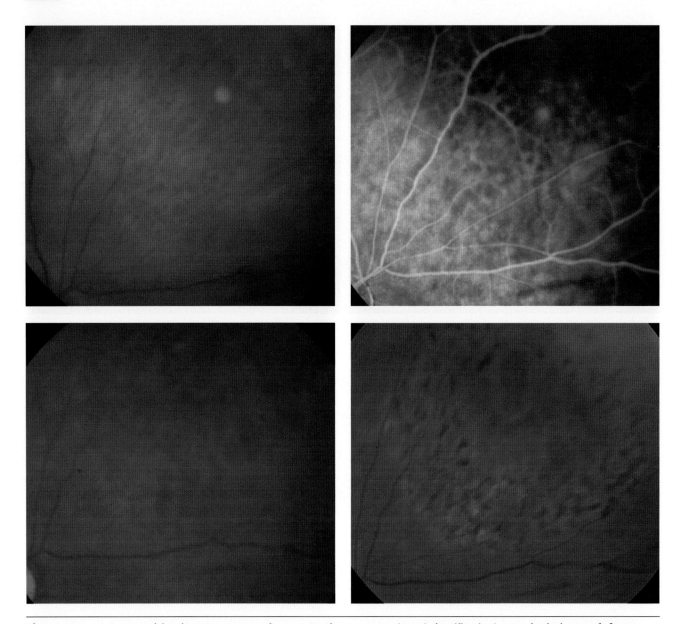

Figure 22-4 Superonasal fundus appearance after surgery for a stage 2 (Gass' classification) macular hole. **Top left:** Two months postoperatively, funduscopy showed honeycomb changes and FAG revealed granular RPE mottling **(top right)**. **Botton left:** Six months later, cystic changes appeared confluent with fibrotic retinal changes. As the retina looked very thin with multiple atrophic holes, prophylactic scatter laser was performed in this area **(bottom right)**.

✦ Risk Factors

◆ *Intraoperative air–fluid exchange* is an important precondition for postvitrectomy VFD.[6] The complication became apparent when MHS became one of the most frequent vitreoretinal procedures performed. Furthermore, eyes with a macular hole usually do not reveal other pathologies. Therefore, postoperative scotomas are most likely caused by the surgery itself **(Figure 22-1)**. When comparing eyes with macular hole (gas tamponade) and ERM (no gas tamponade), the latter one did not show postoperative scotomas.[6] Moreover, the location of VFD usually depends on the placement of the infusion cannula through which the air is infused, which indicates damage to the contralateral retina induced by the flow of air. When positioning the infusion port inferotemporally, scotomas appeared inferotemporally and when located inferonasally, then were present inferonasally.[14,24] The air pressure during air–fluid exchange has been found to influence the rate of VFD. Usually, the air pressure usually is set at 40 to 50 mm Hg. When lowering the air pressure from 50 to 30 mm Hg, the occurrence of VFD decreased significantly.[24]

◆ *Surgical-induced posterior vitreous detachment (PVD)* is an essential part of MHS. Kerrison et al.[2] and Boldt et al.[11] suggested that elevation of the posterior hyaloid causes trauma to the ONH, for example, the peripapillary vasculature or nerve fiber layer. This hypothesis was substantiated by a comparative study (102 eyes, macular holes stage 2 and 3) showing that eyes in which a PVD limited to the macular area was created did NOT show postoperative VFDs, whereas in 22% of those in whom a complete PVD was created develop a scotoma.[15] Contradictorily, VFD have also been reported in stage 4 macular holes in which PVD is not necessary, as the vitreous cortex is already detached.[4,12] Thus, there is some, but no strong evidence, that surgical PVD contributes to the occurrence of postoperative VFD.

◆ More recently, *ICG dye* used to visualize the vitreoretinal interface structures during ERM, and ILM peeling has been found to increase the risk of postvitrectomy scotomas, in particular when high concentrations (0.5%) and long exposure times (e.g., several minutes, applied under air) were used.[7,16–19] The pattern of postoperative visual field loss differs from those observed in eyes without dye application: The nasal sectors are most often affected or extensive constriction may be present,[19,25,26] but the central part is excluded as well **(Figure 22-2)**. A different pathogenic mechanism of retinal damage must be suspected. When comparing a surgical series with and without ICG staining, the group without dye application did not show VFD, whereas those with ICG showed scotomas in 30% to 50% of cases.[16,26]

◆ *Postvitrectomy IOP elevation* is a common problem, particularly in the early postoperative phase, with the subsequent risk of optic nerve damage, even blindness. In all studies on postoperative visual field loss, careful attention was paid to monitor IOP. There was none that provided sufficient data to support IOP peaks as a cause for the VFD described.

Pathogenesis

The Role of Intraoperative Fluid–Air Exchange

Postoperative visual field loss manifested after MHS in which gas tamponade is an indispensable part of surgery. Furthermore, prior to the era of ILM peeling (with/without visualization aids) it was believed that extensive fluid drainage, both from the vitreal cavity and from the macular hole, contributes to high anatomic success rates. Several findings indicate that the mechanism of damage is airflow during fluid–air exchange that causes dehydration injury during this maneuver. First, when comparing eyes after MHS (gas tamponade) and eyes after ERM (no gas), the latter did not reveal any scotoma.[6] Second, the location of the infusion cannula affects the area of VFD (see above).[14,24,27] Third, passing air through water (humidified air) reduces the incidence of postoperative scotomas significantly.[28] Fourth, the duration of airflow and air pressure has a significant impact on the VFD, for example, lower pressure and sclerotomies kept closed correlate with a lower complication rate.[24,29] Finally, the protective effect of a limited vitrectomy that is confined to the posterior pole in MHS has been shown to prevent VFD, presumably by protecting the retinal surface from direct airflow.[28]

Postoperative scotomas correlate with RNFL thinning.[9,10,13] Correspondingly, focal and multifocal ERG of the involved retina have been shown to be normal indicating damage to the inner retina, but sparing the outer retina (photoreceptor cells, bipolar cells).[9,22]

The clinical data is supported by experimental studies. Vitrectomy and air infusion caused retinal damage in rabbit eyes, whereas vitrectomy alone did not. The amount of damage was more prominent at the opposite site from the infusion cannula and more pronounced with higher air pressure.[30,31] Using a modified infusion cannula that was designed to scatter the air by multiple radial openings also reduced retinal damage in an experimental rabbit model.[32] Interestingly, early morphologic findings showed predominantly inner retinal changes,[30] whereas morphologic findings at 4 weeks also revealed photoreceptor thinning and RPE alterations.[31] Those outer retinal changes at a later time indicate that the extent of damage may progress. The experimental data proves mechanical airflow-induced retinal damage that offers an explanation for postoperative scotomas.

The Role of Surgically Induced PVD

Melberg and Thomas[1] first took this pathogenic mechanism into consideration. Occasionally, very firm adhesion of the posterior vitreous cortex to the optic nerve head (ONH) is a well-known observation during surgery, sometimes resulting in petechial hemorrhages at the disk margin. Hypothetically, damage to the peripapillary nerve fiber layer or supplying capillaries by shearing forces is conceivable.[6,10,11] An experimental study in cynomolgus monkeys has shown considerable morphologic changes at the vitreoretinal interface after having performed a surgical separation of the cortical vitreous from the retina/ONH,[33] in particular disruption, breaks and delamination of the ILM, avulsion and breaks in the inner retina, and avulsion of axon bundles of the optic disk. Noteworthy, the lesions detected histologically were not evident to the surgeon. In other words, surgical PVD may cause more pronounced tissue damage than estimated from clinical findings. It is unclear if the experimental data can be applied to the clinical situation. As functional tests (e.g., visual field examination) are not applicable in an experimental setting, the question remains unanswered, whether the traumatic lesions caused by mechanical PVD can directly lead to peripheral VFD or indirectly increase the susceptibility for additional damage by airflow through the vitreous cavity. Postoperative optic disc pallor and reduced peripapillary RNFL thickness are seen in eyes with postoperative VFD, but these findings do not allow drawing conclusions about their pathogenesis (e.g., juxtapapillary vs. peripheral nerve fiber loss).

The Role of ICG-assisted Peeling

ILM removal in MHS undoubtedly has increased anatomic success rates. When ICG was introduced for ILM staining,[34] no data about the biocompatibility of ICG solution was available. Meanwhile, numerous clinical and experimental data hint on ICG toxicity, at least when using high concentrations and long exposure times.[35] Among the complications reported there are postoperative VFDs.[25] Different from the above mentioned etiology of postvitrectomy scotomas, a different pathogenetic mechanism must be assumed, as the pattern and the extent of scotomas are different (more pronounced and usually nasally located).

Several studies support ICG to be the cause for visual field loss: First, ICG-assisted peeling of ERM without the use of a gas tamponade may also generate scotomas.[7] Second, when comparing MHS with and without the use of ICG, the former group had 50% peripheral scotomas, the latter did not show this complications.[16] Third, ICG concentration and exposure to the retina affect the rate of visual field loss, whereas 0.25% solution with immediate washout was not followed by visual defects.[17] In our clinic, we have not detected any cases with postoperative visual field loss following ICG-assisted ILM peeling with a 10-year experience using an isotonic, iso-osmolar 0.1% ICG solution.

Experimental and clinical data on the mechanism of retinal damage by ICG are heterogeneous and controversial, but a dose-dependent toxic effect is verified. Furthermore, ultrastructural findings of ILM specimens obtained during surgery for ERM and MH revealed significant retinal cell debris at the retinal surface of the ILM.[24,25,36]

Similar to eyes that had undergone MHS without dye and develop a postoperative scotoma, cases with ICG-related VFD also show a reduced RNFL thickness as measured by OCT.[23] Noteworthy, all quadrants except the temporal quadrant were affected. When comparing RNFL thickness findings in eyes with VFD after ICG exposure with those after gas–fluid exchange with no ICG use, the latter showed only superonasal thinning in most cases.[9]

To sum up, postoperative visual field loss after ICG-assisted MHS can be differentiated from that without the use of dye by the pattern of scotomas, but thinning of the RNFL is a common feature.

Other Contributing Factors

Few data hint on possible vascular pathologic changes in eyes with postvitrectomy scotomas. Basically, the retinal vessels, choriocapillaris or epipapillary vasculature can be affected.

Focal narrowing of the retinal arteriole extending into the area corresponding to the VFD has been observed.[11,21] FFA has delayed filling in these areas. Intermittent arterial compression and occlusion during gas tamponade were suspected, but not substantiated by further studies.

A choroidal filling delay was also found by ICG-A in areas of visible fundus changes, such as RPE mottling.[20] As these findings were not regularly present and became apparent in the late postoperative course, they might be secondary phenomena.

Hypothetically, peripapillary vessels may be damaged by vigorous PVD. Whether damage to the epipapillary capillaries contributes to the pathogenesis of postvitrectomy visual field loss is not yet clarified. The frequently observed disc pallor is an unspecific symptom that can be explained by several etiologic factors.

Differential Diagnosis

Evident postoperative visual field loss may also be attributed to surgery-independent diseases in few cases. Clinical experience shows that *arterial occlusion* and *nonarteritic ischemic optic neuropathy (NAION)* are the most probable causes. Whether these vascular incidents are purely coincidental or indirectly provoked by cardiovascular instability in the perioperative phase, are difficult to elucidate. NAION after anterior segment surgery is a known phenomenon that may occur within the early postoperative period (mean interval 5 weeks). The rate/frequency is higher than would be expected if there had been no surgery.[37] Taban et al.[38] reported two cases of NAION after macular surgery. Different from VFD after air–fluid exchange or ICG-assisted peeling, ischemic optic disc edema, a RAPD, and altitudinal or arcuate VFDs were present. They concluded that in cases with unexplained visual field loss, those cases with optic disc pathology are likely due to NAION and that the frequency may be underestimated. One of our cases is demonstrated in **Figure 22-5**.

Furthermore, eyes with pre-existing glaucomatous VFD may experience progression after surgery. As usually fluctuation or decompensation of the IOP is present, proper diagnosis can be made easily.

A summary of the characteristic features of postoperative visual field loss is given in Table 22-1.

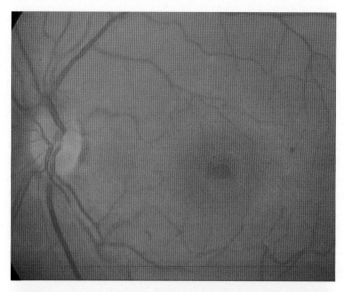

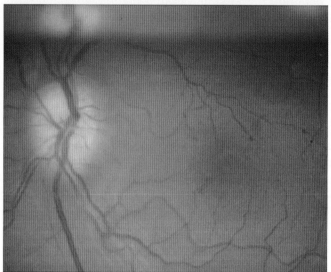

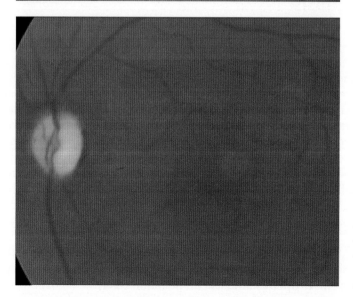

Figure 22-5 A 50-year-old female patient with a macular hole stage 3 based on Gass' classification developed severe AION 3 weeks after MHS with gas tamponade. She noticed sudden visual loss overnight. We could not perform visual field testing, as VA had dropped to hand motions. The eye went blind within a few weeks due to complete optic atrophy.

Table 22-1 • Postvitrectomy Visual Field Loss: Characteristics and Differential Diagnosis

	Vitrectomy/Gas-related VFD	ICG Dye-related VFD	Other VFD: NAION	Other VFD: Artery Occlusion
Etiology (1)	RNFL dehydration by airflow	Direct retinal toxicity	Vascular	Vascular
Etiology (2)	Enhanced by surgical PVD	Increased risk of retinal phototoxicity by the light sources used in green-stained tissues (i.e., following ICG)	Arteritic/nonarteritic	Retinal embolus, vasoconstriction
Risk Factors	Duration/pressure of airflow, open sclerotomies	ICG concentration/exposure time	Cardiovascular disease	Cardiovascular disease
Location/Damage	Opposite to the infusion cannula	Retinal area with contact to ICG	Short posterior ciliary artery blockage	Central, branch arterial occlusion
Pattern of VFD	Wedge-shaped, usually inferotemp. ±adjacent quadrants Macula spared	Nasal quadrants ≥ 90 degrees, constriction	Altitudinal sup./inf. (hemianopia), total	Dependent on the arteriole involved
RAPD	±	±	+	+
ONH	±segmental pallor	Segmental/diffuse pallor	Edema, hem spots > pallor	Segmental/diffuse pallor
RNFL Thickness	↓ (superonasal)	↓ (sup, nasal, temp.)	↓ (segment./diffuse)	↓ (diffuse)

Pearls on How to Prevent It

As several risk factors have been identified, strategies to avoid postvitrectomy VFD are as follows:

◆ Prolonged *airflow* through the vitreous cavity at a high pressure with sclerotomies open should be avoided to prevent dehydration injury to the inner retina, especially the nerve fiber layer. Instead, closure of the sclerotomies when not introducing instruments and limiting the phase of the fluid–air exchange to a minimum are recommended. Today, in the era of routine ILM peeling during MHS with excellent closure rates, extensive drainage of fluid, particularly from the macula hole, is no longer mandatory.

◆ The role of *surgical PVD* in macula surgery for the pathogenesis of postoperative VFD remains controversial. Some surgeons prefer limited (core) vitrectomy in macular cases; others always perform complete vitrectomy. There is no evident clinical data that proves that either method is superior to prevent visual field loss, when obeying the improved surgical strategies mentioned above.

◆ *ICG-assisted membrane and ILM peeling* have definitely the potential to damage the retina by a direct or indirect toxic effect.[35] When using short exposure times (application to the areas of intended peeling, immediate washout, endoillumination kept at a distance from the retina, fast peeling) and low concentrations (0.05% or 0.1%), the risk of postoperative visual field loss appears minimal. In case of doubt, use other dyes, which are available and approved for surgery. Because of the concerns with its toxicity, ICG has been widely replaced by the use of trypan blue and brilliant blue or a combination of both (supplement, Membrane-Dual is meant by this).

◆ As the cause of postoperative *NAION* or arterial vascular occlusion is not known, no preventive measures can be recommended. Careful medical perioperative care with respect to cardiovascular morbidity should be taken.

Pearls on How to Solve It

There is no treatment available to restore visual field once postoperative VFD has manifested.

Expected Outcomes

Various etiologic factors contribute to the risk of postoperative visual field loss. VFDs usually manifest immediately after surgery, and are usually nonprogressive and permanent. Very few articles describe either progression[18,39] or regression.[13] Size and depth of scotomas vary and many remain asymptomatic for the patient.

As several risk factors have been identified, the overall incidence of vitrectomy-associated visual field loss has decreased over the years. In experienced hands this complications should be avoidable. Moreover, it can be expected that the use of small-gauge instrumentation will further reduce the risk. Intraocular flow and turbulence of air during air/fluid exchange is less compared to the conventional 20-gauge approach. Sclerotomy cannulae with valves further reduce high airflow and pressure. To prove this hypothesis, additional studies are warranted. Moreover, ICG-related visual field loss today is of no clinical significance any more, as new nontoxic dyes are available.

Finally, VFDs occurring after an initially uncomplicated course are most likely of vascular origin and must be differentiated from those related to the surgical procedure itself.

REFERENCES

1. Melberg NS, Thomas MA. Visual field loss after pars plana vitrectomy with air/fluid exchange. *Am J Ophthalmol.* 1995;120:386–388.
2. Kerrison JB, Haller JA, Elman M, et al. Visual field loss following vitreous surgery. *Arch Ophthalmol.* 1996;114:564–569.
3. Pendergast SD, McCuen BW 2nd. Visual field loss after macular hole surgery. *Ophthalmology.* 1996;103:1069–1077.
4. Bopp S, Lucke K, Hille U. Peripheral visual field loss after vitreous surgery for macular holes. *Graefes Arch Clin Exp Ophthalmol.* 1997;235:362–371.
5. Kerrison JB, Haller JA, Elman M, et al. Visual field loss following vitreous surgery. *Arch Ophthalmol.* 1996;114:564–569.
6. Yan H, Dhurjon L, Chow DR, et al. Visual field defect after pars plana vitrectomy. *Ophthalmology.* 1998;105:1612–1616.
7. Uemura A, Kanda S, Sakamoto Y, et al. Visual field defects after uneventful vitrectomy for epiretinal membrane with indocyanine green-assisted internal limiting membrane peeling. *Am J Ophthalmol.* 2003;136:252–257.
8. Yang SS, McDonald HR, Everett AI, et al. Retinal damage caused by air–fluid exchange during pars plana vitrectomy. *Retina.* 2006;26:334–338.

9. Hutton WL, Fuller DG, Snyder WB, et al. Visual field defects after macular hole surgery. A new finding. *Ophthalmology*. 1996;103:2152–2158.

10. Ezra E, Arden GB, Riordan-Eva P, et al. Visual field loss following vitrectomy for stage 2 and 3 macular holes. *Br J Ophthalmol*. 1996;80:519–525.

11. Boldt HC, Munden PM, Folk JC, et al. Visual field defects after macular hole surgery. *Am J Ophthalmol*. 1996;122:371–381.

12. Paques M, Massin P, Santiago PY, et al. Visual field loss after vitrectomy for full-thickness macular holes. *Am J Ophthalmol*. 1997;124:88–94.

13. Arima T, Uemura A, Otsuka S, et al. Macular hole surgery-associated peripheral visual field loss. *Jpn J Ophthalmol*. 1998;42:476–483.

14. Takenaka H, Maeno T, Mano T, et al. Causes of visual field defects after vitrectomy. *Nihon Ganka Gakkai Zasshi*. 1999;103:399–403.

15. Cullinane AB, Cleary PE. Prevention of visual field defects after macular hole surgery. *Br J Ophthalmol*. 2000;84:372–377.

16. Gass CA, Haritoglou C, Schaumberger M, et al. Functional outcome of macular hole surgery with and without indocyanine green-assisted peeling of the internal limiting membrane. *Graefes Arch Clin Exp Ophthalmol*. 2003;241:716–720.

17. Kanda S, Uemura A, Yamashita T, et al. Visual field defects after intravitreous administration of indocyanine green in macular hole surgery. *Arch Ophthalmol*. 2004;122:1447–1451.

18. Yamashita T, Uemura A, Kita H, et al. Long-term outcomes of visual field defects after indocyanine green-assisted macular hole surgery. *Retina*. 2008;28:1228–1233.

19. von Jagow B, Höing A, Gandorfer A, et al. Functional outcome of indocyanine green-assisted macular surgery: 7-year follow-up. *Retina*. 2009;29:1249–1256.

20. Malinowski SM, Pesin SR. Visual field loss caused by retinal vascular occlusion after vitrectomy surgery. *Am J Ophthalmol*. 1997;123:707–708.

21. Yonemura N, Hirata A, Hasumura T, et al. Fundus changes corresponding to visual field defects after vitrectomy for macular hole. *Ophthalmology*. 2001;108:1638–1643.

22. Oh KT, Boldt HC, Maturi RK. Evaluation of patients with visual field defects following macular hole surgery using multifocal electroretinography. *Retina*. 2000;20:238–243.

23. Yamashita T, Uemura A, Kita H, et al. Analysis of the retinal nerve fiber layer after indocyanine green-assisted vitrectomy for idiopathic macular holes. *Ophthalmology*. 2006;113:280–284.

24. Hirata A, Yonemura N, Hasumura T, et al. Effect of infusion air pressure on visual field defects after macular hole surgery. *Am J Ophthalmol*. 2000;130:611–616.

25. Haritoglou C, Gandorfer A, Gass CA, et al. Indocyanine green-assisted peeling of the internal limiting membrane in macular hole surgery affects visual outcome: A clinicopathologic correlation. *Am J Ophthalmol*. 2002;134:836–841.

26. Haritoglou C, Gandorfer A, Gass CA, et al. The effect of indocyanine-green on functional outcome of macular pucker surgery. *Am J Ophthalmol*. 2003;135:328–337.

27. Welch JC. Dehydration injury as a possible cause of visual field defect after pars plana vitrectomy for macular hole. *Am J Ophthalmol*. 1997;124:698–699.

28. Ohji M, Nao-I N, Saito Y, et al. Prevention of visual field defect after macular hole surgery by passing air used for fluid–air exchange through water. *Am J Ophthalmol*. 1999;127:62–66.

29. Welch JC. Prevention of visual field defect after macular hole surgery by passing air used for fluid–air exchange through water. *Am J Ophthalmol*. 1999;128:396–397.

30. Hasumura T, Yonemura N, Hirata A, et al. Retinal damage by air infusion during vitrectomy in rabbit eyes. *Invest Ophthalmol Vis Sci*. 2000;41:4300–4304.

31. Yonemura N, Hirata A, Hasumura T, et al. Long-term alteration in the air-infused rabbit retina. *Graefes Arch Clin Exp Ophthalmol*. 2003;241:314–320.

32. Hirata A, Yonemura N, Hasumura T, et al. New infusion cannula for prevention of retinal damage by infusion air during vitrectomy. *Retina*. 2003;23:682–685.

33. Russell SR, Hageman GS. Optic disc, foveal, and extrafoveal damage due to surgical separation of the vitreous. *Arch Ophthalmol*. 2001;119:1653–1658.

34. Kadonosono K, Itoh N, Uchio E, et al. Staining of internal limiting membrane in macular hole surgery. *Arch Ophthalmol*. 2000;118:1116–1118.

35. Rodrigues EB, Meyer CH, Mennel S, et al. Mechanisms of intravitreal toxicity of indocyanine green dye: Implications for chromovitrectomy. *Retina.* 2007;27: 958–970.

36. Schumann RG, Gandorfer A, Priglinger SG, et al. Vital dyes for macular surgery: A comparative electron microscopy study of the internal limiting membrane. *Retina.* 2009;29:669–676.

37. McCulley TJ, Lam BL, Feuer WJ. Nonarteritic anterior ischemic optic neuropathy and surgery of the anterior segment: Temporal relationship analysis. *Am J Ophthalmol.* 2003;136:1171–1172.

38. Taban M, Lewis H, Lee MS. Nonarteritic anterior ischemic optic neuropathy and 'visual field defects' following vitrectomy: Could they be related? *Graefes Arch Clin Exp Ophthalmol.* 2007;245:600–605.

39. Tosi GM, Martone G, Balestrazzi A, et al. Visual field loss progression after macular hole surgery. *J Ophthalmol.* 2009;127:62–66.

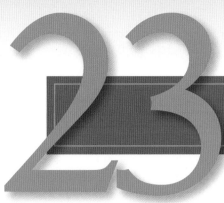

HYPOTONY

Siegfried G. Priglinger and Thomas C. Kreutzer

⬩ The Complication: Definition

Hypotony is usually defined as an intraocular pressure (IOP) of 5 mm Hg or less. Low IOP can adversely impact the eye in many ways, including corneal decompensation, accelerated cataract formation, hypotony maculopathy, choroidal swelling, and discomfort. Clinically significant changes occur more frequently as the IOP approaches 0 mm Hg.

⬩ Risk Factors

Various conditions predisposing eyes for the development of postvitreoretinal surgery hypotony have been described: Myopic eyes with higher axial length and young patients have been reported to be at higher risk for postoperative hypotony.[1] Chronic inflammation in uveitis also increases the risk for postoperative hypotony.[2] Wound leakage is the main reason for an increased risk of postoperative hypotony in eyes with previous vitrectomy in case of reoperation.[3] This has also been shown for pseudophakic as well as aphakic eyes and in cases of combined surgery.[3,4] Preexisting conjunctival scarring is another risk factor leading to a higher incidence of postsurgical wound leakage especially after sutureless vitreoretinal surgery. Furthermore, silicone oil tamponade removal results in high rates of postoperative hypotony, which is mostly transitory.[1]

⬩ Pathogenesis: Why Does It Occur

Postoperative hypotony develops when aqueous outflow exceeds the aqueous production of the ciliary body. Primary reasons may be factors suppressing ciliary body function and/or excessive aqueous leakage. On average, the ciliary body produces 2.5 μL of aqueous humor every minute. In healthy eyes, 90% of aqueous humor exits through the conventional trabecular meshwork–Schlemm canal–episcleral venous route. The remaining 10% exits via the uveoscleral outflow. In case of hypotony, the IOP declines below the episcleral venous pressure (about 9 mm Hg) leading to a predominance of the uveoscleral outflow.

Reasons for **increased aqueous loss** following vitreoretinal surgery

One major reason for postoperative hypotony resulting from a loss of intraocular fluids has emerged from sutureless vitrectomy surgery, which has an increased incidence of possible wound leakage. Risk of wound leakage has been shown to be higher in larger nonsutured wounds (20 gauge >23 gauge >25 gauge >27 gauge) and is correlated to the technique of wound construction.[5,6] Multiple-step sclerotomies seem to be superior concerning passive wound closure compared to single-step approaches.[7,8] While use of intravitreal triamcinolone increases the risk of postoperative hypotony, application of a gas tamponade at the end of surgery seems to increase the likelihood of closed scleral wounds.[3,9] Postoperative hypotony, in general, recovers spontaneously at latest by day 7.

Recurrent posterior retinal detachment similar to long-lasting retinal detachment also can cause postoperative hypotony.[10]

Reasons for ciliary body malfunction

Inflammation plays an important role in ciliary body malfunction. Histopathologic studies in an animal model showed reduced aqueous production presumably caused by breakage of the blood–aqueous barrier.[11] In addition, the interstitial edema of the ciliary muscle causes increased fluid exchange between the anterior chamber and the supraciliary space. This and further decrease of IOP well below 5 mm Hg relatively increase uveoscleral outflow leading to accumulation of choroidal fluid in its potential suprachoroidal space thereby inducing additional ciliary body detachment. This further prevents aqueous production since the newly created suprachoroidal space may act as a barrier. Once choroidal effusion has developed an anterior ring of choroidal fluid, it can dislocate the ciliary body forward, potentiating its inability to produce aqueous humor.

Advanced anterior proliferative vitreoretinopathy (PVR) with persisting tractional elements after vitreoretinal surgery can cause marked hypotony.[12] In anterior PVR, mechanical forces with consecutive traction on the ciliary body led to a detachment of the ciliary body and stoppage of aqueous humor production. Occasionally, even pronounced shrinkage of posterior capsule opacification after combined anterior and posterior segment surgery may lead to significant traction on the ciliary body.

Large retinectomies or comprehensive retinotomies may also yield higher rates of postoperative hypotony caused by increased uveoscleral outflow.[13,14]

There is a very high incidence of postoperative hypotony after silicone oil removal with an incidence up to 60%.[10] Recent studies have shown that postoperative hypotony in most cases seems to be transient and recovers within 1 week postoperatively (94%).[1] Henderer et al.[10] in 1999 found that about 47.6% of patients developed a long-lasting hypotony for up to 1 and 2 years. While number of previous pars plana vitrectomies, extent of remaining PVR, number of preoperative antiglaucoma ophthalmic medications, and duration of silicone oil tamponade seem to have no influence on the incidence of postoperative hypotony after silicone oil removal, patients with long axial length and aphakia have increased odds of developing transient hypotony after silicone oil removal.[1,10]

In the silicone oil study, postoperative hypotony was more frequently found in eyes treated with long-acting gas tamponade than with a silicone oil tamponade suggesting the choice of silicone oil as tamponade in PVR.[15]

⬧ Pearls on How to Prevent It

♦ Efficient primary wound closure in sutureless vitrectomy.

♦ Flatten the conjunctiva and sclera in order to allow entry more parallel to the limbus.

♦ Displace conjunctiva laterally to prevent communication between conjunctival and scleral incisions, a combined holder and conjunctival displacer are helpful **(Figure 23-1)**.

♦ Perform oblique incision for a self-sealing wound **(Figure 23-2)**.

♦ In case of one-step approach **(Figure 23-3)**, bevel-down position (flat side down, **Figure 23-4A**) of the trocar lancet is to be preferred.

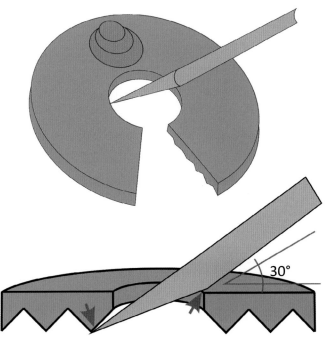

Figure 23-1 Schematic of an eye holder and conjunctival displacer with additional support of correct degree of scleral entry

Two-step oblique

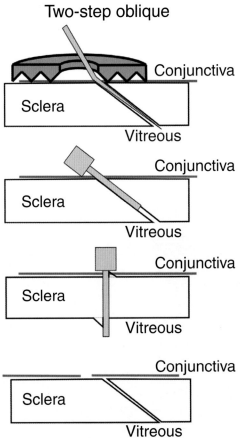

Figure 23-2 Schematic of a two-step oblique scleral entry with conjunctival displacement

Single-step perpendicular

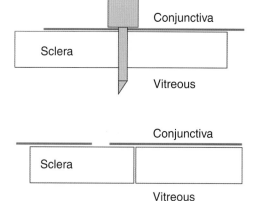

Figure 23-3 Schematic of a one-step perpendicular scleral entry with conjunctival displacement

♦ An incision parallel to the limbus might even decrease stress on scleral tissue during surgery increasing the likelihood of primary wound closure **(Figure 23-4B)**.

♦ Prevent vitreous prolapse by placing an instrument (e.g., light pipe) through the trocar during removal.

♦ Clear benefits should be expected when one decides to remove silicone oil tamponade in eyes with low pressure. Otherwise, the silicone oil tamponade may be left in place. In surgery of significant PVR, primary silicone oil tamponade may result in less frequent postoperative hypotony.

♦ Thorough inspection for wound leakage: Seidel's test, loss of tamponade (e.g., subconjunctival gas bubbles).

♦ Use of a gas or air tamponade at the end of surgery in sutureless vitrectomy and after silicone oil removal.

♦ Increased awareness to pressurize the eye at the end of surgery in aphakic eyes and eyes with higher axial length.

♦ Termination of longer-lasting antiglaucomatous drugs before surgery (e.g., prostaglandine derivates, systemic carbonic acid inhibitors).

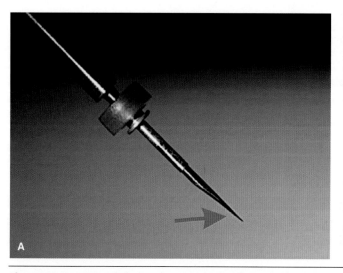
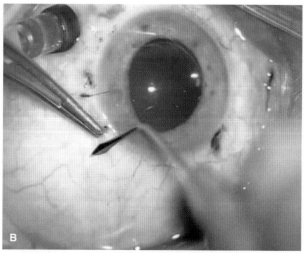

Figure 23-4 A: Bevel-down one-step trocar. **B:** Limbus-parallel entry position in an oblique two-step scleral trocar

Pearls on How to Solve It

◆ Leaking sclerotomy: Suture of the wound, injection of air/gas tamponade.

◆ Increase steroids, when wound leak is ruled out; decrease when it is suspected.

◆ Use medium-lasting cycloplegic medications (e.g., cyclopentolate, scopolamine) to stabilize the iris–lens diaphragm and ciliary body.

◆ Topical application of 2% ibopamine may also increase IOP but its relevance in treatment of prolonged hypotony has yet to be proven.[16,17]

◆ In case of refractory significant hypotony, intracameral application of viscoelastic can be tried, but the effect is often temporary and eye pressure has to be monitored frequently.[2]

◆ In case of persisting tractional anterior forces after complicated vitreoretinal surgery or persisting retinal detachment, repeated vitrectomy with complete vitreous removal and excision of PVR membranes should be performed.

◆ In case of hypotony caused by tractional forces due to anterior and/or posterior capsular fibrosis in pseudophakic or aphakic eyes perform YAG-laser or surgical capsulotomy.

◆ Reoperation with reinjection of a silicone oil tamponade may also be beneficial to end prolonged hypotony especially in cases with otherwise anatomically successfully treated cases.

 ## Expected Outcomes: What Is the Worst-case Scenario

Transient or permanent visual impairment may result from corneal changes, accelerated cataract formation, suprachoroidal fluid, choroidal folds, maculopathy with disturbance of the retinal pigment epithelium (RPE), cystoid macular edema and macular folds, vascular engorgement and tortuosity, and optic disc edema. Hypotony further increases the risk of suprachoroidal hemorrhage, which can result in severe vision loss. In a worst-case scenario, severe chronic hypotony can ultimately lead to phthisis.

In addition, early postoperative hypotony may be one reason for a higher rate of postoperative endophthalmitis in sutureless transconjunctival vitrectomy. In early postoperative hypotony, incomplete wound closure of the unsutured wounds may allow intraocular influx of extraocular fluid and micro-organisms. Modifications in entry technique and preoperative disinfection have reduced this risk. The use of povidone–iodine along the lid margins and perioperative area preoperatively significantly reduces the bacterial flora, thus decreasing the risks of endophthalmitis.[18] Furthermore, placing povidone–iodine for a few seconds near entry sites may further lower the risk as direct application has been demonstrated in well-controlled studies to decrease the microbiologic flora before intraocular surgery.

REFERENCES

1. Kim SW, Oh J, Yang KS, et al. Risk factors for the development of transient hypotony after silicone oil removal. *Retina*. 2010;30:1228–1236.
2. Kucukerdonmez C, Beutel J, Bartz-Schmidt KU, et al. Treatment of chronic ocular hypotony with intraocular application of sodium hyaluronate. *Br J Ophthalmol*. 2009;93:235–239.

3. Bamonte G, Mura M, Stevie Tan H. Hypotony after 25-gauge vitrectomy. *Am J Ophthalmol.* 2011;151:156–160.

4. Tseng JJ, Schiff WM, Barile GR, et al. Influence of postoperative lens status on intraocular pressure in proliferative vitreoretinopathy. *Am J Ophthalmol.* 2009;147:875–885, 885. e1–e2.

5. Oshima Y, Wakabayashi T, Sato T, et al. A 27-gauge instrument system for transconjunctival sutureless microincision vitrectomy surgery. *Ophthalmology.* 2010;117:93–102. e2.

6. Gutfleisch M, Dietzel M, Heimes B, et al. Ultrasound biomicroscopic findings of conventional and sutureless sclerotomy sites after 20-, 23-, and 25-G pars plana vitrectomy. *Eye (Lond).* 2010;24:1268–1272.

7. Shimozono M, Oishi A, Kimakura H, et al. Three-step incision for 23-gauge vitrectomy reduces postoperative hypotony compared with an oblique incision. *Ophthalmic Surg Lasers Imaging.* 2011;42:20–25.

8. Lopez-Guajardo L, Vleming-Pinilla E, Pareja-Esteban J, et al. Ultrasound biomicroscopy study of direct and oblique 25-gauge vitrectomy sclerotomies. *Am J Ophthalmol.* 2007;143:881–883.

9. Yamane S, Kadonosono K, Inoue M, et al. Effect of intravitreal gas tamponade for sutureless vitrectomy wounds: Three-dimensional corneal and anterior segment optical coherence tomography study. *Retina.* 2011;31:702–706.

10. Henderer JD, Budenz DL, Flynn HW Jr, et al. Elevated intraocular pressure and hypotony following silicone oil retinal tamponade for complex retinal detachment: Incidence and risk factors. *Arch Ophthalmol.* 1999;117:189–195.

11. Toris CB, Pederson JE. Aqueous humor dynamics in experimental iridocyclitis. *Invest Ophthalmol Vis Sci.* 1987;28:477–481.

12. Faude F, Lambert A, Wiedemann P. 360 degrees retinectomy in severe anterior PVR and PDR. *Int Ophthalmol.* 1998;22:119–123.

13. Blumenkranz MS, Azen SP, Aaberg T, et al. Relaxing retinotomy with silicone oil or long-acting gas in eyes with severe proliferative vitreoretinopathy. Silicone Study Report 5. The Silicone Study Group. *Am J Ophthalmol.* 1993;116:557–564.

14. Iverson DA, Ward TG, Blumenkranz MS. Indications and results of relaxing retinotomy. *Ophthalmology.* 1990;97:1298–1304.

15. Barr CC, Lai MY, Lean JS, et al. Postoperative intraocular pressure abnormalities in the Silicone Study. Silicone Study Report 4. *Ophthalmology.* 1993;100:1629–1635.

16. Windisch BK, Iliev ME. [Treatment of uveitis-associated refractory ocular hypotony with topical ibopamine]. *Klin Monbl Augenheilkd.* 2006;223:422–424.

17. Ugahary LC, Ganteris E, Veckeneer M, et al. Topical ibopamine in the treatment of chronic ocular hypotony attributable to vitreoretinal surgery, uveitis, or penetrating trauma. *Am J Ophthalmol.* 2006;141:571–573.

18. Ta CN, Singh K, Egbert PR, et al. Prospective comparative evaluation of povidone–iodine (10% for 5 minutes versus 5% for 1 minute) as prophylaxis for ophthalmic surgery. *J Cataract Refract Surg.* 2008;34:171–172.

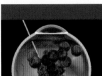

PART F. COMPLICATIONS COMMON TO SCLERAL BUCKLING, PNEUMATIC RETINOPEXY AND PARS PLANA VITRECTOMY— INTRAOPERATIVE COMPLICATIONS

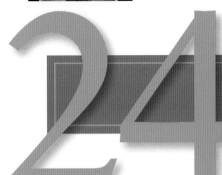

24 PROBLEMS INITIATING SURGERY

SVEN CRAFOORD AND GUY SHANKS

24A Working in Small and Deep Set Eyes

Certain cases will present the surgeon with problems from the very beginning. The anatomy of both the eye and the surrounding tissues may mean that we are forced to adapt our standard approach so as to be able to operate. The anatomy may deviate from the norm due to congenital malformations, injuries, previous pathology including infections, natural variations, to name but a few.[1-4] Often, we cannot change the actual anatomy to facilitate the surgery (although this is possible in a few cases). However, by recognizing the problem before we start the surgery, and being familiar with the possible consequences, we can plan our operation to minimize the negative effects, and hopefully avoid serious complications. The aim of this chapter is to present the most common anatomical hinders, and to give advice on how to cope with subsequent problems.

Working in Small and Deep Set Eyes

Eyes falling into this category are often difficult to access with surgical instruments and maneuverability is restricted. This can affect both the set up of the operating theatre, positioning of the surgeon, and choice of instruments.

The subtitle really covers three separate, but related conditions:

◆ Deep set eyes

◆ Small palpebral fissures

◆ Small globes

Abnormally, deep set eyes may be an extreme anatomical variation without underlying pathology, due to skull malformations, congenital syndromes (e.g., Trisomy 9 Mosaicism),[5] secondary to trauma with orbital fat atrophy,[2] and so on. The salient point in this situation is not the pathogenesis, but rather the importance of recognizing the problem before commencing surgery. Observe that a prominent nasal bridge can result in similar problems with access to the eye, even if the eye is not actually deep set. Acromegaly[6] with prominent brows can give the same effect.

Small palpebral fissures may be seen without underlying pathology, or most commonly as a result of congenital syndromes, for example, blepharophimosis,[7] Edwards syndrome (trisomy 18),[8] and so on. Other syndromes[9–12] may give changes in the soft tissues causing similar problems with accessibility. Examples include the epicanthal folds seen in Down[13] and cri-du-chat syndromes,[14] and the oblique eye fissures, most common again in Down syndrome. Previous trauma can give soft-tissue scarring that may cause problems with access.[2]

Small globes may also be a result of a congenital syndrome, for example, Patau syndrome,[15] but microphthalmos[16] may also be an isolated finding. High hyperopia is often associated with a small globe. Maybe the most common situation where we find ourselves facing a small globe, often behind a small palpebral fissure, is in surgery in premature children, that is, surgery for retinopathy of prematurity.

The situations above give rise to a series of related difficulties:

◆ Choice of entry site, sclerotomy placement, hindered by restricted access to the globe.

◆ Entry site tears in the peripheral retina due to narrow pars plana.

◆ Lens touch: Both the smaller globe and difficulties in maneuvering the instruments will increase the risk of lens touch.

◆ Wide-angle viewing system (WAVS) fogging—deep set eyes give a higher humidity around the eyes' surface and the noncontact viewing system, which can cause fogging.

◆ Contact lens displacement. Smaller palpebral fissures encroach on the contact lenses distorting the view of the surgical field.

◆ Standard-sized instruments too large for smaller globes.

◆ Choroidal detachment in microphthalmic eyes.

◆ Pooling of fluids in and around the eye, the natural runoff being compromised by the surrounding tissues.

◆ Difficulty in angling instruments to access the periphery. The surrounding tissues only allow an acute angle of entry to the eye, making it difficult to traverse the eye with instruments to reach the periphery opposite the entry site (**Figs. 24A-1A,B**).

Individuals with the above anatomical features represent a certain percentage of our patients and will continue to do so. It is of paramount importance that we identify the potential problems involved before we commence surgery, and take measures to minimize the risks.

✦ Possible Solutions

◆ Arrange the setup of the operating theatre to allow the surgeon to sit in the optimal position. A temporal approach often gives a superior access to the eye.

◆ Careful positioning of the patient's head. Hyperextension of the neck when eyebrows are prominent. Angling of the head around the sagittal plane in cases with a protruding nose. The operating table may also be angled to increase the effect (**Figure 24A-2A–G**).

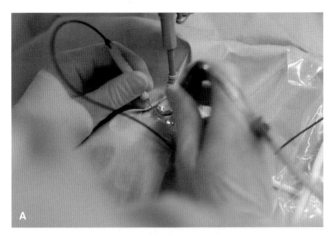 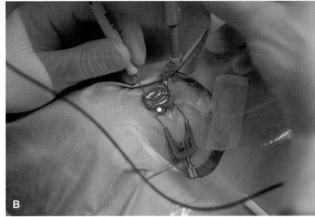

Figure 24A-1 These photos show the crowding that can be a problem while operating on the small eyes of children. The limited size of the surgical field means that the surgeon is forced to approach the eye at a relatively acute angle, making it harder, for example, to reach the opposite periphery with the instruments.

♦ Preparation of the surrounding tissues, including canthotomy, temporary blepharoplasty, and in extreme cases even lateral orbitomy to increase exposure of the globe **(Figure 24A-3A,B)**.

♦ Tractional sutures in the eyelids may help to widen the palpebral fissure in cases where available lid specula give limited help **(Figure 24A-4)**.

♦ Use of appropriately sized instruments, for example, pediatric lid specula may work well in adults with, for example, blepharophimosis.

♦ Retrobulbar injection of, for example, a local anesthetic can displace the globe anteriorly.

♦ Angling of the globe within the orbit to maximize exposure. The eye may be turned sequentially to expose different areas of the sclera when placing the sclerotomies. Tractional sutures in the globe may be useful.

♦ A more anterior placement of sclerotomies **(Figure 24A-5)**. In premature children, pars plicata entry should be used. Smaller gauge instruments, 23 or 25 gauge, can be of benefit.[17–19] In adults, the sclerotomies can be placed as near as 2 mm from the limbus, although such an entry will probably have to be combined with a phaco/IOL, or in appropriate cases, a lensectomy.[20] If left, there will be a high risk of inadvertently damaging the lens. The removal of the lens not only avoids the risk of accidental damage, but also creates more room to work in and easier access to the opposite periphery.

♦ Problems with gaining access via the pars plana have in some cases been accentuated with the increased use of small-gauge transconjunctival instruments which in optimal cases should be angled obliquely. In patients with restricted access to the sclera, it is often hard to find the space to angle the incisions. In these cases, the sclerotomy can be more easily placed perpendicularly to the sclera. These obviously have to be sutured at the end of surgery.

♦ Use of trochars will enable the surgeon to find entry sites, which are often partially hidden by the surrounding tissues, more easily.

In extreme cases, where the vitreous is opaque and the eye small, the surgeon may have to begin surgery in the anterior chamber, placing an anterior chamber maintainer, and then by removing the lens, often by lensectomy. After an anterior

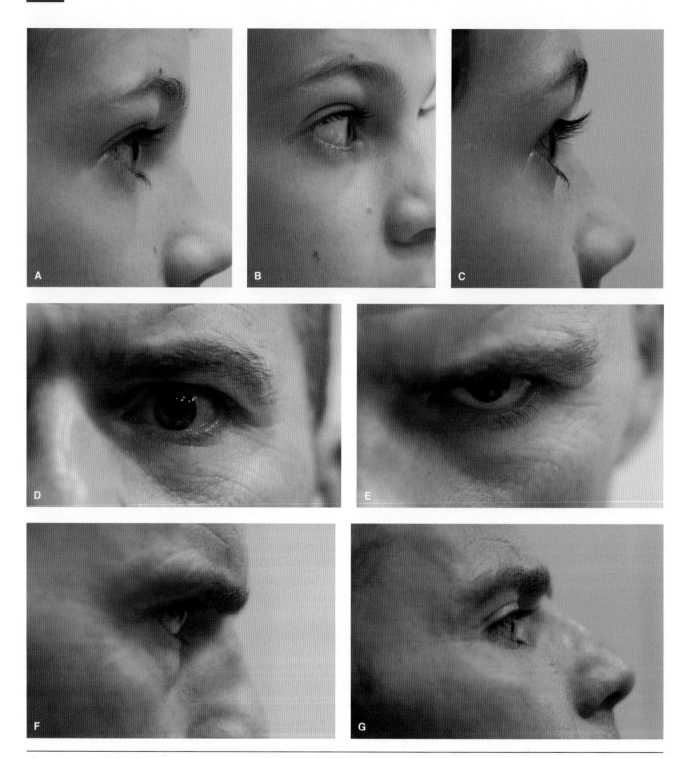

Figure 24A-2 A–C: The photos illustrate the effect of a simple head rotation on the amount of temporal sclera exposed to the surgeon. **D–G:** The photos illustrate the effect of flexion/extension of the patient's head on the area of sclera presented to the surgeon.

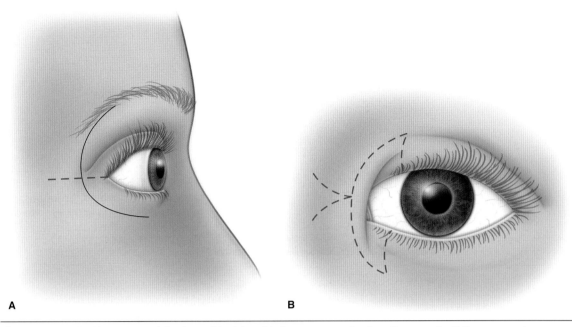

A   B

Figure 24A-3 A: Placement of the lateral incision. **B:** A pronounced epicanthus can limit the surgeon's access to the medial aspect of the sclera. This hinder may be overcome in exceptional cases by a standard epicanthal plasty, the incision lines of which are illustrated. The patient should be counseled preoperatively as to whether or not to remove the epicanthus permanently, or only temporarily for the duration of the surgical period.

vitrectomy to remove, for example, blood or opaque vitreous, the periphery may be indented allowing the surgeon to place their posterior chamber infusion cannula under direct visualization in the microscope, thus avoiding damageto the peripheral retina. This is especially helpful in cases where the retina is detached, and may lay over the pars plana. A typical situation for this kind of approach would be in trauma cases. In easier cases, such as simple vitreous hemorrhage in a small eye, the surgeon may still have to begin in the anterior chamber to ensure that they do not injure the peripheral retina, but they can gain access to the posterior segment by doing a phaco combined with a posterior capsulorrhexis enabling the implantation of an IOL at the end of surgery.

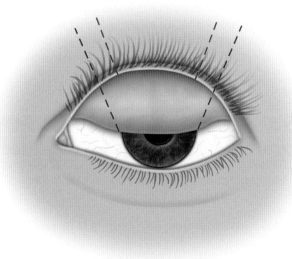

Figure 24A-4 In a few patients, it is hard to achieve the desired opening of the eyelids in spite of the correct use of an adequate lid speculum. The insertion of the speculum may be hindered by a prominent superciliary ridge, or a deep set eye. In these cases tractional sutures in the eyelids can be of use. They can be placed as full-thickness sutures at the ciliary margin (*red line*), or, further in at the margin of the tarsal plates (*blue line*). The latter placement is especially appropriate in patients with concomitant Floppy Eyelid Syndrome whose tissues have a tendency to prolapse into the surgical field. The blue placement of the sutures not only opens the lids, but also acts as a mechanical barrier to such a prolapse.

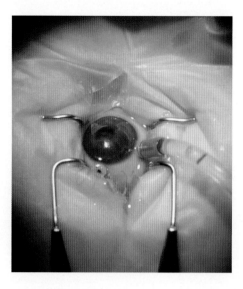

Figure 24A-5 The sclerotomies in this patient are only 1 mm behind the limbus, making this a partly pars plicata entry. In spite of the anterior placement, the trochars barely fit inside the palpebral fissure.

◆ WAVS lenses may be warmed to body temperature to reduce the tendency for fogging. Their surfaces can be treated with commercial antifogging agents (e.g., Ultrastop Promed, Sigma Pharma).

◆ In very deep set eyes, it is difficult to place the WAVS lens sufficiently close to the eye to give appropriate wide-angled viewing. In these cases, a contact lens system can provide a better alternative.

◆ In eyes with a very small palpebral fissure, pediatric contact lenses can be of use.

◆ Concurrent phaco/IOL helps to create space in small eyes. Observe however that special care should be taken in microphthalmic eyes where phaco may not be a simple addition to the surgery, because of the danger of, for example, choroidal effusion.[21–23]

◆ In microphthalmic eyes, relatively high perioperative intraocular pressure can be maintained to avoid tendency for choroidal effusion. The positive effects of this should be weighed against the risks, especially in eyes with glaucoma.

◆ In eyes with a frank choroidal effusion, scleral fenestration.

These cases can be very troubling. There is an increased risk for iatrogenic damage to multiple tissues, including eyelids, conjunctiva, sclera, lens, retina, and choroid. A microphthalmic eye with lens touch, choroidal effusion or hemorrhage, and retinal detachment due to multiple entry site ruptures is not the best start of the day. We can try to minimize the risks involved primarily by recognizing that the situation is problematic, and tailoring our preparation and surgery to the specific case.

REFERENCES

1. Athanasiov PA, Prabhakaran VC, Selva D. Non-traumatic enophthalmos: A review. *Acta Ophthalmol.* 2008;86(4):356–364.
2. Clauser L, Galiè M, Pagliaro F, et al. Posttraumatic enophthalmos: Etiology, principles of reconstruction, and correction. *J Craniofac Surg.* 2008;19(2):351–359.
3. Levin AV. Congenital eye anomalies. *Pediatr Clin North Am.* 2003;50(1):55–76.
4. Guercio JR, Martyn LJ. Congenital malformations of the eye and orbit. *Otolaryngol Clin North Am.* 2007;40(1):113–140.
5. Liyanage S, Barnes J. The eye and Down's syndrome. *Br J Hosp Med (Lond).* 2008; 69(11):632–634.
6. Reddy R, Hope S, Wass J. Acromegaly. *BMJ.* 2010;341:c4189.

7. Allen CE, Rubin PA. Blepharophimosis-ptosis-epicanthus inversus syndrome (BPES): Clinical manifestation and treatment. *Int Ophthalmol Clin.* 2008;48(2): 15–23.
8. Shaw J. Trisomy 18: A case study. *Neonatal Netw.* 2008;27(1):33–41.
9. Chak G, Wang HZ, Feldon SE. Coup de Sabre presenting with worsening diploplia and enophthalmos. *Ophthal Plast Reconstr Surg.* 2011;27(4):e97–e98.
10. Jayaprakasam A, Ghazi-Nouri S. Periorbital fat atrophy—an unfamiliar side effect of prostaglandin analogues. *Orbit.* 2010;29(6):357–359.
11. Hwang TN, et al. Sunken eyes, sagging brain syndrome: Bilateral enophthalmos from chronic intracranial hypotension. *Ophthalmology.* 2011;118(11):2286–2295.
12. Chang BY, Cunliffe G, Hutchinson C. Enophthalmos associated with primary breast carcinoma. *Orbit.* 2002;21(4):307–310.
13. Liyanage S, Barnes J. The eye and Down's syndrome. *Br J Hosp Med (Lond).* 2008; 69(11):632–634.
14. Cerruti Mainardi P. Cri du Chat syndrome. *Orphanet J Rare Dis.* 2006;1:33.
15. Iliopoulos D, Sekerli E, Vassiliou G, et al. Patau syndrome with a long survival(146) months: A clinical report and review of the literature. *Am J Med Genet A.* 2006;140(1):92–93.
16. Shah SP, Taylor AE, Sowden JC, et al. Anophthalmos, microphthalmos, and Coloboma in the United Kingdom: Clinical features, results of investigations, and early management. *Ophthalmology.* 2012;119(2):362–368.
17. Wu WC, Lai CC, Lin RI, et al. Modified 23-gauge vitrectomy system for stage 4 retinopathy of prematurity. *Arch Ophthalmol.* 2011;129(10):1326–1331.
18. Gonzales CR, Singh S, Schwartz SD. 25-gauge vitrectomy for pediatric vitreoretinal conditions. *Br J Ophthalmol.* 2009;93(6):787–790.
19. Kychenthal A, Dorta P. 25-gauge lens-sparing vitrectomy for stage 4A retinopathy of prematurity. *Retina.* 2009;29(1):127.
20. Chaudhry NA, Cohen KA, Flynn HW Jr, et al. Combined pars plana vitrectomy and lens management in complex vitreoretinal disease. *Semin Ophthalmol.* 2003; 18(3): 132–141.
21. Yu YS, Lee JH, Chang BL. Surgical management of congenital cataract associated with severe microphthalmos. *J Cataract Refract Surg.* 2000;26(8):1219–1224.
22. Wladis EJ, Gewirtz MB, Guo S. Cataract surgery in the small adult eye. *Surv Ophthalmol.* 2006;51(2):153–161.
23. Elagouz M, Stanescu-Segall D, Jackson TL. Uveal effusion syndrome. *Surv Ophthalmol.* 2010;55(2):134–145.

24B Managing Scarred and Adherent Conjunctiva

Ocular surface problems can be seen in cases with concurrent ocular pathologies, or following trauma: Mechanical, chemical, thermal, or, most commonly, iatrogenic, after previous surgeries.[1-5] This scarring can complicate safe access to the globe. The conjunctiva may be adherent to the globe, making it hard to displace when setting transconjunctival trochars, or impossible to dissect when performing 20G surgery. Scarred conjunctiva after earlier surgery is often associated with underlying scleral atrophy after sclerotomies, especially where these have been sutured with the risk for a foreign body reaction. These problems must be addressed both at the beginning of surgery to ensure safe access to the globe, but also, at least as important, at the end of surgery. The eye must be left intact, without leakage, preventing infection, and in the optimal situation causing as little extra scarring as possible, in case further operations are necessary.

Extreme scarring may cause malpositioning of the globe, or compromise the extraocular muscles, making them difficult to isolate.[6]

In the era of transconjunctival, small-gauge vitrectomy, one of the new problems we have encountered is a restriction in our ability to indent the sclera as far posteriorly as we would like. The problem is compounded in eyes where scarring has foreshortened the fornices. Scarred conjunctiva may also predispose to abnormal bacterial colonization, increasing the risk for postoperative infection.

Risk Factors

Earlier/concurrent ocular pathology

◆ Systemic diseases, for example, ocular cicatricial pemphigoid (OCP),[2,3] Sjögrens syndrome

◆ Infections, for example, trachoma[4]

◆ Allergy, for example, ligneous, vernal, or atopic keratoconjunctivitis

◆ Graft versus host disease

◆ Other autoimmune reactions, for example, Stevens–Johnson syndrome[7]

◆ Pterygium and associated pathologies

◆ Scleritis

◆ Dry eye

◆ Prolonged use of topical medication[5]

Previous Surgery

◆ Any previous ocular surgeries including strabismus surgery. Fat adherence and anterior displacement of Tenon's are almost exclusively seen after strabismus surgery, and may cause scarring issues.

◆ Buckling surgery, especially including an encircling element, affects large areas of conjunctiva/Tenon's.

◆ Previous vitrectomy(ies). With the advent of small-gauge transconjunctival vitrectomy, cases with massive conjunctival scarring and concurrent scleral atrophy at former sclerotomy sites seem to have decreased. The problem has not, however, totally disappeared.

◆ Glaucoma surgery with filtering blebs or shunt devices presents special problems as these structures have to be avoided in subsequent surgeries.

The use of antimetabolites such as Mitomycin in glaucoma surgery can render parts of the conjunctiva avascular, with atrophy both of the conjunctiva and underlying sclera.

Trauma

◆ Mechanical

◆ Chemical—especially in cases with a profound injury to the limbal stem cells. There is often a progressive scarring, tear deficiency, and corneal problems.

- Thermal
- Radiation

Preventing the Development of Conjunctival Scarring

- Appropriate treatment of systemic conditions at an early, precicatricial.[6] stage: Aggressive treatment before elective ocular surgery is undertaken.

- Careful nontraumatic treatment of conjunctiva/Tenon's in all surgeries to prevent later problems.

- Careful planning in complicated cases to minimize the number of surgeries needed.

- In such cases as above, the use of a tissue fibrin–based glue (e.g., Tiseel Duo Quick, Baxter Medical) may be considered as an alternative to sutures at the end of surgery to minimize future scarring. We find that only very small amounts of these fibrin-based adhesives are necessary to secure the conjunctiva. The adhesive has two components, each in their own 1-mL syringe. Rather than using the mixing cannula provided, we administer a small amount of each component to the dried tissue via 27G cannulae, thus avoiding a large amount of dried glue at the site. The glue components can be applied sequentially while the surgeon keeps the area dry with a microsponge held in the free hand.

- Use of transconjunctival small-gauge technique in vitrectomy cases.

Often, we meet a patient first after the scarring has developed, at which point, we have to make the best of the situation. Much of what we should do, can be gleaned from the preventative measures above. Our aim should be to minimize the stimulant to scarring and optimize the ocular surface before surgery.

Performing Surgery in Eyes with a Scarred Conjunctiva

Preoperative Treatment[6–11]

- Aggressive treatment of coexisting conditions, for example, trachoma, OCP, and so on.

- Topical palliative treatments, artificial tear substitutes, topical antibiotics, and systemic tetracycline to reduce leukocyte migration.

- In extreme cases, the surgical surface may have to be optimized before intraocular surgery is undertaken (e.g., conjunctival rotational flaps to cover sclera, amniotic membrane transplants).

At Surgery

- Careful choice of position of entry sites, utilizing the healthiest areas of conjunctiva/sclera. This may involve an unusual positioning of the surgeon, for example, temporally and/or atypical placement of sclerotomies.

Note the differing anatomy of the pars plana nasally/temporally. The ora serrata typically extends for up to 1 mm more posteriorly and has a more uniform contour on the temporal aspect as compared to the nasal. If the surgeon sits temporally, using the two temporal sclerotomies for instruments, the infusion cannula may be placed nasally. In these cases, it is prudent to remember this fact that the pars plana is narrower nasally. A nasally placed sclerotomy should not be further than 3 mm from the limbus in a normally sized adult eye.

In cases where the patient has a prominent nose, this may compound the difficulties in placing the infusion cannula nasally, and the surgeon can consider placing all three sclerotomies temporally.

◆ In cases with foreshortened fornices due to excessive scarring, it may be difficult to indent the sclera as far posteriorly as wanted. The surgeon can consider opening the conjunctiva allowing access to the sub-Tenon's space, thus allowing freedom to indent at will. The advantages of this method should be balanced against the disadvantage of adding to the subsequent scarring by lifting the conjunctiva, and decided on a case-to-case basis.

◆ At the conclusion of surgery, it is obviously important to close the sclerotomies carefully, without inducing further scarring. It is paramount that the closure is tight to prevent infection. In these eyes, concurrent scleral atrophy can inhibit self-sealing and lead to leakage through suture channels. The use of a fibrin-based tissue glue should be considered to prevent leakage.[12]

◆ Rotational conjunctival flaps may help to cover sclerotomy sites. Similar techniques such as those used in plastic surgery for skin flaps may be used. An advantage is that the conjunctiva is more malleable than skin, and thus easier to manipulate to cover defects. A disadvantage is that the scarred conjunctiva is often exceptionally fragile and may disintegrate on handling. In such cases, it is advisable to use anatomic or even ring forceps, without any form of claws, to avoid further damage.

◆ Autologous conjunctival transplantation from same or fellow eye.

◆ Conjunctival suturing, where needed should involve generous episcleral bites to anchor the conjunctiva adequately and prevent later creeping, or migration.

◆ In unusual cases, especially after alkali burns or, for example, Stevens–Johnson, where extensive deep scarring precludes the use of conjunctiva, amniotic membrane transplantation may help to cover the sclerotomies at the end of surgery.

◆ One should consider carefully the need for an extended postoperative antibiotic treatment.

◆ A sub-Tenon's injection of corticosteroid can be considered at the end of surgery to reduce inflammation.

The vast majority of these cases can be handled with careful planning and preoperative preparation. Special care should be devoted to the treatment of pre-existing infection and inflammation, and the prevention of the same postoperatively.[13,14]

REFERENCES

1. Yamanaka O, Liu CY, Kao WW. Fibrosis in the anterior segment of the eye. *Endocr Metab Immune Disord Drug Targets.* 2010;10(4):331–335.
2. Chang JH, McClusky PJ. Ocular cicatricial pemphigoid: Manifestations and management. *Curr Allergy Asthma Rep.* 2005;5(4):333–338.
3. Saw VP, Dart JK. Ocular mucous membrane pemphigoid: Diagnosis and management strategies. *Ocul Surf.* 2008;6(3):128–142.
4. Burton MJ. Trachoma: An overview. *Br Med Bull.* 2007;84:99–11.
5. Servat JJ, Bernardino CR. Effects of common topical antiglaucoma medications on the ocular surface, eyelids and periorbital tissue. *Drugs Aging.* 2011;28(4):267–282.
6. Chiou AG, Florakis GJ, Kazim M. Management of conjunctival cicatrizing diseases and severe ocular surface dysfunction. *Surv Ophthalmol.* 1998;43(1):19–46.
7. Gregory DG. The ophthalmologic management of acute Stevens–Johnson syndrome. *Ocul Surf.* 2008;6(2):87–95.

8. Fish R, Davidson RS. Management of ocular thermal and chemical injuries, including amniotic membrane therapy. *Curr Opin Ophthalmol.* 2010;21(4):317–321.

9. Nakamura T, Kinoshita S. New hopes and strategies for the treatment of severe ocular surface disease. *Curr Opin Ophthalmol.* 2011;22(4):274–278.

10. Meller D, Pauklin M, Thomasen H, et al. Amniotic membrane transplantation in the human eye. *Dtsch Arztebl Int.* 2011;108(14):243–248.

11. Sangwan VS, Burman S, Tejwani S, et al. Amniotic membrane transplantation: A review of current indications in the management of ophthalmic disorders. *Indian J Ophthalmol.* 2007;55(4):251–260.

12. Batman C, Ozdamar Y, Mutevelli S, et al. A comparative study of tissue glue and vicryl suture for conjunctival and scleral closure in conventional 20-gauge vitrectomy. *Eye (Lond).* 2009;23(6):1382–1387.

13. Cordeiro MF, Chang L, Lim KS, et al. Modulating conjunctival wound healing. *Eye(Lond).* 2000;14(pt 3B):536–547.

14. Yiu SC, Thomas PB, Nguyen P. Ocular surface reconstruction: Recent advances and future outlook. *Curr Opin Ophthalmol.* 2007;18(6):509–514.

24C　Difficulties Isolating Extraocular Muscles

◆ In buckling surgery, especially when setting encircling elements, the extraocular muscles, usually the rectus muscles, need to be identified and isolated.[1–3] This is often relatively easy, but may be complicated in situations where muscles have an anomalous anatomy, or have been affected by pathologic processes such as those listed below.

　　Earlier ocular surgery, especially strabismus surgery, where muscles may be recessed, split, moved, or sutured, and will be fibrotic.

◆ Congenital syndromes, for example, congenital fibrosis of the extraocular muscles, congenital orbital fibrosis, adherence syndrome.

◆ Trauma, including injuries to the orbital contents, but even orbital fractures, for example, ethmoidal avulsion, orbital floor fractures.

◆ Systemic disorders, for example, Graves disease.

◆ Earlier radiotherapy/brachytherapy.

◆ Inflammation, including idiopathic orbital inflammation (IOI).

◆ Infection, for example, earlier orbital cellulitis or postoperative infection.

◆ Earlier neoplasia, for example, rhabdomyosarcoma, metastases from breast cancer, may leave scarred tissues after treatment.

✦ Prevention

In those cases that occur postsurgically, the most one can do to prevent future problems is to use a sterile, atraumatic technique.

　　It is of vital importance that the surgeon realizes the potential problems involved before such patients as listed above reach the operating table. Whereas we cannot magically improve the condition of the muscles involved, the situation can be investigated so as to give an idea of the scope of the pathology, and allow an appropriate preoperative planning.

Our most important tools in the preoperative workup include:

◆ A detailed history to identify the above risk factors.

◆ Radiology, ideally magnetic resonance imaging (MRI), to map the anatomic relationships.

◆ Ocular motility tests including forced duction test.

◆ Consultation with appropriate specialists, for example, oncologist.

◆ Optimal treatment of inflammation and infection before surgery.

On the operating table, we have various alternatives. If it transpires that the dissection and isolation of the extraocular muscles is difficult (and thus risky), the most important step for the surgeon to take is to decide whether or not it is worth the risk, or if the surgery may be done using an alternative method.

In the case of retinal detachment, one of our most powerful tools in this situation is to avoid the need for muscle isolation by performing a vitrectomy.

In cases where a buckle is deemed absolutely necessary, an encircling element can be avoided and segmental buckles placed between the muscle insertions, obviating the need to isolate the muscles. In these cases, the necessary rotation of the eye can be achieved by the use of tractional sutures.

Thus:

◆ Convert to vitrectomy

◆ Segmental buckles

◆ Tractional sutures

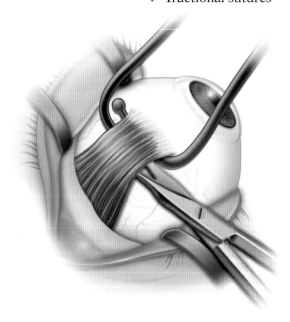

Figure 24C-1 The figure shows two muscle hooks in place under the rectus muscle, maintaining a narrow tunnel. The blunt scissors may be introduced into this tunnel, then the blades are opened carefully to bluntly dissect the adherences between the muscle and the sclera.

In those cases where the surgeon feels that it is absolutely necessary to isolate the muscles, a technique similar to that used by strabismus surgeons during reoperations may be used.[4,5]

In these cases, Tenon's capsule can be incised using small blunt-tipped scissors to expose the scleral surface. This should be done a distance from the expected edge of the muscle. The tip and blades of the scissors should be angled tangentially to the surface of the sclera, tunneling as far back as necessary to come posteriorly to the muscle. The tunneling should progress with small spreading movements, and NO cutting. The scissors can be left under the muscle to allow a muscle hook to follow them under the muscle. With the muscle hook in place, a similar dissection can be performed from the opposite aspect of the muscle to meet the original hook, and a new hook can be placed, giving an isolated muscle over two hooks **(Figure 24C-1)**. Every effort should be made at this point to ensure that the entire muscle is isolated. Special care must be taken in those eyes that have undergone earlier strabismus surgery, as the muscle insertions may be weak, and there is a risk for avulsion. Vascular loops (silicone surgical loops, 1.5 mm diameter, Braun) may provide a less traumatic holding sling for the isolated muscle than, for example, silk sutures **(Figure 24C-2)**.

In summary, isolation of fibrotic, adherent muscles can present severe difficulties for the surgeon. Perforation

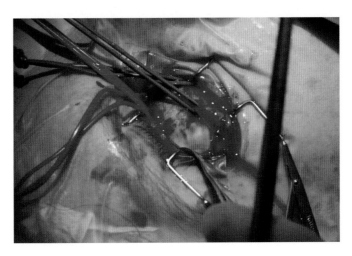

Figure 24C-2 The use of vascular loops to ensnare extraocular muscles during external surgery.

of the globe during the dissection can be a catastrophic event. Even a lost disinserted muscle can be extremely problematic for the patient. The preoperative workup should detail the potential problems as far as possible, to allow the surgeon to make a balanced decision as to whether the potential gains of isolating the extraocular muscles mitigate the risks involved. In many cases, the best solution will be to avoid the situation by using a different surgical technique.

REFERENCES

1. Troutman RC. Microsurgery of the anterior segment of the eye. In: *Introduction in Basic Techniques.* Vol 1. St Louis, MO: CV Mosby; 1974.
2. Eisner G: *Eye Surgery:An Introduction to Operative Technique.* 2nd sub edn. Springer-Verlag Berlin Heidelberg, New York; 1991.
3. Rice TA, Wilkinson CP. *Michels Retinal Detachment.* 2nd edn. St. Louis, MO: Mosby; 1997.
4. Hiles DA. Current concepts in the management of re-operations upon the extraocular muscles. *Ann Ophthalmol.* 1973;5(12):1344–1351.
5. Jampolsky A. Strabismus reoperation techniques. *Trans Sect Ophthalmol Am Acad Ophthalmol Otolaryngol.* 1975;79(5):704–717.

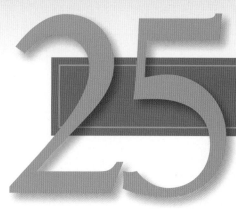

POOR VIEW of the FUNDUS

M<small>ARC</small> D. <small>DE</small> S<small>MET</small>

25A   Lack of Corneal Transparency

✤ Definition

Corneal transparency is essential for adequate visualization of intraocular structures. Lack of transparency will limit the ability to carry out surgery.

✤ Risk Factors

Length of surgery, contact lens systems, inadequate/inappropriate corneal hydration, medical condition (diabetes, glaucoma), combined surgery on the anterior segment, and keratoprosthesis.

✤ Pathogenesis

The cornea is assembled as a compact structure, the transparency of which is as much dependent on its structure as it is on its state of hydration.[1] Lack of corneal transparency arises due to a disruption of this fine assembly leading to excessive light scattering. In the case of prematurity, the corneal structure has not matured sufficiently and requires more time to become transparent.

To the surgeon, backscattered light is particularly bothersome. This is due to light incident onto the corneal surface (as from an indirect ophthalmoscope or the microscope light). Having a source of illumination inside the eye as is most commonly used in vitreoretinal surgery reduces significantly any visual hindrance, and improves visualization 4-fold as compared to external illumination.[2,3] Light coming from the vitreous cavity, particularly when it is directed to anterior vitreous structures, can also; lead to scattering within the cornea. It arises from intense point sources rather than diffuse light. Light reflected from the surface of polished metallic intraocular instruments, or directly from the edge of bullet light sources or the tips of chandelier lights are particularly bothersome. Reducing the intensity of the light source or using a filter can reduce the intensity of scattering. Such physical measures can limit the severity of the problem.

Corneal edema due to a dysfunctional endothelial pump, epithelial instability, or toxicity can lead to increased light scatter. Endothelial pump function may be due to a low endothelial cell count often heralded by the presence of numerous guttatae on the corneal endothelial surface, but it is also found in acute glaucoma and ocular inflammation. It may also develop as a result of prolonged or combined surgery. Stromal edema will lead to striate keratopathy or folds in Descemet's membrane, which limit visibility. Corneal scarring, from an inherited corneal dystrophy or previous trauma, will affect corneal transparency, limiting the visualization of intraocular structures intraoperatively.

Pearls on How to Prevent It

Corneal Edema

◆ Use a noncontact viewing system.

◆ Use viscous gels to maintain corneal hydration and as interface gel for contact lenses.

◆ Avoid gels and topical anesthetics containing preservatives, particularly those which are cell membrane disruptors.

◆ Treat any underlying corneal endothelial dysfunction. Reduce intraocular pressure preoperatively. As corneal turgescence is a function of fluid inflow versus the rate of endothelial-mediated outflow, a reduction in intraocular pressure (infusion pressure) will lead to a more compact cornea, less likely to develop corneal edema. It works best as a preventative measure and should be initiated at the onset of surgery.

◆ Treat any intraocular inflammation with appropriate anti-inflammatory medications.

Corneal Scar

◆ Minimize scar formation by the use of appropriate anti-inflammatory medications.

Pearls on How to Solve It

Corneal Edema

◆ Physical measures to reduce reflected light from the surface of instruments.

◆ Reduce epithelial turgescence: Reduce infusion pressure and use topical hyperosmotic agents such as 100% glycerol.[4] Hypertonic glycerol will lead to decreased epithelial edema, but the improvement is; however, only temporary lasting 10 to 15 minutes. Inject Viscoat in the anterior chamber **(Fig. 25A-1)**.[5]

◆ Remove the corneal epithelium: In many cases, especially in those requiring lengthy surgery, ablation of the corneal epithelium may be needed to obtain adequate visualization of intraocular structures intraoperatively. To remove the epithelium, rub it cautiously using a cotton tip applicator until it separates from Bowman's layer. When the corneal epithelium is edematous, this procedure is easily carried out. Occasionally, a flat blade may be used. It is applied broadside to the cornea so as to sheer the epithelium from its insertion to the cornea. The cornea should not be incised.

◆ In the presence of striate keratopathy or folds in Descemet's membrane, viscoelastic can be injected in the anterior chamber to overcome the reduced clarity from descemet membrane (DM) folds. It will also reduce epithelial edema by providing a barrier to fluid motion into the cornea, and its increased viscosity compared to the corneal stroma may remove some of the fluid already accumulated.[5]

Corneal Opacities

◆ *Band keratopathy:* This can be removed with repeated applications of 3.75% dilution of disodium ethylenediaminetetraacetic acid (EDTA).[6] Other scars will be removed using the backside of a flat blade at the onset of surgery or prior to surgery by Excimer laser.[7]

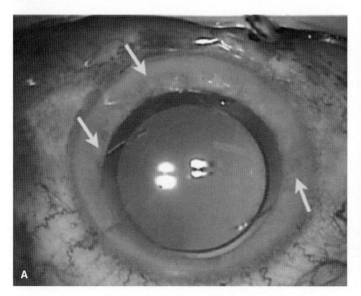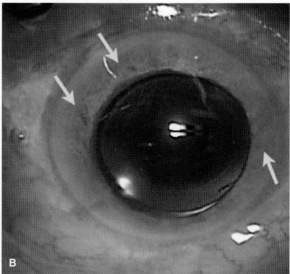

Figure 25A-1 Effect of intracameral Viscoat (within 15 minutes on corneal edema). Details of iris structure become visible. From McCannel CA. Improved intraoperative fundus visualization in corneal edema: The Viscoat trick. *Retina* 2012;32:189–190.

◆ *Stromal scars:* If a corneal scar is centrally located and large enough to hamper visualization of internal structures during preoperative examination, its removal will be required. In many cases a deep lamellar keratoplasty will be sufficient. Descemet's membrane is particularly resilient, and provided that it is left intact, is sufficient to carry out a vitrectomy with or without a keratoprosthesis. Dissection of deeper corneal stromal scarring can be facilitated by injection of Healon or air via a 30G needle or cannula **(Fig. 25A-2)**.[8,9] At the end of surgery a lamellar corneal button without endothelium is sown in place.

◆ *Full thickness corneal scar:* A penetrating keratoplasty with the use of a keratoprosthesis would be required to undertake pars plana vitrectomy under these circumstances. It has the advantage of allowing surgery to proceed in the exact same way as a standard vitrectomy. At the end of surgery, the original corneal button needs to be grafted back on to the eye, or a donor graft is required. Open-sky surgery is also possible particularly when surgery close to the iris root is required. The image remains small, and maneuvers are more difficult than with a keratoprosthesis.[10,11]

◆ An alternative in situations where a corneal transplant is contraindicated and a lamellar keratoplasty is not possible is the use of an endoscope. This allows the surgeon to bypass anterior structures completely.[12,13]

◆ *Corneal immaturity:* In premature infants with lack of corneal clarity, surgery should be delayed until about 32 weeks of age. Use of anti-VEGF agents may help inhibit progression of ROP for days to weeks particularly if combined with laser or cryotherapy.

✥ Expected Outcomes: What Is the Worst-case Scenario

If no visualization through the cornea is possible, the cornea will have to be removed and replaced by a keratoprosthesis. If a keratoprosthesis is not available for any reason, the posterior pole can be approached via an endoscope or using a wide-field contact lens, or the eye can be operated upon using an open-sky approach. It is important in such a case to make sure that a Flieringa ring is secured to the sclera and have a sufficient supply of BSS+ available as the fluid flow will be very high. Under these conditions, the retina will be thrown in folds (chorioretinal folds), which will limit the

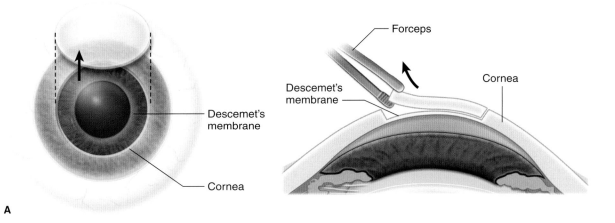

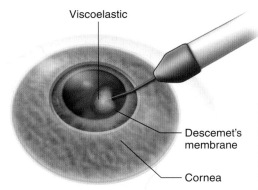

Figure 25A-2 Deep lamellar keratoplasty to expose Descemet's membrane. **A:** Create a lamellar keratoplasty to between 60% and 80% of corneal depth. **B:** Inject air or viscoelastic in the remaining stromal bed to separate the corneal stroma from Descemet's membrane which is loosely adherent to the stroma.

extent of surgery that can be carried out, particularly if peeling is required, but a core vitrectomy as well as elementary manipulations of the retinal surface will be possible.

REFERENCES

1. Meek KM, Boote C. The organization of collagen in the corneal stroma. *Exp Eye Res.* 2004;78:503–512.
2. Saragas S, Krah D, Miller D. Improved visualization through cataracts using intravitreal illumination. *Ann Ophthalmol.* 1984;16:311–313.
3. Salyer DA, Twietmeyer K, Beaudry N, et al. In vitro multispectral diffuse reflectance measurements of the porcine fundus. *Invest Ophthalmol Vis Sci.* 2005;46:2120–2124.
4. Lamberts DW. Topical hyperosmotic agents and secretory stimulants. *Int Ophthalmol Clin.* 1980;20:163–169.
5. McCannel CA. Improved intraoperative fundus visualization in corneal edema: The Viscoat trick. *Retina.* 2012;32:189–190.
6. Najjar DM, Cohen EJ, Rapuano CJ, et al. EDTA chelation for calcific band keratopathy: Results and long-term follow-up. *Am J Ophthalmol.* 2004;137:1056–1064.
7. Jhanji V, Rapuano CJ, Vajpayee RB. Corneal calcific band keratopathy. *Curr Opin Ophthalmol.* 2011;22:283–289.
8. Muraine M, Collet A, Brasseur G. Deep lamellar keratoplasty as surgical management of anterior and posterior segment injuries to the eye. *Cornea.* 2001;20:897–901.
9. Shimmura S, Tsubota K. Deep anterior lamellar keratoplasty. *Curr Opin Ophthalmol.* 2006;17:349–355.
10. Johnston RH, Nguyen R, Jongsareejit A, et al. Clinical study of combined penetrating keratoplasty, pars plana vitrectomy with temporary keratoprosthesis, and pars plana seton implant. *Retina.* 1999;19:116–121.

11. Garcia-Valenzuela E, Blair NP, Shapiro MJ, et al. Outcome of vitreoretinal surgery and penetrating keratoplasty using temporary keratoprosthesis. *Retina.* 1999;19: 424–429.
12. Mura M, de Smet MD: Endoscopically assisted minimally invasive retinal surgery. *Eye.* 2008;22:662–665.
13. de Smet MD, Carlborg E: Management of severe endophthalmitis using an endoscopic approach. *Retina.* 2005;25:976–980.

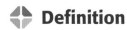

25B   Inadequate Size of the Pupil

Definition

A small pupil limits the visualization of posterior segment structures, particularly the visualization of the peripheral retina. It may seriously hamper or prevent subsequent intraocular maneuvers. Poor dilation can be present at the onset of surgery or may develop in the course of the procedure. Use of preventative measures can reduce the need of additional surgical steps to remedy the problem.

Risk Factors

Structural: Synechiae (anterior or posterior), trauma, and congenital anomalies. Neurogenic: Adie's pupil, syphilis, and age. Pharmacologic: Use of miotics (pilocarpine), preoperative use of mydriatics, and inadequate preoperative dilation. Procedural: Previous recent vitrectomy, duration of surgery (>90 minutes), hypotony, iris manipulation, and fluid–air exchange.

Pathogenesis

Causes of a myotic pupil are listed above. Posterior synechiae initially form at the edge of the pupil. However, with time, synechiae extend along the posterior surface of the iris forming a plaque-like fibrotic scar. It is often visible during the clinical examination as a white membrane protruding beyond the edge of the pupil, or extending on the anterior surface of the iris. Removal of this membrane as described below requires a careful dissection of the scar tissue from the iris proper.

The pharmacology of pupillary dilation and constriction depends on a number of factors listed below. The receptivity of the iris tissue and the level of available pigment determines the initial response to mydriatic agents. Maximal dilation is achieved by providing a sufficient dose of dilatatory agents, best achieved with some form of sustained release mechanism. Tachyphylaxis limits the mydriatic effect as is frequently seen when mydriatics are administered repeatedly in the hours preceding surgery.[1] In the presence of inflammation, miosis will appear more rapidly due to accelerated clearance of the pharmacologic agents occuring as a result of the increased vascular flow present in the uveal tissue, as well as from the release of inflammatory mediators. Neural mechanisms are biphasic in nature and may lead to miosis through a difference in response between the afferent and efferent neural limbs.[1,2] Topical anesthetics, for example, limit surgically induced miosis, while retrobulbar lidocaine does not. Administration of benoxinate or proparacaine, preferably prior to mydriasis, will ensure a more prolonged dilation. Iris manipulation or irritation will release prostaglandins which can lead to miosis . This process can be blocked by the administration of nonsteroidal anti-inflammatory drugs (NSAIDs).[3] Other identified surgical factors are discussed below.

Pearls on How to Prevent It

Mechanical/structural

- *Anterior synechiae:* In the presence of corneal trauma:

  - Meticulous closure of the wound.

  - Avoidance of incarcerated iris tissue in the corneal wound.

  - Adequate mydriasis and anti-inflammatory drops.

- *Posterior synechiae:* In the presence of inflammation:

  - Adequate daily dilation of the pupil is mandatory. The choice of mydriatic depends on the severity of inflammation. For very severe inflammation, atropine 1% is recommended on a daily basis, and for less severe inflammation homatropine 2% once or twice daily will be adequate.

  - If posterior synechiae are present, an attempt at maximal dilation with a cocktail of atropine, cyclopentolate, and epinephrine in a pledget placed adjacent to the sclera may be useful. It should be left in place for 15 to 30 minutes. Alternatively, a Mydriasert (tropicamide/phenylephrine HCl slow release insert; Thea Pharma) associated with atropine may be attempted. These approaches should not be tried within a few days of surgery, as it could limit dilatation once the synechiae are surgically released.

Pharmacologic

- In the days leading up to surgery, it is best to avoid mydriatics as these may limit maximum dilatation.[4]

- Prostaglandin inhibitors are useful in cataract surgery, their role in vitreoretinal surgery is limited to situations where one expects extensive iris manipulation.[2,4,5] In such cases they should be ideally initiated 1 to 2 days prior to surgery.

- Maximal preoperative dilation requires the instillation of a mixture of mydriatic agents, a sufficient number of times, stating a minimum of 30 minutes prior to surgery.[2] Most cocktails will include atropine 1%, homatropine 2%, and/or tropicamide 1%, as well as phenylephrine (2.5%, 5%, or 10%). The latter is particularly effective at achieving a maximal pupillary size.[2]

- The use of sustained release devices such as the Mydriasert (Thea Laboratories) has significantly facilitated the logistics of pupil dilation and its sole use often provides adequate if not better dilation than cocktails.[6] It is particularly useful when dilation is performed on a ward (particularly nonophthalmic). It can be inserted in the conjunctival cul-de-sac as the patient is being transferred to the operation room complex.

- An alternative would be to place a pledget in the cul-de-sac soaked with a mixture of phenylephrine 2.5%, tropicamide 1%, and atropine 1%.[7] Both sustained release procedures tend to provide slightly better dilation than the application of intermittent topical drops.

◆ Procedural: Factors such as the duration of surgery, hypotony, manipulation of the iris, and air–fluid exchange have been associated with miosis.[8]

◆ Adequate surgical planning and avoiding steps associated with miosis until the end of surgery can help reduce its occurrence.

◆ Miosis from an air–fluid exchange is reduced by using humidified air.[8] Since the miosis is likely due to the drying effect of air on the posterior iris surface, preoperative use of NSAIDs might help mitigate this effect.

◆ Scleral buckling as well as extensive cryotherapy may also increase the risk of miosis, but the true risk is difficult to differentiate from the effect of prolonged surgery which in itself is probably the most important factor.[4]

✦ Pearls on How to Solve It

◆ Synechiae can best be dealt with using viscoelastic injected through any remaining opening between the iris and the lens/IOL surface. The viscoelastic separates the two surfaces, allowing release of the synechiae using an iris sweep, a cyclodialysis spatula, or the edge of a blade or needle. Usually upon release, as long as the iris constrictors are still functional, the pupil will dilate.

◆ When dilation is absent, it is likely that a fibrous plaque is present on the posterior surface of the iris. Its removal may require a combination of viscoelastics where possible, and dissection with a von Graefe knife or equivalent since shearing it from the iris surface usually leads to removal of the pupillary dilators **(Fig. 25B-1)**.

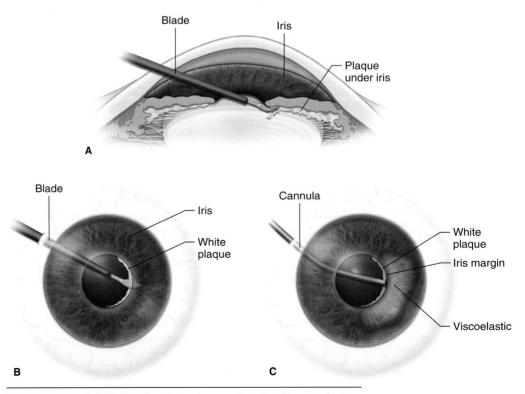

Figure 25B-1 Separating the iris from an underlying fibrous plaque.

◆ If the pupil remains small, a mechanical solution is needed to provide sufficient dilatation. This can be achieved by:

◆ Using 10-0 polypropylene sutures passed through the pars plana and the anterior segment. When overstretching is avoided, this is simple and effective solution **(Fig. 25B-2)**.[9–11]

◆ Iris retractors are also a popular and simple solution.[12] Four to five retractors are inserted short of the limbus through a small paracentesis made with a

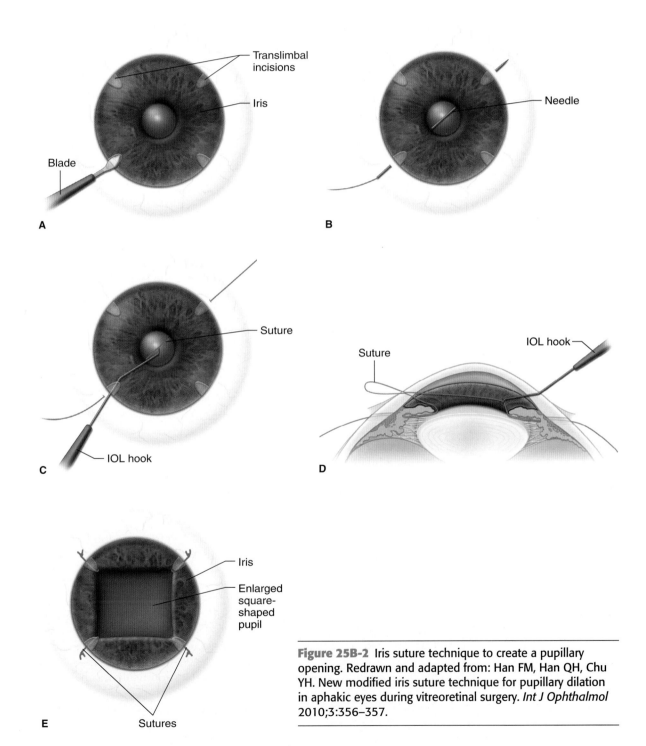

Figure 25B-2 Iris suture technique to create a pupillary opening. Redrawn and adapted from: Han FM, Han QH, Chu YH. New modified iris suture technique for pupillary dilation in aphakic eyes during vitreoretinal surgery. *Int J Ophthalmol* 2010;3:356–357.

needle or a blade angulated in a slightly posterior direction (aiming for the edge of the pupil). They should only be placed after pre-existing synechiae have been severed, and preferably when any retrolenticular membrane has been removed or incised. Iris retractors do not need to be fully stretched to provide an adequate pupillary aperture. In fact, it is best to avoid overstretching the iris as this can lead to sphincter damage and an irregular pupillary margin.[13]

◆ Injection of epinephrine in the anterior chamber may help in redilating a constricted pupil from manipulation or from lack of epinephrine in the infusion solution.[14] A dosage of 1:1,000,000 to 1:500,000 appears sufficient to dilate the pupil when injected intracamerally.

Expected Outcomes: What Is the Worst-case Scenario

In cases in which pupil dilation cannot be established due to an extensive fibrotic scar which precludes dilatation, one would have to proceed to either excision using a combination of the vitreous cutter and scissors or approach the posterior pole via an endoscope.[15,16] This can also be considered as an option if marked miosis occurs late in the surgical procedure and only limited manipulations such as laser are still required.[17]

REFERENCES

1. Ueda N, Muramatsu I, Fujiwara M. Capsaicin and bradykinin-induced substance P-ergic responses in the iris sphincter muscle of the rabbit. *J Pharmacol Exp Ther.* 1984;230:469–473.

2. Duffrin RM, Camras CB, Gardner SK, et al. Inhibitors of surgically induced miosis. *Ophthalmology.* 1982;89:966–979.

3. Mirshahi A, Djalilian A, Rafiee F, et al. Topical administration of diclofenac (1%) in the prevention of miosis during vitrectomy. *Retina.* 2008;28:1215–1220.

4. Smiddy WE, Glaser BM, Michels RG, et al. Miosis during vitreoretinal surgery. *Retina.* 1990;10:42–46.

5. Kim SJ, Lo WR, Hubbard GB, III, et al. Topical ketorolac in vitreoretinal surgery. A prospective, randomized, placebo-controlled, double-masked trial. *Arch Ophthalmol.* 2008;126:1203–1208.

6. Caruba T, Couffon-Partant C, Oliary J, et al. Mydriase préopératoire obtenue par insert ophtalmique versus collyres. *J Fr Ophtalmol.* 2006;29:789–795.

7. McCormick A, Srinivasan S, Harun S, et al. Pupil dilation using a pledget sponge: A randomized controlled trial. *Clin Exp Ophthalmol.* 2006;34:545–549.

8. Cekic O, Ohji M, Hayashi A, et al. Humidified air effect on pupil size during fluid–air exchange. *Retina.* 2001;21:529–531.

9. Niehaus H, Kroll P. Pupillary dilation with Eckardt iris retraction sutures within the scope of vitreoretinal surgery. *Ophthalmologe.* 1993;90:440–442.

10. Eckardt C. Pupillary stretching. A new procedure in vitreoretinal surgery. *Retina.* 1985;5:235–238.

11. Han FM, Han QH, Chu YH. New modified iris suture technique for pupillary dilation in aphakic eyes during vitreoretinal surgery. *Int J Ophthalmol.* 2010;3: 356–357.

12. McCuen B, 2nd, Hickingbotham D, Tsai M, et al. Temporary iris fixation with a micro-incision retractor. *Arch Ophthalmol.* 1989;107:925–927.

13. Tognetto D, Agolini G, Grandi G, et al. Iris alteration using mechanical iris retractors. *J Cataract Refract Surg.* 2001;27:1703–1705.

14. Corbett MC, Richards AB. Intraocular adrenaline maintains mydriasis during cataract surgery. *Br J Ophthalmol.* 1994;78:95–98.

15. de Smet MD, Mura M. Minimally invasive surgery—Endoscopic retinal detachment repair in patients with media opacities. *Eye.* 2007;1–4.
16. de Smet M, Carlborg EAE. Managing severe endophthalmitis with the use of an endoscope. *Retina.* 2005;25:976–980.
17. de Smet MD. Retinal transscleral photocoagulation under endoscopic control. *Retina.* 2000;20:18–19.

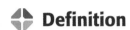

Problems Related to the Lens Capsule

Definition

Capsular opacification can prevent visualization of posterior pole structures. It may be present preoperatively, develop during surgery, or develop in the postoperative period preventing adequate follow-up. Patients with a long-standing cataract or intraocular lens (IOL), or following ocular inflammation, may have thick plaque-like deposits on the posterior capsule which prevent visualization of the posterior pole.

Risk Factors

Lens Touch

Posterior displacement of the lens, hyperopia, lenticular defects (e.g., lentiglobus), and anteriorly located Vitreo-retinal (VR) pathology.

Capsular Opacification

◆ Pre-existing: Prior ocular trauma, ocular inflammation, pediatric cataract, and long-standing IOL.

◆ Predisposed: Diabetic, AIDS, and ocular inflammation.

◆ Induced: Air–fluid exchange and lens touch.

Pathogenesis

Lens touch is usually due to an unfortunate move while inside the vitreous cavity (see also Chapter 10B). Its frequency decreases with experience and adequate surgical planning. With proper orientation inside the eye and the use of certain adjunctive procedures, it is possible to avoid surgical instruments getting in contact with the crystalline lens. It is rarely the tip of the instrument but usually its shaft that touches the posterior capsule, particularly when reaching for a structure across the midline in the far periphery. An arc of a few degrees around the sclerotomy has the highest risk, with the risk increasing proportionally as one gets closer to a position 180 degrees away from the point of insertion into the eye. The outer 60 degrees are safe with little chance of hitting the lens. However, zonules could be weakened if the manipulation is brought sufficiently anterior.

Posterior sub capsular opacification (PSC) occurs as a result of posterior migration and inward displacement of anterior and equatorial lens epithelial cells (see also Chapter 20A). Inflammation and ocular steroids will frequently lead to a visually significant posterior subcapsular cataract (PSC) possibly by mediating the restructuring of extracellular matrix by way of matrix metaloproteases (MMPs).[1] A metaplastic change may also occur in long-standing PSC or following IOL implantation leading to the formation of a collagenous plaque, the excision of which may be quite challenging.[2]

 ## Pearls on How to Prevent It

Lens Touch

◆ Avoid crossing the midline when performing a vitrectomy or manipulating tissues adjacent to the pars plana (see also Chapter 10B).

◆ Single hand manipulations with external indentation to minimize a distal reach.

◆ Use of chandelier light sources kept close to the scleral insertion.

◆ Position initial sclerotomies or trocars along the horizontal axis or create new sclerotomies at 45 degrees from the intended zone of peripheral manipulation.

◆ A small air bubble may help identify the posterior surface of the lens.

◆ Drainage of the anterior chamber will cause an anterior displacement of the lens, allowing easier access to the pars plana region **(Fig. 25C-1)**.

Capsular Opacification

◆ Increasing the amount of glucose in the infusion bottle to 400% its normal concentration will reduce cataract development in patients with diabetes (see also Chapter 20A).[3]

◆ Dry air will cause the posterior lens surface to opacify. Directing the air stream away from the posterior capsule and insuring hydration of the air entering the eye will prevent this complication.

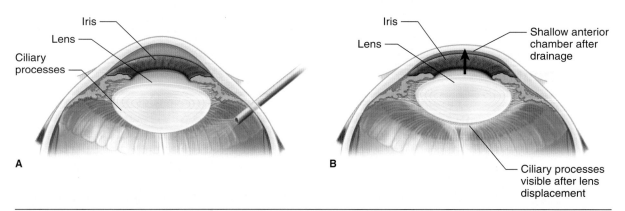

Figure 25C-1 A, B: Draining the anterior chamber leads to an anterior displacement of the lens giving better access to the pars plana region of the eye without significantly affecting vision when using a wide-field viewing system.

◆ A short surgical time with limited exposure to air will limit the risk of developing a cataract and posterior capsule opacification in patients at risk.

 ## Pearls on How to Solve It

Lens Touch

◆ If not severe and off the visual axis, it can be left alone. However, the patient should be followed carefully (see also Chapter 10B). In mild lens touch, where only compression of the overlying vitreous occurred, there will be no sequel. In those cases with a significant indentation, a posterior capsular opacity appears which is associated with a high risk of posterior capsular rupture at the time of cataract surgery.[4,5] Concurrent cataract extraction with IOL implant may be a better solution, or a planned intervention in the following weeks to months before the posterior capsule weakens.

Capsular Opacity

◆ If significant capsular opacity is present, a lens extraction will be required. If present at the onset of surgery, a phacovitrectomy with an IOL implant is the preferred approach. If it develops during surgery, either a phacoemulsification or a pars plana lensectomy can be considered. Since phacoemulsification preserves the capsular bag and allows for the subsequent placement of an IOL, this technique should be chosen whenever possible.

◆ If secondary to air, returning to a liquid state or using oil will improve if not completely restore visualization.

◆ Plaques on the posterior capsule of pseudophakic eyes can in most cases be removed with a vitreous cutter on high suction. Occasionally, it will be necessary to incise the plaque with a blade to create an edge along which the vitreous cutter can aspirate and cut. On rare occasions, a good portion of the plaque will have to be cut using intraocular scissors.

 ## Expected Outcomes: What Is the Worst-case Scenario

If visualization of the posterior segment is not possible and the vitreoretinal procedure cannot progress because of this complication, a combined phacovitrectomy should be carried out even if the IOL power was not determined prior to the intervention. Axial length measurements can be obtained once the eye is rehabilitated, and an IOL can be implanted as a secondary procedure by opening up the capsular bag.[6–8]

REFERENCES

1. Alapure BV, Praveen MR, Gajjar DU,et al. Matrix metalloproteinase-2 and -9 activities in the human lens epithelial cells and serum of steroid induced posterior subcapsular cataracts. *Mol Vis.* 2012;18:64–73.
2. Peng Q, Hennig A, Vasavada AR, et al. Posterior capsular plaque: A common feature of cataract surgery in the developing world. *Am J Ophthalmol.* 1998;125:621–626.
3. Haimann MH, Abrams GW. Prevention of lens opacification during diabetic vitrectomy. *Ophthalmology.* 1984;91:116–121.

4. Asaria RH, Wong SC, Sullivan PM. Risk for posterior capsule rupture after vitreo-retinal surgery. *J Cataract Refract Surg.* 2006;32:1068–1069.
5. Saravanan VR, Singh G, Narendran V. Posterior capsule rupture after vitreoretinal surgery. *J Cataract Refract Surg.* 2007;33:562–563.
6. Chen YJ. Delayed in-the-bag implantation of intraocular lens. *Can J Ophthalmol.* 2009;44:95–97.
7. Chen YJ. Secondary in-the-bag implantation of intraocular lenses in aphakic eyes after vitreoretinal surgeries. *Ophthalmologica.* 2012;227:80–84.
8. Nihalani BR, Vanderveen DK. Secondary intraocular lens implantation after pediatric aphakia. *J AAPOS.* 2011;15:435–440.

25D Difficult View due to the Presence of Tamponade Agents

Definition

The view to the posterior structures is hampered by the presence of a tamponade agent in the anterior chamber, in particular by the formation of multiple small bubbles in the anterior chamber.

Risk Factors

Air or silicone oil can enter the anterior chamber if there is zonular dehiscence, a peripheral iris defect or a full iris defect, and a misdirected infusion line.

Pathogenesis

As air enters the vitreous cavity, the refractive power of the posterior lens surface strongly increases, shifting the refractive power of the eye from +59 to +102 D.[1,2] The presence of air in the anterior chamber will only change this power slightly. However, if the air fill is incomplete, bubbles will create a series of prismatic lenses that can severely distort visibility of posterior structures. Air in the anterior chamber also affects negatively the corneal endothelium particularly if dry air is used. In patients whose endothelial cell count is poor, or after prolonged surgery, folds may appear in the corneal endothelium which will adversely affect visibility.

Silicone oil entering the anterior chamber will also distort the view particularly when filling of the chamber is incomplete. Slight displacement of the eye or of the microscope may allow the edge of the bubble to move away from the visual axis and restore a decent view to the posterior pole. Alternatively, if a large enough bubble is present, its prismatic effect may be utilized to facilitate visualization of posterior structures (this is also true for air bubbles).

Air and oil enter the anterior chamber around the lens or intraocular lens because of weak or damaged zonules, less frequently due to a misdirected infusion line that directs the stream anteriorly to the posterior lens surface and surrounding zonules.

Pearls on How to Prevent It

♦ Before initiating the fluid–tamponade exchange, the exact position of the cannula should be checked. It should direct the flow to the posterior pole and not to anterior structures.

♦ Avoid collapse/pressure on anterior structures of the eye and rotations in the direction of the infusion line that could displace the tamponade agent anteriorly during injection.

♦ When shaving the vitreous base around peripheral tears, avoid as much as possible infusing tamponade agents in the same area.

♦ Use of Viscoat applied to the corneal endothelium reduces the desiccation injury caused by air and prevents/eliminates the folds that interfere with visibility.[3–5]

♦ Leave an air bubble in the anterior chamber to reduce the risk of oil re-entering the chamber.

 ## Pearls on How to Solve It

Air in the Anterior Chamber

♦ It is best to fill the anterior chamber fully and create a single bubble.

♦ In the presence of several endothelial folds, the injection of a small layer of Viscoat can re-establish visibility.

Silicone Oil in the Anterior Chamber

♦ The infusion line should be repositioned or possibly a different infusion site (cannula) should be used to inject oil.

♦ A small oil bubble in the anterior chamber can be left in place until the oil is removed as it is unlikely to affect the view intraoperatively or cause problems postoperatively.

♦ Larger bubbles should be removed during the surgical procedure. These can be sometimes displaced with air infused into the anterior chamber, or by filling the eye with viscoelastic or saline under some pressure to redirect the oil posteriorly.

Expected Outcomes: What Is the Worst-case Scenario

It may be difficult to prevent oil from re-entering the anterior chamber. In such cases, particularly if the oil must be left in the eye for a prolonged period, it may be necessary to reinitiate an oil fill after removing all or part of the oil in the vitreous cavity.

REFERENCES

1. Stefansson E, Tiedeman J. Optics of the eye with air or silicone oil. *Retina.* 1988;8: 10–19.
2. Chalam KV, Shah VA. Optics of wide-angle panoramic viewing system-assisted vitreous surgery. *Surv Ophthalmol.* 2004;49:437–445.
3. Landers MB 3rd. Sodium hyaluronate (Healon) as an aid to internal fluid-gas exchange. *Am J Ophthalmol.* 1982;94:557–559.
4. Çekiç O, Ohji M, Hayashi A, et al. Effects of humidified and dry air on corneal endothelial cells during vitreal fluid-air exchange. *Am J Ophthalmol.* 2002;134:75–80.
5. Çekiç O, Ohji M, Zheng Y, et al. Experimental study of viscoelastic in the prevention of corneal endothelial desiccation injury from vitreal fluid-air exchange. *Am J Ophthalmol.* 2003;135:641–647.

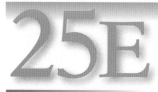

Intraocular Lens "Steaming" During Pars Plana Vitrectomy

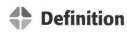

Definition

Steaming (condensation) on the posterior surface of an intraocular lens (IOL) can occur following air–fluid exchange or upon extraction of silicone oil. Lens steaming usually prevents visualization of the posterior segment structures. Any further surgical steps will not be possible until the issue is resolved.

Risk Factors

An opening in the posterior capsule is present in all cases. Certain lens types (PMMA and silicone lenses) have a higher propensity to be covered by condensation. Eyes in which a capsulotomy has been recently performed are more likely to develop this complication. Lens steaming occurs when an air exchange or a silicone oil exchange is being undertaken.

Pathogenesis

Intraoperative condensation on a posterior chamber IOL severely limits a surgeon's view. It occurs upon performing an air–fluid exchange, in the presence of a posterior capsulotomy or a rent in the posterior capsule. The likelihood of experiencing this complication depends on the wetting properties of the lens material (silicone > PMMA > hydrogel), more specifically on the contact angle between the water bead and the lens surface.[1] The more acute the angle, the more wettable is the lens surface. With angles approaching 0, the droplets form a film on the lens surface through which posterior structures can be seen. If wetting properties of the lens material are high, then simply wiping the posterior lens surface (as in hydrogel lenses) will be sufficient to temporarily give a good view to the posterior pole. At the other extreme, with highly hydrophobic surfaces such as silicone, wiping only results in displaced droplets of similar size. One can alter the surface properties of the IOL by applying a film of viscoelastic which as long as it adheres to the posterior lens surface will modify its wetting properties and bring them close to 0.[2] With time the wetting properties of intraocular lenses improve as proteins deposit on the posterior lens surface.

Condensation tends to occur when warm moist air contacts a cool surface. When various IOL materials were tested in a test chamber, condensation could be prevented in all cases when the temperature in the anterior chamber was kept above the temperature of the posterior chamber.[1] The air/gas-filled eye is warm relative to the anterior segment. Air in the posterior segment is warmed by the choroidal circulation while the anterior segment, by its exposure to room temperature, is relatively cold. Clinically, there is often a delay between completion of the air–fluid exchange and the appearance of mist on the posterior lens surface. This interval can be lengthened if cold air is used in the air–fluid exchange instead of air at room temperature.[2]

Misting can also occur when silicone oil is used or removed. Small water droplets have been "trapped" between a silicone IOL and silicone oil. These tend not to be displaced with time, and are best removed immediately at the time of oil tamponade.[3] More frequently observed is the tendency of silicone oil to coat IOL surfaces with thick droplets. It is independent of the viscosity and density of the oil, occurring in 100% of silicone IOLs.[4]

Pearls on How to Prevent It

◆ Avoid a capsulotomy in high risk situations.

◆ Choose or recommend a hydrophylic acrylic lens material with a low contact angle rather than a hydrophobic acrylic or silicone lens in high risk cases.

◆ Raising the temperature of the anterior segment with warmed saline solution may prevent condensation from occurring on the posterior lens surface of any IOL material. The visualization is better than with viscoelastics applied on the posterior lens surface, as these tend to produce an irregular surface hampering visualization of posterior structures.

◆ Drop the temperature of the infused air entering the vitreous cavity and insure venting (lowering the temperature in the vitreous cavity).

Pearls on How to Solve It

◆ Wiping the back surface of the IOL in patients with a hydrophylic lens material may be sufficient to obtain a good view to the posterior pole.

◆ Wiping the back surface of hydrophobic acrylic IOLs (AcrySof) will provide only a temporary view.

◆ Use of viscoelastic injected on the posterior surface of the IOL (as it dries, the viscoelastic will have to be wiped off the posterior surface and replaced with a new film). The film must be kept as shallow as possible to avoid additional prismatic effects.

◆ Increase the surface temperature of the anterior chamber by irrigating with warmed saline solution.

◆ Removal of silicone oil droplets from the surface of IOLs made of materials other than silicone can be achieved by wiping the lens surface and aspirating the residual oil, but the removal is often incomplete.[5] Irrigation with F_4H_5 in which silicone oil is highly soluble is an effective technique.[6] As the solution is injected on the posterior surface of the IOL, the silicone oil rapidly dissolves in the solvent which can be repeatedly injected and aspirated leading to complete removal of the oil from any lens surface.[7]

Expected Outcomes: What Is the Worst-case Scenario

In most cases, the required additional procedures can be carried out under heavy liquid. The vitreous chamber is filled above the pars plana. Saline is allowed to replace the air, with the residual air removed from the anterior vitreous cavity and the remaining steps are carried out in this way. The final fluid–air exchange is carried out by filling the eye completely with perfluorocarbon liquid (PFCL), positioning the tip of the aspirator along the edge of the most anterior tear and aspirating fluid until there is none present either at the edge of the tear or above the optic nerve. If one is unsure if all PFCL has been removed, placing a few drops of saline or BSS onto the "dried" retinal surface can facilitate removal of any residual PFCL droplets. As the added saline or BSS is being aspirated, the few remaining droplets of PFCL will also be aspirated from the retinal surface.

REFERENCES

1. Porter RG, Peters JD, Bourke RD. De-misting condensation on intraocular lenses. *Ophthalmology.* 2000;107:778–782.
2. Francese JE, Christ FR, Buchen SY, et al. Moisture droplet formation on the posterior surface of intraocular lenses during fluid/air exchange. *J Cataract Refract Surg.* 1995;21:685–689.
3. Khawly JA, Lambert RJ, Jaffe GJ. Intraocular lens changes after short- and long-term exposure to intraocular silicone oil. *Ophthalmology.* 1998;105:1227–1233.
4. Yaman A, Saatci AO, Sarioglu S, et al. Interaction with intraocular lens materials: Does heavy silicone oil act like silicone oil? *J Cataract Refract Surg.* 2007;33:127–129.
5. Dick HB, Augustin AJ. Solvent for removing silicone oil from intraocular lenses. Experimental study comparing various biomaterials. *J Cataract Refract Surg.* 2000;26:1667–1672.
6. Stappler T, Williams R, Wong D. F4H5: A novel substance for the removal of silicone oil from intraocular lenses. *Br J Ophthalmol.* 2010;94:364–367.
7. Liang Y, Kociok N, Leszczuk M, et al. A cleaning solution for silicone intraocular lenses: "sticky silicone oil". *Br J Ophthalmol.* 2008;92:1522–1527.

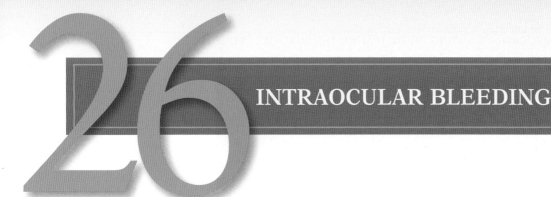

INTRAOCULAR BLEEDING

26A Subretinal Hemorrhage Complicating Retinal Detachment Surgery

MOSTAFA A. ELGOHARY AND ZDENEK J. GREGOR

 ## The Complication: Definition

Subretinal hemorrhage is an accumulation of blood in the subretinal space; that is, between the neurosensory retina and the retinal pigment epithelium (RPE).

In macula-sparing ("macula-on") retinal detachment (RD), subretinal hemorrhage is usually not sight threatening as the blood rarely dissects under the macula. However, in macula-involving ("macula-off") RD, the blood tends to gravitate under the macula and may cause significant visual loss. The following discussion, therefore, will pertain mainly to subretinal hemorrhage in patients with rhegmatogenous macula-off RD and in particular those with submacular hemorrhage (SMH).

Causes and Risk Factors

In rhegmatogenous RD, SMH may occur either during scleral buckling or vitrectomy procedures, or during peribulbar or retrobulbar anesthesia, as a result of injury to the retinal or choroidal vessels. SMH may also result from pre-existing pathologic conditions such as choroidal neovascularization in age-related macular degeneration (ARMD) and high myopia, idiopathic polypoidal choroidal vasculopathy (IPCV), retinal artery macroaneurysms (RAMA), or trauma.

During Scleral Buckling Procedures

Focal injury of the choroidal blood vessels. This may occur in the following instances.

◆ During external drainage of subretinal fluid using either a sharp needle (**Fig. 26A-1**), scleral cut-down or argon laser drainage techniques, for example, as part of the Drainage, Air, Cryotherapy, and Explant (DACE) procedure (see also Chapter 2). This is more likely to happen if the drainage site is posterior to the equator in the horizontal meridians (3- and 9-o'clock positions) as a result of injury to one of the long ciliary vessels or if the drainage site is near one of the vortex veins, for example, by the insertions of the superior or inferior oblique muscles.

◆ As a result of deep scleral suture path during placement of the buckle retaining sutures (see also Chapter 1).

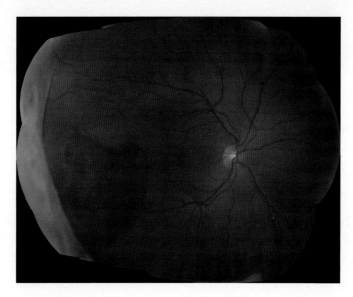

Figure 26A-1 Subretinal hemorrhage as a result of needle drainage of subretinal fluid during a scleral buckling procedure.

Choroidal vessel rupture during cryotherapy. This may occur if the cryotherapy probe is forcibly removed before the ice ball has completely thawed.

During Vitrectomy Procedures

Focal injury to the retinal blood vessels. This may occur in the following instances.

◆ During trimming of the flap or operculum of a retinal tear, particularly if this is associated with intact retinal blood vessels **(Fig. 26A-2A,B)**. If the tear and the RD are in the superior or temporal quadrants, the blood can easily gravitate posteriorly and form a blood clot under the macula.

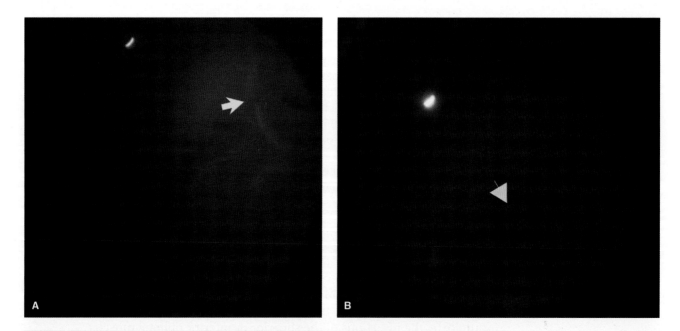

Figure 26A-2 A: Focal retinal injury during trimming of a temporally located tear (*arrow*) in a patient with macula-off RD. **B:** Submacular hemorrhage noticed during fluid–air exchange (*arrow head*). The patient was postured on the left side overnight. Recurrence of RD occurred due to PVR and final VA was 6/24.

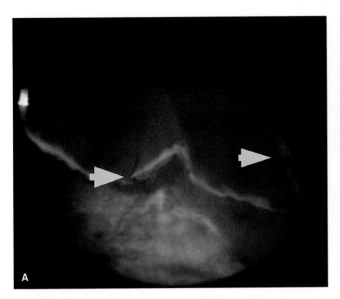
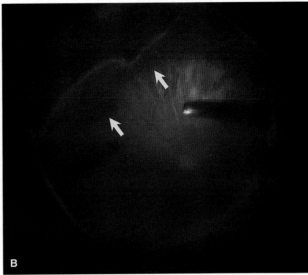

Figure 26A-3 A: Focal retina injury (*thick arrows*) during retinectomy for anterior PVR. **B:** Subretinal hemorrhage (*thin arrows*).

◆ During relieving retinectomy in patients with proliferative vitreoretinopathy (PVR) if adequate closure of the retinal vessels with diathermy has not been achieved **(Fig. 26A-3A,B)**.

◆ During peeling of contracted epiretinal membranes in PVR or delamination of fibrovascular membranes in proliferative diabetic retinopathy.

◆ As a result of hypotony, which increases the risk of spontaneous or uncontrollable bleeding from damaged retinal vessels.

Focal injury to the choroidal blood vessels. This may occur when using the following.

◆ The back-flush (flute) cannula during fluid–air exchange if the tip of the cannula is placed within the retinal defect selected for internal drainage of subretinal fluid (SRF).

◆ The vitrectomy cutter or the retinal microscissors during retinectomy in the presence of shallow SRF **(Fig. 26A-4)**.

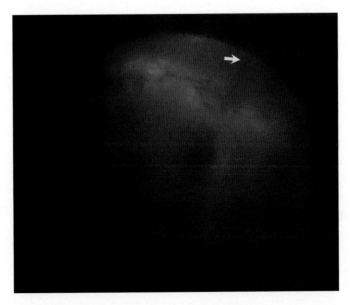

Figure 26A-4 Focal choroidal injury during retinectomy. (Courtesy of Mr. Paul Sullivan.)

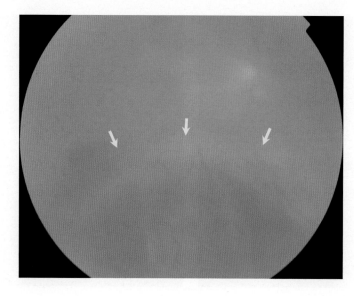

Figure 26A-5 Subretinal and suprachoroidal hemorrhages that developed as a result of transient hypotony in an area where cryotherapy was applied.

As a Result of Suprachoroidal Hemorrhage

◆ Hypotony at any stage during the operation increases the risk of suprachoroidal hemorrhage **(Fig. 26A-5)**.[1] Suprachoroidal blood, however, seldom dissects into the subretinal or submacular space.

Due to Perforation During Peribulbar or Retrobulbar Anesthesia

◆ Scleral perforation during peribulbar or retrobulbar injection of local anesthetic may result in focal choroidal or retinal injury causing severe subretinal and suprachoroidal hemorrhages.

Predisposing Factors for SMH During RD Surgery

Ocular

◆ Degenerative conditions such as ARMD, high myopia, RAMA, angioid streaks, and IPCV.

◆ Choroidal vascular tumors, for example, hemangioma.

◆ Excessive use of cryotherapy. This causes dilatation of choroidal blood vessels and increases the risk of suprachoroidal hemorrhage.

◆ Trauma, including blunt trauma or iatrogenic trauma, for example, laser photocoagulation.

◆ Inflammations, for example, presumed ocular histoplasmosis syndrome (POHS).

◆ Hypotony. This predisposes mainly to suprachoroidal hemorrhage but may increase the risk of bleeding from damaged retinal vessels into the subretinal space.

Systemic

◆ Vascular disorders, for example, atherosclerosis and uncontrolled hypertension.

◆ Hemorrhagic diathesis, for example, thrombocytopenia and hemophilia.

◆ Anticoagulant or antiplatelet medications.

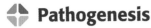 **Pathogenesis**

Visual Loss Following Subretinal and Submacular Hemorrhages

Damage to the Retina and Retinal Pigment Epithelial Cells

In experimental models of SMH,[2,3] irreversible retinal damage, including intracellular edema, disintegration, and pyknosis of the photoreceptors, was noted to begin within the first 24 hours and extensive damage to the outer nuclear layer occurred by the seventh day. The mechanisms of retinal damage include[4]:

Barrier effect. The blood clot acts as a diffusion barrier, impairing access of oxygen and nutrients to the photoreceptors and blocking the transport of metabolites from the outer retinal layers to the choriocapillaris.

Mechanical effect. In experimental models[3,5] fibrin was found to be attached to the photoreceptor outer segments within the first 25 minutes. The shearing force by the contracting blood clot leads to their displacement and separation after 1 hour. Seven days later, extensive degenerative changes occur, involving the outer and inner retinal layers as well as the RPE.

Iron toxicity. This involves a time- and dose-dependent mechanism. The released ferritin molecules are thought to contribute to the damage of the photoreceptors, RPE cells, and inner retinal layers.[2,3,6]

Development of Proliferative Vitreoretinopathy and Subretinal Fibrocellular Membranes

Subretinal blood contains chemoattractants for macrophages and fibroblasts that lead to the formation of contractile subretinal fibrocellular membranes.[7,8] PVR can also develop, especially in the presence of vitreous hemorrhage.[9] Both pathologic changes increase the risk of retinal redetachment.

Increased Intraocular Pressure

Red blood cells (RBCs) can migrate from the posterior segment into the anterior chamber. These may lead to the development of a characteristic grey-greenish colored hyphema (the so-called "khaki hypoyon"). As the RBCs subsequently degenerate, they may block the trabecular meshwork causing increased intraocular pressure (IOP) and secondary open angle glaucoma (ghost cell glaucoma).

Pearls on How to Prevent It

Suggested ways to reduce the risk of SMH during RD surgery include the following.

During Scleral Buckling

- Avoid drainage choroidotomy in the following locations.

  - Anterior to the equator at 3- and 9-o'clock positions (to avoid injury of the long ciliary arteries).

  - Near the vortex veins, for example, next to the oblique muscle insertions. Because of the variable positions and numbers of vortices, careful inspection of the sclera before indentation or placement of the sutures to identify their locations will minimize the risk of their damage.

  - In areas where cryotherapy had been performed.

- Whenever possible, drain in the nasal quadrants. If bleeding occurs, this will reduce the risk of the blood seeping under the macula.

- Consider using diathermy or laser to obliterate the choroidal vessels at the drainage site. Using low-power diathermy to render the drainage area avascular

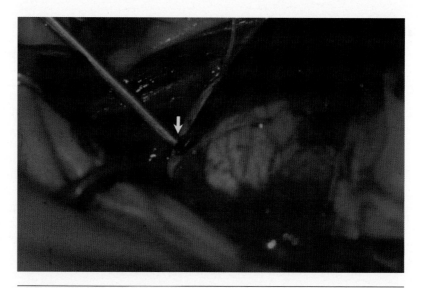

Figure 26A-6 Laser choroidotomy using intraocular laser probe for draining of subretinal fluid during a scleral buckling procedure. (Courtesy of Mr. Bill Aylward.)

before applying high power to vaporize the choroid (choroidotomy) was shown to reduce the risk of hemorrhage.[10] Choroidotomy can also be performed using either the indirect laser delivery or an intraocular laser probe **(Fig. 26A-6)** and this was found to reduce the risk of subretinal hemorrhage.[11,12]

◆ Consider the so-called "controlled drainage" of SRF. This technique involves using a 30G needle attached to either a 1-mL syringe without the plunger or to an extrusion line while visualizing its tip and the drainage site with the indirect ophthalmoscope. This technique was also shown to reduce the risk of subretinal hemorrhage.13

◆ Maintain adequate control of IOP during drainage of SRF. This can be achieved by applying external pressure to the sclera with cotton-tipped applicators or by tightening a preplaced encircling band.[14]

During Vitrectomy

◆ Ensure that adequate diathermy has been applied to retinal vessels prior to their transection, for example, to vessels bridging retinal tears or along the edge of a planned retinectomy.

◆ Place retinotomy or retinectomy as anteriorly as possible.

◆ Decompress retinal bullae before trimming the retinal tears or performing retinectomy by performing "fluid–fluid exchange" (drain subretinal fluid with a back-flush cannula through a pre-existing tear while under fluid to reduce the height of an RD). This will reduce the potential subretinal space and thus the amount of blood settling under the macula should bleeding occur.

◆ Maintain adequate IOP control by plugging the sclerotomy ports or by using valved ports when using smaller (e.g., 23G) cannulae to avoid a sudden reduction of IOP when the instruments are withdrawn from an air-filled eye.

In Degenerative Retinal Conditions

In patients with choroidal neovascular membrane (CNVM) of ARMD, adequate and timely pretreatment with antivascular endothelial growth factor drugs may reduce the risk of SMH.

NATURAL HISTORY

Table 26A-1 summarizes published observational and natural history studies of the outcome of SMH after RD surgery as well as in degenerative conditions. Although in the large majority of patients subretinal hemorrhage absorbs within 3 to 6 months, it may take up to 2 years in some patients with ARMD. It is likely that in patients with RD whose RPE cells and subretinal tissues are healthier, submacular blood will absorb more speedily.

Table 26A-1 • Observational and Natural History Studies of Submacular Hemorrhage

Study	No.	Cause of SMH	Mean Follow-up (Range)	Mean Time to Clearance (Range)	Visual Outcome and Predictors
Bennett et al. (1990)[15] Included subretinal hemorrhage of ≥1 DD Large hemorrhage ≥4 DD Thick hemorrhage: With elevation	29	*ARMD* = 12 *Non-ARMD* = 17 Trauma = 7 POHS = 3 RAMA = 4 Pseudoxanthoma elasticum = 1 Scleral buckle = 1	*ARMD* 37.7 (9–108 months) *Non-ARMD* 35.8 (6–144 months)	NA	*ARMD* VA ≥ 20/400: 25% Improved: 33.3% Same: 33.3% Worse: 33.3% *Non-ARMD* VA ≥ 20/70: 47% Improved: 64.7% Same: 11.8% Worse: 23.5% *Poor VA associated with:* ARMD and thick SMH (size of SMH did not affect VA)
Hayasaka et al. (1990)[17]	24	*Pathologic myopia* (≥8 D) CNVM = 9 *Non-CNVM* = 15	*CNVM* 24 (12–48 months) *Non-CNVM* 10 (4–72 months)	*CNVM* Hemorrhage organized or recurred *Non-CNVM* Within 3 months	*CNVM* Improved: 0% Same: 44.4% Worse: 55.6% *Non-CNVM* Improved: 66.7% Same: 33.3% *Poor VA associated with:* CNVM
Avery et al. (1996)[24]	41	*ARMD*	27 (3–36 months)	NA	*VA at 3 and 6 months* 20/25–20/40: 10% and 13% Mean change in VA: 0.8 and 3.5 lines loss. ≥3 lines increase 13% and 20% <3 lines change 57% and 7% ≥ 3 lines loss 30% and 74% *Poor VA associated with:* Larger size of SMH

(continued)

Table 26A-1 • Observational and Natural History Studies of Submacular Hemorrhage (*continued*)

Study	No.	Cause of SMH	Mean Follow-up (Range)	Mean Time to Clearance (Range)	Visual Outcome and Predictors
Berrocal et al. (1996)[16] Size of SMH: Small < 400 μm Medium 400 μm–2 DD Large > 2 DD Thick hemorrhage, that is, with elevation	31	*ARMD = 20*	*ARMD* 29 (3–36 months)	*ARMD* 8 (3–24 months)	*ARMD* *VA* ≥20/40: 15% ≥20/80: 30% Improved ≥ 2 lines: 40% No change: 30% Worse: 30%
		Non-ARMD = 11 Valsalva retinopathy = 1 Trauma = 1 RAMA = 2 Diabetic retinopathy = 2 CSCR = 1 CRVO=1 Choroidal rupture = 1	Non-ARMD 8 (2–24 months)	Non-ARMD 5 (2–11 months)	*Non-ARMD* *VA* ≥20/40: 45% ≥20/80: 55% Improved ≥ 2 lines: 45% Same: 27.5% Worse: 27.5% *Poor VA associated with:* Subfoveal CNVM (thickness and size did not affect VA)
Scupola et al. (1999)[25]	60	*ARMD*	24 (3–55 months)	6 (2–18 months)	*VA* Worse: 80% *Poor VA associated with:* Larger size and increased thickness of lesion
McCabe et al. (2000)[26]	41	*RAMA*	15.7 (2–87 months)	4.6 (1–14 months)	*VA* ≥20/40: 37% 20/50–20/100: 29% ≤20/400: 34% Improved ≥ 3 lines: 85.4% Same: 2.4% Worse: 0% *Poor VA associated with:* Macular pigment changes after clearance of SMH.
Submacular surgery trial, report no. 11; 2004 (Observation arm)[55]	228	*ARMD*	36 months	Lesion size at 36 months: Smaller or unchanged: 22% Larger: 78%	*VA at 36 months* ≥20/40: 13% 20/50–20/160: 30% 20/200–20/640: 48% Improved ≥2 lines: 20% Unchanged: 27% Worse: 53%

No., number of eyes; DD, disc diameter; ARMD, age-related macular degeneration; POHS, presumed ocular histoplasmosis syndrome; RAMA, retinal artery macroaneurysm; SMH, submacular hemorrhage; CNVM, choroidal neovascular membrane; CSCR, central serous chorioretinopathy; CRVO, central retinal vein occlusion; NA, not available.

Visual Outcome

The determinants of visual outcome in SMH include the following (Table 2).

The cause of hemorrhage. This seems to be the most important predictor of visual outcome. Particularly poor visual outcome has been reported in patients with degenerative conditions, such as CNVM.[15–17]

The duration of hemorrhage. As discussed above, the degree of retinal damage due to subretinal blood is time-dependent. Better final visual acuity was described in patients with SMH of less than 7 to 30 days' duration.[18–22] However, some authors also reported relatively good visual outcome in patients with SMH of longer duration, especially in those with otherwise healthy maculae.[16,17,23]

The extent of hemorrhage. The effect of the size of the total area covered by the SMH on visual outcome varies between different studies, with some reporting larger areas of SMH to be associated with worse outcome[24,25] whereas others reporting no such effect.[15,16]

The thickness of the hemorrhage as observed by ophthalmoscopy or on stereo-fundus images also seems to be predictive of poor visual prognosis.[15,25]

RPE changes. Even when SMH eventually absorbs, the underlying RPE often undergoes atrophy with hypo- or hyperpigmentation, and these signs are often associated with poor visual outcome.[26]

Recurrence of RD

Subretinal hemorrhage, especially if associated with blood in the vitreous cavity, may increase the risk of a recurrence of the RD due to the development of PVR and subretinal fibrosis.[9,27]

⬥ Pearls on How to Treat It

To date, no randomized clinical trial has been conducted to compare the different methods of management of SMH after RD surgery. Thus our recommendations for the management will rely on the evidence derived from our own clinical experience as well as from case series and controlled studies of surgical interventions for the treatment of SMH in RD and other conditions, mainly ARMD, RAMA, and trauma.

Intraoperative Management

During Scleral Buckling

◆ Immediate increase of IOP by applying pressure on the sclera (e.g., with a cotton wool bud) or by pulling on the muscle traction sutures.

◆ Deliberate incomplete drainage of the subretinal fluid combined with appropriate postoperative posturing may encourage the gravitation of the blood away from the macula.

During Vitrectomy

◆ Increasing the bottle height (≥40 cm) or air pump pressure (≥50 mm Hg) for 5 minutes to raise the IOP will minimize bleeding from the retinal vessels. If the bleeding restarts after normalization of the IOP, endodiathermy may be applied to coagulate the bleeding vessels.

◆ Immediate aspiration of the subretinal fluid and blood with the back-flush cannula or the extrusion line may minimize the volume of blood that might otherwise settle under the macula.

◆ If a blood clot is observed during the fluid–air exchange stage, reinfusing the eye with fluid will allow the retina to redetach and to displace or float up the blood clot, thus facilitating its removal, perhaps through the original retinal tear.

Postoperative Management

SMH observed toward the end of the surgery (scleral buckling or vitrectomy) or in the immediate postoperative period can be managed as follows.

Observation

Extramacular subretinal hemorrhage or a thin SMH may be left alone as neither is likely to cause a significant visual loss. Patients with SMH greater than 4 disc diameters (DD) have been found to have worse visual outcome.[15,26]

Surgical intervention

This includes either pneumatic displacement (PD), surgical drainage of SMH or extraction of the blood clots. These techniques can be used in combination with recombinant tissue plasminogen activator (tPA), a thrombolytic agent, to facilitate the liquefaction of the clotted blood.

◆ *Indications.* Surgical intervention may be considered if SMH is associated with high macular elevation and severe reduction in visual acuity (e.g., ≥3 lines).

◆ *Timing of surgery.* There is no clear indication from natural history or interventional studies to the optimum time for surgery in patients with SMH following complicated RD procedures.

◆ *Outcome.* Most of the evidence is derived from studies of patients with CNVM, RAMA, or traumatic RD.

Improvement in visual acuity has been reported in patients who developed SMH during scleral buckling procedures when surgical drainage of SMH was carried out within 1 hour to 30 days.[20,21,28] On the other hand, good visual outcome has also been reported in patients with SMH of longer duration.[16,17,22,23,29] However, surgical removal of clotted blood can be technically difficult or results in incomplete removal, even with the use of tPA,[8,30] and therefore, some authors have recommended delaying treatment by 3 to 7 days in order to allow the blood to liquefy.[31]

Surgical Intervention

Pneumatic Displacement

◆ *Technique.* PD may be performed in an outpatient setting, using 0.3 to 0.4 mL of an expansile gas [100% of sulfur hexafluoride (SF_6) or perfluoropropane (C_3F_8)]. After the injection, patients are advised to maintain partial prone posturing (40 to 60 degrees) during the day and temporal side dependent at night.[32]

◆ *Outcome.* Several case series have shown that partial (>50%) or complete displacement of the blood and improvement in visual acuity (≥2 lines or visual acuity ≥20/200) occurs in the large majority of patients.[32–34]

◆ *Complications.* Some of the reported complications with PD include incomplete displacement of the blood, vitreous hemorrhage, retinal tears, and RD.[31,33,34]

Intravitreal Injection of tPA and PD

◆ *tPA.* This is a thrombolytic agent that activates plasminogen into plasmin.[35,36] Several studies have recently reported its use in the treatment of SMH in combination with PD.[37–43]

◆ *Dose.* 18 to 100 μg in 0.1 to 0.2 mL is injected in the midvitreous cavity using a 25G or 30G needle followed by supine posturing for a few hours before PD is performed.

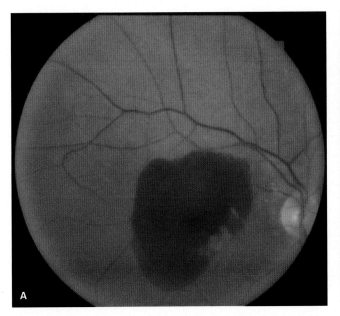
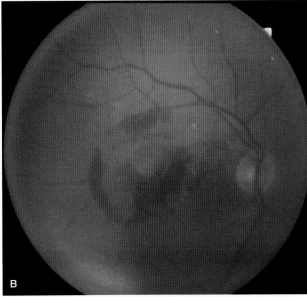

Figure 26A-7 Subretinal hemorrhage before **(A)** and after **(B)** TPA and intraocular gas injection in a patient who had submacular hemorrhage due to neovascular age-related macular degeneration. (Courtesy of Dr. John A. Wells, III.)

◆ *Outcome of tPA and PD* (**Fig. 26A-7**).[19,37,39,40,42–46] Partial or complete displacement of the blood clots has been reported to occur in 52% to 100% and visual improvement in 15% to 100% of patients. In a comparative study, the addition of tPA was a positive predictor of visual improvement of 2 or more lines after PD.[19]

◆ *Complications.* The reported complications with the use of tPA and PD include recurrent subretinal and vitreous hemorrhages, exudative RD, RPE hyperpigmentation, and endophthalmitis.[31,40,47]

Surgical Drainage

◆ *Indications.* Conversion to pars plana vitrectomy and drainage through a posterior retinotomy have been described in patients with large subretinal hemorrhage complicating scleral buckling procedures.[28,48] Indications for surgical removal of extensive subretinal or submacular hemorrhage include hemorrhagic elevation of retinal breaks, and bullous hemorrhagic RD.[8]

◆ *Timing of surgery.* While it is tempting to remove a submacular blood clot immediately, it is often technically difficult and can result in further macular trauma as well as incomplete removal of SMH.[28] Surgery performed a few days after the onset of the hemorrhage (perhaps 7 to 14 days later) when the SMH has sufficiently liquefied may reduce the risk of further damage to the photoreceptors and RPE cells.

◆ *Technique.* One or more large (up to 1 mm) posterior retinotomies are fashioned to remove the blood with an extrusion cannula or submacular forceps followed by intraocular tamponade of either air, nonexpansile concentration of SF_6, C_3F_8, or silicone oil.[8,28,48]

◆ *Outcome.* Table 26A-2 summarizes the studies of surgical drainage of SMH in RD and ARMD patients. It clearly shows that the large majority of patients experienced 2 or more lines of visual improvement.

Table 26A-2 • Outcome of the Surgical Drainage of Submacular Hemorrhage

Study and Design	No.	Causes of SMH	Follow-up Mean (Range)	Surgical Intervention	Anatomical Outcome	Final Visual Outcome
Wade et al. (1990)[45]	14	*Group 1* RRD = 3 Scleral buckling complications = 3 traumatic RD = 1 Perforating injury = 1 Sickle cell retinopathy = 1 *Group 2* ARMD = 5	*Group 1:* 17 (6–36 months) *Group 2:* 6 (2–12 months)	Vitrectomy and internal drainage	*Group 1* Recurrent RD: 55.6% Final reattachment: 88.9% *Group 2* Subretinal fibrosis: 40%	*Group 1* ≥20/400: 8 Improved ≥3 lines: 8 Unchanged: 0 Worse: 1 *Group 2* ≤5/200: 5 Improved ≥3 lines: 3 Unchanged: 1 Worse: 1
Han et al. (1990)[8]	19	*Traumatic hemorrhagic RD* (1) Hemorrhagic elevation of retinal break (*n* = 9) (2) Massive hemorrhagic RD (nonmobile) (*n* = 4) (3) Bullous hemorrhagic RD (*n* = 3) (4) Extramacular subretinal hemorrhage (*n* = 3)	11.2 (6–27 months)	Vitrectomy, internal drainage of subretinal hemorrhage with 20G–24G extrusion cannula or forceps	Reattachment: 68% PVR: 21.1% Globe atrophy: 10.5%	*VA* ≥5/200 (authors defined functional success) Group (1): 33% Group (2): 25% Group (3): 0% Group (4): 67% ≥2 lines (Groups 1–3) Improved: 31.3%/ Unchanged: 56.3% Worse: 6.3%

SMH, submacular hemorrhage; ARMD, age-related macular degeneration; PVR; proliferative vitreoretinopathy.

Submacular tPA Before Surgical Drainage

An injection of tPA into the submacular blood clot can be used to aid its liquefaction and thus minimizing the damage to the photoreceptors and RPE cells in the process.[20,30,49–52]

◆ *Technique.* About 10 to 125 μg of tPA may be injected into the subretinal blood clot through a posterior retinotomy. Ten to forty minutes later, the blood is aspirated using either an irrigation–aspiration cannula or a 30G subretinal cannula attached to the flute cannula or an extrusion line. Reinjection at 10 µg increments of tPA can be done if necessary. Perfluorocarbon liquid "heavy liquid" can help to express the liquefied blood through the retinotomy.[20] Leaving a small amount of subretinal fluid and postoperative posturing may allow any residual submacular blood to displace inferiorly by intraocular air or gas bubble during the postoperative period.

◆ *Outcome.* Although subretinal tPA has been reported to facilitate the removal of SMH in many patients,[49] some reports showed that the clot lysis was variable.[30,53] Improvement in visual acuity also varies between different studies.[30,49]

◆ *Complications.* Complications of surgical drainage of submacular blood include PVR, recurrent RD, macular pucker, vitreous hemorrhage, recurrence of SMH, and in patients with ARMD, submacular fibrosis, and RPE tear.[20,30,49–51]

✛ Management of SMH Associated with Suprachoroidal Hemorrhage

During Scleral Buckling

◆ Increase the IOP either by scleral compression with cotton-tipped applicators or pulling on the muscle traction sutures (see also Chapters 27C and 31).

◆ Once the bleeding has stopped, reform the globe with fluid, air, or an expansile gas bubble in the unlikely event of persistent hypotony.

During Vitrectomy

◆ Increase the IOP either by raising the bottle height or changing the pump pressure settings to 50 or 60 mm Hg and wait for 5 to 10 minutes to allow the blood to coagulate and the bleeding to stop. Check the position of the infusion cannula to ensure that it has not become covered by suprachoroidal hemorrhage. If this appears to be the case, maintain a high infusion pressure via a handheld angled needle inserted into the center of the vitreous cavity through one of the superior sclerotomies.

Postoperatively

◆ If there is only minimal SMH, observation is the best strategy as both suprachoroidal and subretinal blood usually resolve spontaneously.

◆ Drainage of persistent or extensive suprachoroidal hemorrhage (appositional or "kissing suprachoroidal hemorrhage") may be performed 7 to 10 days after its occurrence.[1,54] This time will allow liquefaction of the blood clot to occur. Preoperative ultrasound examination may reveal the degree of clot liquefaction as well as the optimal site of the drainage sclerotomy. The liquefied blood will easily drain either through one or more of the sclerotomy ports, if the patient requires vitrectomy, or via a separate drainage sclerotomy made at the highest point of the hemorrhage while infusing the eye either through the pars plana or the limbus.

◆ Use of perfluorocarbon liquid may help anterior displacement and removal of the suprachoroidal blood.

◆ Intraocular tamponade using either long-acting gas or silicone oil is usually employed at the conclusion of the procedure.

REFERENCES

1. Tabandeh H, Flynn HW Jr. Suprachoroidal hemorrhage during pars plana vitrectomy. *Curr Opin Ophthalmol.* 2001;12(3):179–185.
2. Glatt H, Machemer R. Experimental subretinal hemorrhage in rabbits. *Am J Ophthalmol.* 1982;94(6):762–773.
3. Toth CA, Morse LS, Hjelmeland LM, et al. Fibrin directs early retinal damage after experimental subretinal hemorrhage. *Arch Ophthalmol.* 1991;109(5):723–739.
4. Hochman MA, Seery CM, Zarbin MA. Pathophysiology and management of subretinal hemorrhage. *Surv Ophthalmol.* 1997;42(3):195–213.
5. Johnson MW, Olsen KR, Hernandez E. Tissue plasminogen activator treatment of experimental subretinal hemorrhage. *Retina.* 1991;11(2):250–258.
6. Sanders D, Peyman GA, Fishman G, et al. The toxicity of intravitreal whole blood and hemoglobin. *Albrecht Von Graefes Arch Klin Exp Ophthalmol.* 1975;197(3):255–267.
7. Campochiaro PA, Jerdan JA, Glaser BM. Serum contains chemoattractants for human retinal pigment epithelial cells. *Arch Ophthalmol.* 1984;102(12):1830–1833.
8. Han DP, Mieler WF, Schwartz DM, et al. Management of traumatic hemorrhagic retinal detachment with pars plana vitrectomy. *Arch Ophthalmol.* 1990;108(9):1281–1286.
9. Nagasaki H, Shinagawa K. Risk factors for proliferative vitreoretinopathy. *Curr Opin Ophthalmol.* 1995;6(3):70–75.
10. Saran BR, Brucker AJ, Maguire AM. Drainage of subretinal fluid in retinal detachment surgery with the El-Mofty insulated diathermy electrode. *Retina.* 1994;14(4):344–347.
11. Aylward GW, Orr G, Schwartz SD, et al. Prospective, randomised, controlled trial comparing suture needle drainage and argon laser drainage of subretinal fluid. *Br J Ophthalmol.* 1995;79(8):724–727.
12. Pitts JF, Schwartz SD, Wells J, et al. Indirect argon laser drainage of subretinal fluid. *Eye (Lond).* 1996;10(pt 4):465–468.
13. Charles ST. Controlled drainage of subretinal and choroidal fluid. *Retina.* 1985;5(4):233–234.
14. Jaffe GJ, Brownlow R, Hines J. Modified external needle drainage procedure for rhegmatogenous retinal detachment. *Retina.* 2003;23(1):80–85.
15. Bennett SR, Folk JC, Blodi CF, et al. Factors prognostic of visual outcome in patients with subretinal hemorrhage. *Am J Ophthalmol.* 1990;109(1):33–37.
16. Berrocal MH, Lewis ML, Flynn HW Jr. Variations in the clinical course of submacular hemorrhage. *Am J Ophthalmol.* 1996;122(4):486–493.
17. Hayasaka S, Uchida M, Setogawa T. Subretinal hemorrhages with or without choroidal neovascularization in the maculas of patients with pathologic myopia. *Graefes Arch Clin Exp Ophthalmol.* 1990;228(4):277–280.
18. Vander JF, Federman JL, Greven C, et al. Surgical removal of massive subretinal hemorrhage associated with age-related macular degeneration. *Ophthalmology.* 1991;98(1):23–27.
19. Fang IM, Lin YC, Yang CH, et al. Effects of intravitreal gas with or without tissue plasminogen activator on submacular hemorrhage in age-related macular degeneration. *Eye (Lond).* 2009;23(2):397–406.
20. Kamei M, Tano Y, Maeno T, et al. Surgical removal of submacular hemorrhage using tissue plasminogen activator and perfluorocarbon liquid. *Am J Ophthalmol.* 1996;121(3):267–275.
21. Lewis H. Intraoperative fibrinolysis of submacular hemorrhage with tissue plasminogen activator and surgical drainage. *Am J Ophthalmol.* 1994;118(5):559–568.
22. Gillies A, Lahav M. Absorption of retinal and subretinal hemorrhages. *Ann Ophthalmol.* 1983;15(11):1068–1074.
23. Dellaporta A. Retinal damage from subretinal hemorrhage. *Am J Ophthalmol.* 1983;95(4):568–570.
24. Avery RL, Fekrat S, Hawkins BS, et al. Natural history of subfoveal subretinal hemorrhage in age-related macular degeneration. *Retina.* 1996;16(3):183–189.
25. Scupola A, Coscas G, Soubrane G, et al. Natural history of macular subretinal hemorrhage in age-related macular degeneration. *Ophthalmologica.* 1999;213(2):97–102.

26. McCabe CM, Flynn HW Jr, McLean WC, et al. Nonsurgical management of macular hemorrhage secondary to retinal artery macroaneurysms. *Arch Ophthalmol.* 2000;118(6):780–785.

27. Pastor JC. Proliferative vitreoretinopathy: An overview. *Surv Ophthalmol.* 1998;43(1):3–18.

28. Rubsamen PE, Flynn HW, Jr, Civantos JM, et al. Treatment of massive subretinal hemorrhage from complications of scleral buckling procedures. *Am J Ophthalmol.* 1994;118(3):299–303.

29. Claes C, Zivojnovic R. Subretinal hemorrhage removal. *Bull Soc Belge Ophtalmol.* 1993;250:85–88.

30. Ibanez HE, Williams DF, Thomas MA, et al. Surgical management of submacular hemorrhage. A series of 47 consecutive cases. *Arch Ophthalmol.* 1995;113(1):62–69.

31. Johnson MW. Pneumatic displacement of submacular hemorrhage. *Curr Opin Ophthalmol.* 2000;11(3):201–206.

32. Lincoff H, Kreissig I, Stopa M, et al. A 40 degrees gaze down position for pneumatic displacement of submacular hemorrhage: Clinical application and results. *Retina.* 2008;28(1):56–59.

33. Ohji M, Saito Y, Hayashi A, et al. Pneumatic displacement of subretinal hemorrhage without tissue plasminogen activator. *Arch Ophthalmol.* 1998;116(10):1326–1332.

34. Gopalakrishan M, Giridhar A, Bhat S, et al. Pneumatic displacement of submacular hemorrhage: Safety, efficacy, and patient selection. *Retina.* 2007;27(3):329–334.

35. Ranby M, Bergsdorf N, Nilsson T. Enzymatic properties of the one- and two-chain form of tissue plasminogen activator. *Thromb Res.* 1982;27(2):175–183.

36. Verstraete M, Collen D. Pharmacology of thrombolytic drugs. *J Am Coll Cardiol.* 1986;8(6 suppl B):33B–40B.

37. Mizutani T, Yasukawa T, Ito Y, et al. Pneumatic displacement of submacular hemorrhage with or without tissue plasminogen activator. *Graefes Arch Clin Exp Ophthalmol.* 2011;249(8):1153–1157.

38. Chen SN, Ho CL, Kuo YH, et al. Intravitreous tissue plasminogen activator injection and pneumatic displacement in the management of submacular hemorrhage complicating scleral buckling procedures. *Retina.* 2001;21(5):460–463.

39. Handwerger BA, Blodi BA, Chandra SR, et al. Treatment of submacular hemorrhage with low-dose intravitreal tissue plasminogen activator injection and pneumatic displacement. *Arch Ophthalmol.* 2001;119(1):28–32.

40. Hassan AS, Johnson MW, Schneiderman TE, et al. Management of submacular hemorrhage with intravitreous tissue plasminogen activator injection and pneumatic displacement. *Ophthalmology.* 1999;106(10):1900–1906;discussion 1906–1907.

41. Yang PM, Kuo HK, Kao ML, et al. Pneumatic displacement of a dense submacular hemorrhage with or without tissue plasminogen activator. *Chang Gung Med J.* 2005;28(12):852–859.

42. Hattenbach LO, Klais C, Koch FH, et al. Intravitreous injection of tissue plasminogen activator and gas in the treatment of submacular hemorrhage under various conditions. *Ophthalmology.* 2001;108(8):1485–1492.

43. Hesse L, Schmidt J, Kroll P. Management of acute submacular hemorrhage using recombinant tissue plasminogen activator and gas. *Graefes Arch Clin Exp Ophthalmol.* 1999;237(4):273–277.

44. Hesse L, Schroeder B, Heller G, et al. Quantitative effect of intravitreally injected tissue plasminogen activator and gas on subretinal hemorrhage. *Retina.* 2000;20(5):500–505.

45. Chen CY, Hooper C, Chiu D, et al. Management of submacular hemorrhage with intravitreal injection of tissue plasminogen activator and expansile gas. *Retina.* 2007;27(3):321–328.

46. Tsai SC, Lin JM, Chen HY. Intravitreous recombinant tissue plasminogen activator and gas to treat submacular hemorrhage in age-related macular degeneration. *Kaohsiung J Med Sci.* 2003;19(12):608–616.

47. Vote BJ, Buttery R, Polkinghorne PJ. Endophthalmitis after intravitreal injection of frozen preprepared tissue plasminogen activator (tPA) for pneumatic displacement of submacular hemorrhage. *Retina.* 2004;24(5):808–809.

48. Wade EC, Flynn HW Jr, Olsen KR, et al. Subretinal hemorrhage management by pars plana vitrectomy and internal drainage. *Arch Ophthalmol.* 1990;108(7): 973–978.

49. Hillenkamp J, Surguch V, Framme C, et al. Management of submacular hemorrhage with intravitreal versus subretinal injection of recombinant tissue plasminogen activator. *Graefes Arch Clin Exp Ophthalmol.* 2010;248(1):5–11.

50. Olivier S, Chow DR, Packo KH, et al. Subretinal recombinant tissue plasminogen activator injection and pneumatic displacement of thick submacular hemorrhage in age-related macular degeneration. *Ophthalmology.* 2004;111(6):1201–1208.

51. Humayun M, Lewis H, Flynn HW Jr, et al. Management of submacular hemorrhage associated with retinal arterial macroaneurysms. *Am J Ophthalmol.* 1998;126(3): 358–361.

52. Peyman GA, Nelson NC Jr, Alturki W et al. Tissue plasminogen activating factor assisted removal of subretinal hemorrhage. *Ophthalmic Surg.* 1991;22(10):575–582.

53. Hesse L, Meitinger D, Schmidt J. Little effect of tissue plasminogen activator in subretinal surgery for acute hemorrhage in age-related macular degeneration. *Ger J Ophthalmol.* 1996;5(6):479–483.

54. Chu TG, Green RL. Suprachoroidal hemorrhage. *Surv Ophthalmol.* 1999;43(6):471–486.

55. Hawkins BS, Bressler NM, Miskala PH, et al. Submacular surgery trial group. Surgery for Subfoveal Choroidal Neovascularization in Age-Related Macular Degeneration: Ophthalmic Findings. SST Report No. 11. *Ophthalmology.* 2004;111(11):1967–1980.

26B Bleeding During Pars Plana Vitrectomy

MILTON NUNES DE MORAES-FILHO, J. FERNANDO AREVALO, ANDRE MAIA, AND MAURICIO MAIA

✥ The Complication: Definition

Intraoperative bleeding during pars plana vitrectomy (PPV) is a challenge for the surgeon and has been a matter of debate regarding techniques for controlling these hemorrhages. Massive intraoperative bleeding is correlated to histologic damage due to high degree of hemosiderin deposit into retina.[1] High volumes of blood clot retraction can produce tractional retinal detachment (TRD), retinal holes, and subretinal accumulation of blood.[2]

Bleeding during the surgical procedure may impair the view of the surgical field, thus yielding poor postoperative results including low vision, proliferative vitreoretinopathy (PVR), and secondary retinal detachment. Prevention as well as the correct management of intraoperative bleeding is important to achieve good surgical results. A meticulous surgical technique is essential to prevent intraocular hemorrhage; however, when bleeding occurs it must be promptly controlled. This chapter will discuss causes, management, and prevention of intraoperative bleeding during PPV.

✥ Risk Factors and Causes

Intraoperative hemorrhage may occur either in the anterior or posterior segment and vitreoretinal surgeons must be aware regarding the following causes.

Intraoperative Anterior Segment Bleeding

Iris Hemorrhage

Iris and/or ciliary body (CB) touch during vitrectomy or iris manipulation by instruments during cataract surgery in phacoemulsification associated to vitrectomy may be followed by bleeding in the anterior chamber (AC). Turbidity of AC may impair the intraoperative visualization of intraocular microstructures such as epiretinal and internal limiting membranes (ILMs); this may lead to difficulties performing specific surgical maneuvers. In addition, microscopic hyphema can also occur as a result of hypotony. The bleeding leaves a fine film of red blood cells deposited on the anterior surface of the lens, which can impair the view of the posterior segment.

A good pharmacologic dilation, iris hooks, and other techniques to maintain iris dilation might prevent tissue touch and consequent bleeding. Viscoelastic agents may decrease dispersion of blood and concentrate coagulation factors at the site of bleeding in order to achieve good hemostasis. Injection of viscoelastic in the AC also increases the intraocular pressure (IOP) and stops bleeding from rubeotic iris blood vessels due to many causes.

Care must be taken when performing peripheral inferior iridectomy (PII) in aphakic eyes when silicone oil injection is intended. Intense bleeding may appear from minor and major arterial circles. In cases of intense dilation, miosis using AC carbachol injection before undertaking PII may help the procedure and avoid arterial circles. Particularly, when PII is performed just before perfluorocarbon liquid (PFCL) removal (e.g., during giant retinal tear management), bleeding may occur. In the majority of cases, it would be advisable to wait until complete spontaneous hemostasis after PII has occurred before injecting silicone oil. In some cases, intense bleeding may occur that can be controlled by IOP rising or AC viscoelastic injection.

If PII is not made (or forgotten) before silicone oil injection one needs to be performed at the end of the surgery. If iris bleeding occurs under these circumstances (PII after silicone oil injection), air injection in the AC may be used after silicone oil injection in order to decrease the blood flow and minimize the possibility of bleeding. This maneuver is also important in order to decrease the possibility of silicone oil migrating into the AC and the consequences of oil migration such as corneal endothelial touch.

Conjunctival and Episcleral Bleeding

Large sclerotomies may create enough space for the penetration of blood from episcleral vessels and conjunctiva into the vitreous cavity. A slight and adequate cauterization of localized vessels should be done before making sclerotomies during 20G PPV. However, excessive episcleral cauterization may induce postoperative scleral ectasia, which may lead to subsequent choroidal prolapse.

At the end of PPV procedure, 23G or 25G trocar removal may yield blood inflow from the sclerotomy sites into the vitreous cavity. Careful wound construction with tunneled sclerotomies and/or adequate sclerotomy sutures at the end of the surgical procedure might prevent a blood pathway into the vitreous cavity, minimizing the possibility of postoperative vitreous bleeding.

Intraoperative Posterior Segment Bleeding

Vitreoretinal Bleeding

Vitreous hemorrhage may occur during dissection, segmentation, and delamination of fibrovascular membranes from proliferative diabetic retinopathy (PDR). Focal fibrovascular adhesions have less chance of persistent bleeding as compared to plaques. Bleeding may be controlled using many techniques such as: Raising the IOP, endodiathermy, PFCL, and fluid–air exchange. In addition, a back-flush needle can be used to clear the blood away to get a better view and to discover the bleeding site.

Unimanual bipolar diathermy is routinely applied to sites of persistent bleeding other than the optic nerve. Avoiding delamination of highly vascularized membranes and ensuring that the patient's blood pressure (BP) is normal can reduce the incidence of hemorrhage. Elevation of IOP is used to minimize bleeding during the dissection of vascularized tissue. Particularly, raising IOP for 1 to 2 minutes will frequently stop persistent bleeding in patients with normal values of BP (see later for details).

Any blood on the retina should be removed immediately, before clot formation. Clotted blood should be cautiously stripped from the retina, as it may be tightly adhered. In some instances, scissors, forceps, or vitrectomy tip may be necessary to excise a clot. The anticoagulant heparin sodium into the infusion bottle (10 U/mL) just before dissecting diabetic fibrovascular membranes was used by[3] a fast blood aspiration with a back-flush tip and endodiathermy at bleeding points was performed in order to prevent clot formation; after that, the infusion bottle was replaced with physiologic saline solution with no heparin. Although only a few cases of postoperative vitreous hemorrhage were observed, it is not a currently widely used surgical technique.

Recently, reduction in the intraoperative bleeding was shown by intravitreal injection of anti-vascular endothelial growth factor (VEGF) (ranibizumab or bevacizumab) 3 to 5 days before vitrectomy (see section later) and this is especially performed routinely preoperatively in vitreoretinal surgery for PDR.

Adequate preoperative BP control as well as a normal systemic blood coagulation status are also very important measures to avoid intraoperative bleeding during vitreoretinal surgeries as various indications[4] showed that intraoperative systolic hypertension more than 180 mm Hg had high risk of suprachoroidal hemorrhage. In addition, the use of epinephrine into the infusion bottle may be a helpful maneuver, in cases of well-controlled systemic BP. However, it is not currently used in vitreoretinal surgery worldwide.

The choice of irrigating solution for infusion may have an influence in the bleeding time. Some commercially available solutions have citric acid that has an anticoagulant effect (e.g., balanced saline solution, BSS, Alcon labs, Fort Worth, TX, USA). When intraoperative hemorrhage is expected, solutions without citric acid must be used (e.g., BSS Plus).[5]

Blood in the vitreous cavity may also occur during dissection of PVR starfold membranes. Care must be taken when performing peeling close to major vessels or near to the optic disk. Large vein rupture may cause intense bleeding at the posterior pole, followed by difficulty to remove big clots, mainly in the macula region that may aggravate low vision and PVR during postoperative period.

Some vitrectomy systems have a back-flush option that is also delivered through the vitrectomy probe. It is an important surgical maneuver to remove blood from the fovea. In this technique, a reverse flow from the vitreous probe (reflux) is achieved. The clot is "washed" nicely from the posterior pole using the indirect mechanical flow of balanced salt solution (BSS). (Video 26B-1 shows removal of the blood from the macula using the back-flush technique in order to avoid direct touch over the fovea.)

Some surgeons do prefer to perform a posterior retinotomy at the nasal retina in order to drain subretinal fluid during fluid–air exchange for rhegmatogenous retinal detachment (RD). An adequate retinotomy away from large vessels, endodiathermy of microvessels, and deviation of vitrectomy aperture from large vessels may preclude bleeding either into the vitreous cavity or into the subretinal space. However, the formation of a subretinal clot may be disastrous to the postoperative visual and anatomic prognosis, such as PVR formation and retinal redetachment. Slow and careful aspiration of blood with or without further rising of IOP may prevent its subretinal migration and the size of the clot. After controlling the hemorrhagic process, mechanical removal of blood may be difficult using only one retinotomy site. Particularly, retinectomy and subretinal blood wash out with tissue plasminogen activator (tPA) and aspiration may dissolve and facilitate clot removal, although the toxic dose of intravitreal commercial tPA has not been well established. Severe atrophy of outer retina is reported[6] and may occur in rare cases using 50 μg/0.1 mL.[7] Usually concentrations between 12.5 and 25 μg/0.1 mL in sterile water are employed for submacular hemorrhage due to choroidal neovascularization.[8,9]

Intraoperative control of hemorrhage in penetrating ocular injuries may be a challenge to the surgeon. Some techniques (such as IOP rising, fluid–air exchange, endodiathermy, endophotocoagulation) must be known to be part of the surgical arsenal to avoid such complication.[10,11] The addition of thrombin to the infusion solution may be another alternative; however, it is not a widely utilized procedure during vitreoretinal surgery. Thrombin is a potent agent in platelet aggregation and also converts soluble plasmatic fibrinogen into a fibrin clot. Lyophilized thrombin from bovine plasma is commercially available. The powder is diluted with BSS to a concentration of 100 U/mL into a separate infusion bottle and connected to a three-way stopcock. In situations that require a better hemostatic control, the surgeon can quickly change from the regular infusion bottle to the thrombin mixture bottle. Later, thrombin can be washed out with regular infusion, in order to decrease the risk of potential side effects related to it such as postoperative inflammation and unexpected clot formation.[12] The excessive postoperative intraocular inflammation is due to AC and residual anterior vitreous gel fibrin deposition. In severe cases, sterile hypopyon may occur. If endophthalmitis is suspected, it is advised to tap the vitreous for microbiology and administer antibiotic injections.[13,14]

It is known that thrombin increases production of fibrin and since fibrin has been implicated in PVR formation, it may be particularly prudent to avoid the use of thrombin during rhegmatogenous RD where the subretinal space can be accessed by thrombin.[15]

Ciliary Body Bleeding

This modality of hemorrhage may be very difficult to control because the major arterial circle is located at the apex of the CB. An inadvertent touch by the vitrectomy probe during most anterior vitreous base shavings may induce bleeding from CB. Retinectomy in difficult cases of RD, such as severe anterior PVR (anterior displacement), may lead to trauma to the CB during the removal of the anterior retina from the CB. Lensectomy in phakic eyes can facilitate PVR dissection and retinectomy performance under direct visualization and anterior indentation. This particularly helps avoid repetitive trauma to CB and consequent bleeding. Furthermore, during retinectomy, endodiathermy at the posterior cutting edge may prevent blood migration from retinal vessels.

Choroidal Bleeding

Inadvertent choroidal touch by instruments may induce focal or diffuse bleeding which may be difficult to control. Adequate rising of IOP may relieve choroidal hemorrhage.

Bleeding may come from choroidal detachment. Attempts to raise and maintain high IOP and other measures to prevent/manage hemorrhagic choroidal detachment are crucial to avoid its impairment (see Chapter 26C).

✦ Pearls on How to Manage Intraoperative Posterior Segment Bleeding

There are several ways to control intraocular hemorrhage and all of them follow three basic principles:

- ◆ **Compressive effect over the vessels** by fluids and/or IOP leading to vasoconstriction and clot formation; these maneuvers do not require a direct contact of instruments with the bleeding vessels and are especially useful for hemorrhage in the macular area and optic disc.

◆ **Induction of pharmacologic vasoconstriction** reducing the vascular permeability; these maneuvers do not require a direct contact of instruments with the bleeding vessels and are especially useful for hemorrhage in the macular area and optic disc.

◆ **Direct thermal effect over the blood,** leading to local coagulation of the blood and resulting in a clot formation; these maneuvers require a direct contact of instruments with the bleeding vessels and are especially useful for hemorrhage outside of the macular area and/or optic disc.

On the basis of these principles, the management of intraoperative hemorrhage may be organized in the following didactic ways:

Raising the IOP

This is a rapid and common technique for controlling intraoperative hemorrhage. Thrombosis and hemostasis occur with difficulty under fluid-filled medium. Thus, increasing of IOP is a useful maneuver to compress bleeding vessels and helps to decrease blood flow, resulting in clot formation (**Fig. 26B-1A–C**, Video 26B-2). In hypotonic eyes, the hemorrhage process tends to be a more frequent and complex event. Rising of IOP is achieved by lifting the infusion bottle or preferentially by increasing the pressure in the infusion system using a controlled mechanism (**Fig. 26B-1D–F,** Video 26B-3). Estimated infusion pressure from the first method is not known. Nowadays, vitrectomy systems have enough resources to induce elevation of IOP in a controlled way (e.g., Alcon, vented-gas forced-infusion, VGFI), resulting in better outcomes of vitreoretinal surgeries.

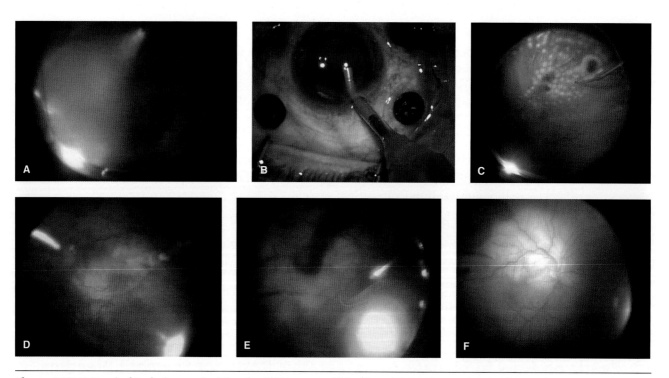

Figure 26B-1 Surgical techniques of raising the IOP to control bleeding. **(A)** Persistent vitreous hemorrhage case submitted to vitrectomy using temporary IOP rise of 60 mm Hg for 3 minutes in order to control bleeding from neovessels due to branch retinal vein occlusion (Video 26B-2). **(B)** Aspiration/irrigation of blood from the AC in order to improve the identification of structures in the vitreous cavity. Note the use of valved trocars (*blue*). **(C)** Endophotocoagulation over the ischemic areas associated to BRVO at the end of the surgery. **(D)** Vitrectomy in vitreous hemorrhage after blunt trauma (Video 26B-3). **(E)** Active bleeding from CB controlled by 3 minutes of high IOP. **(F)** Pale retina inferior to the macula at the end of the surgery showing a case of traumatic sclopetary chorioretinopathy.

There is no safety data about how long and how much IOP elevation must be performed to control intraoperative bleeding during a closed-system vitrectomy. It is advisable to minimize surgical time and achieve the infusion pressure enough to stop or minimize the bleeding process. Particularly, the regular infusion pressure during the entire vitrectomy must be as low as possible and not be routinely set at 30 mm Hg.

Theoretically, it is known that human neural tissue can support until 3 minutes of ischemia. Furthermore, the laboratory test of bleeding time (Duke method) is usually about 1 to 3 minutes. Thus, we recommend adjusting the IOP levels until optic disc venous pulsation is observed, and the hemorrhage management should be performed in about 1 to 2 minutes, depending on the case and variables such as size and number of bleeding sites, vessel caliber, systemic status of blood coagulation as well as BP.

Vitrectomy machines have sound to alert the surgeon about the spent time under high controlled IOP levels[13] that recommend lowering 1 foot (about 30 cm) per minute when lifting of bottle infusion method is used. It is also important to avoid optic disc arterial circulation closure (observed as a pale disc), since postoperative outer retinal and choroidal ischemia may occur.[5,16,17]

Difficulties will be observed in cases where optic disc is not seen (e.g., a big clot over the optic disc, intense fibrovascular membrane over the optic disc, partially opened funnel-shaped RD). In these cases, the use of high infusion pressure levels must be empirically adjusted. We recommend not raising IOP levels more than 60 mm Hg and not exceeding more than 3 minutes. Pallor of retina vessels must help to control the infusion pressure. Independent of the IOP raising technique, if hemostasis is not achieved in less than 3 minutes, the consideration to other techniques for bleeding control becomes necessary (e.g., manual compression of the oozing site, endodiathermy, endolaser).

Maintenance of a closed system is important to keep the high and controlled levels of IOP; to achieve this goal, plugged sclerotomies, avoiding the frequent removal of instruments away from the eye or the preferred valved-trocars systems (Fig. 26B-1B) may help to maintain a steady IOP during the surgery and a reasonable fluidic dynamics. The high IOP technique is especially useful for management of neovascularization at the AC in order to avoid bleeding (Video 26B-4 shows intraoperative view of valved trocars in an eye with neovascular glaucoma undergoing phacoemulsification and PPV with endophotocoagulation, using elevated values of IOP). High IOP values must be used with care to avoid atrophic changes at the optic disc after surgery.

Increased IOP may damage intraocular structures sensitive to ischemia. Particularly, care must be taken in eyes with glaucoma, diabetic retinopathy, and retinopathy of prematurity[18]; in these eyes, the "safe time/length of high IOP" is unknown and should be the shortest possible, enough to control the bleeding process. It is important to know that inadvertent retinal incarceration at sclerotomy sites could happen in retina-detached eyes when the infusion pressure is elevated and instruments are suddenly removed from the sclerotomies. To avoid such complication, IOP should be lowered to normal values before removal of instruments from the eye.

Fluid–Air Exchange

Increasing of IOP values can also be achieved by intraocular air application. The surface tension of an air bubble is higher than that exerted by fluid. So, an intraocular air/gas bubble frequently stops the blood flow[13] and facilitates thrombus formation (Fig. 26B-2, Videos 26B-5 and 26B-6). It is a worldwide surgical technique used during extensive hemorrhage because this maneuver is able to maintain the blood "packed" posteriorly to the fluid–air surface, especially at the posterior pole because the surface tension of air is higher than that of fluid (Fig. 26B-2C). This is a useful

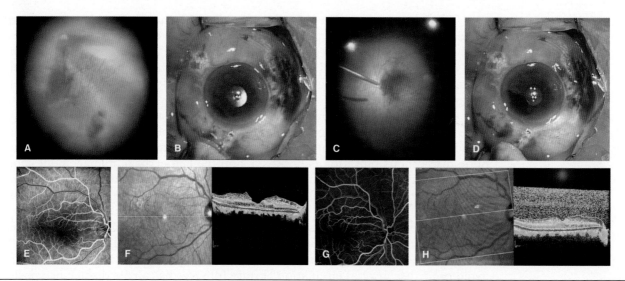

Figure 26B-2 Surgical technique of fluid–air exchange to minimize intraoperative bleeding. **(A)** ILM peeling (after removal of epiretinal membrane—ERM) using brilliant blue dye. Note the bleeding at the initial retinal touch and foveal bleeding by indirect forceps traction of the ILM, despite of high IOP levels. Patient was under anticoagulation therapy for cardiac disease (Video 26B-5). **(B)** Progressive bleeding from iris/CB following trocar removal at the end of the surgery in the same patient under anticoagulation therapy. The eye was submitted to reinsertion of the infusion system. **(C)** Fluid–air exchange and removal of blood from posterior pole. **(D)** Hemostasis caused by the surface tension of air at the vitreous cavity at the end of the surgery. No active bleeding is observed. **(E,F)** Preoperative fluorescein angiogram (FA) and optical coherence tomography (OCT) from an eye with recurrence of ERM (best corrected visual acuity—BCVA = 20/200). FA showing no window defect and dragging of the vessels at the macula. OCT image showing the hyperreflective image and irregularity of the retinal surface in ERM recurrence. Eye was submitted to reoperation including phaco-PPV + ERM and ILM peeling. Bleeding during ILM peeling was controlled by fluid with high IOP and fluid–air exchange (Video 26B-6). **(G,H)** Seventh postoperative day (BCVA = 20/30). FA showing no window defect and no dragging of the vessels at the macula. OCT image showing a normal anatomy.

maneuver to control extensive bleeding from many causes. It is also useful during epiretinal membrane and ILM peeling, especially in patients unable to stop the systemic anticoagulation therapy due to systemic diseases; in these eyes, bleeding in the macular area is very common and must be treated by indirect compression of the clot using high IOP levels instead of endodiathermy to avoid thermal damage to the macular area **(Fig. 26B-2A)**. In addition, in these patients, bleeding from the iris/CB may occur and should be treated by fluid–air exchange and increasing of the IOP **(Fig. 26B-2C)**.

Vitrectomy systems have an air-pump device for fluid–air exchange. It is suggested that flute, back-flush, or especially the soft-tipped cannula be used and connected into the vitrectomy aspiration line or preferentially into an accessory extrusion line. The vitrectomy tip can also be used particularly when progression of hemorrhage is too big to allow instruments change. During the fluid–air exchange, the recently formed little soft clots can be simultaneously removed by aspiration under fluid while the air is injected.

Fluid–air exchange may be a good alternative to improve the visualization of the periphery of retina and to show up bleeding sites. It is worthy particularly in cases where vitreous hemorrhage persisted despite adequate blood aspiration. Once bleeding is controlled, reversal from air to fluid may be done at any moment.[11]

Perfluorocarbon Liquids

The properties of transparency, molecular weight higher than water, and high surface tension have made PFCLs an adjunctive for management of complicated cases in vitreoretinal surgeries. Their property of immiscibility with blood and water and their liquid transparency allow surgeons to identify and stop bleeding sites when injected above the retina. This facilitates the cauterization of bleeding sources. Intraocular perfluorooctane significantly reduced the time to achieve hemostasis.[19]

Injection is performed using a syringe-threaded soft-tipped cannula over the optic disc. To prevent liquid dispersion, the tip must be positioned into the bubble, in order to produce only a single big one.

The technique for "en bloc" PFCL dissection of fibrovascular membranes in PDR and TRD showed good results in preventing intraoperative bleeding.[20] Separation of epiretinal tissues is performed by injecting PFCL between retina and posterior hyaloid. In addition to iatrogenic retinal breaks that may be observed in 7% of patients, care must be taken to avoid PFCL injection into the subretinal space. Moreover, during PFCL injection into the vitreous cavity, the fluid (BSS, blood, subretinal) inside the vitreous cavity must go outside of the eye and the valved-trocar systems may prevent this fluid migration. For this reason, it is very important to turn off the infusion or insert an unconnected, open needle throughout into the trocars. These maneuvers allow the migration of fluid displaced by PFCL through the valved trocars. Furthermore, use of coaxial cannulas (e.g., 20G/25G when performing 20G vitrectomy or 23G/30G when doing 23G surgery) may help PFCL injection in a unique valved trocar without subretinal migration. It allows PFCL to be injected and at the same time allows the fluid to come out of the eye.

Instrument Touch at Bleeding Site

When a punctiform bleeding outside the macular region is encountered, a direct and gentle application of pressure of any blunt-tipped instrument (e.g., silicone tipped, light pipe, vitrectomy tip, Hem-stopper) may be used. It may result in vasoconstriction, thus assisting the natural process of coagulation. It is held in place until blood flow at the bleeding site is stopped and a thrombus is formed. This is a good alternative for the side effects of raised IOP.

Injection of Adrenaline in the Infusion Bottle

This sympathomimetic amine acts as a vasopressor, bronchodilator, and vasoconstrictor. Pharmacologic vasoconstriction may help to contain bleeding. A prospective study showed that 0.5 mL of 1:1,000 (0.5 mg) adrenaline per 500 mL of Hartman's solution had insignificant serum absorption compared to a control group.[21]

However, secondary effects directly on retina are not known. Besides mydriasis, intravenous administration of epinephrine may induce transitory problems with color vision (red-green defect), acute macular neuroretinopathy,[22,23] and may precipitate an ocular vasoconstrictive event such as retinal arterial occlusion and optic nerve ischemia.[24]

Systemic side effects may occur such as headache, sweats, syncope, arrhythmia, tachycardia, palpitations, hypertension, and ventricular extrasystole.[25] It would be advisable not to use epinephrine in patients with unstable systemic BP or carrying medications that could increase it (e.g., tricyclic antidepressants), and heart diseases including arrhythmias. Particularly, ocular features that may predispose to vascular occlusive diseases and previous history of central serous chorioretinopathy may not be good candidates for epinephrine use into posterior segment infusion during vitreoretinal surgery.

Endodiathermy and Cauterization

Protein denaturation and hemostasis occur when resistance of tissues to electric currents are applied by diathermy; it is different from cauterization, in which an electric current heats up the probe tip and results in tissue coagulation[13]; both techniques—endodiathermy and cauterization—require the touch of the tip of the probe at the target tissue.

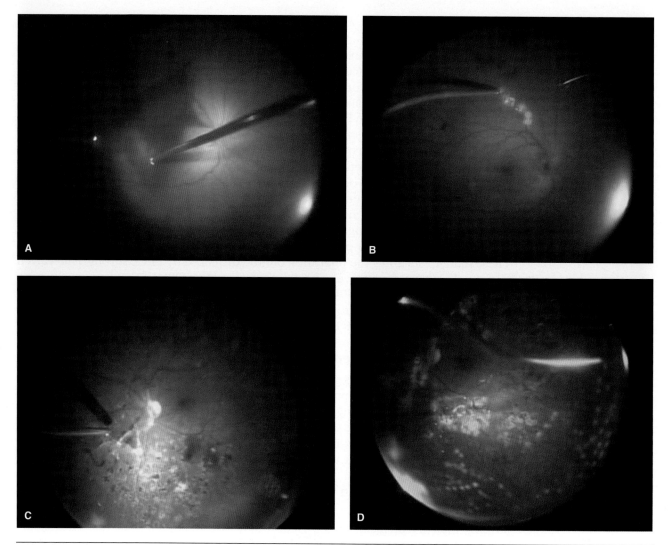

Figure 26B-3 Surgical techniques of endodiathermy for management of intraoperative bleeding. **(A)** Active bleeding from BRVO neovascularization over the posterior pole. It was removed by aspiration using vitrectomy probe (Video 26B-7). **(B)** Endodiathermy probe in the right hand and aspirating vitrectomy probe in the left hand to optimize the procedure of diathermy—"bimanual endodiathermy" technique. **(C)** Dissection/segmentation of proliferative tissue in PDR using 23G vitrectomy probe, 5,000 cuts/minute, aspiration of 200 and 30 mm Hg of infusion pressure (Video 26B-8). **(D)** Bimanual endodiathermy and back-flush techniques were used. Final stage of endodiathermy on bleeding sites. Panretinal endophotocoagulation at the final step of PDR using a flexible/extendable laser probe to avoid lens touch.

The endodiathermy is the preferable technique for many surgeons to manage the bleeding during PPV because it minimizes the epiretinal blood side effects (**Fig. 26B-3,** Videos 26B-7 and 26B-8). Unimanual coaxial bipolar (coaxial probe containing both electrodes connected) endodiathermy probes are available for 20G, 23G, and 25G systems. They can be used to coagulate active bleeding retinal neovascularization (**Fig. 26B-3B),** to assist retinotomies for subretinal fluid drainage, and to coagulate neovascularization in diabetic fibrovascular membrane dissection/segmentation (Video 26B-8). The bimanual endodiathermy technique (that employs connected electrodes to two intraocular electrical conductor instruments) is especially useful to treat elevated islands of fibrovascular membranes grasped between instruments.

Endodiathermy should be avoided at the fovea as well as over the optic nerve and papillomacular bundle. For better control of the hemostasis procedure, this technique should be performed using a pedal that contains a progressive control of the intensity. It avoids iatrogenic heating, retinal shortening, and tears especially if the bleeding site is close to the fovea or optic disc. In case of inadvertent avulsion of retinal vessel or iatrogenic retinal tears, complementary techniques (e.g., IOP increasing, PFCL, air–fluid exchange) should be used to establish visualization and control of bleeding. In addition, elevated disc neovascularization must be treated very carefully with low energy and maximum distance from optic nerve surface to prevent damage to nerve fiber layer and vascular supplies.

Laser Photocoagulation

Laser energy absorbed by the hemoglobin in the bleeding vessel can induce thermal denaturation of proteins followed by hemostasis (Fig. 26B-4). This has similar effect to intraocular diathermy.[13] Green laser could be initiated using power of 200 mW and exposure time at 200 ms. Delivery should be applied to flat areas and not under direct contact.

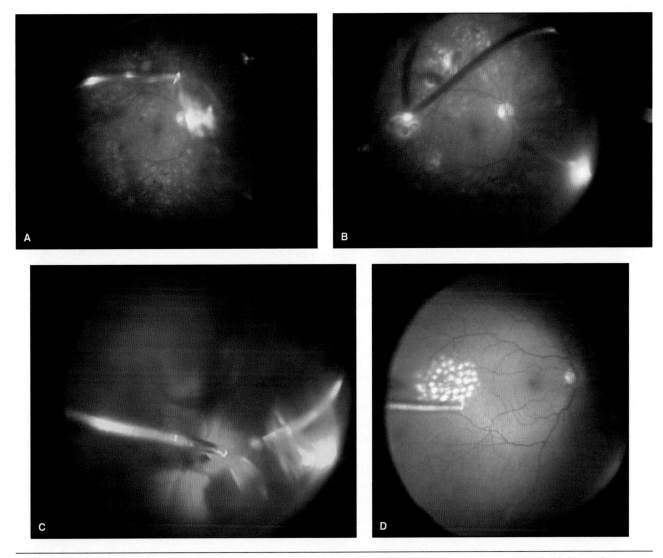

Figure 26B-4 Surgical techniques of laser for intraoperative bleeding. **(A)** Initial stage of posterior hyaloidal detachment in PDR submitted to 1.25 mg of intravitreal bevacizumab injection 3 days before PPV. **(B)** Endolaser performed over the bleeding sites in the same case. **(C)** Core vitrectomy in vitreous hemorrhage due to branch retinal vein obstruction (BRVO) neovascularization. **(D)** Endophotocoagulation at the site of BRVO. **(E)** Fluorescein angiography on the 7th postoperative day of right eye submitted to vitrectomy in vitreous hemorrhage in BRVO **(C,D)**. Macula and optic disk showed normal vessels perfusion and no leakage. BCVA improved from hand motions to 20/20. **(F,G)** FA showing the laser scars and hypofluorescent image at early phase **(F)** and late phase **(G)**. (*continued*)

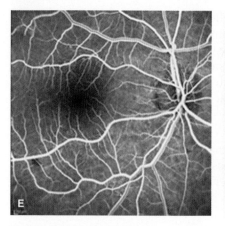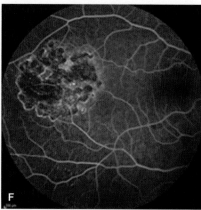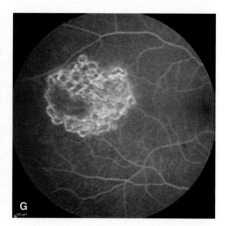

Figure 26B-4 (*continued*)

Alternative instruments with coupled aspiration could be useful in cases of active bleeding.[26–28] Those aspirating laser probes have practical ability to improve visualization and make local hemostasis without the need to exchange instruments.

Laser photocoagulation is useful for minimal amount of active bleeding (**Fig. 26B-4B,D**) around the attached retina; and in eyes with intraocular foreign body incarcerated into the retina may help to prevent bleeding progression during its removal.

◈ Pearls on How to Prevent It: Preoperative Procedures to Minimize the Possibility of Intraoperative Bleeding

Blood Pressure Control

Preoperative BP control could aid in preventing intraoperative bleeding during vitrectomy. Particularly, strict BP control is necessary to achieve minimal hemorrhage during TRD dissection from PDR, despite the use of additional techniques for bleed hemostasis. Recommended systolic and diastolic BPs must be 130 and 80 mm Hg or lower, respectively.

Intravitreal Injection of Anti-VEGF before Surgery in Proliferative Diabetic Retinopathy

Recent studies have shown the benefit of anti-VEGF therapy 3 to 5 days before vitrectomy for PDR. Regression of neovascularization resulting in less intraoperative bleeding contributes to an easier procedure in PDR (**Fig. 26B-5**, Videos 26B-9 and 26B-10). Intravitreal bevacizumab administration 2 to 11 days prior to PPV reported a reduction of intraoperative bleeding during PPV in patients with advanced PDR[29–32] (**Fig. 26B-5A,B**). The gap between bevacizumab administration and PPV should be less than 7 days in order to reduce the risk of increased vitreoretinal traction due to excessive fibrosis in patients with advanced PDR; the possible risk factors for progression of TRD are: Uncontrolled systemic diabetes, previous TRD, type I diabetes, and attached hyaloid to the retina[20] (**Fig. 26B-5E,F**).

Minimal intraoperative bleeding in 85% of cases was reported when 1.25 mg of bevacizumab was injected 1 week prior to vitrectomy.[33] Lowest dose of bevacizumab (0.16 mg) was as effective as the standard dose (1.25 mg) in reducing intraoperative hemorrhage when administered 3 days before surgery.[34] A recent meta-analysis showed that the incidence of intraoperative bleeding and frequency of endodiathermy were considerably lower following intravitreal bevacizumab injection before the surgery in PDR compared to surgery without previous anti-VEGF injection.[35] Nowadays it is suggested that 1.25 mg of intravitreal bevacizumab injection be performed 3 days before the vitrectomy in PDR **(Fig. 26B-5A,B)**. This preoperative technique allows the surgical procedure to be performed even in complex surgical cases **(Fig. 26B-5E,F)**.

Differences were also observed when injecting ranibizumab (0.5 mg) 7 days before vitrectomy for TRD. Incidence of intraoperative hemorrhage was decreased by 65% when compared to sham group.[36]

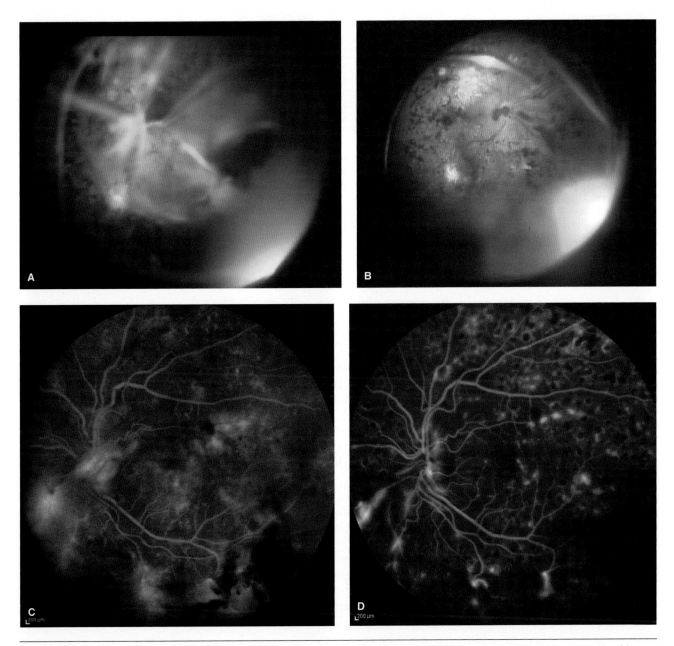

Figure 26B-5 Intraoperative bleeding control in PDR (using several surgical techniques) 3 days following 1.25 mg of intravitreal bevacizumab injection. **(A)** Posterior hyaloidal detachment using the vitrectomy probe. The hyaloid is extremely thick and adherent and no bleeding is observed (Video 26B-9). **(B)** Vitreous base removal to avoid PDR anterior proliferation. Minimal bleeding is observed. **(C)** Preoperative FA from the same case showing leakage of vessels in macula. **(D)** FA on the 7th postoperative day showing no vitreous bleeding and minimal residual leakage nasal to the optic disc/arcades. BCVA improved from counting fingers at 1 m to 20/40. *(continued)*

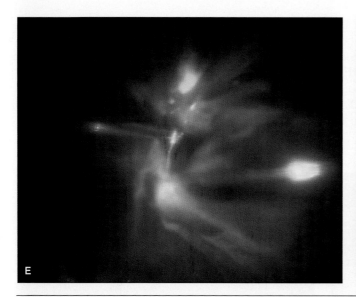
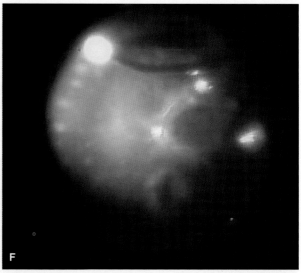

Figure 26B-5 *(continued)* **(E)** Complicated TRD in a 26-year-old patient. Bimanual dissection and segmentation of proliferative membranes. Minimal bleeding is observed following preoperative bevacizumab injection. **(F)** Fluid–air exchange to reattach the retina and to minimize bleeding. Panretinal endophotocoagulation after vitreous base removal to avoid anterior PDR followed by silicone oil injection (Video 26B-10).

Antiplatelets and Anticoagulants

Is It Necessary to Discontinue before Surgery?

Warfarin, the most used anticoagulant, inhibits vitamin-K–dependent clotting factors (II, VII, IX, and X) and needs the International Normalized Ratio (INR) between 2 and 3 to maintain optimal anticoagulation (e.g., atrial fibrillation, valvular heart disease, and thromboembolic diseases). There are two main platelet aggregation pathways to be inhibited. Clopidogrel inhibits adenosine diphosphate–produced platelet aggregation. Aspirin works through the inhibition of the cyclooxygenase pathway and frequently has been used in combination with warfarin, although with less therapeutic efficacy than clopidogrel. The most common indication for antiplatelet therapy in vitrectomy candidates is cardiac stent, coronary artery bypass grafting, and history of transient ischemic attack.[37] Use of antiplatelet agents has increased in patients undergoing vitreoretinal surgery.[38]

However, there is no unified consensus regarding the risks of systemic anticoagulation or platelet inhibition during ocular surgery and whether continuation of such medication is appropriate.[37] Fu et al.[39] studied 25 cases receiving warfarin during vitreoretinal surgery. Only one patient submitted to scleral buckling and external drainage of subretinal fluid had intraoperative subretinal hemorrhage. The authors concluded that continuation of anticoagulation does not increase the risk of hemorrhage during the operation.[40] However, they suggested that aspirin should not be stopped prior to retinal detachment surgery. Warfarin may be stopped if the patient's thromboembolic risk is low, because of high possibilities of either intraoperative and/or postoperative bleeding.

Many studies have observed no anesthesia-related or intraoperative hemorrhagic complications during repair of retinal detachment, epiretinal membrane, and diabetic retinopathy.[37,40–43] Additional attention must be given in diabetic patients. A recent study revealed significantly worse final visual acuity in patients using warfarin.[42] Naturally, each case must be evaluated individually. Particularly, if a PDR patient with highly active neovascularization and TRD has a high risk of thromboembolic event, anticoagulation may be continued. Preoperative use of anti-VEGF[35] and a fast as well as good-quality small-gauge surgery[37] may contribute to achieving lower rates of hemorrhagic events.

REFERENCES

1. Sanders D, Peyman GA, Fishman G, et al. The toxicity of intravitreal whole blood and hemoglobin. *Albrecht Von Graefes Arch Klin Exp Ophthalmol.* 1975;197(3):255–267.

2. Ehrenberg M, Thresher RJ, Machemer R. Vitreous hemorrhage nontoxic to retina as a stimulator of glial and fibrous proliferation. *Am J Ophthalmol.* 1984;97(5):611–626.

3. Imamura Y, Kamei M, Minami M, et al. Heparin-assisted removal of clotting preretinal hemorrhage during vitrectomy for proliferative diabetic retinopathy. *Retina.* 2005;25(6):793–795.

4. Tabandeh H, Sullivan PM, Smahliuk P, et al. Suprachoroidal hemorrhage during pars plana vitrectomy. Risk factors and outcomes. *Ophthalmology.* 1999;106(2):236–242.

5. Chow DR, Bustros S. Ch 143: Control of perioperative bleeding in vitreoretinal surgery. In: Ryan SJ, Hinton DR, Schachat AP, Wilkinson CP, eds. *Retina.* 4th ed. Mosby; 2006:2451–2462.

6. Johnson MW, Olsen KR, Hernandez E. Tissue plasminogen activator thrombolysis during surgical evacuation of experimental subretinal hemorrhage. *Ophthalmology.* 1992;99(4):515–521.

7. Chen SN, Yang TC, Ho CL, et al. Retinal toxicity of intravitreal tissue plasminogen activator: Case report and literature review. *Ophthalmology.* 2003;110(4):704–708.

8. Sandhu SS, Manvikar S, Steel DH. Displacement of submacular hemorrhage associated with age-related macular degeneration using vitrectomy and submacular tPA injection followed by intravitreal ranibizumab. *Clin Ophthalmol.* 2010;4:637–642.

9. Wong KL. Chapter 10: Surgery for submacular hemorrhage. In: Bhavsar AR, ed. *Retina and Vitreous Surgery.* 1st ed. Saunders Elsevier, Philadelphia, PA, USA; 2009;125–129.

10. De Bustros S. Intraoperative control of hemorrhage in penetrating ocular injuries. *Retina.* 1990;10(suppl 1):S55–S58.

11. Ambler JS, Meyers SM. Management of intraretinal metallic foreign bodies without retinopexy in the absence of retinal detachment. *Ophthalmology.* 1991;98(3):391–394.

12. Thompson JT, Glaser BM, Michels RG, et al. The use of intravitreal thrombin to control hemorrhage during vitrectomy. *Ophthalmology.* 1986;93(3):279–282.

13. Chou F, Kertes PJ. Chapter 23: Control of intraocular hemorrhage during vitrectomy. In: Peyman GA, Meffert SA, Conway MD, eds. *Vitreoretinal Surgical Techniques.* 2nd ed. Informa Healthcare, London, England; 2007:213.

14. Verdoon C, Hendrikse F. Intraocular human thrombin infusion in diabetic vitrectomies. *Ophthalmic Surg.* 1989;20:278–279.

15. Vidaurri-Leal JS, Glaser BM. Effect of fibrin on morphologic characteristics of retinal pigment epithelial cells. *Arch Ophthalmol.* 1984;102:1376–1379.

16. Gass JD, Parrish R. Outer retinal ischemic infarction–a newly recognized complication of cataract extraction and closed vitrectomy. Part 1. A case report. *Ophthalmology.* 1982;89:1467–1471.

17. Parrish RK, Gass JD, Anderson DR. Outer retina ischemic infarction—a newly recognized complication of cataract extraction and closed vitrectomy. Part 2. An animal model. *Ophthalmology.* 1982;89:1472–1477.

18. van Heuven WA, Kiel JW. ROP surgery and ocular circulation. *Eye (Lond).* 2008;22(10):1267–1272. Epub 2008 .

19. Moreira Júnior CA, Uscocovich CE, Moreira AT. Experimental studies with perfluoro-octane for hemostasis during vitreoretinal surgery. *Retina.* 1997;17(6):530–534.

20. Arevalo JF, Maia M, Flynn HW Jr, et al. Tractional retinal detachment following intravitreal bevacizumab (Avastin) in patients with severe proliferative diabetic retinopathy. *Br J Ophthalmol.* 2008;92:213–216.

21. Heyworth P, Bourke R, Moore C, et al. The systemic absorption of adrenaline from posterior segment infusion during vitreoretinal surgery. *Eye (Lond).* 1998;12(Pt 6):949–952.

22. O'Brien DM, Farmer SG, Kalina RE, et al. Acute macular neuroretinopathy following intravenous sympathomimetics. *Retina.* 1989;9:281–286.

23. Desai UR, Sudhamathi K, Natarajan S. Intravenous epinephrine and acute macular neuroretinopathy. *Arch Ophthalmol.* 1993;111:1026–1027.

24. Savino PJ, Burde RM, Mills RP. Visual loss following intranasal anesthetic injection. *J Clin Neuroophthalmol.* 1990;10(2):140–144.

25. Fraunfelder FT, Fraunfelder FW, Chambers WA. *Clinical Ocular Toxicology.* 1st ed. Saunders, Philadelphia, PA, USA; 2008:165–166.

26. Peyman GA, D'Amico DJ, Alturki WA. An endolaser probe with aspiration capability. *Arch Ophthalmol.* 1992;110:718.

27. Chang S. Multifunction endolaser probe. *Am J Ophthalmol.* 1992;114:648–649.

28. Charles S, Chang S, McCuen BW. New techniques for hemostasis during diabetic vitrectomy. *Retina.* 2003;23(1):120–122.

29. Avery RL, Pearlman J, Pieramici DJ, et al. Intravitreal bevacizumab (Avastin) in the treatment of proliferative diabetic retinopathy. *Ophthalmology.* 2006;113:1695. e1–e15.

30. Chen E, Park CH. Use of intravitreal bevacizumab as a preoperative adjunct for tractional retinal detachment repair in severe proliferative diabetic retinopathy. *Retina.* 2006;26:699–700.

31. da R Lucena D, Ribeiro JA, Costa RA, et al. Intraoperative bleeding during vitrectomy for diabetic tractional retinal detachment with versus without preoperative intravitreal bevacizumab (IBeTra Study). *Br J Ophthalmol.* 2009;93:688–691.

32. Ishikawa K, Honda S, Tsukahara Y, et al. Preferable use of intravitreal bevacizumab as a pretreatment of vitrectomy for severe proliferative diabetic retinopathy. *Eye (Lond).* 2009;23:108–111.

33. Abdelhakim MA, Macky TA, Mansour KA, et al. Bevacizumab (Avastin) as an adjunct to vitrectomy in the management of severe proliferative diabetic retinopathy: A prospective case series. *Ophthalmic Res.* 2011;45(1):23–30. Epub 2010 Aug 11.

34. Hattori T, Shimada H, Nakashizuka H, et al. Dose of intravitreal bevacizumab (Avastin) used as preoperative adjunct therapy for proliferative diabetic retinopathy. *Retina.* 2010;30(5):761–764.

35. Zhao LQ, Zhu H, Zhao PQ, et al. A systematic review and meta-analysis of clinical outcomes of vitrectomy with or without intravitreal bevacizumab pretreatment for severe diabetic retinopathy. *Br J Ophthalmol.* 2011;95(9):1216–1222. Epub 2011.

36. Ribeiro JA, Messias A, de Almeida FP, et al. The effect of intravitreal ranibizumab on intraoperative bleeding during pars plana vitrectomy for diabetic traction retinal detachment. *Br J Ophthalmol.* 2011;95(9):1337–1339. Epub 2011.

37. Mason JO 3rd, Gupta SR, Compton CJ, et al. Comparison of hemorrhagic complications of warfarin and clopidogrel bisulfate in 25-gauge vitrectomy versus a control group. *Ophthalmology.* 2011;118(3):543–547. Epub 2010.

38. Oh J, Smiddy WE, Kim SS. Antiplatelet and anticoagulation therapy in vitreoretinal surgery. *Am J Ophthalmol.* 2011;151(6):934–939.e3. Epub 2011 Mar 16.

39. Fu AD, McDonald HR, Williams DF, et al. Anticoagulation with warfarin in vitreoretinal surgery. *Retina.* 2007;27:290–295.

40. Narendran N, Williamson TH. The effects of aspirin and warfarin therapy on haemorrhage in vitreoretinal surgery. *Acta Ophthalmol Scand.* 2003;81(1):38–40.

41. Dayani PN, Grand MG. Maintenance of warfarin anticoagulation for patients undergoing vitreoretinal surgery. *Arch Ophthalmol.* 2006;124(11):1558–1565.

42. Brown JS, Mahmoud TH. Anticoagulation and clinically significant postoperative vitreous hemorrhage in diabetic vitrectomy. *Retina.* 2011;31(10):1983–1987. doi: 10.1097/IAE.0b013e31821800cd.

43. Chandra A, Jazayeri F, Williamson TH. Warfarin in vitreoretinal surgery: A case controlled series. *Br J Ophthalmol.* 2011;95(7):976–978. Epub 2010 Nov 11.

26C Intraoperative Suprachoroidal Hemorrhage

EHAB ABDELKADER, DAVID WONG, AND NOEMI LOIS

The Complication: Definition

Suprachoroidal hemorrhage (SCH) relates to the accumulation of blood into the suprachoroidal space, which is the potential space between the choroid and the sclera. It differs from choroidal detachment in that, in the latter, there is effusion of fluid, but not blood, into the suprachoroidal space.

SCH is a rare but dreaded complication of vitreoretinal (VR) surgery. The incidence of SCH in vitrectomy surgery has been reported to range between 0.17% and 1.9%.[1-4] Machemer and Laqua[5] reported an incidence of 4.3% in vitrectomy for complex cases. Hawkins and Schepens[4] reported an incidence of 1% in cases of sclera buckling. SCH can develop intraoperatively with expulsion of the intraocular contents through the surgical wound, which is known as expulsive hemorrhage, very rare nowadays with the use of microsurgical incisions, or postoperatively, often shortly following surgery.[2] Ishida and Takeuchi[6] reported 0.09% incidence of intraoperative SCH in vitrectomy surgery.

Risk Factors

Several systemic, ocular, and operative risk factors have been implicated in the occurrence of SCH. Systemic risk factors include advanced age,[7] atherosclerosis,[8] hypertension,[9] coagulation defects,[10] and diabetes mellitus.[11] It is not clear whether or not anticoagulants such as warfarin increase the risk of SCH. Chandra et al.[12] found no increased incidence of SCH in patients on warfarin undergoing vitrectomy, when compared to those not using this drug. The INR in their groups of patients using warfarin ranged between 0.94 and 4.6 (median 2.3). Chapter 27B gives more insight on the issue of the use of anticoagulants in VR surgery. Ocular risk factors include glaucoma,[8] myopia,[1,8,9,13,14] aphakia and pseudophakia,[1,14] recent intraocular surgery,[7] previous trauma to the eye,[15] intraocular inflammation,[16,17] presence of retinal detachment,[13] and previous retinal detachment surgery.[13] Idiopathic polypoidal choroidal vasculopathy (IPCV) has been associated with the occurrence of spontaneous SCH and SCH following photodynamic therapy.[18,19] Thus, it is possible that IPCV may pose an increased risk of SCH in retinal surgery.

Intraoperative risk factors include sudden drop of intraocular pressure (IOP),[9,15] Valsalva maneuvers,[9,20] and rise of blood pressure.[9,13] Certain intraoperative maneuvers have been reported to be associated with increased risk for SCH including broad posterior scleral buckling, cryotherapy, external drainage of subretinal fluid, and prolonged surgical time.[1,13,16] Other possible risk factors for the development of SCH have been described below (see Pathogenesis). In 23G and 25G vitrectomy, slippage or of the infusion cannula into the suprachoroidal space was reported to cause suprachoroidal effusion and SCH.[21,22]

Pathogenesis

In general, ocular hypotony is believed to be the initial step in the development of SCH with abnormal transluminal pressure in the choroidal vascular bed with high choroidal vascular pressure or low IOP.[23,24] Several risk factors have been linked to increased fragility of the choroidal vessels, which would predispose them to an easy rupture, including old age, atherosclerosis, hypertension, diabetes as well as axial myopia, and glaucoma.[2,11,13,14] Manschot[24] postulated that glaucoma results in degeneration of the choroidal vascular wall predisposing to SCH. It is also suggested that axial myopia predisposes to SCH based on vascular fragility.[25] Some histopathology studies on human eyes with SCH demonstrated ruptured necrotic posterior ciliary arteries.[24,26] Beyer et al.[23] experimented the sequence of events of SCH in healthy rabbit eyes. In their study they induced increased pressure on the vortex veins and reduced the IOP. As a result, the following sequence of events occurred: Engorgement of the choriocapillaris, choroidal effusion, tearing of the ciliary vessels at the base of ciliary body, and massive extravasation of blood from the torn blood vessels followed by expulsion of blood from the surgical wound. In retinal surgery, additional mechanisms may also explain the pathogenesis of SCH. For instance, obstruction of the vortex veins can result from scleral buckling and may be associated with SCH, as shown in animal models.[27] Direct damage of the choroidal vessels may also be the precipitating cause of SCH, such as during drainage of SRF, inadvertently by cryofracture of the choroid result of an early removal of the cryoprobe while the choroid is still frozen, or by needle punctures while placing scleral sutures.[13,25] Separation of the choroid from the sclera by the SCH may shear more choroidal vessels traversing the suprachoroidal space with the subsequent increased bleeding. If the globe is open, like during phaco-vitrectomy, this may push the intraocular contents out of the wound. If it is closed, the rise of the IOP and blood clotting may limit its further extension. SCH can compromise visual outcome by a number of mechanisms including secondary retinal degeneration, causing retinal breaks and retinal detachment, subretinal hemorrhage with damage to photoreceptors, vitreous hemorrhage, glaucoma, and persistent ocular hypotony.[25]

✦ Clinical Findings

Clinical signs of intraoperative SCH include sudden rise of IOP, shallowing of the anterior chamber, loss of red reflex, anterior movement of the iris and lens (or intraocular lens in pseudophakic eyes), dark brown convexity at the retinal periphery with visualization of the ora serrata or pars plana, and bleeding into the subretinal space or the vitreous cavity. Prolapse of the vitreous into the sclerotomies or through the corneal wound can also be a sign of SCH developing during pars plana vitrectomy or combined phaco-vitrectomy, respectively. Ocular ultrasound is useful to confirm the diagnosis in patients that have experienced this complication as well as it usually helps in the planning of subsequent surgical intervention. It also allows determining the site and extension of the SCH as well as whether a concomitant retinal detachment is present. Initially, A-scan ultrasonography demonstrates a double-peaked high-reflective spike (from the retina and choroid underneath) followed by low reflective spikes representing the blood in the suprachoroidal space. On B-scan, SCH appears as a single dome-shaped lesion, if in one quadrant, or multiple dome-shaped lesions, if in more than one quadrant. When highly elevated and touching, the term "kissing choroids" is applied (Fig. 26C-1). As compared to choroidal effusion that shows echo-silent interior structure, SCH shows internal echoes within the dome(s) of various intensities, distribution, and kinetic features depending on the density of the blood and the duration of the SCH. US can determine if the SCH is liquefied when echoes become mobile during kinetic examination.

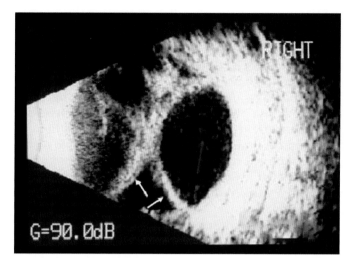

Figure 26C-1 Ultrasound scan obtained from a patient with a suprachoroidal hemorrhage and kissing choroidals. Two thick bands are seen in the vitreous cavity touching each other (*white arrows*). High reflective echoes can be also detected between the detached choroidal band and the ocular wall representing blood in the suprachoroidal space (*red arrow*). (Courtesy of Dr. Hatem Atta.)

 Pearls on How to Prevent It

Care should be taken to control all modifiable risk factors for SCH to avoid the occurrence of this complication as follows.

Preoperatively

◆ Good control of blood pressure in hypertensive patients (systolic pressure below 150 mm Hg).[8]

◆ In patients using anticoagulants (warfarin), the authors prefer to keep the INR levels between 2 and 3 if surgical intervention is planned, especially when operating in high-risk groups (see above). Although some surgeons may opt to stop antiplatelet drugs (aspirin, clopidogrel) before undertaking planned vitreoretinal surgery, this is not the common practice of the authors as there is no evidence in the literature to support this action (see also Chapter 27B).

◆ If possible, avoid operating on eyes with high IOP or with active inflammation. These factors need to be controlled well prior to surgery.

◆ If operating in patients with pre-existing SCH it is important to evaluate whether risk factors (as outlined above) for its occurrence were present when this complication occurred; if so, they should be controlled as best as possible before undertaking further surgery. If the complication occurred in a previous surgery, it would be important to understand the possible reason for its occurrence, for instance, whether it related to a particular maneuver performed during the surgery with the plan of avoiding it when further surgery is undertaken. Preventing marked changes in IOP and hypotony peroperatively and postoperatively would be recommended. It may be reasonable to work with higher IOP than under normal circumstances and, despite of lacking evidence to support it, to stop anticoagulants/antiplatelet drugs, if possible, prior to surgery.

Intraoperatively

◆ Care should be taken to avoid slippage of the infusion cannula into the suprachoroidal space. Taping the infusion line with sterile strips would stabilize it and prevent possible pulling during intraoperative maneuvers, such as when inserting and removing the indirect viewing systems from the operating field. Care also should be taken when indenting the sclera close to the infusion site.

♦ Avoid sudden reduction of IOP. During pars plana vitrectomy and with current vitrectomy systems, this is now possible by using the automated infusion through the machine, which allows maintaining constant IOP throughout the surgery. During sclera buckling procedures, a reduction of IOP following intentional or nonintentional drainage of subretinal fluid should be avoided by applying external pressure to the globe while subretinal fluid is drained. This maneuver, however, is only possible to be undertaken by surgeons who use transscleral needle puncture techniques to drain subretinal fluid but not for those that use the scleral cut-down approach. This can be done with the fingers or by keeping tightly supported the globe by holding the muscle insertions. If high amounts of subretinal fluid are drained, intraocular injection of air (it can be easily done through the vitrectomy machine) may be used to maintain good IOP. Alternatively, the scleral buckle should be raised immediately after or concomitantly to the drainage of subretinal fluid, to avoid a reduction in IOP.

♦ Avoid removing the cryoprobe before it thaws. Warm balance salt solution (BSS) can be used intraoperatively to speed up the process of thawing.

♦ Avoid excessive pressure on the globe, for example, during scleral indentation, especially in eyes with friable sclera such as high myopes and, importantly, be careful, slow, and gentle when letting it go on the indentation.

♦ Make sure that all sclerotomies (as well as the corneal tunnel in cases of combined phaco-vitrectomy) are well closed and not leaking at the end of the surgery. In order to test whether the sclerostomies and corneal wound are competent and well closed, if the conjunctiva has been opened, fluorescein drops can be used to test for a positive Seidel test with wash-out of the fluorescein by the fluid leaking through the sclerostomy/corneal wound. This test may still be done even if a conjunctival peritomy has not been performed, as when doing small-bore vitrectomy, by using a thin cannula (like an anterior chamber cannula) attached to a syringe containing fluorescein which is then injected through the conjunctival slits made at the beginning of the surgery, at the time of trocar insertion. A slow and mild positive Seidel test under these circumstances, however, may be difficult to detect. If air/gas had been inserted, bubbles will form and be seen when fluid is injected over the sclerostomies.

♦ Avoid leaving the eye soft at the end of the surgery, especially if the surgery is performed under general anesthesia (see later); it is better to leave the eye with an IOP on the higher side than on the lower side postoperatively.[15]

♦ Avoid Valsalva maneuvers in patients under general anesthesia. Laryngeal masks offer a good alternative to endotracheal tubes that might cause straining of the patient during recovery.

♦ In eyes with pre-existing SCH, some surgeons may prefer to complete the surgery leaving the eye with a liquid (saline or silicone oil) rather than air/gas as liquids are incompressible and may limit the extension of further bleeding if it were to occur.

Pearls on How to Solve It

Intraoperatively

♦ Check quickly if the infusion line is not blocked; make sure that the infusion cannula is in place, and that the infusion bag is full.

♦ If the tip of the infusion cannula cannot be seen and suprachoroidal infusion is suspected, another infusion line should be placed immediately through a different sclerostomy site and the previously existing one should be stopped at the same time. In cases of SCH due to slippage of the infusion cannula into the suprachoroidal space, insertion of another infusion cannula may help to maintain the IOP and limit the SCH.[21]

♦ Increase the infusion pressure through the vitrectomy machine or raise the bag immediately, should the former function not being available/in use, once it is assured that the infusion cannula is in the vitreous cavity.

♦ Close the sclerostomy ports with plugs initially and wait for some minutes to allow stabilization of the IOP. Indirect ophthalmoscopy may be useful to monitor the stabilization of the SCH before removing the trocars when small-gauge vitrectomy is being performed or before suturing the sclerostomies if 20G vitrectomy is being used.

♦ Avoid any Valsalva maneuvers in patients undergoing general anesthesia when the patient is recovering. Smooth extubation and avoiding struggling of the patient is recommended.

Postoperatively

The management of SCH depends on the site and extent of SCH as well as the associated complications.

♦ Localized SCH not involving the macula with no other VR complications: Observation. Frequent topical, in addition to systemic, steroids may be added to the regular treatment regime to reduce inflammation as much as possible.

♦ In the presence of large SCH, rhegmatogenous or tractional retinal detachment, break through vitreous hemorrhage, vitreous incarceration into the wound, or retained lens fragments, surgical intervention should be considered.[25]

♦ If intervention is required, the surgeon may proceed with one of the two following surgical approaches or both sequentially: (1) drainage of the SCH and (2) VR surgery.

When drainage of the SCH is considered, a decision should be made with regard to the timing for this intervention. Liquefaction of clotted blood in the suprachoroidal space usually takes place between 7 and 14 days from the onset of SCH.[28–31] Liquefaction can be assessed by ultrasonography when mobile echoes are seen in the suprachoroidal space on kinetic examination. As soon as early liquefaction of the clot is observed, surgical intervention may be undertaken. Drainage of the liquefied blood can often be achieved through the sclerostomies made for the vitrectomy. Only if this attempt fails, radial sclerotomies at the dependent part of the quadrant(s) involved by SCH could be opened. This is usually combined with the injection of BSS[32] or viscoelastic[33] material in the anterior chamber to maintain the IOP and to force the blood in the suprachoroidal space out. The drainage sclerotomy can be held open with a forceps until the fluid in the suprachoroidal space is out and then sutured. Alternatively, early intervention may be considered in an attempt to reduce the damage caused by the blood in retinal structures, especially on the retinal pigment epithelium and photoreceptors, especially in cases with macular involvement. Thus, Murata et al. (Murata T, Shiraga F, and Ishibashi T. tPA-assisted surgical drainage of massive SCH in a globe rupture leading to excellent visual recovery. Presented at the XXVIIth Meeting of the Club Jules Gonin, Kyoto, Japan, 3–6 November 2010) proposed the use of tissue plasminogen activator (tPA) into the clot to achieve its liquefaction, allowing early removal. They used it in three eyes of three patients with massive SCH with excellent visual results. tPA was injected (40,000 IU) from the scleral side followed by vitrectomy in a case with massive kissing hemorrhagic choroidal detachment and subretinally during vitrectomy in two other cases with massive suprachoroidal and subretinal hemorrhages with excellent results. Following injection of tPA into the clot, 15 to 25 minutes should be waited to allow lysis of the clot prior to removal of the liquefied blood.

VR surgery may be needed, in addition to the drainage of the SCH. This is usually indicated in cases with retinal detachment, vitreous hemorrhage, or retained lens fragments. Even in the absence of these additional complications, some surgeons may opt to perform this surgery. When a PPV is undertaken at the same time as the drainage of the SCH, the latter is usually done first, in the early stages of the procedure with concomitant injection of BSS in the anterior chamber or vitreous cavity. The former is usually preferred in aphakic cases whereas the latter is used in pseudophakic and phakic cases. If a pars plana approach is used, care should be taken to make sure that the tip of the infusion cannula is inside the vitreous cavity, and not under the retina or in the suprachoroidal space. Long cannulas (6 mm) may be used in these cases, although care is needed with these to avoid damage to the retina, especially in cases with bullous RD. Perfluorocarbon liquid (PFCL) can also be used instead or in addition to BSS.[32,34] The former has the advantage of allowing flattening of the retina, floating any retained lens fragments as well as forcing the blood out of the sclerotomies. It is advisable to remove peripheral vitreous, especially at the sclerostomy areas, prior to the injection of PFCL to prevent vitreous incarceration into the sclerostomy sites with the subsequent risk of peripheral retinal tear development. Associated VR complications such as retinal detachment are then dealt with. The PFC can be removed at the end of the surgery by a PFC–air exchange and then air–gas[35] or air–oil[36] exchange or by direct PFC–oil exchange. Ultrasonography prior to the surgical procedure (or intraoperatively) with the patient lying flat (as during surgery) is very useful as it allows determining areas not involved by the SCH or where the SCH may be less elevated and where no retinal detachment is present (or is shallower), which may be the most convenient ones to place the infusion, minimizing the risk of infusing fluid into the suprachoroidal or subretinal space. Similarly, it will help to determine the area of maximal elevation of the SCH when planning to inject tPA into the clot or the site of external drainage.

Recently, a new surgical approach has been proposed by Nadarajah et al.[37] for the treatment of massive SCH, defined as that in which near or actual retinal apposition is present. In none of the 10 cases presented the SCH occurred in the context of a VR procedure. As described, the surgery involves the performance of a 180-degree inferior conjunctival peritomy followed by isolation of the medial, inferior, and lateral rectus muscles. Then two full-thickness triangular scleral flaps, measuring $3 \times 3 \times 3$ mm are created at the equator one in each inferonasal and inferotemporal quadrants; these flaps are left unsutured at the end of the procedure, although the conjunctiva overlying it is closed with sutures. Partial drainage of SCH can be attempted intraoperatively prior to closure of the conjunctiva. Intravitreal injection of 100% perfluoropropane gas (C_3F_8) is then performed, with a maximal volume of 0.3 mL. Excellent visual results were obtained using this technique; importantly, in 7/10 early intervention (≤3 days) was undertaken.[37]

Given that the photoreceptor/retinal pigment epithelium cell loss related to the presence of blood, that will likely break through from the suprachoroidal space into the subretinal pigment epithelium and subretinal space, is likely to occur within 3 to 7 days or earlier following the event,[38,39] early intervention would be expected to achieve better visual outcomes and, thus, would be recommended. Similarly, attempts should be made to remove all blood present, if possible.

✦ Expected Outcomes

The prognosis of cases of SCH is variable depending on the location and severity of the condition as well as the associated complications. Favorable visual outcomes ($\geq6/60$) may occur in localized SCH not involving the posterior pole.[13,25] Cases with expulsive (massive) hemorrhage are expected to have severe visual loss in the majority of them.[7,16,29] Several reports recorded a less than 50% chance to recover >6/60 vision despite surgical intervention.[2,13,28,32] The majority of those cases with poor visual outcomes had kissing choroids, associated retinal detachment, 360-degree SCH. Murata et al., however, reported very good outcomes in three cases of massive SCH (see above) following trauma with visions of 0.8, 0.4, and 0.5 (Snellen equivalent of 6/7.5, 6/15, and 6/12, respectively) following treatment.

What Is the Worst-case Scenario

NPL has been reported to occur in 12% to 57% of cases of SCH despite secondary intervention.[1,3,13,28] In cases of massive intraoperative SCH, around 86% of eyes ended up with no light perception.[16] Factors reported to carry a poor visual prognosis include initial retinal detachment, duration of retinal apposition, vitreous incarceration into the wound, 360-degree SCH, and involvement of the posterior pole.[2,13,29,40] The main causes of poor final visual outcome are persistent retinal detachment, secondary glaucoma, or hypotony.[25]

REFERENCES

1. Sharma T, Virdi DS, Parikh S, et al. A case-control study of suprachoroidal hemorrhage during pars plana vitrectomy. *Ophthalmic Surg Lasers.* 1997;28(8):640–644.
2. Piper JG, Han DP, Abrams GW, et al. Perioperative choroidal hemorrhage at pars plana vitrectomy. A case-control study. *Ophthalmology.* 1993;100(5):699–704.
3. Speaker MG, Guerriero PN, Met JA, et al. A case-control study of risk factors for intraoperative suprachoroidal expulsive hemorrhage. *Ophthalmology.* 1991;98(2): 202–209;discussion 210.
4. Hawkins WR, Schepens CL. Choroidal detachment and retinal surgery. *Am J Ophthalmol.* 1966;62(5):813–819.
5. Machemer R, Laqua H. A logical approach to the treatment of massive periretinal proliferation. *Ophthalmology.* 1978;85(6):584–593.
6. Ishida M, Takeuchi S. Vitrectomy for the treatment of expulsive hemorrhage. *Jpn J Ophthalmol.* 2000;44(5):571.
7. Moshfeghi DM, Kim BY, Kaiser PK, et al. Appositional suprachoroidal hemorrhage: A case-control study. *Am J Ophthalmol.* 2004;138(6):959–963.
8. Obuchowska I, Mariak Z, Stankiewicz A. [The risk factors for massive suprachoroidal hemorrhage in the material of the Department of Ophthalmology, Medical Academy in Bialystok from 1990 to 2000]. *Klin Oczna.* 2002;104(2):89–92.
9. Romero Aroca P, Salvat Serra M, Mendez Marin I. [Suprachoroidal bleeding: review and description of eight cases]. *J Fr Ophtalmol.* 2003;26(2):164–168.
10. Maguluri S, Bueno CL, Fuller IB, et al. Delayed suprachoroidal hemorrhage and factor VIII deficiency. *Am J Ophthalmol.* 2005;139(1):195–197.
11. Haring G, Behrendt S, Wiechens B, et al. [Severe intra- and postoperative suprachoroid hemorrhage. Risk factors, therapy, results]. *Ophthalmologe.* 1999;96(12):822–828.
12. Chandra A, Jazayeri F, Williamson TH. Warfarin in vitreoretinal surgery: A case controlled series. *Br J Ophthalmol.* 2011;95(7):976–978.
13. Tabandeh H, Sullivan PM, Smahliuk P, et al. Suprachoroidal hemorrhage during pars plana vitrectomy. Risk factors and outcomes. *Ophthalmology.* 1999;106(2):236–242.
14. Ghoraba HH, Zayed AI. Suprachoroidal hemorrhage as a complication of vitrectomy. *Ophthalmic Surg Lasers.* 2001;32(4):281–288.
15. Mei H, Xing Y, Yang A, et al. Suprachoroidal hemorrhage during pars plana vitrectomy in traumatized eyes. *Retina.* 2009;29(4):473–476.
16. Lakhanpal V, Schocket SS, Elman MJ, et al. Intraoperative massive suprachoroidal hemorrhage during pars plana vitrectomy. *Ophthalmology.* 1990;97(9):1114–1119.
17. Kapamajian M, Gonzales CR, Gupta A, et al. Suprachoroidal hemorrhage as an intraoperative complication of 25-gauge pars plana vitrectomy. *Semin Ophthalmol.* 2007;22(3):197–199.

18. Ojima Y, Tsujikawa A, Otani A, et al. Recurrent bleeding after photodynamic therapy in polypoidal choroidal vasculopathy. *Am J Ophthalmol.* 2006;141(5):958–960.
19. Tan CS, Wong HT, Lim BA, et al. Polypoidal choroidal vasculopathy causing massive suprachoroidal haemorrhage. *Eye (Lond).* 2007;21(1):132–133.
20. Pollack AL, McDonald HR, Ai E, et al. Massive suprachoroidal hemorrhage during pars plana vitrectomy associated with Valsalva maneuver. *Am J Ophthalmol.* 2001; 132(3):383–387.
21. Ooto S, Kimura D, Itoi K, et al. Suprachoroidal fluid as a complication of 23-gauge vitreous surgery. *Br J Ophthalmol.* 2008;92(10):1433–1434.
22. Chen CJ, Satofuka S, Inoue M, et al. Suprachoroidal hemorrhage caused by breakage of a 25-gauge cannula. *Ophthalmic Surg Lasers Imaging.* 2008;39(4):323–324.
23. Beyer CF, Peyman GA, Hill JM. Expulsive choroidal hemorrhage in rabbits. A histopathologic study. *Arch Ophthalmol.* 1989;107(11):1648–1653.
24. Manschot WA. The pathology of expulsive hemorrhage. *Am J Ophthalmol.* 1955; 40(1):15–24.
25. Tabandeh H, Flynn HW Jr. Suprachoroidal hemorrhage during pars plana vitrectomy. *Curr Opin Ophthalmol.* 2001;12(3):179–185.
26. Wolter JR. Expulsive hemorrhage: A study of histopathological details. *Graefes Arch Clin Exp Ophthalmol.* 1982;219(4):155–158.
27. Zauberman H. Expulsive choroidal haemorrhage: An experimental study. *Br J Ophthalmol.* 1982;66(1):43–45.
28. Chu TG, Cano MR, Green RL, et al. Massive suprachoroidal hemorrhage with central retinal apposition. A clinical and echographic study. *Arch Ophthalmol.* 1991;109(11):1575–1581.
29. Reynolds MG, Haimovici R, Flynn HW Jr, et al. Suprachoroidal hemorrhage. Clinical features and results of secondary surgical management. *Ophthalmology.* 1993;100(4):460–465.
30. Gloor B, Kalman A. [Choroidal effusion and expulsive hemorrhage in penetrating interventions–lesson from 26 patients]. *Klin Monbl Augenheilkd.* 1993;202(3):224–237.
31. Le Quoy O, Girard P. [Postoperative choroidal hemorrhage. Surgical indications]. *J Fr Ophtalmol.* 1995;18(2):96–105.
32. Wei W, Yang W, Wang J. [Secondary surgical management of massive suprachoroidal hemorrhage]. *Zhonghua Yan Ke Za Zhi.* 1998;34(6):408–410, 26.
33. Ruderman JM, Harbin TS Jr, Campbell DG. Postoperative suprachoroidal hemorrhage following filtration procedures. *Arch Ophthalmol.* 1986;104(2):201–205.
34. Desai UR, Peyman GA, Chen CJ, et al. Use of perfluoroperhydrophenanthrene in the management of suprachoroidal hemorrhages. *Ophthalmology.* 1992;99(10):1542–1547.
35. Becquet F, Caputo G, Mashhour B, et al. Management of delayed massive suprachoroidal hemorrhage: A clinical retrospective study. *Eur J Ophthalmol.* 1996; 6(4):393–397.
36. Lee SC, Lee I, Koh HJ, et al. Massive suprachoroidal hemorrhage with retinal and vitreous incarceration; a vitreoretinal surgical approach. *Korean J Ophthalmol.* 2000; 14(1):41–44.
37. Nadarajah S, Kon C, Rassam S. Early controlled drainage of massive suprachoroidal hemorrhage with the aid of an expanding gas bubble and risk factors. *Retina.* 2011;32(3):543–548.
38. Glatt H, Machemer R. Experimental subretinal hemorrhage in rabbits. *Am J Ophthalmol.* 1982;94(6):762–773.
39. Toth CA, Morse LS, Hjelmeland LM, et al. Fibrin directs early retinal damage after subretinal hemorrhage. *Arch Ophthalmol.* 1991;109(5):723–729.
40. Scott IU, Flynn HW Jr, Schiffman J, et al. Visual acuity outcomes among patients with appositional suprachoroidal hemorrhage. *Ophthalmology.* 1997;104(12):2039–2046.

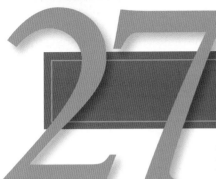

27

REFRACTIVE CHANGES ASSOCIATED with VITREORETINAL SURGERY

DAVID STEEL

Although not a primary objective of vitreoretinal surgery, refractive changes occur to greater or lesser extents with a number of vitreoretinal procedures and are important to consider.

The Complication

How to Avoid It/How to Reduce It

Refractive Changes Associated with Scleral Buckles

Scleral buckling clearly alters the shape of the globe, but the degree of refractive change after scleral buckling surgery is related to the type of scleral buckle used.

Encirclement using scleral resection or sutures to provide the indentation effect will result in axial length shortening with a hypermetropic shift. The more common technique of encirclement using a buckle that is shortened to produce the desired indentation will lengthen an eye with inducement of 2.5 to 3 diopters (D) of myopia per 1 mm of axial length elongation resulting in approximately 1.5 D of myopia in most cases. The amount of induced myopia is said to be greater in phakic eyes compared to aphakic ones secondary to anterior displacement of the lens; however, some studies have not found this.[1] There is also a variable degree of irregular astigmatism induced which usually decreases somewhat over time. Segmental buckles have been variably associated with induced astigmatism with the axis of the induced change corresponding to the position of the buckle. The degree of induced change is greater as the buckle becomes more anterior particularly for radial sponges. The astigmatic effect reduces over time in cases where there is no encircling band as the indentation effect fades.[2,3]

It has been observed that there is greater irregular corneal astigmatism and higher-order aberrations induced by segmental buckles than encirclement on its own, with the direction of coma aberration again corresponding to the scleral buckle position. The degree of higher-order aberration change is approximately equal to that occurring when using spherical IOLs during cataract surgery.[4]

Interestingly, in a study from Japan on children undergoing encircling scleral buckling surgery with diathermy, there was a reduction in myopic shift in the years following surgery compared to the fellow nonoperated eyes in children under 10 years old. The authors hypothesized that this was probably due to impeded ocular growth.[5]

Refractive Changes Associated with Pars Plana Vitrectomy

A steepening in corneal topography is reported in the first week following 20G vitrectomy most marked in the meridians of the sclerostomies (and related to suturing), which normalizes however by week 12. 23G surgery is associated with approximately half as much and 25G by approximately quarter as much as 20G surgery. Astigmatic changes normalize by 1 month after 25G surgery compared to 2 to 3 months for 20G surgery. Gas tamponade appears to have no effect on the steepening observed.[5-10]

Refractive Changes Associated with Vitrectomy Prior to or After Phacoemulsification

For refractive changes associated with phacovitrectomy, see Chapter 20D.

Vitrectomy Prior to Phacoemulsification

Although some work suggests the possibility of a small positive shift secondary to increased anterior chamber depth in contradistinction to phacovitrectomy, there is no clear evidence of any shift in refraction when phacoemulsification is performed after vitrectomy compared to nonvitrectomized eyes.[11-13]

Vitrectomy After Phacoemulsification (Vitrectomy in Pseudophakic Eyes)

There is scarce evidence suggesting a small myopic shift in refraction after 20G vitrectomy with scleral tunnels in pseudophakic eyes. No changes were seen in the anterior chamber depth and it was hypothesized that the myopic shift could be secondary to increased axial length with scleral stretch. In support of this, the author has observed that a myopic shift does not occur in pseudophakic eyes after narrow gauge vitrectomy.[14]

Refractive Changes Related to Sulcus Positioned Intraocular Lenses

The necessity to place a posterior chamber intraocular lens (IOL) in the ciliary sulcus supported by the anterior lens capsule as opposed to the regular in the bag placement is a common scenario for VR surgeons, particularly, after dropped nucleus surgery or after lensectomy. Due to the more anterior position of the IOL, the "effective power" of the IOL increases and the IOL power has to be decreased to achieve the desired refraction. Eyes with an average axial length of approximately 23 mm require a reduction of IOL power of 1 D in most studies.[15,16] Several useful nomograms and tables are published to allow calculation of the power adjustment necessary to achieve the desired refraction (http://doctor-hill.com/iol-main/bag-sulcus.htm). Power reduction is predicted to increase as IOL power increases ranging from a 0.5D reduction in IOLs under 16 D to a reduction of 1.5 D in IOLs greater than 29 D (i.e., approximately a reduction of 1/20 of the bag IOL power as Cartwright et al.[17] have observed). However, others have suggested that the power needed to be removed does not vary as much as theory suggests, and removal of fixed values from 0.5 D[18] to, 1.25 to 1.5 D[19] in all cases have been suggested. It seems that the effective IOL position changes more in myopic eyes than predicted and the relationship between the anterior chamber depth and axial length is variable. Optic capture of the IOL in the remaining anterior capsulorhexis, if present, might be expected to reduce the power reduction required. Similarly, IOL design and material may influence parameters such as angulation and size of the haptics that can affect the postoperative refraction obtained. Personalized audit data with the sulcus IOL normally used is required for optimum results.

Refractive Changes Occurring Following the Use of Silicone Oil

Silicone oil tamponade, having a higher refractive index than that of vitreous, alters the refractive power of an eye. The degree of refractive change depends on the type of oil used and the lens status of the eye. Different tamponade agents are associated with different speeds of transmission of light and hence have different refractive indices. The refractive index of 1,300 cs oil has been quoted as 1.405; 5,000 cs oil, 1.3990; and 5,700 cs oil, 1.3985 (Compared with 1.3346 for vitreous). In an aphakic eye, oil forms a convex shape at the pupil resulting in a positive lens effect of 6 to 8 D and a refractive change often enough to provide a near emmetropic refraction in an aphakic, previously myopic eye. In phakic eyes, the oil forms a concave lens effect against the posterior surface of the lens with a hypermetropic shift in refraction of 5 to 8 D. The situation is more complex in pseudophakic eyes as it depends on the IOL geometry. Silicone oil insertion in patients with biconvex IOLs, the commonest type in use, results in a refractive change of approximately 3 to 5 D so that the patient is 3 to 5 D more hypermetropic when the oil is in and has a 3 to 5 D myopic shift when it is removed. The refractive effect will also vary with the type of oil used and the completeness of the oil fill.[20–25]

How to Avoid/Reduce Refractive Errors When Selecting the Intraocular Lens Power in Eyes with Silicone Oil

IOL Power Calculation Prior to Combined Cataract Extraction and Oil Removal

When A-scan ultrasonography is used to measure axial length in silicone-filled eyes, an artifactually long value is obtained because of the reduction in the speed of ultrasound through the oil. The easiest solution to this problem is perhaps to measure all eyes before oil insertion; there are a many reasons; however, why this may not have been done or done accurately (e.g., if it was done following scleral buckling surgery or in the presence of a retinal detachment etc.). Values from the fellow eye are occasionally used but significant error can result. Nepp et al. found that 26% of fellow eyes were greater than 1 mm different (= 2.5 to 3 D) in axial length to the operative eye.[26] A variety of approaches have thus been adopted to solve this problem when planned cataract extraction combined with oil removal is to be undertaken.

The length of the silicone oil-filled vitreous cavity can be calculated separately and added to the other measurements. The correct measurement of each eye-length component can be calculated by using the ratio of the correct sound velocity in the medium being measured by the velocity assumed by the machine.[27] Siddiqui et al.[28] have recently published a useful list of speeds of transmission of A-scan ultrasound through different tamponade agents which can be used to calculate true lengths (Table 27-1). So, in practice, the eye is measured using the aphakic sound velocity settings (measured using an assumed velocity of 1,532 m/s). The scan is then used to measure the individual components—anterior chamber depth, lens thickness, and vitreous length (as well as any retrosilicone space, if present). Each individual true length is then calculated and the results added to provide a true axial length for IOL calculation (see Figure 27-1 for an example). The scan must be done in the upright posture and as perpendicular to the eye as possible. Time must also be taken to allow the oil to settle into a stable position. Larkin et al.[29] used a conversion factor of 0.64 for the vitreous cavity length; however, this does not take into account any fluid-filled retrosilicone space and also does not take into account different oil types.

Murray et al.[30] simplified the calculation by using a conversion factor of 0.71 on the measured axial length value from ultrasound in standard phakic mode using 1,300 cs oil and achieved an acceptable average mean error in achieved versus predicted IOL power of 0.74 D with 71% within 0.5 D. Again other viscosities of oil would require different conversion factors based on their relative refractive indices.

Other authors have avoided these calculations by simply measuring the axial length following oil removal prior to IOL insertion and Gupta et al.[31] achieved a mean absolute prediction error (MAE) of 0.74 D using this technique compared to 1.34 D using the conversion factor of 0.71 D suggested by Murray et al.[30] Indeed

Table 27-1 • Correct Measurement = (Vc/Vm) × measurement (Where Vc = Correct Velocity in the Medium Being Measured; Vm = Aphakic Velocity in Aqueous of 1,532 m/s)	
1,000 cs oil[a]	976 m/s[a]
5,000 cs oil[a]	970 m/s[a]
Oxane HD	930 m/s
Densiron	914 m/s
Perfluorodecalin	645 m/s
Human lens	1,641 m/s
PMMA	2,718 m/s
Silicone IOL	980 m/s
Acrylic IOL	2,120 m/s

Adapted from Siddiqui MA, Awan MA, Fairhead A, et al. Ultrasound velocity in heavy ocular tamponade agents and implications for biometry. *Br J Ophthalmol.* 2011;95(1):142–144.

All values given at 37 c.

[a]Please note the exact value may vary with brand used—the 1,000 cs and 5,000 cs oil used for these values was from Medicel AG, Widnau, Switzerland. Other papers quote values of 1,040 for 5,000 cs oil.

El-Baha and Hemeida[32] have shown that refractive results as accurate as partial coherence interferometry (PCI) can be achieved using intraoperative biometry following oil removal.

Optical biometry using PCI and the IOL master (Carl Zeiss, Germany) allows easy calculation of IOL power if accurate fixation is possible and the cataract is not too dense. Internal algorithms adjust the measured axial length when "silicone-filled eye" in the axial length settings are selected (http://doctor-hill.com/iol-main/silicone.htm). Habibabadi et al.[33] achieved a mean postoperative prediction error of −0.30 D using this system with 54% of patients within 0.5 D and 70% within 1 D. The authors noted, however, that PCI could not be performed in 38% of patients, either because of a dense cataract or because of technical problems. Clinical results suggest that the settings do not need to be changed with heavy silicone oil.[34]

A further alternative is a simple technique recently described by Patwardhan et al.[35] using intraoperative retinoscopy. Retinoscopy was performed using a vertex

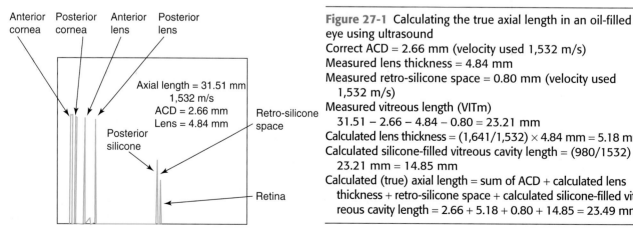

Figure 27-1 Calculating the true axial length in an oil-filled eye using ultrasound
Correct ACD = 2.66 mm (velocity used 1,532 m/s)
Measured lens thickness = 4.84 mm
Measured retro-silicone space = 0.80 mm (velocity used 1,532 m/s)
Measured vitreous length (VITm)
    31.51 − 2.66 − 4.84 − 0.80 = 23.21 mm
Calculated lens thickness = (1,641/1,532) × 4.84 mm = 5.18 mm
Calculated silicone-filled vitreous cavity length = (980/1532) × 23.21 mm = 14.85 mm
Calculated (true) axial length = sum of ACD + calculated lens thickness + retro-silicone space + calculated silicone-filled vitreous cavity length = 2.66 + 5.18 + 0.80 + 14.85 = 23.49 mm

distance of 13 mm and distance of 50 cm. All eyes had in-the-bag implantation of a foldable IOL with an A-constant of 118.4. The IOL power was calculated using the Lanchulev formula as follows: R × 2.0145. The postoperative refractive error was within ±0.50 D in four eyes (33.3%) and within ±1.00D in all eyes.

Finally, CT scanning and MRI can be used to give results of similar accuracy to ultrasonography. Fine slices are needed to maximize accuracy and assess the foveal position. Good head and eye orientation is also needed to make the scan as sagittal as possible. This would certainly be an option in situations where PCI and ultrasound are either impossible or unreliable, for example, dense cataracts, silicone emulsification, silicone underfill, or myopic eyes with posterior staphylomas.[36,37]

A potential source of error in IOL calculation in this situation is that some authors have found a reduction in axial length following oil removal[38]; however, others have found an increase[39] but overall most surgeons have found no change.

IOL Calculation in Oil-Filled Eyes When Cataract Extraction Is Planned and Oil Is to Be Left in Place

If silicone oil is to remain in the eye, then the IOL power needs to be adjusted to prevent significant postoperative hypermetropia. The two effects that need to be considered are the following:

1. Oil has a higher refractive index than that of vitreous and hence a higher-power IOL is needed to achieve the same intended postoperative refraction. This can be calculated using the following formula:

Power to be added to IOL ("ΔP") = (Refractive index of oil – refractive index of vitreous) **divided by** (true or calculated axial length – anterior chamber depth) **multiplied by** 1,000.

The anterior chamber depth is that supplied by the IOL manufacturer for the IOL used. The distance required is from the anterior cornea to the posterior surface of the IOL. If not available, the ACD can be estimated by the formula:

ACD = (0.292 multiplied by axial length) – 2.93 + IOL thickness
(= ~4.8 mm for an average length eye)

Meldrum et al.[40] have provided common values for this:

Axial Length (mm)	Approximate Power to Be Added (Diopters)
20	4
23	3.5
25	3.25
28	3

2. The refractive power of the posterior surface of the IOL/oil interface will also be altered. If a standard biconvex IOL is used, then the effect of the reduced power of the posterior surface needs to be allowed for: a 20-D biconvex IOL could lose between one-third and one-fourth of its power in this situation. Again, Meldrum et al. have provided an equation to calculate this. An important point here is that some IOLs have fixed anterior curvatures and alter the posterior curvature to change power (e.g., Alcon MA50BM)—while other IOLs use a fixed posterior curvature for a limited range of IOL powers and alter the anterior curvature to change the power within that range (e.g., Alcon MA60AC). The situation is hence quite complex.

Table 27-2 • An Example of Working Out IOL Power in an Oil-Filled Eye When Cataract Extraction Is Planned and Oil Is to Be Left in Place

True axial length = 23.49 mm

Acrylic folding biconvex IOL to be used

Supplied ACD = 4.8 mm

Back radius of IOL in dioptric range considered = 25 mm
(see http://www.google.com/patents/US20110242482?printsec=drawing#v=onepage&q&f=false for data for an Alcon MA60AC IOL)

5,000 cs oil used (In this particular instance the manufacturer quotes a refractive index of 1.399)

Planned postoperative refraction in vitreous-filled eye = 0 with a 22 D IOL in a normal eye

1) Power to be added to IOL("ΔP") = refractive index of oil (1.399) – refractive index of vitreous (1.336) **divided by** (true or calculated axial length (23.49) – anterior chamber depth (4.8) **multiplied by** 1,000 = 3.37 D

2) Adjustment needed (a negative value in the case of a biconvex IOL) "ΔI" = refractive index of oil (1.399) – refractive index of vitreous (1.336) **divided by** back radius of IOL (R) in millimeters **multiplied by** 1,000 = −2.52 D

Total adjustment = 3.33 + (−2.52) = +0.86D

So if a 22-D lens had been planned, a 23-D one should be inserted.

Adjustment needed (a negative value in the case of a biconvex IOL) "ΔI" = Refractive index of oil – refractive index of vitreous **divided by** back radius of IOL (R) in millimeters **multiplied by** 1,000 (Note: R is negative for a biconvex IOL and positive for a meniscus IOL).

Hence the total power = $\Delta P + \Delta I$ + IOL power for desired refraction with a normal vitreous (see Table 27-2 for an example).

Certain IOL formulas (including the Holladay IOL Consultant) will usefully, automatically adjust for the type of IOL used in this situation.

A PMMA convex–plano IOL with the plano side facing the oil has been recommended (http://doctor-hill.com/iol-main/silicone.htm) (PMMA has a refractive index close to that of oil: 1.491 vs. 1.403). If this type of lens is used, then the change in power will be less effected by oil in the vitreous cavity but some adjustment will still be needed. Light entering the IOL will be convergent after refraction from the anterior IOL surface and cornea—these convergent rays will be diverged as they pass through the posterior IOL and into the oil resulting in a relative hypermetropic shift and a reduction in IOL power.

McCartney et al.[41] showed that a meniscus (convex–concave) IOL produces the lowest hyperopic shift with oil. Indeed, recently Baraki and Peterson[42] used a meniscus-type IOL (where the posterior radius of curvature matched the vitreous cavity length) with optic capture posteriorly through a posterior capsulorhexis. They found a difference in refraction of only 0.22 D with and without oil making this type of IOL especially suitable for cases where the question of long-term oil tamponade is uncertain (e.g., the hydrophilic three-piece CT 59RET from Carl Zeiss).

It should be noted that these discussions and calculations assume a 100% oil fill—an oil fill of less than this will result in variations in the contact of the oil with the back surface of the IOL and a less predictable and variable refraction.

REFERENCES

1. Smiddy WE, Loupe DN, Michels RG, et al. Refractive changes after scleral buckling surgery. *Arch Ophthalmol.* 1989;107(10):1469–1471.
2. Abdullah AS, Jan S, Qureshi MS, et al. Complications of conventional scleral buckling occurring during and after treatment of rhegmatogenous retinal detachment. *J Coll Physicians Surg Pak.* 2010;20(5):321–326.
3. Li YM, Xu YS, Shen LP, et al. [Anterior corneal topographic changes after scleral buckling surgery] Zhongguo Yi Xue Ke Xue Yuan Xue Bao. 2005;27(6):734–738.
4. Okamoto F, Yamane N, Okamoto C, et al. Changes in higher-order aberrations after scleral buckling surgery for rhegmatogenous retinal detachment. *Ophthalmology.* 2008;115(7):1216–1221.
5. Sato T, Kawasaki T, Okuyama M, et al. Refractive changes following scleral buckling surgery in juvenile retinal detachment. *Retina.* 2003;23(5):629–635.
6. Kim YK, Hyon JY, Woo SJ, et al. Surgically induced astigmatism after 23-gauge transconjunctival sutureless vitrectomy. *Eye (Lond).* 2010;24(5):799–804.
7. Galway G, Drury B, Cronin BG, et al. A comparison of induced astigmatism in 20- vs 25-gauge vitrectomy procedures. *Eye (Lond).* 2010;24(2):315–317.
8. Avitabile T, Castiglione F, Bonfiglio V, et al. Transconjunctival sutureless 25-gauge versus 20-gauge standard vitrectomy: correlation between corneal topography and ultrasound biomicroscopy measurements of sclerotomy sites. *Cornea.* 2010;29(1):19–25.
9. Park DH, Shin JP, Kim SY. Surgically induced astigmatism in combined phacoemulsification and vitrectomy; 23-gauge transconjunctival sutureless vitrectomy versus 20-gauge standard vitrectomy. *Graefes Arch Clin Exp Ophthalmol.* 2009;247(10):1331–1337.
10. Citirik M, Batman C, Bicer T, et al. Keratometric alterations following the 25-gauge transconjunctival sutureless pars plana vitrectomy versus the conventional pars plana vitrectomy. *Clin Exp Optom.* 2009;92:416–420.
11. Yang SJ, Kim TI, Jo BJ et al. Effect of vitreous on the anterior chamber depth after cataract surgery. *J Korean Ophthalmol Soc.* 2004;45:1446–1450.
12. Lee NY, Park SH, Joo CK. Refractive outcomes of phacoemulsification and intraocular lens implantation after pars plana vitrectomy. *Retina.* 2009;29(4):487–491.
13. Manvikar SR, Allen D, Steel DH. Optical biometry in combined phacovitrectomy. *J Cataract Refract Surg.* 2009;35(1):64–69.
14. Byrne S, Ng J, Hildreth A, et al. Refractive change following pseudophakic vitrectomy. *BMC Ophthalmol.* 2008;8:19.
15. Suto C, Hori S, Fukuyama E, et al. Adjusting intraocular lens power for sulcus fixation. *J Cataract Refract Surg.* 2003;29(10):1913–1917.
16. http://doctor-hill.com/iol-main/bag-sulcus.htm (accessed 14/8/11).
17. Knox Cartwright NE, Aristodemou P, Sparrow JM, et al. Adjustment of intraocular lens power for sulcus implantation. *J Cataract Refract Surg.* 2011;37(4):798–799.
18. Spokes DM, Norris JH, Ball JL. Refinement of lens power selection for sulcus placement of intraocular lens. *J Cataract Refract Surg.* 2010;36(8):1436–1437.
19. Bayramlar H, Hepsen IF, Yilmaz H. Myopic shift from the predicted refraction after sulcus fixation of PMMA posterior chamber intraocular lenses. *Can J Ophthalmol.* 2006;41(1):78–82.
20. Stefansson E, Anderson MM Jr, Landers MB 3rd, et al. Refractive changes from use of silicone oil in vitreous surgery. *Retina.* 1988;8:20–23.
21. Smith RC, Smith GT, Wong D. Refractive changes in silicone filled eyes. *Eye.* 1990;4:230–234.
22. Seo MS, Lim ST, Kim HD, et al. Changes in refraction and axial length according to the viscosity of intraocular silicone oil. *Korean J Ophthalmol.* 1999;13(1):25–29.
23. Song WK, Kim SS, Kim SE, et al. Refractive status and visual acuity changes after oil removal in eyes following phacovitrectomy, intraocular lens implantation, and silicone oil tamponade. *Can J Ophthalmol.* 2010;45(6):616–620.
24. Dick HB, Schwenn O, Pavlovic S, et al. Effect of head position on refraction in aphakic and phakic silicone-filled eyes. *Retina.* 1997;17(5):397–402.

25. Murray DC, Potamitis T, Good P, et al. Biometry of the silicone oil-filled eye. *Eye (Lond)*. 1999;13:319–324.

26. Nepp J, Krepler K, Jandrasits K, et al. Biometry and refractive outcome of eyes filled with silicone oil by standardized echography and partial coherence interferometry. *Graefes Arch Clin Exp Ophthalmol*. 2005;243(10):967–972.

27. Chi-Wah Yung. IOL determination in eyes with silicone oil. http://eyeatlas.medicine. iu.edu/wp/residents/ (accessed 21/7/11).

28. Siddiqui MA, Awan MA, Fairhead A, et al. Ultrasound velocity in heavy ocular tamponade agents and implications for biometry. *Br J Ophthalmol*. 2011;95(1):142–144.

29. Larkin GB, Flaxel CJ, Leaver PK. Phacoemulsification and silicone oil removal through a single corneal incision. *Ophthalmology*. 1998;105:2023–2027.

30. Murray DC, Durrani OM, Good P, et al. Biometry of the silicone oil-filled eye: II. *Eye (Lond)*. 2002;16:727–730.

31. Gupta C, Shroff CM, Singh AK, et al. To evaluate the accuracy of conversion factor 0.71 proposed by Murray et al to calculate axial length vs intra operative axial length measurement in silicone oil filled eyes. *AIOS*. 2008 http://www.aios.org/proceed08/ papers/RV-I/RV-I2.pdf (accessed 14/7/11).

32. El-Baha SM, Hemeida TS. Comparison of refractive outcome using intraoperative biometry and partial coherence interferometry in silicone oil-filled eyes. *Retina*. 2009;29(1):64–68.

33. Habibabadi HF, Hashemi H, Jalali KH, et al. Refractive outcome of silicone oil removal and intraocular lens implantation using laser interferometry. *Retina*. 2005; 25(2):162–166.

34. Roessler GF, Huth JK, Dietlein TS, et al. Accuracy and reproducibility of axial length measurement in eyes with silicone oil endotamponade. *Br J Ophthalmol*. 2009;93(11):1492–1494.

35. Patwardhan SD, Azad R, Sharma Y, et al. Intraoperative retinoscopy for intraocular lens power estimation in cases of combined phacoemulsification and silicone oil removal. *J Cataract Refract Surg*. 2009;35(7):1190–1192.

36. Bencic G, Vatavuk Z, Marotti M, et al. Comparison of A-scan and MRI for the measurement of axial length in silicone oil-filled eyes. *Br J Ophthalmol*. 2009;93(4): 502–505.

37. Takei K, Sekine Y, Okamoto F, et al. Measurement of axial length of eyes with incomplete filling of silicone oil in the vitreous cavity using x ray computed tomography. *Br J Ophthalmol*. 2002;86(1):47–50.

38. Wang K, Yuan MK, Jiang YR, et al. Axial length measurements before and after removal of silicone oil: A new method to correct the axial length of silicone-filled eyes for optical biometry. *Ophthalmic Physiol Opt*. 2009;29(4):449–457.

39. Parravano M, Oddone F, Sampalmieri M, et al. Reliability of the IOLMaster in axial length evaluation in silicone oil-filled eyes. *Eye (Lond)*. 2007;21(7):909–911.

40. Meldrum ML, Aaberg TM, Patel A, et al. Cataract extraction after silicone oil repair of retinal detachments due to necrotizing retinitis. *Arch Ophthalmol*. 1996;114(7): 885–892.

41. McCartney DL, Miller KM, Stark WJ, et al. Intraocular lens style and refraction in eyes treated with silicone oil. *Arch Ophthalmol*. 1987;105(10):1385–1387.

42. Baraki H, Petersen J. [How can the shift of refraction due to vitreous substitutes be avoided? Posterior chamber intraocular lens for patients suffering from diabetic retinopathy]. *Ophthalmologe*. 2011;108(7):683–636.

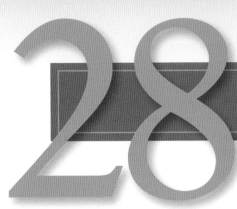

28 DIPLOPIA AND STRABISMUS

HOWARD YING AND DAVID GUYTON

The Complication: Definition

The complication addressed here is diplopia and/or strabismus after vitreoretinal surgery. Diplopia is the simultaneous perception of two images of a single object. The two images may originate from the same eye (monocular diplopia) or from misregistration of both eyes (binocular diplopia). Common causes of monocular diplopia include an irregular refractive error, media opacity, corneal irregularity, an iris defect, cataract, crystalline lens subluxation, and a warped or subluxated intraocular lens implant. Binocular diplopia is caused by loss of normal binocular retinal correspondence, which in turn, results either from misalignment of the eyes (or misalignment of just the foveas), or from aniseikonia. Foveal misalignment may arise from impaired function of the extraocular muscles, from mechanical scarring of the extraocular muscles or of the connective tissue surrounding the eye, from retinal distortion allowing peripheral fusion but with foveal misalignment, or from sensory mechanisms triggered by prolonged monocular occlusion after vitreoretinal surgery. Aniseikonia (different image sizes appreciated by the brain) may arise from monocular retinal distortion or from large differences in refractive error. For cases with retinal distortion, there is usually both micropsia (smaller distorted image size) and diplopia that is heterogeneous across the affected area.[1] If the retina is folded or contracted, rather than stretched, the distorted image will be larger than normal because the optical image covers more photoreceptors.

Unintentional displacement of the retina after otherwise successful rhegmatogenous retinal detachment repair may be detected using fundus autofluorescence (FAF) imaging. FAF imaging may show hyperfluorescent lines which appear to correspond to areas of retinal pigment epithelium with increased metabolic activity that were shielded from the light by major retinal vessels preoperatively. Retinal displacement after primary vitrectomy was found in 27 of 43 eyes studied (63%) and was more often associated with larger or macula-involving detachments. None of the patients in this series, however, had symptomatic diplopia.[2] Displacement of retinal vessels has also occurred after a scleral buckling procedure and resulted in symptomatic diplopia in 3 of 5 eyes in another series. Postoperative visual acuity measured 20/20 to 20/60 at the 6-month follow-up visit, indicating that such displacement is not always associated with poor visual acuity outcome[3] and is consistent with the observation that symptomatic diplopia is often associated with better visual acuity.

Risk Factors

Risk factors identified by population-based epidemiologic studies would be reliable, but no population-based longitudinal studies have included a significant number of patients undergoing vitreoretinal surgery, so population-based risk factor analysis of diplopia and strabismus in such patients has not been useful. Risk factors mechanistically related to the specific etiology in prospective case-control series are more prone to bias and confounding factors but constitute the bulk of the available data. For example, strabismus incidence is 4% to 43% following scleral buckling procedures[4–6] and occurs after both scleral buckling (30%) and vitrectomy (24%) procedures.[7,8] Case-control risk factors for strabismus after vitreoretinal surgery include: Pre-existing or latent misalignment, sensory deviations, local anesthetic myotoxicity, direct muscle injury, scleral buckling (mechanical effects, secondary scarring, anisometropia from myopic shift, mal-repositioning of a detached muscle, or capture of an oblique muscle), and retinal distortion and/or torsion from macular translocation procedures. Retrospective review of these risk factors has shown that scleral buckling under general anesthesia is much less likely to cause strabismus than scleral buckling under local anesthesia, consistent with local anesthetic myotoxicity being a major etiologic factor.[9] We shall describe in detail the pathogenesis, strategies for prevention, solutions, and expected outcomes below.

PRE-EXISTING OR LATENT STRABISMUS

Pathogenesis

2.1% to 3.3% of people in the United States develop strabismus in childhood,[10,11] and adults can develop strabismus from diseases such as thyroid eye disease, myasthenia gravis, cranial nerve palsies, phoria decompensation, and acquired foveal dystopia. All of these patients are at high risk for manifest, symptomatic strabismus after vitreoretinal surgery. Other diseases, such as pathologic myopia,[12] retinopathy of prematurity,[13–15] and diabetes,[16,17] confer increased risk for both strabismus and the need for vitreoretinal surgery. Vitreoretinal disease often causes poor vision, possibly rendering a pre-existing strabismic condition asymptomatic by the patient and overlooked by the vitreoretinal surgeon so that the problem becomes apparent only after the successful vitreoretinal procedure when there is improvement in vision in the affected eye.[18] Sensory mechanisms resulting from intraocular tamponade and prolonged occlusion in the convalescent period may unveil latent strabismus.[19–21] Finally, a significant change in the angle of strabismus may move the object of regard out of a suppression scotoma and cause pre-existing strabismus to become symptomatic.[22]

Pearls on How to Prevent It

◆ Preoperative recognition by retinal surgeons or referral to strabismus specialists.

◆ Obtain ophthalmic history of prior patching or strabismus therapy.

◆ Observe head tilt currently and in old photographs.

◆ Perform forced ductions during surgery to diagnose subclinical restrictive pathology as in thyroid eye disease.

◆ Perform prompt vitreoretinal surgery to prevent sensory deviations.

Pearls on How to Solve It

◆ Inform the patient of the pre-existing condition.

◆ Provide prompt referral to a strabismus specialist.

◆ Treat the strabismus with Fresnel prisms for temporary relief of small angles of deviation, orthoptic training to improve control of the deviation, botulinum toxin injection, or extraocular muscle surgery to restore muscle balance.

The expected outcome is treatment of the strabismus as above. The worst-case scenario is constant central diplopia despite central alignment (horror fusionis) or persistence of central misalignment and diplopia despite superimposition and fusion of the peripheral visual fields (the dragged-fovea diplopia syndrome). In either case, the patient may require occlusion of the vision of one eye in the direction(s) of gaze where the diplopia is most symptomatic.

LOCAL ANESTHETIC MYOTOXICITY

Pathogenesis

Peribulbar and retrobulbar injections of local anesthetic agents for both the anterior segment and posterior segment eye surgeries in the modern era are associated with the same pattern of muscle involvement, suggesting a common mechanism for postoperative strabismus.[23] Peribulbar and retrobulbar injections of local anesthetics may increase the risk for postoperative strabismus through several possible mechanisms: (1) direct mechanical damage from tearing muscle fibers with the needle,[24] (2) palsy from damage to an ocular motor nerve,[25] (3) ischemia from laceration of anterior ciliary vessels,[26] (4) compartment syndrome from intramuscular hematoma,[26] and (5) myotoxicity from the local anesthetic agent itself.[27] Local anesthetics, such as bupivacaine, cause inflammation and necrosis in a dose-dependent fashion when injected directly into the extraocular muscles.[28] Subsequently, the inflammation and necrosis lead to variable proportions of hypertrophy and fibrosis of the injected muscle. This results in an early underaction followed by a late overaction of the involved muscle as hypertrophy and fibrosis occur. If this process is segmental, or primarily hypertrophy, overaction develops. If the process is primarily fibrosis involving a large portion of the muscle, restrictive strabismus occurs.[29] Scott et al.[30] have exploited this myotoxicity to increase the action of the lateral rectus muscle as a treatment for esotropia.

Pearls on How to Prevent It

◆ Retinal surgeons should recognize anesthetic myotoxicity as a potential problem and use the minimum amount of local anesthetic required.

◆ Avoid local anesthesia by using topical or general anesthesia instead.

◆ Avoid the muscle bellies with the retrobulbar needle by strict adherence to placing the needle at the border of the middle and lateral thirds of the lid margin.

◆ Use sub-Tenon's infusion to reduce the possibility of injection into an extraocular muscle.[31]

Pearls on How to Solve It

◆ Prescribe Fresnel prisms for temporary relief or small angles of deviation.

◆ Use orthoptic training to improve control of the deviation.

◆ Recess the fibrosed or overactive muscle, using adjustable sutures.

Spontaneous resolution may occur, but persistence beyond 2 months usually requires strabismus surgery for resolution. The worst-case scenario is persistent diplopia that is so incomitant that it is not amenable to prism therapy or strabismus surgery.

MECHANICAL EFFECTS OF SCLERAL BUCKLING AND/OR SECONDARY SCARRING

✥ Pathogenesis

Mechanical effects of scleral buckling and/or secondary scarring from vitreoretinal surgery may cause strabismus by changing the shape of the eye,[32] changing the vector force of the muscle from the buckle material,[33] myoscleral adhesions,[34] the fat adherence syndrome,[18] direct muscle injury, and mal-repositioning of a detached muscle. Restrictive fibrosis with both myoscleral adhesions and the fat adherence syndrome is associated with silastic implants and use of diathermy, but has been reported after all retinal reattachment surgeries.[35] Larger and circumferential buckles are associated with greater restriction in motility.[36,37] Direct muscle injury during surgery by blunt dissection with cotton-tip applicators,[38] prolonged stretching or twisting by traction sutures or muscle hooks, cryo application on a muscle, erosion of the tendon by anteriorly placed exoplants, accidental tenotomy, and mal-repositioning of a detached muscle have all been reported.

✥ Pearls on How to Prevent It

◆ Use smaller or segmental buckle elements and properly placed buckle elements at least 2 mm from muscle insertions.

◆ Avoid excessive cryo applications or diathermy.

◆ Refine technique to minimize operative trauma, including careful muscle dissection and traction, preservation of Tenon's capsule and muscle sleeves to prevent fat adherence,[31] avoidance of blunt dissection with cotton-tip applicators,[38] avoidance of cryo application directly to the muscle,[33] and careful repositioning of detached muscles.

◆ In cases where larger and circumferential buckles are unavoidable or after direct muscle injury has been recognized, instillation of an adjuvant to decrease postoperative fibrosis or inflammation is sensible; however, various agents, including sodium hyaluronate, mitomycin-C, 5-fluorouracil, triamcinolone, hydroxypropyl methylcellulose, and others have been used to limit scarring in a rabbit model without success. Systemic administration of corticosteroids, anecdotally, also appears to be ineffective in secondary prevention of this complication.

✥ Pearls on How to Solve It

◆ Freeing of adhesions is difficult because of uncertainty regarding which particular area of scar tissue caused the mechanical restriction,[39] the subsequent excitation of worse inflammatory fibrosis,[40] and increased risk for scleral perforation.[41]

◆ Removal of the scleral buckle may correct the inciting mechanism but is usually not sufficient to correct the strabismus.[42]

◆ Botulinum toxin injection to balance the muscle forces and neutralize the deviation may prove useful if the risk for retinal redetachment is high and buckle manipulations are to be avoided.[43,44] Selective injection into the belly of an extraocular muscle in the setting of marked orbital fibrosis, however, may prove challenging.

◆ Muscle recession/resection with adjustable sutures may be required for definitive correction of strabismus and is our treatment of choice. Note that one can leave the buckle in place and still recess or resect muscles either by using a nonabsorbable suture over the top of the buckle, or preferably, by threading the detached muscle under the buckle from the posterior edge so that the buckle itself helps to hold the muscle against the globe for proper healing.[9]

The expected outcome for large deviations is extraocular muscle surgery with or without scleral buckle removal. The worst-case scenario is retinal redetachment during extraocular muscle surgical manipulations (fortunately uncommon).

DRAGGED-FOVEA DIPLOPIA SYNDROME
Pathogenesis

The dragged-fovea diplopia syndrome most commonly occurs from retinal distortion near the fovea from an epiretinal membrane, a retinal scar, or retinal reattachment in a distorted manner. Peripheral fusion dominates so that if the fovea in one eye is displaced due to foveal dragging, central diplopia results. Symptoms may appear as a consequence of visual acuity improvement after peeling of a long-standing epiretinal membrane (the membrane decreased vision so much preoperatively that the distortion and central diplopia were not noted). This condition cannot be treated with prisms (diplopia returns within seconds to minutes). Likewise, it cannot be treated with eye muscle surgery. Peripheral fusion continues to win out over less strong central fusion, with persistent, recurring central diplopia. This is rarely seen with central vision worse than about 20/50, because then the brain is usually able to suppress the second image from that eye. The dragged-fovea diplopia syndrome, most often from an epiretinal membrane, should be suspected whenever there is a small, relatively comitant deviation, most always with a vertical component, not uncommonly occurring 1 to 3 years after intraocular surgery such as cataract surgery or laser retinopexy, most always with at least some distortion on Amsler grid testing, and only temporary response to trial prisms held before the eye. The diagnosis is most easily proven with the "lights on/off test." This test involves the use of a small-field central fusion target, such as a single white 20/70 letter on a black monitor screen. With the room lights on in a rich visual environment, the patient will see the single letter as double. When the room lights are suddenly extinguished, a positive result is recorded if the doubled letter becomes single, usually in 2 to 10 seconds. We found that this test is universally positive in patients with a central versus peripheral fusion conflict and a deviation within the patient's fusional range.[45]

Pearls on How to Prevent It

◆ Prompt epiretinal membrane peeling before retinal distortion becomes significant.

Pearls on How to Solve It

◆ Monocular occlusion

Expected outcome is selective occlusion using Scotch Satin (gift-wrap) tape on the rear surface of the spectacle lens.[45] Worst-case scenario is a complication from attempted surgical management of the diplopia.

ANISOMETROPIA AND ANISEIKONIA
Pathogenesis

Vitreoretinal procedures causing anisometropia, such as silicone oil tamponade, aphakia, and scleral buckling, may result in aniseikonia and loss of fusion.[40]

Pearls on How to Prevent It

◆ Use scleral imbrication rather than circumferential tightening to achieve high buckle height.

Pearls on How to Solve It

◆ Use contact lens correction, intraocular lens exchange, or remove silicone oil.

◆ Lower the buckle to reduce myopic shift.

◆ Convert glasses to monovision correction in applicable cases.

Expected outcome is restoration of refractive correction and binocular vision after vitreoretinal procedures are completed. Worst-case scenario is so much interference with binocular function that a full-time eye patch is required.

CAPTURE OF THE SUPERIOR OBLIQUE TENDON OR INFERIOR OBLIQUE MUSCLE BY THE SCLERAL BUCKLE

 Pathogenesis

Capture of the superior oblique tendon by the scleral buckle placed superior to it, moving its course too far forward, may alter the course of the superior oblique tendon and result in Brown syndrome with intorsion and hypotropia.[46,47] Capture of the inferior oblique muscle by the scleral buckle placed inferior to it can similarly cause anteriorization with restrictive hypotropia and extorsion.[48] These cyclovertical tropias are usually not amenable to prisms, orthoptic training, or botulinum toxin injections.

 Pearls on How to Prevent It

◆ Refinement of technique for proper buckle placement inferior to the superior oblique tendon and superior to the inferior oblique muscle, that is, the buckle should be adjacent to the globe without inadvertently looping the oblique muscles or their tendons around the buckle. Proper buckle placement can be verified by inspection for tissue trapped between the buckle and the globe.

 Pearls on How to Solve It

◆ Restoration of oblique muscle anatomic position usually with scleral buckle removal to free up the scarred tendon. Cutting the tendon and reattaching it by passing it over the buckle is very difficult with an intact buckle. If the buckle is loose, it might as well be removed.

◆ Cyclovertical strabismus surgery involving horizontal transposition of the vertical rectus muscles may be helpful.[41]

Expected outcomes are the need for extraocular muscle surgery or occlusion therapy. Worst-case scenario is persistent disabling torsional diplopia.

DISTORTION AND TORSIONAL STRABISMUS CAUSED BY MACULAR TRANSLOCATION

 Pathogenesis

Traditional macular translocation procedures resulted in a high incidence of proliferative vitreoretinopathy and intractable torsional diplopia.[49,50] Normal binocular vision cannot be restored in these cases, even though large rotational procedures of the globe have been tried. The rotational surgery interfered with the normal planes of eye movement, making adaptation by the patients difficult or impossible. Patients were left only with the option of monocular occlusion, with no hope of fusing. Limited macular translocation (macular detachment followed by scleral imbrication) produced smaller angles of torsional misalignment (0–16 degrees) and caused symptomatic diplopia in only 5.2% of cases,[51] consistent with Guyton's observation that in the absence of horizontal and vertical strabismus, a moderate amount of torsional disparity can be fused by sensory means alone.[52]

◈ Pearls on How to Prevent It

◆ Avoid full macular translocation procedures.

◈ Pearls on How to Solve It

◆ Prisms or extraocular muscle surgery to neutralize the deviation as much as possible and monocular occlusion if diplopia persists.

Expected outcome is persistent cyclotropia for significant macular translocations.

REFERENCES

1. Ugarte M, Williamson TH. Horizontal and vertical micropsia following macula-off rhegmatogenous retinal-detachment surgical repair. *Graefes Arch Clin Exp Ophthalmol.* 2006;244(11):1545–1548.
2. Shiragami C, Shiraga F, Yamaji H, et al. Unintentional displacement of the retina after standard vitrectomy for rhegmatogenous retinal detachment. *Ophthalmology.* 2010;117(1):86–92. e1.
3. Pandya VB, Ho IV, Hunyor AP. Does unintentional macular translocation after retinal detachment repair influence visual outcome? *Clin Experiment Ophthalmol.* 2012; 40(1):88–92.
4. Klainguti G, Castella A, Chamero J, et al. Extraocular muscle complications in retinal detachment surgery. In: Kaufmann H, ed. *Transactions of the XIX Meeting of ESA.* Crete, Greece: European Strabismological Association; 1991:125–130.
5. Smiddy WE, Loupe D, Michels RG, et al. Extraocular muscle imbalance after scleral buckling surgery. *Ophthalmology.* 1989;96(10):1485–1489; discussion 1489–1490.
6. Mets MB, Wendell ME, Gieser RG. Ocular deviation after retinal detachment surgery. *Am J Ophthalmol.* 1985;99:667–672.
7. Wright LA, Cleary M, Barrie T, et al. Motility and binocularity outcomes in vitrectomy versus scleral buckling in retinal detachment surgery. *Graefes Arch Clin Exp Ophthalmol.* 1999;237(12):1028–1032.
8. Kasbekar SA, Wong V, Young J, et al. Strabismus following retinal detachment repair: A comparison between scleral buckling and vitrectomy procedures. *Eye (Lond).* 2011;25(9):1202–1206.
9. Yadarola MB, Pearson-Cody M, Guyton DL. Strabismus following posterior segment surgery. *Ophthalmol Clin North Am.* 2004;17(4):495–506.
10. Multi-ethnic Pediatric Eye Disease Study Group. Prevalence of amblyopia and strabismus in African American and Hispanic children ages 6 to 72 months: The multiethnic pediatric eye disease study. *Ophthalmology.* 2008;115:1229–1236.
11. Friedman DS, Repka MX, Katz J, et al. Prevalence of amblyopia and strabismus in white and African American children aged 6 through 71 months: The Baltimore Pediatric Eye Disease Study. *Ophthalmology.* 2009;116:2128–2134.
12. Tanaka A, Ohno-Matsui K, Shimada N, et al. Prevalence of strabismus in patients with pathologic myopia. *J Med Dent Sci.* 2010;57(1):75–82.

13. VanderVeen DK, Bremer DL, Fellows RR, et al. Prevalence and course of strabismus through age 6 years in participants of the Early Treatment for Retinopathy of Prematurity randomized trial. *J AAPOS.* 2011;15(6):536–540.

14. Repka MX, Tung B, Good WV, et al. Outcome of eyes developing retinal detachment during the Early Treatment for Retinopathy of Prematurity study. *Arch Ophthalmol.* 2011;129(9):1175–1179.

15. Quinn GE, Dobson V. Outcome of prematurity and retinopathy of prematurity. *Curr Opin Ophthalmol.* 1996;7(3):51–56.

16. Sharpe JA, Wong AM, Fouladvand M. Ocular motor nerve palsies: Implications for diagnosis and mechanisms of repair. *Prog Brain Res.* 2008;171:59–66.

17. Cheung N, Mitchell P, Wong TY. Diabetic retinopathy. *Lancet.* 2010;376(9735):124–136.

18. Hwang JM, Wright KW. Combined study on the causes of strabismus after retinal surgery. *Korean J Ophthalmol.* 1994;8(2):83–91.

19. Brodsky M. Marlow occlusion: Does it create or eliminate artifact? *Strabismus.* 2005;13(3):149–150; author reply 151–152.

20. Marlow FW. The prolonged occlusion test. *Br J Ophthalmol.* 1930;14(8):385–393.

21. Hwang JM, Guyton DL. The Lancaster red-green test before and after occlusion in the evaluation of incomitant strabismus. *J AAPOS.* 1999;3(3):151–156.

22. Peduzzi M, Campos EC, Guerrieri F. Disturbances of ocular motility after retinal detachment surgery. *Doc Ophthalmol.* 1984;58(1):115–118.

23. Guyton DL. Strabismus complications from local anesthetics. *Semin Ophthalmol.* 2008;23(5):298–301.

24. Hamed LM, Helveston EM, Ellis FD. Persistent binocular diplopia after cataract surgery. *Am J Ophthalmol.* 1987;103(6):741–744.

25. Hunter DG, Lam GC, Guyton DL. Inferior oblique muscle injury from local anesthesia for cataract surgery. *Ophthalmology.* 1995;102(3):501–509.

26. Hamed LM. Strabismus presenting after cataract surgery. *Ophthalmology.* 1991;98(2):247–252.

27. Salama H, Farr AK, Guyton DL. Anesthetic myotoxicity as a cause of restrictive strabismus after scleral buckling surgery. *Retina.* 2000;20(5):478–482.

28. Zhang C, Phamonvaechavan P, Rajan A, et al. Concentration-dependent bupivacaine myotoxicity in rabbit extraocular muscle. *J AAPOS.* 2010;14(4):323–327.

29. Capó H, Guyton DL. Ipsilateral hypertropia after cataract surgery. *Ophthalmology.* 1996;103(5):721–730.

30. Scott AB, Alexander DE, Miller JM. Bupivacaine injection of eye muscles to treat strabismus. *Br J Ophthalmol.* 2007;91:146–148.

31. Hansen EA, Mein CE, Mazzoli R. Ocular anesthesia for cataract surgery: A direct sub-Tenon's approach. *Ophthalmic Surg.* 1999;21(10):696–699.

32. Wolff S. Strabismus after retinal detachment surgery. *Trans Am Ophthalmol Soc.* 1983;81:182–192.

33. Farr AK, Guyton DL. Strabismus after retinal detachment surgery. *Curr Opin Ophthalmol.* 2000;11(3):207–210.

34. Muñoz M, Rosenbaum A. Long-term strabismus complications following retinal detachment surgery. *J Pediatr Ophthalmol Strabismus.* 1987;24:309–314.

35. Portney GL, Campbell LH, Casebeer JC. Acquired heterotropia following surgery for retinal detachment. *Am J Ophthalmol.* 1972;73:985–990.

36. Sewell JJ, Knobloch WH, Eifrig DE. Extraocular muscle imbalance after surgical treatment for retinal detachment. *Am J Ophthalmol.* 1974;78(2):321–323.

37. Spencer AF, Newton C, Vernon SA. Incidence of ocular motility problems following scleral buckling surgery. *Eye (Lond).* 1993;7:751–756.

38. Wright KW. The fat adherence syndrome and strabismus after retina surgery. *Ophthalmology.* 1986; 93(3):411–415.

39. Rosenbaum AL. Strabismus following retinal detachment surgery. *Am Orthoptic J.* 2001;51:47–53.

40. Seaber JH, Buckley EG. Strabismus after retinal detachment surgery: Etiology, diagnosis, and treatment. *Semin Ophthalmol.* 1995;10(1):61–73.

41. Cooper LL, Harrison S, Rosenbaum AL. Ocular torsion as a complication of scleral buckle procedures for retinal detachments. *JAAPOS.* 1998;5:279–284.

42. Fison PN, Chignell AH. Diplopia after retinal detachment surgery. *Br J Ophthalmol.* 1987;71(7):521–525.

43. Lee J, Page B, Lipton J. Treatment of strabismus after retinal detachment surgery with botulinum neurotoxin A. *Eye (Lond).* 1991;5:451–455.

44. Petitto VB, Buckley EG. Use of botulinum toxin in strabismus after retinal detachment surgery. *Ophthalmology.* 1991;98(4):509–512.

45. De Pool ME, Campbell JP, Broome SO, et al. The dragged-fovea diplopia syndrome: Clinical characteristics, diagnosis, and treatment. *Ophthalmology.* 2005;112(8): 1455–1462.

46. Kushner BJ. Superior oblique tendon incarceration syndrome. *Arch Ophthalmol.* 2007;125(8):1070–1076.

47. Price R, Pederzolli A. Strabismus following retinal detachment surgery. *Am Orthoptic J.* 1982;32:9–17.

48. Kushner BJ. Unexpected cyclotropia simulating disruption of fusion. *Arch Ophthalmol.* 1992;110:1415–1418.

49. Ninomiya Y, Lewis JM, Hasegawa T, et al. Retinotomy and foveal translocation for surgical management of subfoveal choroidal neovascular membranes. *Am J Ophthalmol.* 1996;122(5):613–621.

50. Seaber JH, Machemer R. Adaptation to monocular torsion after macular translocation. *Graefes Arch Clin Exp Ophthalmol.* 1997;235(2):76–81.

51. Buffenn AN, de Juan E, Fujii G, et al. Diplopia after limited macular translocation surgery. *JAAPOS.* 2001;5(6):388–394.

52. Guyton DL, von Noorden GK. Sensory adaptation to cyclodeviations. In: Reinecke R, ed. *Strabismus.* New York, NY: Grune and Stratton; 1978:399–403.

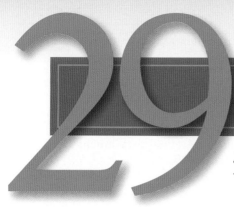

SEROUS CHOROIDAL DETACHMENT

JUSTIN GOTTLIEB AND ANDREW M. HENDRICK

⬥ The Complication

The choroid is the pigmented, highly vascularized tissue that forms the posterior aspect of the uveal tract. Choroidal detachment (also known as choroidal effusion, suprachoroidal effusion, supraciliary effusion) is the development of serous fluid in the potential space between the sclera and the uvea. It appears clinically as a pigmented dome-shaped convex lesion typically anterior to the equator although there is significant variation in appearance. Progression of choroidal detachment can extend circumferentially to the point of retinal–retinal apposition known as "kissing choroidals," and can lead to vision loss, serous retinal detachment, angle-closure glaucoma, and suprachoroidal hemorrhage.

Serous choroidal detachments have been described to occur spontaneously,[1] in association with nanophthalmos,[2] inflammation,[3] intraocular tumors,[4,5] systemic medications,[6] and carotid–cavernous fistula.[7] As a surgical complication, choroidal detachments can occur both intra- or postoperatively with seemingly any intraocular surgery including cataract surgery,[8] penetrating keratoplasty,[9] panretinal photocoagulation,[10] glaucoma filtration, and glaucoma shunting procedures.[8] It is notable that choroidal detachment has even been described as a complication of an intravitreal injection with a 30G needle.[11] For purposes of this chapter, we will consider how choroidal detachment impacts vitreoretinal surgery including scleral buckling and pars plana vitrectomy.

Serous choroidal detachment is an uncommon complication of pars plana vitrectomy and in the last two decades the incidence has remained stable. According to a retrospective analysis of medicare beneficiary data, the rate of choroidal detachment from 1994 to 1995 was 0.5%, from 1999 to 2000 was 0.4%, and from 2004 to 2005 was 0.4%.[12] However, it is possible that these results are biased toward underreporting complications. Alternative analyses have demonstrated higher rates of postoperative choroidal detachment.

The impact of small-gauge surgery and improved techniques and instrumentation on the incidence of serous choroidal detachment is unknown. Small-gauge vitrectomy is gaining popularity although many vitreoretinal surgeons are concerned that so-called "sutureless" techniques may increase the risk of hypotony and increase the risk of developing endophthalmitis and choroidal detachment.[13] One large retrospective case series of 23G pars plana vitrectomies only had 1/831 (0.1%) choroidal detachment.[13] Similarly, two separate retrospective analyses of 23G vitrectomies described serous choroidal detachment occurring at a rate of 1.8%.[14,15] Comparatively, rates using 20G instrumentation were historically slightly higher. Two studies reported an incidence of 3.9% in case series of nearly 400 patients each.[16,17]

Scleral buckling involves a heterogeneous group of surgical maneuvers, including the use of encircling versus segmental elements, cryopexy versus laser retinopexy, use of intravitreal gas tamponade or not, as well as the drainage or not of subretinal fluid. Thus, multiple components of the scleral buckling procedure have been identified that could relate to the development of choroidal detachment. The relative risk of each component is debated.

In general, scleral buckling is associated with a higher risk of choroidal detachment than pars plana vitrectomy. A very large historic case series described clinically evident serous choroidal detachment occurring in 348/1,485 (23%) of cases undergoing scleral buckling.[18] In this series, choroidal detachment appeared on the first or second postoperative day and was located at the equator with anterior extension. The authors described the choroidals most frequently adjacent to or opposite from the buckling site, and it was rare for the choroidal detachment to become prominent over the convexity of the buckle. Approximately 10% of their cases of serous choroidal detachments involved all four quadrants. Spontaneous resolution most often occurred over a 2-week period after a crescendo in size between postoperative days 2 and 4. They additionally describe a diffuse pigmentary proliferation in the sites of previous choroidal detachment that may resemble demarcation lines (Fig. 29-1).

Diagnostic ultrasonography reveals subclinical choroidal detachment following scleral buckling that is even more common than noted ophthalmoscopically. In a prospective series, high-frequency ultrasound biomicroscopy (UBM) revealed ciliary body effusions in 12 of 15 (80%) eyes examined at the 1-week postoperative visit.[19] Only one of their patients had a clinically detectable choroidal detachment. UBM was used similarly in another series in which 22 of 35 (67%) eyes had ciliary body detachment at the first postoperative visit.[20] Only 3/35 (9%) had clinically visible choroidal detachment. Encircling elements were associated with higher rates

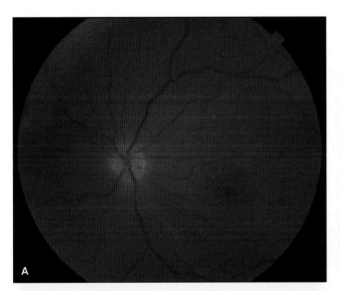

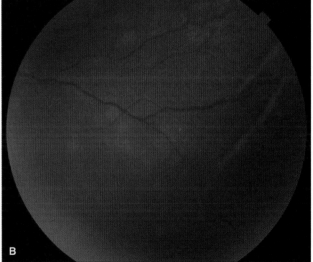

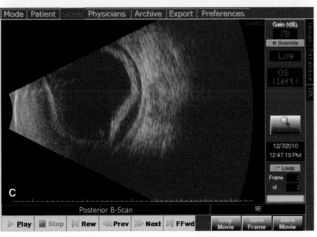

Figure 29-1 A–C: An 11-year-old female with diffuse choroidal hemangioma 4 months postoperatively from a valved glaucoma tube shunt implantation complicated by combined serous retinal detachment and serous choroidal detachment, conservatively managed. Her intraocular pressure was never low in the postoperative recovery. Note the extensive subretinal pigment deposition and characteristic appearance on ultrasonography.

of ciliary body detachment than segmental buckles (80% vs. 55%). Another series prospectively examined 46 consecutive eyes undergoing scleral buckling techniques with ultrasound undertaken postoperatively to examine the presence of ciliary thickening, choroidal detachments, and anterior chamber depth.[21] The overall rate of choroidal detachment in all patients was 30%. Choroidal detachment occurred in 47% of patients with an encircling element and 18% with segmental buckling. Heterogeneity aside, it can be concluded that after scleral buckling subclinical ciliary body detachments are fairly common, tend to be benign, and less commonly progress to clinical choroidal detachment.

◆ Risk Factors and Pathogenesis

The important patient characteristics in developing this postoperative complication vary between studies. Patient age has been shown to consistently be a risk.[18] This may relate to a progressive thinning of the choroid with age[22] and greater vascular permeability and incompetence.[18] A similar mechanism may explain why myopia is consistently associated with development of suprachoroidal hemorrhage, which is considered a disastrous complication that is often preceded by choroidal detachment (see also Chapters 26C and 30).[23]

The main surgical factors consistently associated with onset of choroidal detachment are hypotony, inflammation, extent of scleral buckling, and damage to the vortex veins. When choroidal detachments occur intraoperatively, it is often associated with hypotony.[18,24] Low intraocular pressure is believed to lead to a shift in the Starling equilibrium between the venous pressure and the extravascular space.[25,26] This gradient then favors fluid accumulation in the normally only potential suprachoroidal space. As such, techniques to minimize the risk of hypotony are paramount in preventing this surgical complication. This is particularly important during sutureless small-gauge vitrectomy where no buckling is employed, no vortex veins are damaged, and inflammation is minimal.

During pars plana vitrectomy, attention to the position of the infusion cannula is of the utmost importance. The first cases of intraoperative choroidal detachment were described during 23G vitrectomy either during either scleral depression or accidental lid speculum displacement both leading to infusion cannula slippage.[24] This was subsequently investigated in cadaveric eyes examining the technique of trocar placement and likelihood of cannula slippage. Insertion techniques utilizing a lower angle of incidence increase the likelihood of spontaneous wound closure due to the longer tunneling. However, when the infusion cannula was inserted at 15 degrees, only 1 mm of retraction was necessary to displace the infusion tip into the suprachoroidal space.[14] Routine scleral depression in the inferotemporal quadrant or nearby deforms the globe and may easily lead to cannula slippage, especially when an inexperienced assistant is utilized.

Inflammation alone can to lead to spontaneous choroidal detachment.[3] Greater intraoperative proinflammatory maneuvers such as laser retinopexy, panretinal photocoagulation **(Fig. 29-2)**, and cryopexy are associated with a higher risk of choroidal effusion and detachment. Some authors suggest retinal detachments themselves as proinflammatory which is why choroidal detachment is common during retinal detachment repair.[23,24] Similarly, other series have noted that the extent of retinal detachment correlates with the incidence of choroidal detachment and a higher incidence occurs in patients with giant retinal tears.[18] It is suspected that the vascular permeability of the choroidal vessels increases when inflamed leading to increased colloid leakage into the suprachoroidal space.[26] As such, proper postoperative management of all intraocular surgeries includes the use of topical steroids to be tapered on the basis of clinical response. When postoperative choroidal detachment occurs, the surgeon should consider adjunctive periocular or oral steroids.

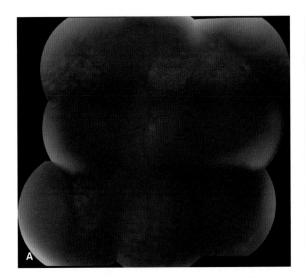
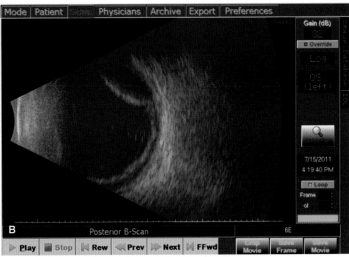

Figure 29-2 A, B: Postoperative choroidal detachment. This is a 63-year-old male who underwent 23G pars plana vitrectomy 2 days for proliferative diabetic retinopathy with nonclearing vitreous hemorrhage. This eye was naive to panretinal photocoagulation which was completed intraoperatively. Postoperative day 1 intraocular pressure was 8 mm Hg and improved to 10 mm Hg on the day of the photograph. Note the fresh panretinal photocoagulation (PRP) laser and characteristic pigmented dome-shaped peripheral convexities. Ultrasonography confirms choroidal effusion with diffuse extent not visible ophthalmoscopically. Choroidal detachment clinically resolved within 1 week.

Specifically during retinal detachment repair, scleral buckling posterior to the equator is more likely to obstruct vortex venous flow and increase the likelihood of development of choroidal detachment.[24] Direct damage to the vortex veins via cautery, avulsion, or cryopexy increases the likelihood of this complication.[18] Encircling bands lead to greater amounts of ciliary body edema and higher rates of choroidal detachment than segmental buckles.[21]

The choroid is firmly attached to the sclera only at the scleral spur, the exit points of vortex veins and optic nerve. Thus, with an accumulation of fluid, detachment of the choroid demonstrates a characteristic quadrantic dome-shaped configuration. Perfusion to the choroid originates from both the long and short posterior ciliary arteries in addition to the perforating anterior ciliary arteries in a highly anastomotic network. Capillaries in this system are fenestrated and nearly four times the diameter of normal capillary.[26] The majority of venous flow is drained via the vortex veins and obstruction of these veins increases the risk of development of choroidal detachment.[27] Analysis of suprachoroidal fluid demonstrates electrolyte balance similar to plasma with a protein concentration 60% lower than plasma, consistent with theories that choroidal detachment results from an imbalance in the Starling equilibrium.[26] This theory, additionally, explains why arterial hypertension is a risk of the development of choroidal detachments,[20] that is, the perfusion pressure into the choroidal vasculature overwhelms the capillary system, especially in a state of relative hypotony or with vortex vein compromise or increased episcleral venous pressure.

◆ Pearls on How to Prevent It

Postoperatively, topical cycloplegia and steroids are routinely used to reduce inflammation and facilitate optimal healing conditions and patient comfort. Postoperative activity levels are often limited following retinal detachment repair and macular hole surgery simply due to positioning requirements; however, physical limitations should always be emphasized. Patients are given an eye shield to prevent direct trauma while sleeping; they are additionally advised to avoid eye rubbing, lifting greater than 10 lbs for 2 weeks, and strict avoidance of Valsalva maneuvers.

Pars Plana Vitrectomy

◆ Avoid hypotony, especially rapid changes in intraocular pressure.

  ◆ Maintain constant infusion when possible.

  ◆ Avoid aggressive aspiration rates especially when performing an air–fluid exchange; or with expanded sclerotomies, allowing efflux around instruments.

  ◆ Exchange instruments one at a time when performing an air–fluid exchange.

◆ Infusion insertion technique that employs a 30- to 45-degree angle of insertion.

◆ Visualize the tip of the infusion cannula before opening/unclamping it.

◆ Secure the infusion cannula tubing to the drape to prevent inadvertent displacement.

◆ Orient the infusion cannula perpendicular to the globe.

◆ Careful scleral depression by a skilled assistant especially near the infusion cannula.

◆ Plug trocars that are not in use.

◆ Suture sclerotomies when in doubt regarding wound closure.

◆ Fill the vitreous cavity with air rather than fluid allowing the bubble surface tension to assist wound closure at conclusion of the case.

◆ Avoid heavy or redundant laser treatments/cryotherapy and titrate spot intensity.

Scleral Buckling

◆ Avoidance of hypotony, especially rapid changes in intraocular pressure.

  ◆ Avoid excessive pressure on eye during initiation of external drainage.

  ◆ Maintain digital pressure or multiple cotton-tip applicators can be used during drainage of subretinal fluid to prevent hypotony.

  ◆ Allow subretinal fluid to passively drain to maintain a constant stream of fluid release, utilizing massage at conclusion of drainage only.

  ◆ After drainage of subretinal fluid rapid tightening of buckle or instillation of tamponade into the vitreous cavity immediately is possible if a needle technique for drainage is used.

◆ Avoid buckle placement posterior to the equator if possible.

◆ Consider segmental elements for appropriate retinal detachments.

◆ Identification of vortex veins in all four quadrants to avoid inadvertent cauterization, cryopexy, or direct compression with the encircling element when possible.

◈ Pearls on How to Solve It

  ◆ Prompt recognition of intraoperative serous choroidal detachment can have a significant impact on the success of the case (see above). A choroidal detachment appears as a dome-shaped peripheral pigmented elevation that tends to

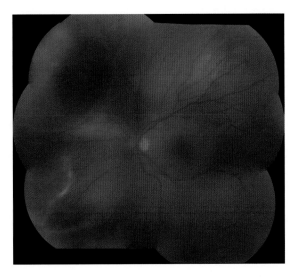

Figure 29-3 Postoperative choroidal detachment (composite photography). This is a 28-year-old male referred after scleral buckling revision for retinal detachment with recurrent retinal detachment associated with choroidal detachment. Note the characteristic pigmented dome-shaped peripheral convexity superonasally.

progressively occupy more of the intravitreal space if left unattended **(Fig. 29-3)**. It may be more common during scleral depression, especially with an unskilled assistant near the infusion cannula during vitrectomy. However, subtle changes may be recognized if the extent of choroidal detachment is limited and not bullous. For example, the surgeon may note relatively increased uptake with laser when photocoagulating the area. If the retina is detached over the choroidal detachment, it may tend to slip posteriorly and achieving proper position of the retina for further retinopexy may be difficult.

◆ During pars plana vitrectomy, if an intraoperative serous choroidal detachment is visualized, first check if the eye is hypotonous and ensure that the infusion tubing is not kinked and is opened. The next maneuver should be to clearly visualize a patent microcannula tip inside the eye without removing instruments from the eye. The assistant may be able to manipulate the microcannula into view especially under wide-angle viewing conditions. If the cannula is visualized and the eye is hypotonous, vitreous or intravitreal contents (protein, hemorrhage, white blood cells) may be occluding the infusion tip. Care should be taken to normalize the intraocular pressure first. A 27G cannula fits nicely into any trocar and can be used to inject balanced salt solution into the vitreous cavity. Subsequently, priority should be given to the vitreous surrounding the infusion cannula. If the cannula tip is not adequately visualized, the infusion cannula should be clamped to prevent potential further infusion into the suprachoroidal space. Instruments should be removed one by one and the sclerotomies/trocars promptly plugged. The intravitreal location of the tip may be directly visualized through the pupil with external pressure on the infusion cannula or indirect ophthalmoscopy performed to more easily visualize the peripherally located cannula tip. If uncertain despite these methods, the infusion cannula is easily swapped to an alternate pre-existing trocar in small-gauge vitrectomy. The questionable trocar should then be removed and replaced to an alternate position avoiding the area of choroidal detachment. The surgeon may note spontaneous egress of suprachoroidal fluid with removal of the infusion trocar. During a 20G vitrectomy, longer infusion tips are available and should be employed. Lastly, if the case is combined with phacoemulsification, the anterior segment wound needs to be assessed and should always be sutured.[28] Consequently, the remainder of the case can progress but may be difficult. Priority should be placed to prompt conclusion of all imperative operative goals with limited extraneous manipulations. If repairing a retinal detachment, an expansile concentration of gas tamponade should be considered due to the intraocular volume the choroidal detachment occupies. Postoperative laser retinopexy can be applied in the clinic through the gas bubble although this may prove challenging. No matter which gauge was utilized, all cases with an intraoperative choroidal detachment should have sclerotomies sutured closed. Finally, favoring a minor amount of ocular hypertension is preferable to hypotony in these circumstances.

◆ In cases in which a thickened choroid or a choroidal detachment may be present preoperatively, such as following failed scleral buckle, the choice of infusion cannula is very important. A longer infusion cannula may be chosen as well as a selection of an area with less choroidal elevation. If an infusion cannula appears to slip beneath the pars plana pigment epithelium, the surgeon may carefully use an micro vitreoretinal (MVR) blade or the light pipe to push the epithelium from the infusion tip. Alternatively, the infusion may be completely replaced to another, safer quadrant.

◆ Patients should always be informed that they have had a complication that requires extra care and monitoring. Patients with choroidal detachments must be especially aware how serious the consequences can be. Adequate analgesia and antiemetics should be provided to prevent Valsalva maneuvers. Postoperative serous choroidal detachment is a condition that is best managed conservatively in most circumstances since limited choroidal detachments often self-resolve without consequence.[14]

◆ Surgical drainage is rarely indicated for a serous choroidal detachment, and the timing of this is controversial.[29] Medical therapy should be attempted, including cycloplegia, aggressive control of intraocular inflammation, and management of intraocular pressure as needed, unless circumstances progress to the loss of anterior chamber with iridocorneal or lenticulocorneal touch leading to progressive corneal edema which may necessitate surgical drainage.[6] Other surgeons consider "kissing choroidal" to be an indication for surgery due to concerns of retinal–retinal apposition.[30,31] No matter the indication, the cause should be established and addressed prior to, or at the time of attempted surgical drainage. For proper surgical drainage the surgeon must first establish an infusion cannula to overcome the induced hypotony with drainage. This cannula may be placed into the anterior chamber with a Lewicky cannula or via the pars plana over a quadrant without choroidal detachment.[32] If diffuse detachment is present, pars plana infusion cannula insertion technique should be adjusted to a more anterior position. Conjunctival peritomy is then performed in the quadrant with the most suprachoroidal fluid and careful limited full thickness sclerotomy is made over the highest area of accumulation. Careful manipulation of adjacent areas with a cotton tip may be used to express more fluid to the sclerotomy. Some surgeons place a cyclodialysis spatula into the suprachoroidal space to assist fluid drainage although this may increase risk of hemorrhage. The sclerotomy may be sewn closed or left open to allow additional drainage of accumulated fluid but the conjunctiva should always be reapproximated. Alternative techniques have been described by vitreoretinal surgeons. This includes cannulating the suprachoroidal space using a flat-angled insertion to the standard small-gauge trocar system and allowing the infusion to push the fluid out the trocar.

Depending on the extent of serous choroidal detachment, visual outcomes may not be impaired.[14] However, they can be associated with development of serious consequences including vision loss, endophthalmitis,[18,25] angle-closure glaucoma, and suprachoroidal hemorrhage.

Angle-closure glaucoma can lead to severe pain, delayed postoperative visual recovery, or even permanent visual loss. The rate of postoperative angle-closure glaucoma approximates 4% from scleral buckling.[33] This risk may be slightly higher in the presence of choroidal detachment.[18] It is important to recognize the mechanism of this complication to be a posterior pushing mechanism rather than pupillary block. With ciliary body detachment, progressive fluid accumulation rotates the ciliary body forward, thereby compromising the angle. Unless pupillary block is concomitantly present, a peripheral iridotomy will not treat this mechanism and relieve the high pressure. Proper treatment involves intraocular pressure lowering via osmotic, diuretics, aqueous suppressants, and enhancing outflow. Topical cycloplegics may help to deepen the anterior chamber and reduce discomfort. The surgeon should use oral analgesics and consider using oral steroids.

❖ Expected outcomes: What Is the Worst-case Scenario

Serous choroidal detachment is believed to be a final common pathway that can lead to suprachoroidal hemorrhage. The extent of involvement may be limited or expulsive depending on proper recognition and management of the situation. Expulsive suprachoroidal hemorrhage is one of the worst complications that an ophthalmologist will encounter. Development of suprachoroidal hemorrhage increases the likelihood of additional surgery and vision loss.[27]

REFERENCES

1. Velzeboer CM. Spontaneous choroidal detachment: Report of two cases. *Am J Ophthalmol.* 1960;49:898–903.
2. Brockhurst RJ. Nanophthalmos with uveal effusion: A new clinical entity. *Trans Am Ophthalmol Society.* 1974;72:371–403.
3. McGrand JC. Choroidal detachment in aphakic uveitis. *Br J Ophthalmol.* 1969;53: 778–781.
4. Palamar M, Thangappan A, Shields CL, et al. Necrotic choroidal melanoma with scleritis and choroidal effusion. *Cornea.* 2009;28:354–356.
5. Kreiger AE, Meyer D, Smith TR, et al. Metastatic carcinoma to the choroid with choroidal detachment. A case presenting as uveal effusion. *Arch Ophthalmol.* 1969; 82:209–213.
6. Parikh R, Parikh S, Das S, et al. Choroidal drainage in the management of acute angle closure after topiramate toxicity. *J Glaucoma.* 2007;16:691–693.
7. Guerry D III, Harbison JW, Wiesinger H. Bilateral choroidal detachment and fluctuating proptosis secondary to bilateral dural arteriovenous fistulas treated with transcranial orbital decompression with resolution: Report of a case. *Trans Am Ophthalmol Soc.* 1975;73:64–73.
8. Maumenee AE, Schwartz MF. Acute intraoperative choroidal effusion. *Am J Ophthalmol.* 1985;100:147–154.
9. Purcell JJ Jr, Krachmer JH, Doughman DJ, et al. Expulsive hemorrhage in penetrating keratoplasty. *Ophthalmology.* 1982;89:41–43.
10. Zamir E, Anteby I, Merin S. Choroidal effusion causing transient myopia after panretinal photocoagulation. *Arch Ophthalmol.* 1996;114:1284–1285.
11. Meyer CH, Brinkman CK, Helb HM. Choroidal detachment after an uneventful intravitreal injection. *J Ocul Pharmacol Ther.* 2010;26:305–307.
12. Stein JD, Zacks DN, Grossman D, et al. Adverse events after pars plana vitrectomy among medicare beneficiaries. *Arch Ophthalomol.* 2009:127:1656–1663.
13. Parolini B, Prigione G, Romanelli F, et al. Postoperative complications and intraocular pressure in 943 consecutive cases of 23-gauge transconjunctival pars plana vitrectomy with 1-year follow-up. *Retina.* 2010;30:107–111.
14. Tarantola RM, Folk JC, Shah SS, et al. Intraoperative choroidal detachment during 23-gauge vitrectomy. *Retina.* 2011;31:893–901.
15. Ooto S, Kimura D, Itoi K, et al. Suprachoroidal fluid as a complication of 23-gauge vitreous surgery. *Br J Ophthalomol.* 2008;92:1433–1434.

16. Fujikawa A, Kitaoka T, Miyamura N, et al. Choroidal detachment after vitreous surgery. *Ophthalmic Surg Lasers.* 2000;31:276–281.

17. Benillouche P, Bonnet M. [Postoperative choroid detachment following microsurgery for rhegmatogenous retinal detachment]. *J Fr Ophthalmol.* 1998;21:397–402.

18. Hawkins WR, Schepens CL. Choroidal detachment and retinal surgery. *Am J Ophthalmol.* 1966;62:813–819.

19. Pavlin CH, Rutnin SS, Devenyi R, et al. Supraciliary effusions and ciliary body thickening after scleral buckling procedures. *Ophthalmology.* 1997;104:433–438.

20. Maruyama Y, Tuuki T, Kimura Y, et al. Ciliary detachment after retinal detachment surgery. *Retina.* 1997;17:7–11.

21. Kawana K, Okamoto F, Hiraoka T, et al. Ciliary body edema after sclera buckling surgery for rhegmatogenous retinal detachment. *Ophthalmology.* 2006;113:36–41.

22. Fujiwara T, Imamura Y, Margolis R, et al. Enhanced depth imaging optical coherence tomography of the choroid in highly myopic eyes. *Am J Ophthalmol.* 2009;148:445–450.

23. Tabandeh H, Sullivan PM, Smahliuk P, et al. Suprachoroidal hemorrhage during pars plana vitrectomy. *Ophthalmology.* 1999;106:263–242.

24. Aaberg TM. Experimental serous and hemorrhagic uveal edema associated with retinal detachment surgery. *Invest ophthalmol.* 1975;14:243–246.

25. Bellows AR, Chylack LT Jr, Hutchinson BT. Choroidal detachment. Clinical manifestation, therapy and mechanism of formation. *Ophthalmology.* 1981;88:1107–1115.

26. Brubaker RF, Pederson JE. Ciliochoroidal detachment. *Surv Ophthalmol.* 1983;27:281–289.

27. Hayreh SS, Baines JAB. Occlusion of the vortex veins. *Br J Ophthalmol.* 1973;57:217–238.

28. Wong RW, Kokame GT, Mahmoud TH, et al. Complications associated with clear corneal cataract wounds during vitrectomy. *Retina.* 2010;30:850–855.

29. Kuhn F, Morris R, Mester V. Choroidal detachment and expulsive choroidal hemorrhage. *Ophthalmol Clin North Am.* 2001;14:639–650.

30. Berrocal JA. Adhesion of the retina secondary to large choroidal detachment as a cause of failure in retinal detachment surgery. *Mod Probl Ophthalmol.* 1979;20:51–52.

31. Weinberg DV, Rosenberg LF. Retina to retina adhesions following suprachoroidal hemorrhage. *Br J Ophthalmol.* 1996;80:674.

32. Krishnan MM, Baskaran RK. Management of postoperative choroidal detachment. *Indian J Ophthalmol.* 1985;33:217–220.

33. Perez RN, Phelps CD, Burton TC. Angle-closure glaucoma following sclera buckling operations. *Trans Sect Ophthalmol Am Acad Ophthalmol Otolaryngol.* 1976;81:247–252.

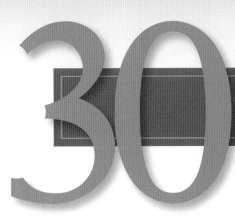

POSTOPERATIVE SUPRACHOROIDAL HEMORRHAGE

EHAB ABDELKADER, DAVID WONG, AND NOEMI LOIS

✦ The Complication: Definition

The definition of suprachoroidal hemorrhage (SCH) has been included in Chapter 26C. This chapter will discuss SCH when occurring as a postoperative complication.

✦ Risk Factors and Pathogenesis

Postoperative risk factors for SCH include Valsalva maneuvers, ocular hypotony, or trauma. Some studies reported a higher incidence of SCH in cases with general anesthesia which could be attributed to coughing on the endotracheal tube.[1,2] Others, however, failed to show such a relationship.[3] Aspirin (antiplatelet therapies and anticoagulants) and Warfarin intake were reported to be associated with spontaneous SCH.[4,5] Thus, they could be a predisposing factor for SCH in VR surgery. Coughing, straining, vomiting, or a rise of blood pressure in the perioperative period may precipitate the rupture of the weak choroidal vessel by increasing the choroidal venous pressure. Leaking sclerotomies following pars plana vitrectomy and leaking corneal wounds following phacovitrectomy may lead to postoperative hypotony and the development of SCH.

The pathogenesis of postoperative SCH should be essentially the same as intraoperative SCH; this has been discussed in Chapter 26C.

Clinical Findings

Postoperative SCH usually presents with sudden ocular pain that may be accompanied with headache, nausea, and vomiting. The anterior chamber is shallow with high intraocular pressure (IOP), loss of red reflex, and a dome-shaped dark choroidal lesion. The vision is usually severely reduced, especially, if the macula is involved. In severe cases, the SCH may markedly elevate the choroid giving the appearance of kissing choroidals.

Ocular ultrasonography (US) is an important tool to confirm the diagnosis especially if the media are opaque. It is also a valuable tool for the follow-up helping on deciding whether surgical intervention for SCH should be considered.

✦ Pearls on How to Prevent It

◆ Prevent marked changes in blood pressure intraoperatively and postoperatively (i.e., low blood pressure intraoperatively, followed by high postoperative blood pressure).

◆ Any Valsalva maneuver such as that associated with coughing, straining, and vomiting, and which may occur following surgery, most commonly under general anesthesia, should be avoided in the early postoperative period.[2]

◆ Avoid leaving the eye with low IOP following surgery; especially in eyes with risk factors (see also Chapter 26C).

◆ Protect the eye from trauma during the early postoperative period with a shield.

✦ Pearls on How to Solve It and Expected Outcomes

Pearls on how to treat SCH and its expected outcomes have been provided in Chapter 26C.

REFERENCES

1. Taylor DM. Expulsive hemorrhage. *Am J Ophthalmol.* 1974;78(6):961–966.
2. Pollack AL, McDonald HR, Ai E, et al. Massive suprachoroidal hemorrhage during pars plana vitrectomy associated with Valsalva maneuver. *Am J Ophthalmol.* 2001; 132(3):383–387.
3. Speaker MG, Guerriero PN, Met JA, et al. A case-control study of risk factors for intraoperative suprachoroidal expulsive hemorrhage. *Ophthalmology.* 1991;98(2): 202–209; discussion 10.
4. Chak M, Williamson TH. Spontaneous suprachoroidal haemorrhage associated with high myopia and aspirin. *Eye (Lond).* 2003;17(4):525–527.
5. Chandra A, Barsam A, Hugkulstone C. A spontaneous suprachoroidal haemorrhage: A case report. *Cases J.* 2009;2:185.

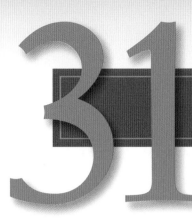

EPIMACULAR MEMBRANE

RICHARD M. AHUJA AND SRILAKSHMI MAGULURI

The Complication: Definition

An epimacular membrane (EMM) may develop after retinal surgery: Scleral buckling, pneumatic retinopexy or pars plana vitrectomy for retinal detachment, or cryotherapy for retinal breaks without retinal detachment.

EMMs, also termed epiretinal membranes, premacular fibrosis, epimacular proliferation, or macular pucker, are avascular, fibrocellular membranes that proliferate on the inner surface of the retina within the retinal temporal vascular arcades. They may contribute to metamorphopsia and visual changes secondary to their effect on the underlying retina.[1] The overall incidence of EMMs at autopsy was found to be 5.4% by Roth and Foos,[2] increasing from 2% at age 50 to over 20% at age 75. Frequently, when no underlying associated ocular condition is found, they are considered idiopathic.[1] EMMs can also be seen in association with ocular conditions such as posterior vitreous detachment, ocular inflammation, ocular trauma, retinal vascular occlusive disease, vitreous hemorrhage, or ocular surgery.[1,3] Clinically significant EMMs occur in 3% to 8.5% of eyes after successful primary retinal detachment surgery.[4–7] Strategies to prevent the occurrence and maximize successful treatment of EMMs after retinal reattachment surgery and treatment of retinal breaks without retinal detachment (RD) will be discussed in this chapter.

Risk Factors

◆ Time of onset after retinal reattachment surgery: EMMs typically develop between the first and the sixth postoperative month.[7]

◆ Preoperative retinal signs: Patients noted to be at the greatest risk for EMMs are those with preoperative signs of proliferative vitreoretinopathy (PVR), including rolled retinal edges, star folds, and equatorial ridges.[5]

◆ Other risk factors include the following: Older age, larger retinal breaks, preoperative vitreous hemorrhage obscuring the fundus, macula-involved detachments, and detachments of longer duration and multiple operations.[4–11]

◆ Subretinal fluid (SRF) drainage versus nondrainage: One study of 312 cases with SRF drainage noted a higher frequency of EMMs in eyes that underwent SRF drainage (7.1%) as compared to those that had nondrainage procedures (3.2%), though the difference was not statistically significant.[12] Uemura et al. reviewed a consecutive series of 277 eyes (268 patients) with macular-spared retinal detachment where no preretinal membrane had been present preoperatively. Postoperatively, 17 eyes (6.1%) developed obvious macular pucker; 260 eyes (93.9%) did not. In eyes with SRF drainage performed, 5 eyes developed an EMM and 93 eyes did not; SRF drainage was not found to be statistically associated with the development of EMM.[6]

◆ Laser or cryotherapy: The risk of EMM development in eyes that have undergone cryotherapy or laser photocoagulation for treatment of retinal tears with or without associated retinal detachment may be difficult to quantify because one cannot precisely determine whether the cellular dispersion was due to the retinal break itself or the subsequent therapy. In vitro and in vivo studies have shown higher rates of dispersion of viable RPE cells in eyes after cryotherapy and a greater breakdown of the blood–retinal barrier with cryotherapy in comparison to eyes that have undergone argon laser photocoagulation.[13–15] Krausher and Morse found no significant data with respect to the incidence of EMM following laser therapy versus cryotherapy in 103 eyes that had prophylactic treatment of retinal breaks. Saran and Brucker[17] conducted a retrospective study of the incidence of EMMs after treatment of retinal breaks without retinal detachment and found no significant difference between cryotherapy, laser photocoagulation, or combined treatment (range 10% to 18%). However, with respect to the influence of the method of adhesion used in repair of retinal detachment, the literature contains conflicting data. A clinical case series of 277 eyes that underwent scleral buckling with either diathermy or cryotherapy found a higher incidence of EMM formation with cryotherapy.[6] A prospective study of 132 eyes following successful operations for repair of retinal detachment by Kraushar and Morse[16] found a statistically significant higher incidence of EMM formation in eyes that had undergone scleral buckling surgery with cryotherapy compared to diathermy. Conversely, Lobes and Burton[5] and Tannenbaum et al.[18] concluded that the formation of EMMs was unrelated to the specific method used to produce the chorioretinal adhesion in patients that had undergone scleral buckling surgery. Hagler and Aturaliya,[4] in a study of 1,071 patients that underwent scleral buckling for repair of retinal detachment, found a higher incidence of EMM formation after diathermy (5%) than with cryotherapy (3%). In the only prospective randomized controlled study comparing scleral buckling with transcleral diode laser to scleral buckling with cryotherapy in the management of rhegmatogenous retinal detachment, the incidence of macular EMM was 10% in the diode group and 5% in the cryotherapy group; this difference, however, was not statistically significant.[19] Sabates et al.[7] also did not find a significant difference in the incidence of EMMs between scleral buckling with either diathermy or cryotherapy. In Silicone Oil Report 8, neither cryotherapy nor laser was associated with an increased prevalence of EMMs.[20]

◆ Silicone oil or gas tamponade: The rate of EMM formation after pars plana vitrectomy with or without scleral buckling for PVR has been reported to range between 15% and 30%.[21,22] In patients that underwent primary vitrectomy and/or scleral buckling for repair of retinal detachments with severe PVR, the Silicone Oil Study Report 8 did not find an association between the rate of postoperative EMM formation and the type of intraocular tamponade used or the extent of its application at 6 months postoperatively.[20]

◆ Retinotomy: Cox et al.[20] in Silicone Oil Study Report 8 did find a 1.4 times increased risk of EMM formation with longer radial relaxing retinotomies. However, they did not find an increased incidence of EMMs with posterior drainage retinotomies.

◆ Pathogenesis

Idiopathic EMMs arise from dehiscences in the retinal inner limiting membrane which permit glial cell migration and proliferation on the retinal surface.[23] EMMs associated with retinal breaks, previous retinal detachments, or retinal cryopexy may be caused by release of viable retinal pigment epithelial (RPE) cells into the vitreous cavity through the retinal break.[23–25] However, histopathologic studies of secondary EMMs have shown a mixed cellular composition. RPE cells were evident in association with retinal detachment though they were not necessarily the principal cell type.[23] Other cell types included macrophages, fibrocytes, fibrous astrocytes, and myofibroblast-like cells that had mostly the characteristics of fibrocytes, and occasionally of RPE cells or fibrous astrocytes.[23,24] Epiretinal membranes that occur following retinal surgery using long-term tamponade agents such as silicone oil and perfluorohexyloctane have architectural features more like those of PVR membranes. These include a mixed fibrocellular population including glial cells, RPE, fibroblasts, and inflammatory cells, particularly macrophages laden with the tamponade agent itself.[26,27] Though the cellular constituents may vary in different types of EMMs, the formation of collagen and the development of cells with myofibroblast-like properties are common features of EMMs and seem to be the basis for their contractile properties.[24]

◈ Pearls on How to Prevent It

◆ Detachment or retinal break variables: Factors such as large size breaks, PVR, macular detachment, vitreous hemorrhage, prior operations, and duration of retinal detachment are preoperative risk factors that have been implicated in the development of postoperative EMMs. These occur prior to patient seeking care and cannot be modified.[5,9,10,18,20,27,28]

◆ Patient-associated variables: Age is a factor that cannot be addressed. Preoperative lens status may be a factor with higher incidence of EMMs in pseudophakic and aphakic eyes, though not all studies support this finding.[16,20]

◆ Vitrectomy variables: Complete vitrectomy with attention to removal of traction at the retinal tear and complete hyaloid disinsertion from the posterior pole would remove any potential scaffold for the formation of the EMM. In order to better visualize the vitreous, Sakamoto et al.[29] used triamcinolone acetonide intraoperatively. This technique improved the visibility of the hyaloid and reduced the breakdown of the blood–ocular barrier as measured by an aqueous laser flare meter. Frequent associated side effects of intraocular steroids include cataract progression and intraocular pressure rise. However, this study only enrolled pseudophakes, and only one of 33 eyes developed a rise in intraocular pressure.[29]

◆ Endophotocoagulation and intraocular cryotherapy variables: Use of endophotocoagulation rather than cryotherapy may reduce postoperative EMM formation; though, there is considerable variability in the literature with respect to the risks of cryotherapy in this regard.[13–15,18–22] Some surgeons advocate the use of intraocular cryotherapy or endophotocoagulation in an air-filled eye during vitrectomy to minimize the dispersion of pigment. However, the use of this technique may inadvertently cause greater retinal damage. Landers et al.[30] compared the histologic appearance of 6-week-old argon laser endophotocoagulation in vitrectomized rhesus monkey eyes to argon laser lesions placed by a standard slit lamp delivery system. They found primarily outer retinal damage in all sections but with more pigment dispersion extending into the neurosensory retina in the vitrectomized eyes.[30] In another histologic study, Johnson et al. found that in an air-filled human eye both cryopexy lesions and argon laser lesions showed full-thickness retinal necrosis. They explain this finding by the absence of the heat-sink effect that a fluid-filled eye would normally provide allowing for more effective heat dissipation in the retina, reduced temperatures in the overlying vitreous cavity, and prevention of thermal spread and retinal damage.[31]

◆ Scleral buckling and pneumatic retinopexy variables: SRF drainage may increase the risk of EMM formation.[12] To help reduce this risk, perform drainage only in cases of total RD, highly elevated RD, or a chronic inferior RD. Care should also be taken in placing scleral sutures to prevent inadvertent scleral perforation. The relationship of EMM formation and cryotherapy is controversial in the literature, and this is discussed in the section on risk factors (see above).[4,5,7,12–18] However, certain techniques are agreed upon to help prevent excessive pigment dispersion. While performing cryotherapy, limiting the freeze time to the first appearance of retinal whitening and treating only the edges of the break, not bare RPE, can help prevent excessive pigment dispersion. In pneumatic retinopexy, a staged procedure can be performed in which intraocular gas injection is done first to flatten the retina followed by argon laser photocoagulation instead of cryotherapy to treat the retinal break. However, sometimes localization of small breaks can be difficult through a gas bubble. The D-ACE procedure, first described by Gilbert and McLeod,[32] involves SRF drainage (D), injection of air (A) or an air–gas mixture, transscleral cryotherapy (C) and finally a silicone explants (E). In the original description, it was recommended to treat bullous retinal detachments complicated with multiple, often equatorial, retinal breaks. In this surgical sequence, the retina is flattened first by doing SRF drainage. This is immediately followed by the injection of air, which not only restores the intraocular pressure but also allows neuroretina–RPE apposition and break closure minimizing the amount of cryotherapy required and the possible dispersion of RPE cells in the vitreous cavity. Then, the scleral buckle (explants) is placed. In their series of 50 patients, Gilbert and McLeod achieved primary retinal reattachment (retinal reattachment with a single surgery) in 90% of cases. Significant hemorrhage including choroidal hemorrhage and subretinal hemorrhage occurred in six eyes.[32] Needle techniques for draining SRF appear to be associated with lower risk of bleeding (see also Chapter 2).

✛ Pearls on How to Solve It

◆ Pars plana vitrectomy with membrane peel is the accepted method of treatment. Timing of the surgery depends upon the extent of visual compromise and severity of the EMM.

◆ Three major steps are involved.

Step 1: Core and peripheral vitrectomy.

◆ A core vitrectomy is performed to remove any vitreous opacities, and the posterior hyaloid is removed to the retinal periphery.[33]

◆ Care must be taken to avoid the natural lens if the patient is phakic and trauma to chorioretinal tissue elevated on a prior scleral buckle, if present.

◆ There is usually a posterior vitreous separation present. If not, any vitreous attachments to the EMM must be removed.[34]

Step 2: Two major techniques have been reported in membrane peeling.

◆ The out-to-in technique

◆ Creating an edge: The surgeon creates a liftable edge of the membrane by engaging one area, preferably the thickest and away from the fovea, with a barbed microvitreoretinal (MVR) blade.[35] If no edge is present, a straight cutdown on the EMM surface can be made with an MVR blade over the thickest part of the EMM to create a slit.

◆ Lifting the EMM: Once an edge is elevated, the membrane can be dissected from the retinal surface with a blunt pick. Alternatively, the membrane can also be elevated with use of a soft-tipped extrusion cannula at a site away from the fovea. The suction should be applied to the thickest portion of the membrane, and care should be taken to avoid direct contact of the retinal surface.[36] Multifunction tissue manipulators or combination pick and fluted needles have also been used to engage the EMM.[37]

♦ Removing the EMM: Fine-tipped, end-gripping intraocular forceps can then be used to engage the EMM at multiple sites pulling the edges toward the foveal center. Peeling should be done tangentially, not in an anteroposterior direction. It is usually necessary to engage the membrane sequentially from various points and directions to avoid shredding of the membrane. Once free from the foveal surface, the distal portions of the EMM can then be stripped centrally, and the entire EMM can be freed entirely from the retinal surface.[35]

♦ Recurrent EMMs: EMMs that occur after retinal reattachment surgery are more tightly adherent and thicker than the idiopathic variety.[35] These often overly a crater-like depression between tractionally elevated edges of retina. A blunt pick or fine-curved scissors can be passed through the trough to engage and/or transect the EMM after which it can be lifted from the retinal surface with fine-tipped, end-gripping forceps.

♦ Removal of the internal limiting membrane (ILM): Attached ILM is often found in surgically removed EMMs.[24,38] The purposeful removal of ILM during EMM removal has not been definitively shown to improve postoperative vision but may help prevent recurrence of the EMM.[38–41] Stains such as trypan blue and indocyanine green have also been reported to be useful in facilitating removal of the ILM in EMM surgery. Small, noncontrolled, interventional case series using these dyes have shown visual improvement and a lower EMM recurrence rate.[42,43]

♦ The in-to-out technique

♦ A 25-gauge end-gripping ILM forceps are used to directly engage the EMM at the thickest portion near the fovea.[44] The center of the EMM is identified by the orientation of the radial macular striae and grasped with the forceps tangentially. With this technique there can be a greater chance for producing iatrogenic posterior pole retinal breaks. To minimize this, it is important to always observe the fovea during the peeling process.

Step 3: Inspection of peripheral retina and intraocular tamponade.

♦ A careful inspection of the peripheral retina with scleral depression should be performed at the end of the surgery. If peripheral retinal breaks are found, they should be surrounded with endophotocoagulation. An air–fluid exchange followed by air–gas with SF6 gas should be performed. Though not needed routinely, postoperative intraocular gas tamponade and prone positioning may also prove beneficial in patients with significant retinal folds.[45]

Expected Outcomes: What Is the Worst-case Scenario

The worst-case scenario in postsurgical EMMs is irreversible vision loss. Secondary EMMs can cause significant limitation of vision in an otherwise successful surgery.[38,46] Though spontaneous visual improvement in EMMs is rare, vision can remain stable even without surgical intervention. In a study by Appiah and Hirose,[3] 55% of mostly postsurgical secondary EMMs that were simply observed had stable vision over a mean follow-up period of 44 months; however, there was greater visual improvement with surgery than with observation (54% vs. 16%), particularly in patients with initial vision worse than 20/100. Postsurgical visual improvement is possible in greater than 80% of eyes.[47,48] Katira et al.[49] reported an average visual improvement of 5.6 Snellen lines after vitrectomy for removal of secondary EMMs. Secondary EMMs do not necessarily have a worse visual outcome than idiopathic EMMs.[47,48] Preoperative prognostic factors include preoperative visual acuity and the duration of blurred vision before surgery.[47,48] Eyes that had better than 20/100 vision preoperatively had slightly better postoperative vision; although eyes with worse preoperative vision tended to have the most visual improvement after surgery.[3,27,47,48] Listed are the common postoperative complications and their incidences related to surgical removal of the EMM.[38,45,47,50-55]

◆ Progression of nuclear sclerotic cataract (12% to 47%)

◆ Retinal breaks (4% to 5.5%)

◆ Retinal detachment (1.2% to 5%)

◆ Recurrent EMM (3% to 5%)

◆ Cystoid macular edema (3%)

◆ Endophthalmitis (0.05%)

REFERENCES

1. Wise GN. Clinical features of idiopathic preretinal macular fibrosis. Schoenberg Lecture. *Am J Ophthalmol.* 1975;79:349–357.
2. Roth AM, Foos RY. Surface wrinkling retinopathy in eyes enucleated at autopsy. *Trans Am Acad Ophthalmol Otolaryngol.* 1971;75:1047–1058.
3. Appiah AP, Hirose T. Secondary causes of premacular fibrosis. *Ophthalmology.* 1989;96:389–392.
4. Hagler WS, Aturaliya U. Macular puckers after retinal detachment surgery. *Br J Ophthalmol.* 1971;55:451–457.
5. Lobes LA Jr, Burton TC. The incidence of macular pucker after retinal detachment surgery. *Am J Ophthalmol.* 1978;85:72–77.
6. Uemura A, Ideta H, Nagasaki H, et al. Macular pucker after retinal detachment surgery. *Ophthalmic Surg.* 1992;23:116–119.
7. Sabates NR, Sabates FN, Sabates R, et al. Macular changes after retinal detachment surgery. *Am J Ophthalmol.* 1989;108:22–29.
8. Gass JDM. *Stereoscopic Atlas of Macular Diseases: Diagnosis and Treatment,* 4th ed. St Louis, MO: CV Mosby; 1997:938–951.
9. Cherfan GM, Smiddy WE, Michels RG, et al. Clinicopathologic correlation of pigmented epiretinal membranes. *Am J Ophthalmol.* 1988;106:536–545.
10. Bellhorn MB, Friedman AH, Wise GN, et al. Ultrastructure and clinicopathologic correlation of idiopathic preretinal macular fibrosis. *Am J Ophthalmol.* 1975;79:366–373.
11. Foos RY. Vitreoretinal juncture; epiretinal membranes and vitreous. *Invest Ophthalmol Vis Sci.* 1977;16:416–422.
12. Francois J, Verbraeken H. Relationship between the drainage of the subretinal fluid in retinal detachment surgery and the appearance of macular pucker. *Ophthalmologica.* 1979;179:111–114.
13. Campochiaro P, Kaden IH, Vidaurri-Leal J, et al. Cryotherapy enhances intravitreal dispersion of viable retinal pigment epithelial cells. *Arch Ophthalmol.* 1985;103:434–436.
14. Jaccoma EH, Conway BP, Campochiaro PA. Cryotherapy causes extensive breakdown of the blood–retinal barrier. A comparison with argon laser photocoagulation. *Arch Ophthalmol.* 1985;103:1728–1730.
15. Glaser BM, Vidaurri-Leal J, Michels RG, et al. Cryotherapy during surgery for giant retinal tears and intravitreal dispersion of viable retinal pigment epithelial cells. *Ophthalmology.* 1993;100:466–470.

16. Kraushar MF, Morse PH. The relationship between retinal surgery and preretinal macular fibrosis. *Ophthalmic Surg.* 1988;19:843–848.

17. Saran BR, Brucker AJ. Macular epiretinal membrane formation and treated retinal breaks. *Am J Ophthalmol.* 1995;120:480–485.

18. Tannenbaum HL, Schepens CL, Elzeneiny I, et al. Macular pucker following retinal detachment surgery. *Arch Ophthalmol.* 1970;83:286–293.

19. Steel DHW, West J, Campbell WG. A randomized controlled study of the use of transscleral diode laser and cryotherapy in the management of rhegmatogenous retinal detachment. *Retina.* 2000;20:346–357.

20. Cox MS, Azan SP, Barr CC, et al. Macular pucker after successful surgery for proliferative vitreoretinopathy. Silicone Study Report 8. *Ophthalmology.* 1995;102:1884–1891.

21. Federman JL, Schubert HD. Complications associated with the use of silicone oil in 150 eyes after retina-vitreous surgery. *Ophthalmology.* 1988;95:870–876.

22. Lopez R, Chang S. Long-term results of vitrectomy and perfluorocarbon gas for the treatment of severe proliferative vitreoretinopathy. *Am J Ophthalmol.* 1992;113:424–428.

23. Bellhorn MB, Friedman AH, Wise GN, et al. Ultrastructure and clinicopathologic correlation of idiopathic preretinal macular fibrosis. *Am J Ophthalmol.* 1975;79:366–373.

24. Green WR, Kenyon KR, Michels RG, et al. Ultrastructure of epiretinal membranes causing macular pucker after retinal re-attachment surgery. *Trans Ophthalmol Soc UK.* 1979;99:65–77.

25. Kampik A, Kenyon KR, Michels RG, et al. Epiretinal and vitreous membranes: Comparative study of 56 cases. *Arch Ophthalmol.* 1981;99:1445–1454.

26. Hiscott P, Magee RM, Colthurst M, et al. Clinicopathological correlation of epiretinal membranes and posterior lens opacification following perfluorohexyloctane tamponade. *Br J Ophthalmol.* 2001;85:179–183.

27. Heidenkummer HP, Messmer EM, Kampik A. [Recurrent vitreoretinal membranes in intravitreal silicon oil tamponade. Morphologic and immunohistochemical studies]. *Ophthalmologe.* 1996;93:121–125.

28. Bonnet M. Macular changes and fluorescein angiographic findings after repair of proliferative vitreoretinopathy. *Retina.* 1994;14:404–410.

29. Sakamoto T, Miyazaki M, Hisatomi T, et al. Triamcinolone-assisted pars plana vitrectomy improves the surgical procedures and decreases the postoperative blood–ocular barrier breakdown. *Graefes Arch Clin Exp Ophthalmol.* 2002;240:423–429.

30. Landers MB 3rd, Trese MT, Stefansson E, et al. Argon laser intraocular photocoagulation. *Ophthalmology.* 1982;89:785–788.

31. Johnson RN, Irvine AR, Wood IS. Endolaser, cryopexy, and retinal reattachment in the air-filled eye. *Arch Ophthalmol.* 1987;105:231–234.

32. Gilbert C, McLeod D. D-ACE surgical sequence for selected bullous retinal detachments. *Br J Ophthalmol.* 1985;69:733–736.

33. Michels RG, Gilbert HD. Surgical management of macular pucker after retinal reattachment surgery. *Am J Ophthalmol.* 1979;88:925–929.

34. Ciulla TA, Pesavento RD. Epiretinal fibrosis. *Ophthalmic Surg Lasers.* 1997;28:670–679.

35. McDonald HR, Johnson RN, Ai Everett. Vitreoretinal surgery for idiopathic epiretinal membranes. In: Peyman GA, ed. *Vitreoretinal Surgical Techniques.* London: Martin Duntz; 2001:327–337.

36. Garretson BR, de Bustros S, Packo K. Suctional elevation of epiretinal membranes. *Arch Ophthalmol.* 1992;110:449.

37. Peyman GA. A combination pick and flute needle. *Arch Ophthalmol.* 1989;107:1687.

38. Michels RG. A clinical and histopathologic study of epiretinal membranes affecting the macula and removed by vitreous surgery. *Trans Am Ophthalmol Soc.* 1982;80:580–656.

39. Bovey EH, Uffer S, Achache F. Surgery for epimacular membrane: Impact of retinal internal limiting membrane removal on functional outcome. *Retina.* 2004;24:728–735.

40. Sivalingam A, Eagle RC, Duker JS, et al. Visual prognosis correlated with the presence of internal-limiting membrane in histopathologic specimens obtained from epiretinal membrane surgery. *Ophthalmology.* 1990;97:1549–1552.

41. Park DW, Dugel PU, Garda J, et al. Macular pucker removal with and without internal limiting membrane peeling: Pilot study. *Ophthalmology.* 2003;110:62–64.

42. Kwok AKH, Lai TYY, Li WWY, et al. Indocyanine green- assisted internal limiting membrane removal in epiretinal membrane surgery: A clinical and histologic study. *Am J Ophthalmol.* 2004;138:194–199.

43. Kwok AKH, Lai TYY, Li WWY, et al. Trypan blue- and indocyanine green-assisted epiretinal membrane surgery: Clinical and histopathological studies. *Eye.* 2004;18:882–888.

44. Charles S. Epimacular membranes and vitreomacular traction syndrome. In: Charles S, ed. *Vitreous Microsurgery.* 5th ed. Baltimore: Williams & Wilkins; 2011:157–163.

45. Margherio RR, Cox MS, Trese MT, et al. Removal of epimacular membranes. *Ophthalmology.* 1985;92:1075–1083.

46. de Bustros S, Rice TA, Michels RG, et al. Vitrectomy for macular pucker: Use after treatment of retinal tears or retinal detachment. *Arch Ophthalmol.* 1988;106: 758–760.

47. Council MD, Shah GK, Lee HC, Sharma S. Visual outcomes and complications of epiretinal membrane removal secondary to rhegmatogenous retinal detachment. *Ophthalmology.* 2005;112:1218–1221.

48. Rice TA, de Bustros S, Michels RG, et al. Prognostic factors in vitrectomy for epiretinal membranes of the macula. *Ophthalmology.* 1986;93:602–610.

49. Katira RC, Zamani M, Berinstein DM, et al. Incidence and characteristics of macular pucker formation after primary retinal detachment repair by pars plana vitrectomy alone. *Retina.* 2008;28:744–748.

50. de Bustros S, Thompson JT, Michels RG, et al. Nuclear sclerosis after vitrectomy for idiopathic epiretinal membranes. *Am J Ophthalmol.* 1988;105:160–164.

51. Maguire AM, Smiddy WE, Nanda SK, et al. Clinicopathologic correlation of recurrent epiretinal membranes after previous surgical removal. *Retina.* 1990;10: 213–222.

52. Sjaarda RN, Glaser BM, Thompson JT, et al. Distribution of iatrogenic retinal breaks in macular hole surgery. *Ophthalmology.* 1995;102:1387–1392.

53. Rizzo S, Belting C, Genovesi-Ebert F, et al. Incidence of retinal detachment after small-incision, sutureless pars plana vitrectomy compared with conventional 20-gauge vitrectomy in macular hole and epiretinal membrane surgery. *Retina.* 2010;30:1065–1071.

54. McDonald HR, Verre WP, Aaberg TM. Surgical management of idiopathic epiretinal membranes. *Ophthalmology.* 1986;93:978–983.

55. Joondeph BC, Blanc J-P, Polkinghorne PJ. Endophthalmitis after pars plana vitrectomy: A New Zealand experience. *Retina.* 2005;25:587–589.

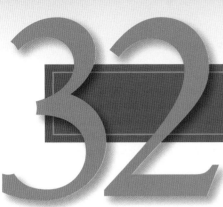

32 POSTOPERATIVE MACULAR EDEMA

LYNDON DA CRUZ AND KUNAL K. DANSINGANI

 The Complication: Definition

Macular edema represents a pathologic state in which there is an increase in macular thickness due to accumulation of intracellular and extracellular fluids within the neurosensory retina. The anatomical changes are usually accompanied by a decrease in visual acuity, with or without distortion. The extent of visual impairment can vary but in certain pathologies it correlates with the degree of edema and its chronicity, both of which can impair retinal function.

Macular thickening may be localized (focal) or diffuse and may take a cystic configuration. These structural findings are usually detectable biomicroscopically. Subclinical macular edema may be demonstrated by fluorescein angiography or optical coherence tomography (OCT).

Postoperative macular edema was first described by Irvine[1] in 1953 following cataract surgery, and macular edema in this subgroup is now referred to as Irvine–Gass syndrome. This chapter covers the pathogenesis, risk factors, and management of macular edema focusing on the vitreoretinal postoperative context.

 Pathogenesis

Macular edema has been described as the "final common pathway" of a diversity of ocular pathologies including genetic (e.g., retinitis pigmentosa and dominant cystoid macular edema (CME)), inflammatory, vascular, and tractional.[2,3] Although the precise mechanisms that lead to the formation of edema are incompletely understood, most cases can be explained in terms of microvascular permeability changes. Retinal edema develops when the ingress of fluid into the extravascular extracellular compartment overwhelms the capacity of scavenger mechanisms to reabsorb that fluid. Macular edema is therefore a dynamic state.

The concept of the blood–retinal barrier (BRB) encapsulates a number of anatomical and functional features of the retina that collectively ensure that excess fluid does not accumulate in the extracellular space of healthy retina. The outer BRB correlates with tight junctions between the cells of the retinal pigment epithelium (RPE) and the inner BRB correlates with tight junctions between endothelial cells of the retinal capillary bed.

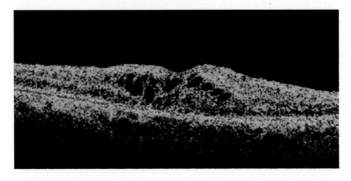

Figure 32-1 Persistent cystoid macular edema 9 months following epiretinal membrane peel.

Traction at the vitreoretinal interface applies mechanical forces on retinal blood vessels. This is especially evident in patients with vitreomacular traction or epiretinal membrane. The internal limiting membrane may also serve to transmit tractional forces. Tractional forces may induce edema either by direct effect on blood vessels, or by altering the cytokine environment through mechanical effects on neuronal and glial cells. It has been shown that the presence of epiretinal membrane can reduce microvascular flow velocities in the retinal capillary bed.[4]

Vascular permeability is increased by various cytokines and vasoproliferative factors. The most influential and consistent is vascular endothelial growth factor (VEGF), which can cause phosphorylation of tight junction proteins. The vitreous of diabetic eyes contains, in addition, elevated levels of angiotensin II, angiotensin-converting enzyme (ACE), platelet-derived growth factor (PDGF), and fibroblast growth factor β (FGF-β), all of which are thought to contribute to increased vascular permeability.[2] Vitreous serves as a depot within which cytokines and other mediators may accumulate to exert a more sustained influence.

Risk Factors and Prevention

Risk factors for developing macular edema may be classified as surgical or pathologic (Table 32-1).

Prevention

Surgically induced macular edema may be prevented by:

◆ Addressing pathologic risk factors prior to surgery (e.g., treating pre-existing uveitis).

Table 32-1 • Risk Factors and Preventive Measures for Postoperative Macular Edema

Surgical	Surgery without intraoperative complication	The incidence of angiographically demonstrable cystoid macular edema following uncomplicated cataract surgery is reported to be as high as 20%.[5–7] However, only about 1% of patients have clinically significant findings (impaired vision or biomicroscopically evident CME).[8,9]
		Although CME following vitrectomy is well recognized, a literature search on the subject yields very little data. Angiographic macular edema has been reported to occur in 80% of eyes undergoing macular hole surgery with internal limiting membrane (ILM) peel, and in this cohort the edema persisted for an average of 4 mos.[10]
		Kim et al.[11] have tried to quantify the phenomenon by OCT in patients operated for epiretinal membrane, vitreous hemorrhage, and macular hole. Their data suggest that at 1 mo postop macular thickness is greater in eyes that have undergone epiretinal membrane (ERM) peel than in eyes treated for MH or VH. The degree of postoperative anterior segment inflammation on day 1 also appears to correlate with macular thickness.
	Prolonged or complicated surgery	Prolonged surgery predisposes to postoperative uveitis. Inflammatory mediators may diffuse from the anterior segment and accumulate in the vitreous, resulting in cystoid macular edema.
		Anterior segment surgery that compromises the capsule and requires anterior vitrectomy significantly increases the risk of clinically significant CME (12–20%). This is especially the case if the posterior hyaloid is still attached and the vitreous is incarcerated in the surgical wound, or if severe iris trauma occurred during surgery.[12,13]
	Vitrectomy	Macular edema arising *de novo* after *pars plana* vitrectomy is uncommon, probably due to the absence of a tractional medium as well as the absence of a depot of inflammatory mediators in the vitrectomized eye. The literature on the subject is sparse, and generally addresses macular edema following vitrectomy **with macular surgery**.

Table 32-1 • Risk Factors and Preventive Measures for Postoperative Macular Edema (*continued*)		
Pathologic		Pre-existing macular edema can persist or increase after vitreoretinal surgery (Fig. 32-1).
	Retinal vascular disease	Macular edema occurring in retinal microvascular disease is a manifestation of capillary decompensation due to cumulative damage. When capillary damage is mild, a degree of functional reversibility may exist (compensation) as in limited branch retinal vein occlusion. However, capillary damage is often irreversible, and, in the case of diabetic maculopathy, tends to be progressive. Diabetic retinopathy and retinal vein occlusion are both well-recognized risk factors for developing postoperative macular edema.
	Macular traction	Macular edema may be associated with tractional macular pathology. Macular edema associated with vitreomacular traction or epiretinal membrane may persist after vitrectomy, even if traction has been relieved during surgery. The incidence for postoperative macular edema (based on OCT central subfield thickness criteria) at 1 mo after epiretinal membrane peel is of the order of 64%.[11] Macular edema can occur associated with retinal vascular disease (diabetic retinopathy) and macular traction and in these cases relief of the tractional component may be beneficial. In patients with diabetic macular edema refractory to macular laser/anti-VEGF therapy and coexisting epiretinal membrane, vitrectomy and internal limiting membrane peel can result in reduction of retinal thickness and may be performed. However, any improvement in visual acuity appears to be limited.[14] Visual acuity improvements due to surgical posterior hyaloid separation and internal limited membrane peeling appear to be more significant in eyes with taut posterior hyaloid, provided the macula in these cases is not ischemic.[15] Following surgery, macular edema may still be present. The time for resolution of macular edema is not clear from the literature on diabetic macular traction. In nondiabetic eyes undergoing internal limiting membrane peel for macular hole, macular edema resolved by 4 mos on average.[10] It may therefore be reasonable to form a judgment about the patient's clinical course by 2–4 mos postop, and then determine whether additional treatment is required.
	Retinal detachment	Although retinal edema usually resolves to a great extent after successful reattachment surgery, macular edema may be observed postoperatively.
	Endophthalmitis	Postoperative or endogenous endophthalmitis can give rise to aggressive posterior segment inflammation, of which cystoid macular edema is a feature. Epiretinal membrane or necrotic macular hole can further complicate the picture. Endophthalmitis can rapidly damage macular function, which may remain poor even after resolution of the infection and inflammatory process.

◆ Optimizing surgical technique to limit operating time and minimize complications.

◆ Ensuring that macular traction is relieved by the end of a posterior segment procedure.

Management and Prognosis

The management of macular edema involves diagnosis, determination of clinical significance, and treatment.

Diagnosis is often clinical, but several imaging modalities are sensitive for CME. Fluorescein angiography and OCT are most popular.

A number of options are available for the treatment of macular edema. These vary in invasiveness and risk and are therefore often invoked in a stepwise escalation (Table 32-2).[16]

Although a number of modalities are available for the treatment of macular edema, each patient is likely to require a tailored strategy due to the heterogeneity

Table 32-2 • Treatment Options for Postoperative Macular Edema

Approach	Comments	Complications
Conservative	In the context of uncomplicated cataract surgery, CME usually occurs within 3–12 wks of surgery, with an incidence of up to 5%.[17] In 80% of cases, spontaneous resolution occurs within 3–12 mos.[18] In vitrectomized eyes, CME is often self-limiting lasting on average 4 mos.[10]	• Irreversible macular damage if CME is prolonged
Topical NSAIDs	The main topical nonsteroidal preparations that are widely used are: • Ketorolac 0.4%, • Diclofenac 1%, and • Indomethacin 1% Administered qid or tid together with a topical steroid, they may be used to lower the production of prostaglandins in the anterior segment. Topical NSAIDs may also be used prophylactically when risk factors for CME have been identified. However, indications for preemptive administration are more relevant to anterior segment surgery than vitreoretinal surgery. Nepafenac is a relatively new NSAID in prodrug form. It is metabolized to amfenac, which is a potent COX-2 inhibitor. Nepafenac has been shown to have significantly better posterior segment permeation than either ketorolac or diclofenac in rabbits, being bio-activated in all parts of the uveal tract.[19] In human subjects, ketorolac has been found to reach higher vitreous concentrations than nepafenac or amfenac.[20] Anecdotal reports suggest that nepafenac may have a role in treating macular edema that is nonresponsive to ketorolac. Nepafenac is normally dosed as 0.1% topical solution administered three or four times per day.	Side effects • Ocular surface irritation • Mydriasis • Corneal melting
Corticosteroids	Topical steroids form the mainstay of anti-inflammatory in most postoperative regimens. They inhibit the production of arachidonic acid by phospholipase A2 and reduce prostaglandin and leukotriene synthesis. Corticosteroids also inhibit VEGF gene expression.[21] Topical steroids are particularly effective in treating macular edema when anterior segment inflammation is the driving factor. Following anterior segment surgery, topical steroids have been shown to act synergistically with NSAIDs to treat macular edema.[22,23] Commonly used topical steroids are dexamethasone 0.1% and prednisolone 0.5% or 1%. Periocular administration of steroid allows the administration of a large bolus of drug with sustained release and with limitation of systemic side effects. The drug may be delivered by subtenons or orbital floor injection and diffuses through the sclera. In animal models scleral penetration has been shown to be greater in inflamed eyes, and periocular steroids have a particular role in treating macular edema secondary to uveitis.[24]	Complications Topical • Ocular hypertension • Cataract • Herpetic keratitis Periocular • Orbital hemorrhage • Globe penetration • Fat atrophy • Ptosis

Table 32-2 • Treatment Options for Postoperative Macular Edema (*continued*)		
Approach	**Comments**	**Complications**
	Commonly used preparations and doses are: • Triamcinolone 40 mg (subtenon) • Methylprednisolone 40 mg (orbital floor) • Betamethasone 4 mg (orbital floor) In retinal vascular disease, intravitreal steroids can be administered to give a high concentration of drug close to the site of desired action. The usual dose for intravitreal triamcinolone is 4 mg. In the absence of chronic retinal vascular disease, a single injection may yield a lasting reduction in CME. However, the beneficial effects tend to be limited to 4–6 mos in patients with diabetic macular edema or branch retinal vein occlusion. Jonas et al.[25–27] have reported that the duration of effect of an increased dose of 20–25 mg triamcinolone in diabetic macular edema is limited to 6–8 mos; after this period, macular edema recurs and repeat injections are required. Moreover, over a third of patients experience raised intraocular pressures. A rebound of macular edema has also been observed after treatment of pseudophakic macular edema with intravitreal triamcinolone 8 mg.[28] When macular edema occurs or persists after surgical removal of epiretinal membrane, intravitreal administration of triamcinolone 4 mg may accelerate postoperative reduction in retinal thickness. Moreover, reduction in macular thickness appears to correlate with improvement in visual acuity.[11] It has also been suggested that intravitreal triamcinolone 4 mg administered at the time of epiretinal membrane surgery may speed up resolution of macular edema and increase the proportion of cases that have physiologic macular thickness at final follow-up.[29] Ozurdex is an intravitreal implant containing dexamethasone 0.7 mg. It has been shown to have a beneficial effect in modifying the clinical course following retinal vein occlusion, both in terms of central subfield thickness and visual acuity.[30] The potential role for Ozurdex in treating postoperative macular edema has not been studied in trial, but has been reported anecdotally.[31] Systemic steroids are frequently used in the treatment of posterior uveitis and are effective in bringing the inflammatory process under control in the acute setting. Administration is often indicated by visual loss due to macular edema and is usually in the form of oral prednisolone or, less frequently, intravenous methylprednisolone. Side effects are considerable, and if prolonged action is required, steroid sparing agents should be considered for maintenance. A literature search does not reveal evidence regarding the use of systemic steroids to treat postvitrectomy CME.	Intravitreal • Endophthalmitis • Ocular hypertension • Cataract • Triamcinolone crystalline maculopathy • Systemic • Cataract • Weight gain • Endocrinopathy (including diabetes and Cushing syndrome) • Osteoporosis • Psychosis

(*continued*)

Table 32-2 • Treatment Options for Postoperative Macular Edema (*continued*)

Approach	Comments	Complications
Carbonic anhydrase inhibitors (CAIs)	CAIs have been shown to enhance the absorption of fluid across the retinal pigment epithelium.[32,33] Their use in clinical practice is well established, and oral acetazolamide has been used in conjunction with topical NSAIDs to treat cystoid macular edema.[34] CAIs are more effective in treating macular edema due to RPE dysfunction, and less effective if the accumulation of fluid is due to retinal capillary hyperpermeability.[34,35] Mutations in the carbonic anhydrase IV (CA IV) gene have been found in patients with autosomal dominant retinitis pigmentosa.[36,37] Interestingly, CAIs are particularly beneficial in treating cystoid macular edema secondary to retinitis pigmentosa. Knowledge of the precise mechanism is incomplete, but prolonged treatment is marked by a tachyphylaxis which is reversible after a period of discontinuation of treatment.[38] Typical administration for oral acetazolamide is 500 mg daily in divided doses over 1 mo,[39] usually in conjunction with a topical steroid and a topical NSAID. With prolonged use, electrolyte balance should be monitored and oral potassium supplementation may be indicated.	Side effects • Paresthesia • Nausea • Dizziness • Hypokalemia
Intravitreal anti-VEGF	Intravitreal agents that target VEGF have become established in the treatment of macular edema due to a number of etiologies, including retinal vein occlusion, diabetes mellitus, uveitis, and retinitis pigmentosa.[40–45] Efficacy of VEGF blockade has also been demonstrated in the treatment of Irvine–Gass syndrome, albeit in small studies.[46,47] The effects on anti-VEGF therapy may be enhanced by combination with intravitreal triamcinolone or macular laser, depending on coexisting pathology.	Complications • Endophthalmitis • Vitreous hemorrhage • Exacerbation of tractional retinal detachment (TRD) • Macular ischemia
Nd-YAG laser	YAG laser anterior vitreolysis can be an effective method for relieving traction due to vitreous incarceration in an anterior segment surgical wound.[48] The laser should be applied to a vitreous strand where it is at a maximum distance from the corneal endothelium and the iris stroma, to minimize collateral damage. The method is effective for vitreous strands of very narrow caliber which can be lysed with up to 3–4 pulses. Sheets of incarcerated vitreous would require surgical anterior vitrectomy.	Complications • Corneal endothelial damage • Iris stromal disruption • Anterior uveitis
Green laser (argon or frequency-doubled YAG: 532 nm)	Focal or grid laser photocoagulation has been the main treatment for diabetic macular edema ever since the findings of the ETDRS. Its mechanism of action is incompletely understood. A number of hypotheses have been suggested, varying from RPE damage-and-repair, to altering oxygen demand by photoreceptor disruption, to microaneurysm photocoagulation. Laser treatment may be effective in treating postoperative macular edema if this is associated with retinal microvascular disease, most notably diabetes and branch retinal vein occlusion. Due to the potentially destructive effect of laser, it would have to be applied to extrafoveally distributed macular edema. Argon laser is not a recognized treatment for postoperative cystoid macular edema.	Complications • Macular burn • Central scotoma • CNVM

Table 32-2 • Treatment Options for Postoperative Macular Edema (*continued*)

Approach	Comments	Complications
Photodynamic therapy (PDT)	PDT with verteporfin is not routinely considered for Irvine–Gass syndrome or postvitrectomy macular edema but some efficacy has been demonstrated for radiation retinopathy refractory to laser photocoagulation.[49] PDT has also been used to treat macular edema associated with choroidal neovascular membranes (CNVM) arising after laser photocoagulation for macular edema.[50] These reports predate the advent of anti-VEGF therapy.	
Surgical treatments	Anterior vitrectomy is often a definitive intervention for macular edema caused by vitreomacular traction due to incarcerated vitreous strands after anterior segment surgery. It may be considered a first-line intervention, though pharmacologic treatments may be prescribed concurrently. Pars plana vitrectomy has been shown to be beneficial as a treatment for macular edema in certain situations, including uveitis and retinitis pigmentosa. In the postvitrectomy setting, macular edema which is attributable to residual vitreomacular traction (VMT) or preretinal membranes may be addressed by further macular surgery.	Complications Vitrectomy • Retinal detachment • Cataract • Vitreous hemorrhage • CME

of risk factors and possible combinations of circumstances. Literature review provides some information as to the expected outcome with each modality, but cannot prescribe a treatment protocol. Factors to be considered include:

◆ Whether macular edema is purely surgical in etiology or whether there is contributory copathology

◆ Duration and extent of edema: If surgery is recent and CME is mild, it may resolve with observation

◆ Suitability of the patient for a particular treatment option

◆ Risk versus benefit: For example, an eye with mild tractional macular edema due to epiretinal membrane would have a different risk–benefit ratio compared to one in which macular edema has been sufficiently gross and longstanding to disrupt neurosensory architecture. In the latter, macular surgery may yield an anatomical result but probably without functional benefit.

If there is residual macular edema after successful ERM peeling, then there is a sequence of options to consider. The authors prefer to initially wait 8 to 12 weeks as resolution may still occur, provided that there is no clinical or OCT evidence of residual traction or membrane. If edema persists, a 4- to 6-week course of combined topical steroid and nonsteroidal drops would be recommended. If there is no response to this treatment intravitreal steroids can be considered, either ozurdex or triamcinolone. If there were evidence of residual traction or the ILM was not peeled in the first surgery, reoperation would be advisable.

Prognosis

The prognosis of macular edema is difficult to quantify globally. This is because the potential contributing factors are so numerous and it is often impossible to elucidate the significance of each one. Moreover, successful resolution of macular edema does not always correlate with improvement in vision.

In discussing prognosis with a patient, it is helpful to explain that outcomes lie on a spectrum, and that a number of factors can influence where on the spectrum the individual patient will end up. Factors to be discussed include:

◆ Potential reversibility of macular edema: Mild CME is likely to be reversible, end-stage ischemic diabetic maculopathy is not. The degree to which macular architecture has been disrupted and the duration of this disruption can both be informative.

◆ Reversibility of macular edema does not necessarily constitute visual recovery.

◆ Recovery of visual acuity may still leave the patient symptomatic if there is residual distortion or decreased contrast sensitivity.

REFERENCES

1. Irvine SR. A newly defined vitreous syndrome following cataract surgery. *Am J Ophthalmol.* 1953;36(5):499–619.
2. da Cruz L, Gregor MZ. Surgery in the treatment of cystoid macular oedema. In: Ryan SJ, Hinton DR, Schachat AP, Wilkinson CP, eds. *Retina.* 4th ed. Elsevier/Mosby (USA): 2006;2633–2644.
3. Tranos PG, Wickremasinghe SS, Stangos NT, et al. Macular edema. *Surv Ophthalmol.* 2004;49(5):470–490.
4. Kadonosono K, Itoh N, Nomura E, et al. Capillary blood flow velocity in patients with idiopathic epiretinal membranes. *Retina.* 1999;19(6):536–539.
5. Peterson M, Yoshizumi MO, Hepler R, et al. Topical indomethacin in the treatment of chronic cystoid macular edema. *Graefes Arch Clin Exp Ophthalmol.* 1992;230(5): 401–405.
6. Ursell PG, Spalton DJ, Whitcup SM, et al. Cystoid macular edema after phacoemulsification: Relationship to blood-aqueous barrier damage and visual acuity. *J Cataract Refract Surg.* 1999;25(11):1492–1497.
7. Wright PL, Wilkinson CP, Balyeat HD, et al. Angiographic cystoid macular edema after posterior chamber lens implantation. *Arch Ophthalmol.* 1988;106(6):740–744.
8. Jampol LM, Sanders DR, Kraff MC. Prophylaxis and therapy of aphakic cystoid macular edema. *Surv Ophthalmol.* 1984;28(suppl):535–539.
9. Stark WJ Jr, Maumenee AE, Fagadau W, et al. Cystoid macular edema in pseudophakia. *Surv Ophthalmol.* 1984;28(suppl):442–451.
10. Staudt S, Miller DW, Unnebrink K, et al. [Incidence and extent of postoperative macular edema following vitreoretinal surgery with and without combined cataract operation]. *Ophthalmologe.* 2003;100(9):702–707.
11. Kim SJ, Martin DF, Hubbard GB 3rd, et al. Incidence of postvitrectomy macular edema using optical coherence tomography. *Ophthalmology.* 2009;116(8):1531–1537.
12. Frost NA, Sparrow JM, Strong NP, et al. Vitreous loss in planned extracapsular cataract extraction does lead to a poorer visual outcome. *Eye (Lond).* 1995;9(pt 4): 446–451.
13. Bergman M, Laatikainen L. Cystoid macular oedema after complicated cataract surgery and implantation of an anterior chamber lens. *Acta Ophthalmol (Copenh).* 1994;72(2):178–180.
14. Rosenblatt BJ, Shah GK, Sharma S, et al. Pars plana vitrectomy with internal limiting membranectomy for refractory diabetic macular edema without a taut posterior hyaloid. *Graefes Arch Clin Exp Ophthalmol.* 2005;243(1):20–25.
15. Pendergast SD, Hassan TS, Williams GA, et al. Vitrectomy for diffuse diabetic macular edema associated with a taut premacular posterior hyaloid. *Am J Ophthalmol.* 2000;130(2):178–186.

16. Zur D, Fischer N, Tufail A, et al. Postsurgical cystoid macular edema. *Eur J Ophthalmol.* 2010;21(S6):62–68.

17. Spaide RF, Yannuzzi LA, Sisco LJ. Chronic cystoid macular edema and predictors of visual acuity. *Ophthalmic Surg.* 1993;24(4):262–267.

18. Bradford JD, Wilkinson CP, Bradford RH Jr. Cystoid macular edema following extra-capsular cataract extraction and posterior chamber intraocular lens implantation. *Retina.* 1988;8(3):161–164.

19. Lindstrom R, Kim T. Ocular permeation and inhibition of retinal inflammation: an examination of data and expert opinion on the clinical utility of nepafenac. *Curr Med Res Opin.* 2006;22(2):397–404.

20. Heier JS, Awh CC, Busbee BG, et al. Vitreous nonsteroidal antiinflammatory drug concentrations and prostaglandin E2 levels in vitrectomy patients treated with ketorolac 0.4%, bromfenac 0.09%, and nepafenac 0.1%. *Retina.* 2009;29(9):1310–1313.

21. Nauck M, Karakiulakis G, Perruchoud AP, et al. Corticosteroids inhibit the expression of the vascular endothelial growth factor gene in human vascular smooth muscle cells. *Eur J Pharmacol.* 1998;341(2–3):309–315.

22. Heier JS, Topping TM, Baumann W, et al. Ketorolac versus prednisolone versus combination therapy in the treatment of acute pseudophakic cystoid macular edema. *Ophthalmology.* 2000;107(11):2034–2038;discussion 2039.

23. Wittpenn JR, Silverstein S, Heier J, et al. A randomized, masked comparison of topical ketorolac 0.4% plus steroid vs steroid alone in low-risk cataract surgery patients. *Am J Ophthalmol.* 2008;146(4):554–560.

24. McCartney HJ, Drysdale IO, Gornall AG, et al. An autoradiographic study of the penetration of subconjunctivally injected hydrocortisone into the normal and inflamed rabbit eye. *Invest Ophthalmol.* 1965;4:297–302.

25. Jonas JB, Kreissig I, Sofker A, et al. Intravitreal injection of triamcinolone for diffuse diabetic macular edema. *Arch Ophthalmol.* 2003;121(1):57–61.

26. Jonas JB, Degenring RF, Kamppeter BA, et al. Duration of the effect of intravitreal triamcinolone acetonide as treatment for diffuse diabetic macular edema. *Am J Ophthalmol.* 2004;138(1):158–160.

27. Jonas JB, Spandau UH, Kamppeter BA, et al. Repeated intravitreal high-dosage injections of triamcinolone acetonide for diffuse diabetic macular edema. *Ophthalmology.* 2006;113(5):800–804.

28. Benhamou N, Massin P, Haouchine B, et al. Intravitreal triamcinolone for refractory pseudophakic macular edema. *Am J Ophthalmol.* 2003;135(2):246–249.

29. Konstantinidis L, Berguiga M, Beknazar E, et al. Anatomic and functional outcome after 23-gauge vitrectomy, peeling, and intravitreal triamcinolone for idiopathic macular epiretinal membrane. *Retina.* 2009;29(8):1119–1127.

30. Haller JA, Bandello F, Belfort R Jr, et al. Randomized, sham-controlled trial of dexamethasone intravitreal implant in patients with macular edema due to retinal vein occlusion. *Ophthalmology.* 2010;117(6):1134–1146.e1133.

31. Meyer LM, Schonfeld CL. Cystoid macular edema after complicated cataract surgery resolved by an intravitreal dexamethasone 0.7-mg implant. *Case Report Ophthalmol.* 2011;2(3):319–322.

32. Marmor MF, Abdul-Rahim AS, Cohen DS. The effect of metabolic inhibitors on retinal adhesion and subretinal fluid resorption. *Invest Ophthalmol Vis Sci.* 1980;19(8):893–903.

33. Marmor MF, Maack T. Enhancement of retinal adhesion and subretinal fluid resorption by acetazolamide. *Invest Ophthalmol Vis Sci.* 1982;23(1):121–124.

34. Cox SN, Hay E, Bird AC. Treatment of chronic macular edema with acetazolamide. *Arch Ophthalmol.* 1988;106(9):1190–1195.

35. Tripathi RC, Fekrat S, Tripathi BJ, et al. A direct correlation of the resolution of pseudophakic cystoid macular edema with acetazolamide therapy. *Ann Ophthalmol.* 1991;23(4):127–129.

36. Alvarez BV, Vithana EN, Yang Z, et al. Identification and characterization of a novel mutation in the carbonic anhydrase IV gene that causes retinitis pigmentosa. *Invest Ophthalmol Vis Sci.* 2007;48(8):3459–3468.

37. Datta R, Waheed A, Bonapace G, et al. Pathogenesis of retinitis pigmentosa associated with apoptosis-inducing mutations in carbonic anhydrase IV. *Proc Natl Acad Sci U S A*. 2009;106(9):3437–3442.

38. Thobani A, Fishman GA. The use of carbonic anhydrase inhibitors in the retreatment of cystic macular lesions in retinitis pigmentosa and X-linked retinoschisis. *Retina*. 2011;31(2):312–315.

39. Wolfensberger TJ. The role of carbonic anhydrase inhibitors in the management of macular edema. *Doc Ophthalmol*. 1999;97(3–4):387–397.

40. Arevalo JF, Sanchez JG, Wu L, et al. Primary intravitreal bevacizumab for diffuse diabetic macular edema: The Pan-American Collaborative Retina Study Group at 24 months. *Ophthalmology*. 2009;116(8):1488–1497, 1497.e1481.

41. Acharya NR, Hong KC, Lee SM. Ranibizumab for refractory uveitis-related macular edema. *Am J Ophthalmol*. 2009;148(2):303–309.e302.

42. Brown DM, Campochiaro PA, Bhisitkul RB, et al. Sustained benefits from ranibizumab for macular edema following branch retinal vein occlusion: 12-month outcomes of a phase III study. *Ophthalmology*. 2011;118(8):1594–1602.

43. Cervantes-Castaneda RA, Giuliari GP, Gallagher MJ, et al. Intravitreal bevacizumab in refractory uveitic macular edema: One-year follow-up. *Eur J Ophthalmol*. 2009;19(4):622–629.

44. Ahmadieh H, Ramezani A, Shoeibi N, et al. Intravitreal bevacizumab with or without triamcinolone for refractory diabetic macular edema; a placebo-controlled, randomized clinical trial. *Graefes Arch Clin Exp Ophthalmol*. 2008;246(4):483–489.

45. Artunay O, Yuzbasioglu E, Rasier R, et al. Intravitreal ranibizumab in the treatment of cystoid macular edema associated with retinitis pigmentosa. *J Ocul Pharmacol Ther*. 2009;25(6):545–550.

46. Barone A, Russo V, Prascina F, et al. Short-term safety and efficacy of intravitreal bevacizumab for pseudophakic cystoid macular edema. *Retina*. 2009;29(1):33–37.

47. Arevalo JF, Maia M, Garcia-Amaris RA, et al. Intravitreal bevacizumab for refractory pseudophakic cystoid macular edema: The Pan-American Collaborative Retina Study Group results. *Ophthalmology*. 2009;116(8):1481–1487, 1487.e1481.

48. Steinert RF, Wasson PJ. Neodymium:YAG laser anterior vitreolysis for Irvine-Gass cystoid macular edema. *J Cataract Refract Surg*. 1989;15(3):304–307.

49. Bakri SJ, Beer PM. Photodynamic therapy for maculopathy due to radiation retinopathy. *Eye (Lond)*. 2005;19(7):795–799.

50. Bakri SJ, Beer PM. Photodynamic therapy with verteporfin for classic choroidal neovascularization secondary to focal laser photocoagulation for radiation retinopathy. *Ophthalmic Surg Lasers Imaging*. 2003;34(6):475–477.

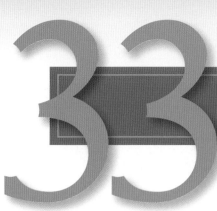

33 POSTOPERATIVE MACULAR HOLE FORMATION

Lyndon da Cruz and Kunal K. Dansingani

The Complication: Definition

The term macular hole describes a group of disorders characterized by a partial or full-thickness defect in the neurosensory fovea. The degree of visual disturbance, ranging from mild distortion to frank central scotoma with poor acuity, is related to the precise nature of foveal disruption. Macular hole may be classified by etiology or by anatomical findings.

Pathogenesis and Risk Factors

Although the understanding of the pathogenesis of primary idiopathic macular hole is incomplete, mechanical aspects of the process are well described from a number of angles. These angles include the following.

◆ The original Gass classification, clinically describing lesion formation and natural history.[1]

◆ Additional evidence from the subsequent advent of optical coherence tomography (OCT).

◆ Success rates of surgical intervention.

Traction

Vitreomacular traction (VMT) occurs in eyes that do not have a complete posterior vitreous detachment (PVD). VMT is implicated in macular hole formation, and relieving VMT has been shown to increase hole closure rates.[2] VMT is also thought to mediate acute macular hole formation following trauma, Yttrium aluminium garnet (YAG) vitreo-disruption, or cataract surgery (Fig. 33-1). In the latter scenario it has been suggested that forces arising from surgical fluctuations in anterior chamber depth may be transmitted directly to the macula. An alternative hypothesis is that removal of the crystalline lens allows forward displacement of the vitreous, exacerbating vitreomacular traction in a more chronic manner.

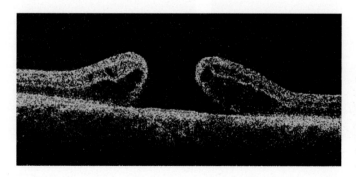

Figure 33-1 Macular hole following YAG vitreo-disruption for symptomatic floaters. The configuration of the hole reflects the etiologic role of traction.

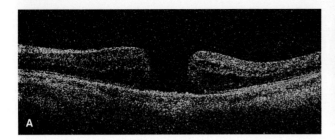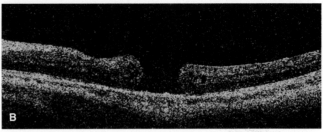

Figure 33-2 OCT sections demonstrating macular hole. **(A)** Detected 6 weeks after vitrectomy with gas tamponade for macula-involving rhegmatogenous retinal detachment. **(B)** Persistence of macular hole with "flat-open" configuration, 6 months after ILM peel. (Acknowledgments: Marie-Hélène Errera and Paul Sullivan.)

Tangential traction at the macula can give rise to foveal dehiscence and contribute to macular hole nonclosure. Tangential traction may arise from focal shrinkage of prefoveal cortical vitreous.[1,3]

Epiretinal membrane, if present, may also contribute to tangential traction and may be a causative factor for lamellar or full-thickness macular hole; the role of the internal limiting membrane in macular hole formation is unclear, but internal limiting membrane (ILM) peeling has been shown to improve closure rates for primary macular hole.

Macular hole formation as a sequel to vitreoretinal surgery is well-recognized, but infrequently reported **(Fig. 33-2)**. The mechanism is incompletely understood. Residual tangential traction is likely to be a contributing factor. In eyes vitrectomized for retinal detachment, it has been shown that residual cortical vitreous can persist at the macula, only to be detected during ensuing macular hole surgery.[4] Further surgery to peel the ILM can result in hole closure, and may do so by enabling complete clearance of residual premacular cortical vitreous.[5] **Figure 33-3** illustrates

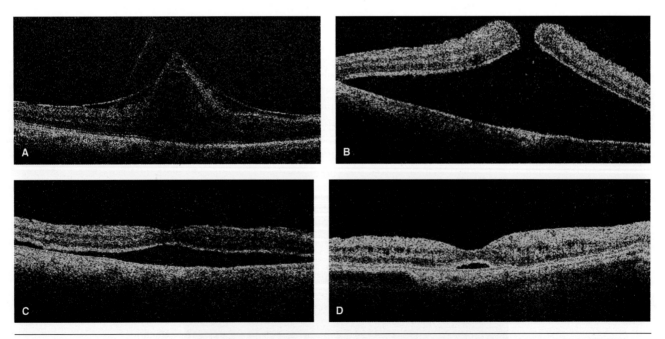

Figure 33-3 A: Vitreomacular traction syndrome. **B:** Macular hole with extensive subretinal fluid and elevated edges 1 month after vitrectomy. **C:** Macular hole closed with persistent subretinal fluid 6 weeks after SF6 tamponade. **D:** Residual submacular fluid at 1 year follow-up. (Acknowledgments: Marie-Hélène Errera and Paul Sullivan.)

Table 33-1 • Nontractional Factors Contributing to Postoperative Macular Hole Formation	
Lamellar hole and CMO	Lamellar foveal defects can be associated with vitreomacular traction or with cystoid macular edema. Both situations give rise to mechanical fragility at the umbo.
	Vitrectomy with ILM peel for lamellar hole may be complicated by full-thickness macular hole formation with a corresponding drop in visual acuity.
	Cystoid macular edema predisposes to macular hole formation through thinning of the inner wall of the cyst. Cyst rupture can occur spontaneously, usually in association with vitreomacular traction, leading to lamellar hole formation. Iatrogenic deroofing of a macular cyst may also occur following epiretinal membrane peeling. The risk of deroofing a cyst may be greater if ILM peel is attempted in such cases.
Inflammation	Intraocular inflammation can lead to macular hole formation through three mechanisms: 1. Cystoid macular edema leading to cyst rupture. 2. Epiretinal membrane formation with tangential pucker. 3. Foveal necrosis (e.g., in endophthalmitis)
Myopia	In myopic eyes, the central retina is thinner than in an emmetropic eye. The combination of vitreomacular traction, retinal thinning, and posterior staphyloma predisposes to foveal schisis with or without a frank macular hole.

iatrogenic macular hole formation after vitrectomy for vitreomacular traction syndrome, and subsequent hole closure with SF_6 tamponade.

Although most cases of postoperative macular hole present within 6 months of the initial surgery, Lipham and Smiddy[6] report that the timeframe can be as long as 5½ years. Moreover, they report that during ensuing surgery, premacular cortical vitreous was absent. They suggest that other factors may be implicated in facilitating spontaneous umbo dehiscence.

In addition to traction therefore, the factors shown in Table 33-1 may be relevant.

Pearls on how to prevent it

Based on an understanding of the mechanisms that contribute to formation of macular holes, a number of surgical precautions may be undertaken to minimize the risk of iatrogenic macular hole as follows.

1. Care during cataract surgery or other forms of intraocular surgery to minimize fluctuations in intraocular pressure, particularly in eyes without posterior vitreous separation.

2. Careful case selection and a modified surgical technique for macular peel surgery, to avoid deroofing cysts or exacerbating lamellar defects. Thus, in cases where there is a foveal cyst or marked vitreomacular traction there is a concern about deroofing the cyst or inducing a full thickness macular hole. In these cases it is useful to stain the vitreous with triamcinolone to visualize the vitreofoveal

Table 33-2 • Case Selection Criteria for Macular Hole Surgery

Favorable		Unfavorable
<500 μm	Size	>500 μm
Elevated edges ("cuff" of subretinal fluid)	Morphology	"Flat open" (no subretinal fluid)
Treatable VMT or tangential traction	Traction	PVD (e.g., Gass stage 4)
Recent onset	Chronicity	Longstanding (e.g., >1 yr)
Dominant eye	Symptoms	Nondominant eye or asymptomatic

attachment. The PVD is always induced on the nasal side of the disc to avoid traction on the cyst. When the PVD is present the vitreous can be peeled toward but not off the fovea. It can then be trimmed back to the fovea. Similarly the ILM can be peeled to the edge of the fovea and then trimmed. Where there are extensive cysts it is sometimes better not to peel the ILM. This minimizes the chance of damaging the fovea. As a precaution, air or gas and face-down posturing can be used to compress the fovea and close any induced macular dehiscence. The use of microplasmin in the future may help in these specific cases to reduce direct surgical traction on the macular surface.

3. Very careful case selection when attempting YAG vitreo-disruption for patients with symptomatic floaters, particularly when the posterior hyaloid is attached.

Pearls on how to treat it

The principles of management of macular hole consist of:

1. Case selection (see Table 33-2).

2. Relief of A-P traction (*pars plana* vitrectomy or biochemical vitreolysis).

3. Relief of tangential traction (ILM peel).

4. Manipulation of the edges of the hole to approximate them.

5. Tamponade with or without posture.

Each of these measures serves to increase the probability of hole closure. Within this list, a large number of permutations exist. In a vitrectomized eye, surgical intervention would typically include all of steps 3 to 4, in an effort to maximize the chance of success.

Expected outcomes

Prognosis for treatment of primary idiopathic macular holes has been well characterized, and surgery has been shown to be superior to observation.[7]

Surgical prognosis for postoperative macular hole is less well characterized. Rahman et al.[5] have reported a series of five cases of macular hole formation following vitrectomy with gas tamponade for rhegmatogenous retinal detachment. One patient declined further surgery. The remaining four all experienced macular hole closure following ILM peel, and C_3F_8 tamponade, with final visual acuity ranging from 6/18 to 6/60.

Conclusion and Future Directions

Macular edema and macular hole are well-described direct complications of intraocular surgery that lead to visual loss. In keeping with the multiple etiologies that contribute to macular edema, a number of treatment modalities are available. The pathogenesis of macular hole is mechanical and surgical treatment is directed at relieving residual traction at the macula. Although surgery to relieve macular traction is relevant to both macular edema and macular hole, the advent of biochemical vitreolysis may prove beneficial as a less invasive alternative to surgery or as an adjunct to surgery.[8]

REFERENCES

1. Gass JD. Idiopathic senile macular hole. Its early stages and pathogenesis. *Arch Ophthalmol.* 1988;106(5):629–639.
2. Altaweel M, Ip M. Macular hole: Improved understanding of pathogenesis, staging, and management based on optical coherence tomography. *Semin Ophthalmol.* 2003;18(2):58–66.
3. Johnson RN, Gass JD. Idiopathic macular holes. Observations, stages of formation, and implications for surgical intervention. *Ophthalmology.* 1988;95(7):917–924.
4. Kimura H, Kuroda S, Nagata M. Premacular cortical vitreous in patients with a rhegmatogenous retinal detachment. *Retina.* 2004;24(2):329–330.
5. Rahman W, Georgalas I, da Cruz L. Macular hole formation after vitrectomy for retinal detachment. *Acta Ophthalmol.* 88(4):e147–e148.
6. Lipham WJ, Smiddy WE. Idiopathic macular hole following vitrectomy: Implications for pathogenesis. *Ophthalmic Surg Lasers.* 1997;28(8):633–639.
7. Ezra E, Gregor ZJ. Surgery for idiopathic full-thickness macular hole: Two-year results of a randomized clinical trial comparing natural history, vitrectomy, and vitrectomy plus autologous serum: Morfields Macular Hole Study Group RAeport no. 1. *Arch Ophthalmol.* 2004;122(2):224–236.
8. Stalmans P, Delaey C, de Smet MD, et al. Intravitreal injection of microplasmin for treatment of vitreomacular adhesion: Results of a prospective, randomized, sham-controlled phase II trial (the MIVI-IIT trial). *Retina.* 2010;30(7):1122–1127.

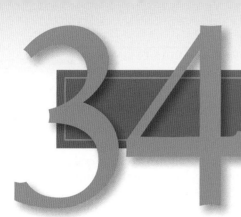

PERSISTENT LOCALIZED SUBRETINAL FLUID

HEINRICH HEIMANN

The Complication: Definition

Persistent localized subretinal fluid refers to collection of subretinal fluid following retinal detachment surgery despite closure of all retinal breaks. Clinically it occurs either as a persistent shallow detachment or as loculated collections of subretinal fluid sometimes referred to as "blebs." Although a spontaneous reabsorption of the persistent fluid can be observed in the majority of cases, this may take several months to years in exceptional cases (Figs. 34-1 through 34-3).[1] Persistent subretinal fluid has to be differentiated from new or recurrent subretinal fluid associated with surgical failure. This is caused by insufficiently closed breaks, missed breaks, new breaks, or vitreoretinal traction (see Chapters 4A, 4B, 16, 35A, 35B and 35C). Persistent localized subretinal fluid can be observed after every type of retinal

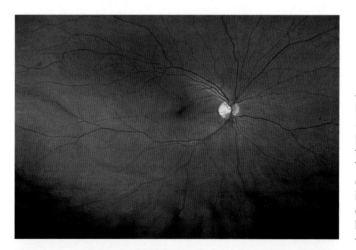

Figure 34-1 Right eye of a 35-year-old female myopic patient with bilateral asymptomatic retinal detachments. The detachments were associated with small round holes in peripheral lattice degeneration and were presumably long-standing.

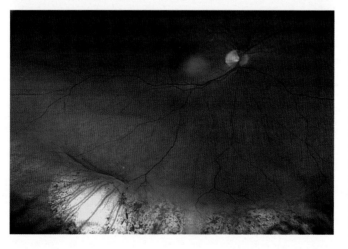

Figure 34-2 Right eye 3 months after nondrainage scleral buckling surgery. Note the regression of the retinal detachment and the persistent subretinal fluid central to the scleral buckle with a concave configuration of its central edge. All breaks were sealed following cryotherapy and were adequately supported by the scleral buckle.

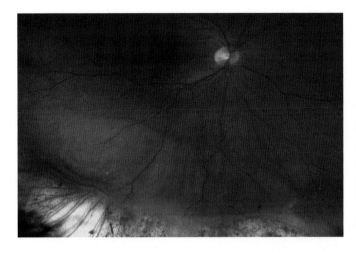

Figure 34-3 Same eye as in Figures 34-2 and 34-3, but now 6 months postoperatively. Note the persistent subretinal fluid central to the buckle and its minimal regression compared to 3 months postoperatively.

detachment surgery. It can be subclinical and detected only by ultrasound or optical coherence tomography. When it occurs under the macular area it may lead to delayed or incomplete visual recovery. It is thought to occur more commonly following nondrainage scleral buckling procedures **(Figs. 34-1** through **34-6)**, pneumatic retinopexy, and in cases with long-standing retinal detachments.[1-5] It may have a significant effect on visual recovery. The diagnosis is established postoperatively with indirect ophthalmoscopy. Relative or absolute scotomata can usually be found in the affected areas. When the posterior pole is involved, decreased visual acuity, impaired color vision, metamorphopsia, micropsia, or macropsia may be noticed. These deficits can be reversible once the subretinal fluid has been reabsorbed.[1] However, the final visual function can also be permanently altered by this complication once the fluid has regressed.

It is important to distinguish between persistent and recurrent subretinal fluid. The latter is a sign of surgical failure caused by insufficiently closed breaks, missed breaks, new breaks, or vitreoretinal traction (Chapters 4A, 4B, 16, 35A, 35B and 35C). It is not always straightforward to differentiate these two complications. As a rule, persistent fluid will decrease, whereas recurrent fluid will increase over time **(Figs. 34-1** through **34-6)**. In cases with persistent subretinal fluid, the central border of the detached retina typically has a concave contour **(Figs. 34-2** and **34-5)**, whereas in recurrent fluid it is convex. Persistent subretinal fluid can also appear as a band of retina that spans between a high buckle and the surrounding attached retina **(Fig. 34-7)** or in an area of retina that is well supported by a buckle and has been treated completely with retinopexy.

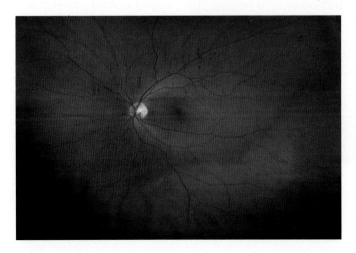

Figure 34-4 Fellow left eye of the patient in Figures 34-1 to 34-3. Asymptomatic inferior retinal detachment caused by multiple small round holes in lattice degenerations.

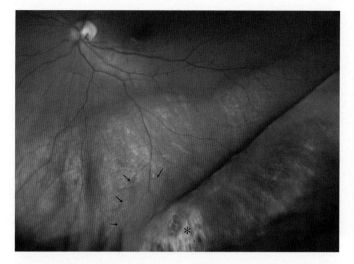

Figure 34-5 Left eye 2 months following nondrainage scleral buckling surgery. All breaks including one larger round hole (*asterisk*) are sealed by the indent and cryotherapy. Note a small collection of persistent subretinal fluid at the inferior edge of the buckle (*arrows*).

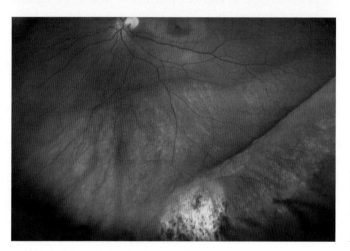

Figure 34-6 Left eye 4 months postoperatively. The residual subretinal fluid has been reabsorbed.

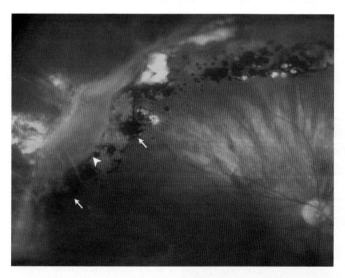

Figure 34-7 Persistent subretinal in a 45-year-old female patient with Stickler's syndrome following scleral buckling surgery. A small pocket of persistent subretinal fluid despite closure and adequate support of all breaks with an encircling band could be noticed postoperatively. A laser retinopexy along the central edge of the persistent subretinal fluid was performed 4 weeks postoperatively. This photograph was taken 6 years after the surgery and additional laser. The persistent subretinal fluid has not been reabsorbed (*arrowhead*) and also has not extended across the border of the chorioretinal scar following laser retinopexy (*arrows*). No patent break or residual vitreoretinal traction is present.

Risk Factors

◆ Long-standing retinal detachments are associated with a higher incidence of persistent subretinal fluid. Clinical signs that may point at a long-standing nature of retinal detachments are demarcation lines, subretinal precipitates, small round holes, and lattice degeneration (Figs. 34-1 and 34-4).[1,5]

◆ Malfunctioning of the retinal pigment epithelium.[6]

◆ Some authors have found an association of persistent subretinal fluid with increasing age,[7] but this could not be observed in other series.[3,4]

◆ Most surgeons share the view that this complication occurs more frequently following scleral buckling surgery (in particular if nondrainage techniques are used) and pneumatic retinopexy. In larger series, persistent subretinal fluid was found in 21% of cases following nondrainage scleral buckling surgery or pneumatic retinopexy.[1–3] After primary vitrectomy, persistent subretinal fluid is less common and usually a short-term phenomenon. This is most likely explained by a more extensive drainage of subretinal fluid during this procedure. The subretinal fluid may also be mixed with and "diluted" by the infusion fluid during intraocular manipulations, resulting in a less viscous mixture that is more easily reabsorbed postoperatively. Some authors argue that persistent subretinal fluid can also frequently be detected following primary vitrectomy and that the increased incidence following scleral buckling surgery may be more likely due to case selection bias, with those at a higher risk more likely to be treated with scleral buckling surgery.[6]

◆ Other intra- and postoperative risk factors that have been associated with persistent subretinal fluid are heavy use of cryotherapy, choroidal ischemia induced by scleral buckling, and choroidal effusion.[1,6]

Pathogenesis: Why Does It Occur

Persistent subretinal fluid can be observed if the active and passive forces that maintain dehydration of the subretinal space are unable to significantly reduce the amount of the remaining subretinal fluid.[8] This is caused by incomplete drainage, a significantly altered composition of the subretinal fluid, and/or malfunctioning retinal pigment epithelium.[6,8] In vivo, these factors are difficult to assess. Current theories to explain persistent subretinal fluid are based on the consideration of clinical and intraoperative risk factors, biochemical analysis of externally or internally drained subretinal fluid, and animal models.

The major reason for delayed absorption of subretinal fluid, in particular in long-standing cases, is thought to be a consequence of changed composition of the subretinal fluid compared to cases with recent onset of retinal detachment. The key differences are an increase in the cellularity and cellular debris (photoreceptors, retinal pigment epithelial cells, macrophages, and red blood cells), the biochemical composition, and the physical properties.[6,8] As a result, the subretinal fluid often appears thickened and more viscous. Its consistency during external or internal drainage resembles more that of viscoelastics rather than being of a more serous, watery composition that is commonly seen in fresh cases.[6] Such fluid is more difficult to drain externally or internally. In addition, this fluid will take longer to be reabsorbed if significant amounts are left in the subretinal space compared to the much faster postoperative reabsorption of the serous subretinal fluid in fresh cases.

The time needed for reabsorption of residual subretinal fluid is difficult to predict, as it depends mainly on factors that cannot be assessed routinely or that are not fully understood to date.[8] Given a similar volume of subretinal fluid, shallow detachments over a larger area of retinal pigment epithelium are reabsorbed more quickly than highly bullous detachments with a smaller base diameter.[8]

✛ Pearls on How to Prevent It

◆ In many cases, persistent subretinal fluid is a "benign" complication that can be part of the expected healing process, for example, in nondrainage scleral buckling surgery of long-standing, localized inferior retinal detachments **(Figs. 34-1** through **34-6).** If only the peripheral retina is affected, it is not essential to prevent its occurrence. Disproportionate measures to avoid persistent subretinal fluid at all costs may be more harmful.

◆ If scleral buckling with external drainage is employed, maximizing the amount of drained subretinal fluid will reduce the volume of residual and potentially persistent subretinal fluid.

◆ There are many variations regarding the technique of external drainage of sub-retinal fluid, all potentially affecting the drainage flow and the amount of fluid drained. The major variations include scleral incision over the drainage site, diathermy of the exposed choroid, type of needle used (electrode, conventional sharp needles for injection, and suture needle), size of the needle, oblique versus straight needle path, and suture of the drainage site.

◆ A quick and complete drainage of subretinal fluid is not always desirable. Potential disadvantages are hypotony with the risks of choroidal hemorrhage or detachment in cases with a large amount of subretinal fluid, excessive drainage of preretinal fluid through the break and vitreal or retinal incarceration in the drainage site.

◆ To maximize external drainage and when a needle technique for drainage is used, try to maintain the outflow through the drainage site by increasing the intraocular pressure with indentation and massage with one or two cotton buds.

◆ Try to prevent clogging of the drainage site by maintaining an uninterrupted flow of subretinal fluid. This is achieved by applying pressure on the side of the drainage needle path to keep the opening patent.

◆ If possible, chose a drainages site in the area with the highest detachment. Conversely, drainage near the edge of the detachment may become covered quickly by reattached retina, preventing further drainage of subretinal fluid.

◆ If the eye is soft and there is a significant amount of persistent subretinal fluid, increase the intraocular pressure by intravitreal injection of balanced salt solution (BSS) or air and continue draining.

◆ A new concept is subretinal fluid lavage. The viscous subretinal fluid is diluted and washed out with a subretinal injection of BSS. A 27G needle is introduced transsclerally into the subretinal space. This is connected to a 3-way tap and two 5 cc syringes, one filled with BSS. The BSS is injected into the subretinal space and then, after turning the 3-way tap, withdrawn again. The resulting mixture of subretinal fluid and BSS is easier to drain and residual fluid will be reabsorbed more quickly.[6,9] This concept can be used in scleral buckling surgery as well as in primary vitrectomy.

◆ When performing pneumatic retinopexy, the "steamroller" positioning of the patient is thought to prevent persistent subretinal fluid at the posterior pole. Immediately following the surgery, the patient is positioned face down for 15 minutes.[10] In this position, subretinal fluid should be drained internally through the break into the vitreous cavity. Then, the position of the head is slowly changed until the break is in the uppermost position and sealed by the gas bubble. When performing pneumatic retinopexy in cases with highly bullous detachments, consider also external drainage.[11]

◆ In cases at risk for clinically significant persistent subretinal fluid (inferior long-standing detachments) with presumed long-standing subretinal fluid at the posterior pole, it may be feasible to use primary vitrectomy. Drainage of subretinal fluid is easier and more controlled with this method compared to scleral buckling surgery. This does not apply to long-standing inferior detachments without macular involvement. These are often successfully treated with scleral buckling surgery.

◆ When performing primary vitrectomy, try to achieve complete drainage of subretinal fluid. In challenging cases, this can be facilitated by enlarging existing retinal breaks for easier active or passive drainage. Other options are to perform a peripheral retinotomy and drain the subretinal fluid by unfolding the retina with heavy liquid or to use a more posterior retinotomy for drainage during fluid–air exchange.[12]

◆ In cases with residual subretinal fluid anterior to the retinal break, this can be drained through the break. First unfold the retina with heavy liquid up to the posterior edge of the break. Second perform a limited fluid–air exchange down to the level of the break. Using passive suction in the area of the break, this will force the anteriorly displaced subretinal fluid into the preretinal space through the retinal break.

◆ In cases with thick subretinal fluid, a repeated cycle of internal drainage and influx of BSS from the infusion under the detached retina before fluid–air exchange can help to wash out the more viscous original subretinal fluid.[6] Residual BSS will be absorbed more quickly.

Pearls on How to Solve It

◆ If only a limited amount of persistent subretinal fluid is present in the retinal periphery, there is no need for active treatment (Figs. 34-1 through 34-6). A laser barrier along the edge of the persistent subretinal fluid has been advocated by some authors to prevent the possible extension of the subretinal fluid (Figure 34-7).[13] A grid-coagulation over the affected area with the aim to promote absorption has had limited success.[1] Other groups have suggested selective laser treatment to the retinal pigment epithelium. This is a new type of laser treatment that utilizes a frequency-doubled Q-switched Nd:YLF laser, with a wavelength of 527 nm in a 100-Hz pulsed mode. The idea behind this concept is to treat the retinal pigment epithelium without damaging the photoreceptors. A quick reabsorption of persisting subretinal fluid could be observed in three cases treated with this method.[14]

◆ The effect of pharmacologic agents to promote reabsorbtion of subretinal fluid has so far been disappointing and plays no role in clinical practice today.

Expected Outcomes: What Is the Worst-case Scenario

The worst-case scenario is permanent damage to the retina caused by a prolonged separation of neuroretina and retinal pigment epithelium. This can result in permanently impaired visual function in the affected area. However, in the majority of cases, visual function will improve once the subretinal fluid has reabsorbed, although this may take many months and up to years in selected cases.[1]

REFERENCES

1. Desatnik H, Alhalel A, Treister G, et al. Management of persistent loculated subretinal fluid after pneumatic retinopexy. *Br J Ophthalmol.* 2001;85(2):189–192.
2. Chan CK, Wessels IF. Delayed subretinal fluid absorption after pneumatic retinopexy. *Ophthalmology.* 1989;96(12):1691–1700.
3. Chignell AH, Talbot J. Absorption of subretinal fluid after nondrainage retinal detachment surgery. *Arch Ophthalmol.* 1978;96(4):635–637.
4. Leaver PK, Chester GH, Saunders SH. Factors influencing absorption of subretinal fluid. *Br J Ophthalmol.* 1976;60(8):557–560.
5. Robertson DM. Delayed absorption of subretinal fluid after scleral buckling procedures. *Am J Ophthalmol.* 1979;87(1):57–64.
6. Veckeneer M, Derycke L, Lindstedt EW, et al. Persistent subretinal fluid after surgery for rhegmatogenous retinal detachment: Hypothesis and review. *Graefes Arch Clin Exp Ophthalmol.* 2012;250(6):795–802.
7. O'Connor PR. Absorption of subretinal fluid after external scleral buckling without drainage. *Am J Ophthalmol.* 1973;76(1):30–34.
8. Quintyn JC, Brasseur G. Subretinal fluid in primary rhegmatogenous retinal detachment: Physiopathology and composition. *Surv Ophthalmol.* 2004;49(1):96–108.
9. Veckeneer M. Subretinal fluid lavage: A novel concept in retinal detachment surgery. *Acta Ophthalmol.* 2011;89:248.
10. Yanyali A, Horozoglu F, Bayrak YI, et al. Steamroller versus basic technique in pneumatic retinopexy for primary rhegmatogenous retinal detachment. *Retina.* 2007; 27(1):74–82.
11. Gunduz K, Gunalp I. Pneumatic retinopexy with drainage of subretinal fluid. *Int Ophthalmol.* 1994;18(3):143–147.
12. Heimann H, Bopp S. Retinal folds following retinal detachment surgery. *Ophthalmologica.* 2011;226(Suppl 1):18–26.
13. Wong YM, Lois N. Demarcation laser therapy in the management of macular-sparing persistent subretinal fluid after scleral buckling procedures. *Graefes Arch Clin Exp Ophthalmol.* 2006;244(8):1039–1042.
14. Koinzer S, Elsner H, Klatt C, et al. Selective retina therapy (SRT) of chronic subfoveal fluid after surgery of rhegmatogenous retinal detachment: Three case reports. *Graefes Arch Clin Exp Ophthalmol.* 2008;246(10):1373–1378.

RETINAL REDETACHMENT

35A — Due to Missed Breaks

Manoharan Shunmugam and Alistair Laidlaw

✣ The Complication: Definition

Most cases of failure of primary retinal detachment surgery arise from undetected breaks.[1,2] Excluding new breaks, uncertain breaks, and breaks in previously attached retina, undetected breaks accounted for 60% of all redetachments in one series.[3] New breaks induced peroperatively are considered distinct from this group and shall be discussed in Chapter 35B.

Up to 20% of rhegmatogenous retinal detachments (RRDs) have no break visualized preoperatively in spite of a thorough retinal examination.[4,5] This may be a high estimate, and careful per operative searching will reveal the causative breaks in about 95% of cases.[6,7] As always, finding the primary break intraoperatively is important as it not only allows appropriate treatment and management but also increases the likelihood of a primary success than when none is found.[8] The surgeon should also ensure that the break corresponds to Lincoff's rules and fits the configuration of the RRD to confirm that it is in fact the primary break.[9] It is important to point out that more than one break is present in the majority (61%; $n = 289$) of cases and finding a break that corresponds to the detachment configuration does not exclude the presence of others (authors' unpublished observation).

The reasons for failing to identify a break are numerous and may be due to the size and position of breaks or other intraoperative factors.[10] An obvious cause for missing breaks prior to surgery includes fundus-obscuring vitreous hemorrhage (VH). There is strong evidence to suggest that early intervention is prudent in cases with VH as almost half of the eyes (46.4%) in a published series had tractional tears which were missed on preoperative fundoscopy and B-mode ultrasound.[11]

Macular holes are sometimes the causative break in myopic eyes with RRD but may occasionally present secondarily with RRDs when the fovea is detached and if this is not anticipated, could be missed.[12–14] As a secondary break however, they rarely require further intervention unless it occurs postoperatively.[15]

✣ Risk Factors

Modern wide-angle intraoperative visualization systems which afford variable zoom and a panoramic view of the fundus during vitrectomy have undoubtedly contributed to the reduction in the number of "no-break" RRDs encountered more contemporaneously.[10,16] In spite of this, media opacities still give rise to difficulties during surgery and can pose a problem when searching for retinal breaks. For example, corneal epithelial edema may be easily overcome with debridement; however, stromal scarring or decompensation may require more elaborate planning with anterior segment surgery to facilitate safe vitreoretinal intervention. Alternatively, an endoscopic vitrectomy may be considered if corneal surgery is not an option.

Cataracts can usually be easily removed if they cause a problem but pre-existing pseudophakia sometimes has also its disadvantages. Even when cataract surgery is uncomplicated, pseudophakic RRDs are frequently associated with smaller, more anterior breaks making them easier to miss.[17] Furthermore, the intraocular lens (IOL) implant can occasionally impair peripheral retinal visualization due to capsular fibrosis, IOL optical aberrations, and any remaining lens remnants.

Retinal, and especially foveal thinning, has been demonstrated on OCT scanning in patients with posterior staphylomas which may then progress to breaks.[18] These breaks are sometimes very difficult to detect as they contrast poorly against the pale fundi of pathologic myopic changes such as posterior staphylomas, retinal, and choroidal atrophy.

Pathogenesis: Why Does It Occur

By its very definition, the true incidence of missed breaks would be impossible to estimate though a thorough anterior retinal inspection, either external or internal, would minimize its occurrence and improves retinal reattachment rates.[2]

The pathophysiology of retinal redetachments are similar to that of primary RRDs and requires a full-thickness break in the retina with or without traction and the presence of fluid currents in the eye. An RRD develops when these forces acting on the retina exceed the physiologic hydrostatic forces, which maintain an attached retina. The presence of a tamponade such as oil or gas would therefore prevent a retinal redetachment. As the tamponades reduce in volume however, a redetachment may manifest when there is no further sustained contact between the missed break and the tamponade. This would therefore provide the examiner a clue to the position of the missed break, which would be at the fluid–tamponade interface at the time of manifestation of the redetachment.

Pearls on How to Prevent It

The fundamental principle of preventing redetachments secondary to missed breaks involves detecting and treating them in the first instance. This involves a thorough retinal search with the best possible fundal view. The following points emphasize this and provide a few strategies to circumvent commonly encountered difficulties but are by no means exhaustive.

◆ In pseudophakic eyes, the edge of the IOL can blur the view of the anterior retina and obscure small peripheral breaks. A wide-field indirect contact lens is useful in eliminating this blur and should be considered at assessment especially when no primary break is detected.[19]

◆ Use laser photocoagulation to mark small breaks in RRD preoperatively if these are not visible on indirect ophthalmoscopy.[20] This may be accomplished with a small laser spot-size and moderate energy levels to create retinal blanching only in the vicinity of the break. The aim is not to create retinal adhesion, but only to facilitate rapid intraoperative localization of tiny breaks so that accurate treatment or buckle placement may be achieved.[20] When using this strategy however, caution should be exercised to ensure additional breaks are not created with excessive laser energy.

◆ When performing an internal search, it is important to use the right technique and apply some basic anatomy. Tears occur on the back edge of the vitreous base. This is usually 2 mm behind the ora serrata, but this varies. One can often identify the vitreous base in attached retina by a white (or more realistically mild grey) with pressure reaction. This arises because the collagen strands in the vitreous base insert perpendicularly into the ora. In detached retina there is often a transition line or fold visible at the back edge of the vitreous base. The combination of vitreous traction and a tear mean that the flap will often stand up when rolled. We use an empty plug forceps or squint hook for this and roll in a posteroanterior fashion up to ora then anteroposteriorly across the whole vitreous base.[7] The aim is to create an indent with the surgeons' line of sight tangential to the retina. Often, small breaks are seen better on the slope of an indent rather than at the apex and as the indent moves posteriorly the break rolls up and then down onto, and off the indent and will frequently stand out in the process. The important point is that it involves dynamic rolling as well as indentation combined with endoillumination.[7] Granules of pigment in the peripheral vitreous close to back edge of the vitreous base should also be treated with great suspicion as they often mark the position of a break.

◆ Optimum use of noncontact wide angle viewing systems such as the Oculus BIOM, Topcon Resight, or Volk Merlin can make a massive difference to the peripheral vitrectomy. There are three principles but the process is iterative and involves all four limbs at once, a bit like flying a helicopter! First, the lens must be close enough to the eye with the correct depth of focus. Ensure that the edge of the iris cannot be seen in the surgeons' view; if anything other than an iris edge is visible the lens is not close enough. For fine-tuning, move the suspended lens down further until a grey patch appears in your view, and then back off just enough to have a full field again. That gives maximum intraocular field. (Unfortunately with some lenses and systems there can be corneal lens contact before the grey patch can be seen.) Second, it is important to roll the eye *as far as you can* using both the cutter and light pipe, this involves quite a push. One then "catches up" with the wide-angle viewing system using the "X–Y"' shift on the microscope. It is also possible to take advantage of the (leading) lens edge to provide a prismatic effect at these extreme peripheral views. Third, rolling the eye results in it sinking in the orbit, so the microscope needs to be lowered further (Z-plane) in order to recapture lost field. The reverse of this is that you have to retract the microscope when rolling the eye back to the primary position. Practicing this results in a better view and faster, better surgery.

◆ Where a cataract significantly obscures the fundal view, strongly consider performing a simultaneous cataract extraction and IOL implant. This may prolong surgery slightly, but saves the patient at least one further procedure and makes the internal search far easier to perform.

◆ In the presence of small (poorly dilating) pupils which are unresponsive to pharmacologic dilatation (including intracameral phenylephrine instillation), consider the following:

   ◆ Iris hooks or other mechanical dilators in pseudophakes.

   ◆ Ophthalmic viscoelastic devices to viscodilate phakic eyes, but ensure it is carefully removed at the end of surgery to avoid postoperative ocular hypertension or cataract formation.

◆ In pseudophakes with posterior capsular opacification, a YAG laser capsulotomy or surgical capsulectomy may be necessary. Following a capsulectomy, you may encounter IOL bedewing during air–fluid exchange. Applying a little noncohesive viscoelastic such as hydroxypropyl-methyl-cellulose (HPMC) to the posterior surface of the IOL or simply wiping it with a soft-tipped cannula solves this problem quite effectively.[21,22] Highly cohesive viscoelastics such as sodium hyaluronate (Healon) form a convex lens rather than a layer on posterior lens surface with severe view impairment.

◆ Ensure there is adequate illumination during your search for retinal breaks— at this time, avoid illuminating the macula unnecessarily. Ensure all optical filters (e.g., laser filters) are disengaged to provide yourself the best possible view. Some light-source manufacturers feature filtered illumination of different wavelengths and claim improved contrast during certain maneuvers but this remains unproven for retinal break detection.

◆ In high myopes especially, if possible, perform a preoperative (or even intraoperative) OCT to confirm the presence or absence of a macular hole if no peripheral break is found.

◆ Pearls on How to Solve It

In cases where no break has been identified intraoperatively, some authors have adopted the following strategies when operating on RRDs:

◆ It has been described that placing an encircling buckle (with no concomitant vitrectomy) anterior to the equator with 360 degrees retinopexy with either cryotherapy or visible or infrared laser with or without subretinal fluid drainage could be used to treat patients with no identified retinal breaks. Studies report primary success rates of up to 85%.[1,23,24]

◆ In patients having a pars plana vitrectomy (PPV) in an RRD with unseen breaks, the addition of a scleral buckle has not been shown to improve outcomes compared to patients with no additional buckles.[1,24,25] Furthermore, the addition of a buckle during PPV increases the risk of complications.[24]

◆ Meticulous peripheral vitreous base dissection augmented with triamcinolone acetonide staining and perfluorocarbon liquids (PFCLs) has been reported to reveal the break in the vast majority of patients with unseen retinal breaks preoperatively.[5,10]

◆ Inserting PFCLs aids in changing the contour of retinal detachments, causing occult breaks to pout as subretinal fluid (SRF) is extruded through it. Schlieren frequently indicates the position of the break as the SRF mixes with the infusion fluid in the vitreous cavity.[26]

◆ In cases in which no break is visualized in spite of a thorough internal search with the above strategies, the dye extrusion technique (DE-Tech) is a valuable adjunctive maneuver.[27,28] In a series evaluating the safety and efficacy of this technique, only 5 of the 47 eyes (11%) with "unseen break" RRDs remained undetected following DE-Tech.[28]

◆ Expected Outcomes: What Is the Worst-case Scenario

It is difficult to estimate the actual incidence of missed breaks causing complications as it is not improbable that small undetected breaks may not cause sequelae in eyes which have had RRD repairs and especially if traction has been relieved during a PPV. As reported however, most redetachments are caused by undetected retinal breaks.[3,29] These mostly require repeated surgery, usually with good final outcomes.

More serious complications of undetected breaks occur as sequelae of retinal redetachments and are similar to that of primary RRDs. These include persistent detachment, proliferative vitreoretinopathy, glaucoma, postoperative uveitis, pthisis, and blindness to name a few.

REFERENCES

1. Salicone A, Smiddy WE, Venkatraman A, et al. Management of retinal detachment when no break is found. *Ophthalmology.* 2006;113:398–403.
2. Norton EW. Retinal detachment in aphakia. *Trans Am Ophthalmol Soc.* 1963;61:770–789.
3. Gartry DS, Chignell AH, Franks WA, et al. Pars plana vitrectomy for the treatment of rhegmatogenous retinal detachment uncomplicated by advanced proliferative vitreoretinopathy. *Br J Ophthalmol.* 1993;77:199–203.
4. Ho PC, Tolentino FI. Pseudophakic retinal detachment. Surgical success rate with various types of IOLs. *Ophthalmology.* 1984;91:847–852.
5. Martinez-Castillo V, Boixadera A, Garcia-Arumi J. Pars plana vitrectomy alone with diffuse illumination and vitreous dissection to manage primary retinal detachment with unseen breaks. *Arch Ophthalmol.* 2009;127:1297–1304.
6. Speicher MA, Fu AD, Martin JP, et al. Primary vitrectomy alone for repair of retinal detachments following cataract surgery. *Retina.* 2000;20:459–464.
7. Rosen PH, Wong HC, McLeod D. Indentation microsurgery: internal searching for retinal breaks. *Eye (Lond).* 1989;3(Pt 3):277–281.
8. Wong D, Billington BM, Chignell AH. Pars plana vitrectomy for retinal detachment with unseen retinal holes. *Graefes Arch Clin Exp Ophthalmol.* 1987;225:269–271.
9. Bartz-Schmidt KU, Kirchhof B, Heimann K. Primary vitrectomy for pseudophakic retinal detachment. *Br J Ophthalmol.* 1996;80:346–349.
10. Brazitikos PD, D'Amico DJ, Tsinopoulos IT, et al. Primary vitrectomy with perfluoro-n-octane use in the treatment of pseudophakic retinal detachment with undetected retinal breaks. *Retina.* 1999;19:103–109.
11. Tan HS, Mura M, Bijl HM. Early vitrectomy for vitreous hemorrhage associated with retinal tears. *Am J Ophthalmol.* 150:529–533.
12. Moshfeghi AA, Salam GA, Deramo VA, et al. Management of macular holes that develop after retinal detachment repair. *Am J Ophthalmol.* 2003;136:895–899.
13. Brown GC. Macular hole following rhegmatogenous retinal detachment repair. *Arch Ophthalmol.* 1988;106:765–766.
14. Greco GM, Bonavolonta G. Treatment of retinal detachments due to macular holes. *Retina.* 1987;7:177–179.
15. Ah Kine D, Benson SE, Inglesby DV, et al. The results of surgery on macular holes associated with rhegmatogenous retinal detachment. *Retina.* 2002;22:429–434.
16. Laatikainen L, Tolppanen EM. Characteristics of rhegmatogenous retinal detachment. *Acta Ophthalmol (Copenh).* 1985;63:146–154.
17. Lois N, Wong D. Pseudophakic retinal detachment. *Surv Ophthalmol.* 2003;48:467–487.
18. Baba T, Ohno-Matsui K, Futagami S, et al. Prevalence and characteristics of foveal retinal detachment without macular hole in high myopia. *Am J Ophthalmol.* 2003;135:338–342.
19. Lincoff H, Kreissig I. Finding the retinal hole in the pseudophakic eye with detachment. *Am J Ophthalmol.* 1994;117:442–446.
20. Yeo JH, Michels RG. Preoperative laser photocoagulation to mark tiny retinal breaks in eyes with retinal detachment. *Retina.* 1985;5:161–162.
21. Jaffe GJ. Management of condensation on a foldable acrylic intraocular lens after vitrectomy and fluid–air exchange. *Am J Ophthalmol.* 1997;124:692–693.
22. Porter RG, Peters JD, Bourke RD. De-misting condensation on intraocular lenses. *Ophthalmology.* 2000;107:778–782.
23. Griffith RD, Ryan EA, Hilton GF. Primary retinal detachments without apparent breaks. *Am J Ophthalmol.* 1976;81:420–427.

24. Tewari HK, Kedar S, Kumar A, et al. Comparison of scleral buckling with combined scleral buckling and pars plana vitrectomy in the management of rhegmatogenous retinal detachment with unseen retinal breaks. *Clin Experiment Ophthalmol.* 2003;31:403–407.
25. Wu WC, Chen MT, Hsu SY, et al. Management of pseudophakic retinal detachment with undetectable retinal breaks. *Ophthalmic Surg Lasers.* 2002;33:314–318.
26. Friberg TR, Tano Y, Machemer R. Streaks (schlieren) as a sign of rhegmatogenous detachment in vitreous surgery. *Am J Ophthalmol.* 1979;88:943–944.
27. Jackson TL, Kwan AS, Laidlaw AH, et al. Identification of retinal breaks using subretinal trypan blue injection. *Ophthalmology.* 2007;114:587–590.
28. Wong R, Gupta B, Aylward GW, et al. Dye extrusion technique (DE-TECH): occult retinal break detection with subretinal dye extrusion during vitrectomy for retinal detachment repair. *Retina.* 2009;29:492–496.
29. Norton EW. Retinal detachment in aphakia. *Am J Ophthalmol.* 1964;58:111–124.

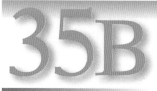

Due to New Breaks

Jose Lorenzo

The Complication: Definition

Occasionally, patients who underwent otherwise successful surgery for vitreoretinal diseases may present with postoperative retinal detachments due to the development of new retinal tears. Most of the time postoperative retinal detachments occur unexpectedly, surprising both doctors and patients. Analysis of new retinal breaks involves distinguishing those derived from the surgical intervention from those occurring as part of the natural history of the disease. They may be the consequence of the ongoing primary disease process when the initial condition is a rhegmatogenous retinal detachment or a retinal tear. However, new retinal breaks may also occur secondary to any intraocular procedure such as transcleral injections, laser-therapy, and pars plana vitrectomy. Pars plana vitrectomy has been advocated increasingly to treat many primary vitreoretinal diseases and complications derived from other ocular conditions such as cataract surgery, eye-trauma, uveitis, retinal vascular diseases, or tumors. When a postoperative retinal detachment occurs in this setting, it often results in a worse scenario than the initial preoperative condition. The occurrence of new retinal tears is reported as the most important cause of retinal detachment in patients undergoing vitrectomy either for macular diseases[1] or retinal detachment.[2] New retinal tears may develop soon after the initial procedure; under this circumstance it may be difficult to differentiate them from missed retinal tears present before the surgical procedure which were not detected intraoperatively or alternatively, iatrogenically caused during the procedure itself. Though they are substantially different, many published reports do not distinguish clearly between these different subtypes of "new retinal tears." This chapter will discuss retinal breaks that develop newly once the initial procedure was successful, whether they may be consequence of the ongoing primary process or secondary to the surgical procedure itself. On the other hand, postoperative proliferative vitreoretinopathy (PVR) is known to be one of the most prevailing and adverse causes of failed vitreoretinal surgery. It is related to the appearance of new tractional retinal tears. This topic, however, is covered in Chapter 35C and, thus, will not be discussed in the current chapter.

Risk Factors

Given that the pathogenesis of new retinal break formation after a vitreoretinal procedure is not fully understood, it is probably better to consider that certain risk factors (as listed below) have been associated to the occurrence of new retinal tears, although the association may not be necessary casual.

Prophylactic Treatment of Retinal Breaks

Development of new retinal tears following prophylactic treatment of a primary retinal break is not uncommon. Between 7% and 14% of eyes treated prophilactically for retinal tears will develop new retinal tears. On one hand, more than one-third of these new retinal tears will lead to a retinal detachment (Table 35B-1). On the other hand, approximately, one-half of retinal detachments that develop despite prophylactic treatment is caused by new retinal breaks and the other half is due to ineffective treatment of the original retinal break(s).[3–5] New retinal breaks or retinal detachment develop in most eyes within few months after prophylactic treatment; however, they may occur also several months or years after

Author	Year	Design	Follow-up (Months)	Nº Eyes Developing New Retinal Breaks/Nº Eyes	Nº Eyes Developing RD/Nº Eyes	Risk Factors
Smiddy[3]	1991	Retrospective	20 mos	24/171 (14%)	8/171 (5%)	Aphakia/ pseudophakia Acute symptoms Peripheral or retinal abnormalities in fellow eye
Combs and Welch[6]	1982	Retrospective	6 mos–22 y	13/177 (7.3%)	8/177 (4.5%)	Aphakia
Kanski and Daniel[5]	1975	Retrospective	≥6 mos	53/520 (13.8%)	33/701 (4.7%)	NA
Robertson and Norton[4]	1973	Retrospective	6 mos– 9 y	25/301 (8.3%)	8/301 (2.6%)	Lattice
Goldberg and Boyer[8]	1980	Retrospective	1 wk–95 mos	8/83 (9.6%)	0	N/A
Boniuk et al.[7]	1974	Retrospective	≥6 mos	40/474 (8.4%)	17/474 (3.5%)	N/A
Mastropasqua et al.[11][a]	1999	Prospective	36–132 mos	NA	5/100 (5%)	N/A
Sharma et al.[10]	2004	Retrospective	3–157 mos	19/155 (12.2%)	5/155 (3.2%)	N/A

Table 35B-1 • Development of New Retinal Tears and Retinal Detachment after Prophylactic Treatment of Retinal Breaks

[a]This study considered high-risk fellow eyes of eyes with retinal detachment.

N/A, not available.

the initial treatment.[6] Most of them develop away from the originally treated retinal break.[3,5] However, when new breaks occur in close proximity to the previously treated tear there appears to be an increased risk for retinal detachment.[4] Retinal detachments tend to occur later when they are caused by new retinal tears elsewhere than when they are caused by the original retinal break(s), which failed to seal adequately following treatment.[3,7,8] Whether prophylactic treatment favors the development of new retinal tears or whether these are the consequence of the ongoing process of posterior vitreous detachment is controversial, but it is probable that excessive treatment may contribute to their development in some cases. Against this hypothesis, Davis[9] observed 9% incidence of additional break formation in his series of eyes with untreated retinal breaks. The incidence reached 23.5% when the initial retinal break was a symptomatic horse-shoe retinal tear. Therefore, development of new retinal breaks might also be part of the ongoing process of posterior vitreous detachment. It is remarkable that a significant proportion of those who develop retinal tears within the first year do so without symptoms.[10]

Retinal Detachment

Buckling surgery: Scleral buckle is still, for many vitreoretinal surgeons, the gold standard for repairing certain types of rhegmatogenous retinal detachments. This procedure achieves anatomical reattachment and preservation of central vision in the majority of eyes at 20 years' follow-up.[12] Retinal tears develop newly after successful buckling surgery and cause retinal redetachment in approximately 2% to 25% of cases (Table 35B-2).[13–19] Most of the early recurrent retinal detachments, which occur within the first 6 weeks postoperatively, are caused by missed breaks, PVR, or inadequate treatment.[13] However, late recurrent retinal detachment, defined as detachments occurring 6 or more weeks postoperatively, are caused mostly by

Table 35B-2 • Retinal Redetachment Due to New Retinal Breaks after Primary Retinal Attachment Surgery

Author	Year	Design	Follow-up	Surgery	Nº Eyes	Redetachments Due to New Retinal Breaks/ Total Nº of Redetachments	Risk Factors
Lincoff and Kreissig[28]	1996	Retrospective	N/A	Scleral balloon	500	7/46 (15%)	N/A
Heimann et al.[2]	2006	Retrospective	14 mos	PPV ± buckling	512	48/150 (32%)	N/A
Tornambe and Hilton[29]	1989	Prospective	≥6 mos	Pneumo-retinopexy	103	20/28 (71%)	Aphakia/ pseudophakia
Tornambe and Hilton[29]	1989	Prospective	≥6 mos	Encircling + segmental buckling	95	12/95 (12%)	Aphakia/ pseudophakia
Rachal and Burton[13]	1979	Retrospective	N/A	Encircling + segmental buckling	863	20/259 (7.7%)	N/A

Table 35B-2 • Retinal Redetachment Due to New Retinal Breaks after Primary Retinal Attachment Surgery (*continued*)

Author	Year	Design	Follow-up	Surgery	N° Eyes	Redetachments Due to New Retinal Breaks/ Total N° of Redetachments	Risk Factors
Haritoglou et al.[30]	2010	Retrospective	≥6 mos	Encircling + segmental buckling	524	35/85 (41.6%)	Aphakia/ pseudophakia
Mendrinos et al.[31]	2008	Prospective	12 mos	PPV (peudosphakic)	100	2/8 (25%)	N/A
Ahmadieh et al.[32]	2005	Prospective	6 mos	PPV (aphakic or pseudophakic)	99	1/37 (2.7%)	N/A
Ahmadieh et al.[32]	2005	Prospective	6 mos	Segmental + encircling buckle (aphakic or pseudophakic)	126	1/40 (2.5%)	N/A
Sharma et al.[33]	2005	Prospective	6 mos	Segmental + encircling buckle (pseudophakic)	25	1/6 (16.6%)	N/A
Sharma et al.[33]	2005	Prospective	6 mos	PPV (pseudophakic)	25	3/4 (75%)	N/A
Campo et al.[34]	1999	Prospective	6 mos	PPV (pseudophakic)	294	17/34 (50%)	N/A
Lai et al.[35]	2008	Retrospective	8 mos	PPV 25G	52	6/14 (43%)	N/A
Johansson et al.[36]	2006	Retrospective	3–14 mos	PPV	131	4/17 (23.5%)	N/A
Mura et al.[37]	2009	Retrospective	1 mo	PPV (25G)	N/A	3/10 (30%)	N/A
Goezinne et al.[21]	2010	Retrospective	50 mos	Scleral buckling	436	9/104(8.6%)	N/A
Wickham et al.[38]	2010	Prospective	6 mos	PPV ± buckling	615	48/79(60%)	Preop. PVR "C," Extent of RD.
Hilton et al.[39]	1981	Prospective	6 mos	Segmental or encircling buckles	120	2/8 (25%)	N/A
Azad et al.[40]	2007	Prospective	6 mos	PPV	30	3/6 (50%)	N/A
Azad et al.[40]	2007	Prospective	6 mos	Segmental + encircling buckle	31	4/6 (66%)	N/A

Pars plana vitrectomy (PPV).

new retinal breaks.[20–22] Although PVR is a common cause of early recurrent retinal detachment, there is relatively little information about its participation in late recurrent retinal detachment. In this setting, PVR is probably a secondary process accompanying new retinal tears.[19,23] Overall, half of retinal redetachments occurs before 6 weeks, and the other half develops thereafter, even years later.[23] According to large retrospective studies, the overall incidence of recurrent retinal detachment presenting more than 6 months after successful primary retinal attachment varies from 1.34% to 6.5%.[19,22,24] Half of the cases of late retinal detachments are caused by single new retinal tears. These new tears may appear equally in areas not treated previously such as areas of normal-looking retina without apparent sings of retinal degeneration or they may occur close to the retinopexy scar or over the slopes of the indented buckle. Most new retinal tears are located in the temporal quadrants, especially in the superior one. Certain types of retinal breaks are more frequently responsible for recurrent retinal detachment: Isolated microholes, fingernail-like tears **(Fig. 35B-1)**—which usually appear close to the chorioretinal scar—and small- or medium-sized horse-shoe tears are the most prevalent.[25,26] Commonly, they appear at the same distance from the limbus as the original breaks.[26] Placement of an encircling band does not seem to help prevent late retinal redetachments.[19,26] In addition, eyes requiring cataract surgery after the initial procedure have a higher risk of retinal redetachment due to new retinal tears.[19,27]

Vitrectomy: In recent years, there has been a growing trend toward vitrectomy with or without additional external encircling elements becoming the procedure of choice for most primary rhegmatogenous retinal detachments. Prospective studies of primary retinal reattachment surgery (including either external buckling or vitrectomy techniques) states that new and missed retinal tears are the main cause of failure of primary surgery.[38,41] New retinal tears causing retinal redetachment develop more frequently in eyes undergoing vitrectomy than in eyes undergoing scleral buckling procedures.[19] Vitrectomy also increases the risk for PVR comparatively to scleral buckling surgery.[19,42–44] This assumption is not accepted uniformly by some other authors who point to PVR as the main cause of new retinal breaks and failure after vitrectomy for retinal attachment.[35,45] Pre-existing conditions modify

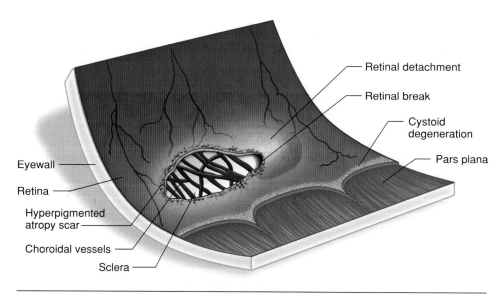

Figure 35B-1 Fingernail-like tears occurring close to the previous treated area are frequently the cause of recurrent retinal detachments. Overtreatment of retinal tears or degenerations may lead to retractions at the boundaries of the scar.

Table 35B-3 • Retinal Detachment after Vitrectomy for Macular Diseases and Retained Lens Fragments

Author	Year	Design	Follow-up	Surgery	Detachments Due to New Retinal Breaks/ Nº Eyes	Risk Factors
Le Rouic[64]	2011	Retrospective	21 mos	Macular hole PPV: (20G, 23G)	7/95 (7.3%)	20G
Le Rouic[64]	2011	Retrospective	20 mos	Epiretinal membrane	11/487 (2.3%)	20G
Guillaubey et al.[72]	2007	Retrospective	28 mos	Epiretinal membrane	9/362 (2.5%)	
Guillaubey et al.[72]	2007	Retrospective	28 mos	Macular hole	18/272 (6.6%)	
Tan et al.[75]	2009	Retrospective	≥3 mos	PPV (MH, MP)	1/218 (0%)	
Chang et al.[104]	1999	Retrospective	≥6 mos	PPV (MH)	23/174 (13.2%)	
Chang et al.[104]	1999	Retrospective	≥6 mos	PPV + encircling (MH)	9/152 (5.9%)	
Passemard[60]	2010	Retrospective	37 mos	PPV 20G (MH)	10/135 (7.4%)	
Chung et al.[82]	2009	Retrospective	≥6 mos	PPV (ERM)	0	
Chung et al.[82]	2009	Retrospective	≥6 mos	PPV (MH)	3/137 (2.2%)	Induction of PVD
Ramkissoon et al.[118]	2010	Retrospective	12 mos	PPV 20G All except RD	11/645 (1.7%)	Intraoperative retinal breaks
Rizzo et al.[69]	2010	Retrospective	6 mos	PPV (20G) (MH, ERM)	3/570 (0.5%)	
Rizzo et al.[69]	2010	Retrospective	6 mos	PPV (25G) (MH, ERM)	21/1580 (1.3%)	
Rizzo et al.[69]	2010	Retrospective	6 mos	PPV (23G) (MH)	2/164 (1.2%)	
Romero-Aroca et al.[119]	2009	Prospective	18 mos	PPV 25G + Phaco (VR diseases other than RD)	0/486 (0%)	
Romero-Aroca et al.[119]	2009	Prospective	18 mos	PPV 20G + Phacofragmentation (VR diseases other than RD)	7/501 (1.39%)	PPV + phacofragmentation
Merani et al.[77]	2007	Retrospective	20 mos	PPV (retained lens fragments)	9/223 (4%)	Delayed surgery
Ho et al.[120]	2009	Retrospective	20 mos	PPV (retained lens fragments)	4/166 (2.4%)	
Moore et al.[58]	2003	Retrospective	8 mos	PPV (retained lens fragments	19/343 (5.5%)	Poor VA, presence of RT pre- or intraoperatively

the risk for postoperative PVR: Thus, aphakia, ruptured posterior capsule and pre-operative PVR make postoperative PVR more likely.[46] Interestingly, the scleral buckling versus primary vitrectomy in rhegmatogenous retinal detachment (SPR) study showed that combining an encircling band with PPV was helpful in pseudophakic cases but not in phakic cases. This combined method diminished the incidence of PVR from 22% to 11% in pseudophakic patients whereas paradoxically increased significantly the PVR incidence from 10% to 20% in phakic patients. However, this conclusion was achieved after subanalysis of the data was undertaking.[47]

While missing breaks is one of the most relevant causes of failure of primary buckling surgery, it plays a lesser role in vitrectomy. Current vitreoretinal techniques employing wide-field viewing systems, scleral indentation, and internal illumination allow for intraoperative identification of small and peripheral retinal breaks which otherwise would go undetected. Both standard 20-gauge and small-gauge vitrectomy yield similar results regarding postoperative incidence of new retinal tears.[48] Postoperative breaks seem to locate mainly in previously normal looking retina. Most of them develop at less than 3 months after the initial operation.[2,42] Most of them are identified at the posterior edge of the vitreous base, unrelated to sclerostomies. Probably, they are secondary to retraction of the residual vitreous skirt over areas of increased vitreoretinal adherence. However, when new retinal breaks are located near to the scleral entry sites, it suggests that they are originated by tangential vitreous contraction which arise from vitreous becoming incarcerated in the wound **(Fig. 35B-2)**.[18,42,43,35,36] This topic is further discussed in Chapter 15A.

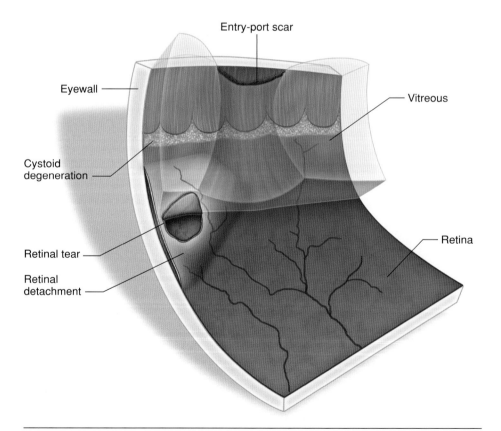

Figure 35B-2 Entry-site retinal breaks are located along the posterior border of the vitreous base and they tend to occur generally in the superior quadrants and later in time. They originated by tangential vitreous contraction which arise from vitreous becoming incarcerated in the wound.

Regardless of their origin, PVR accompanies the formation of new retinal breaks in half of cases after vitrectomy.[2] Distinguishing the contributory role of each to the development of the other is difficult.

Pneumatic retinopexy. Both pneumatic retinopexy and temporary Lincoff balloon buckle are associated with higher incidence of new retinal breaks than standard scleral buckle.[29,49,50] Retinal redetachment occurring after initially successful pneumatic retinopexy is due largely to the development of new retinal tears. New retinal breaks are reported to occur from 7% to 23%, which exceeds what is expected for the standard treatment with scleral buckling.[50-54] Though most of the new retinal tears develop within the first postoperative month, it is not uncommon for new retinal tears to develop in the first 24 hours.[29,50] It is believed generally, that most new retinal tears occur at locations far from the original break; however, prospective studies do not support this.[52,55] Prospective randomized trials comparing pneumatic retinopexy with scleral buckling show that new retinal breaks also developed more frequently in eyes that had supplementary gas injected at the time of scleral buckling procedure than those which had not. Unrelieved tractional forces are perhaps exacerbated by the gas bubble, even in the presence of a scleral buckle. This study showed that new breaks developed in both the scleral buckling and pneumatic retinopexy groups with similar predisposition in the superior two-thirds of the fundus, within 3 clock hours of the original break, within the first 30 days and in aphakic or pseudophakic eyes alike.[29,54] Patients who were aphakic or pseudophakic at the time of either pneumatic retinopexy or scleral buckling surgery were at higher risk for developing new retinal tears. For further information on the subject of new retinal tears following pneumatic retinopexy, see also Chapter 8.

Aphakia and Pseudophakia

Cataract surgery not only increases the risk of retinal detachment but also decreases the rate of successful retinal attachment surgery.[56] One of the reasons for the increased rate of failure is that adequate examination of the peripheral fundus is impeded frequently by capsular opacification or narrow pupils, and hence, peripheral retinal breaks may be missed. A prospective randomized trial revealed that retinal redetachment due to new retinal tears occur more frequently in aphakic or pseudophakic patients.[29] To the same extend, patients who were otherwise successfully treated for retinal breaks or retinal detachment but will require cataract surgery will be at increased risk for new retinal tears and retinal detachment thereafter.[7,12,27,57] Eyes treated prophilactically for retinal tears and lattice degeneration experience retinal detachment following cataract surgery in 13.6% of cases, this represents an additional increase to the 3.6% that would otherwise occurred without cataract surgery.[7] Grand's report based on 124 patients who underwent cataract surgery after successful treatment of retinal detachment found that 4% of patients experienced a retinal redetachment due to new retinal tears. The author states that encircling procedures have a protective role as 2.8% of patients who had a 360-degree band developed a retinal redetachment compared with 18.2% of those who had not. This difference suggests that employing encircling elements would have a protective role; however this hypothesis remains to be proved. Encircling elements supposedly counteract residual peripheral vitreoretinal traction and close unseen breaks in the vitreous base region. Frequently, iatrogenic retinal breaks are found intraoperatively during PPV in phakic eyes. This fact may reflect a higher risk of vitreous base traction when sclerotomies are placed more posteriorly or when peripheral vitreous is removed incompletely.[58]

Macular Surgery

Retinal detachment is the most sight-threatening complication of macular surgery. Retrospective studies have shown that retinal detachment complicates the course of idiopathic full-thickness macular hole (FTMH) surgery in 1% to 14% of patients (Table 35B-3).[59–65] The rate of postoperative retinal detachment is higher after vitrectomy for stage 2 and stage 3 than for stage 4 FTMH, probably because of the forceful separation of the posterior vitreous.[66,67] Most new retinal breaks originated after FTMH surgery are single tears causing macula off retinal detachments.[63,67,68] Both retinal detachment and responsible breaks often are located inferiorly.[65,66] A prospective study with 1 year follow-up found that 11% of patients had a retinal detachment after macular hole surgery, most of them occurring in the early postoperative period (mean, 6.7 weeks). This study reported that none of the eyes in which inferior breaks developed had a complete posterior vitreous detachment before surgery.[65] Whenever the retinal detachment occurs coincident with the disappearance of the gas bubble, it can be assumed that causative retinal tears were created during the surgery or during the tamponade. Otherwise, new retinal breaks are thought to be secondary to progressive contracture of the peripheral vitreous skirt. Though they can be sometimes originated close to the sclerotomy sites, more often they are not related.[69] Entry-site retinal breaks are located along the posterior border of the vitreous base and they tend to occur generally in the superior quadrants and later in time (**Fig. 35B-2**).[63] It has been suggested that combined surgery, with sclerotomies placed more anteriorly, leads to a more complete vitrectomy, thus reducing both the entry-site complications and the volume of residual vitreous.[58,70,71] However, the differences between the rates of retinal detachment in phakic, pseudophakic, and combined procedures are not significant; therefore, the lens status does not seem to influence the rate of RD.[60,72] Axial length did neither influenced the incidence of postoperative RD in that series.[72] Some retrospective studies suggest that small gauge vitrectomy with 23 gauge and 25 gauge are associated with lower risk for postoperative retinal detachment.[65,73–75] However this assumption is not supported by other authors.[69] Macular surgery for epimacular membranes is complicated by retinal detachment due to new retinal tears in approximately 0% to 2.3% with a mean delay of 3 months (range: 14 to 225 days) (Table 35B-3).[64,69,72] Two-thirds of retinal detachments occurring after PPV for epiretinal membranes have superior breaks, and most of them are macula "on." In most cases, the extent of retinal detachments is limited to the area around the retinal breaks.[72]

Vitrectomy for Removal of Retained Lens Fragments

Removal of retained lens fragments by pars plana vitrectomy is mandatory to reduce secondary glaucoma and improve visual acuity. Retinal detachment can occur either before, intraoperative and postoperative after pars plana vitrectomy. The total estimated incidence with pooled data is about 15%; being 7.1% the rate before or during vitrectomy, and 7.5% the rate after vitrectomy.[76] Retinal detachment occurs with a median delay of 8 weeks (range: 20 days to 3 years) (Table 35B-3). Poor visual acuity at presentation and the presence of a retinal tear discovered either before or during the vitrectomy are associated with higher incidence of retinal detachment after vitrectomy. Longer time interval between both surgeries is also correlated to increased risk for postvitrectomy retinal detachment. Most cases of retinal detachments are due to single retinal tears that often are located in the superior peripheral retina. However, attempts at rescuing retained lens fragments during the cataract procedure may promote development of retinal tears and/or dialysis at the opposite meridian from the corneal incision. Neither presenting intraocular inflammation nor elevated intraocular pressure put the eye to a higher risk for retinal detachment after vitrectomy.[77]

Pathogenesis: Why Does It Occur

New retinal tears, developing after successful vitreoretinal surgery, have different pathogenesis according to both the primary disease and the procedure that the surgeon has undertaken to cure the primary disease.

The Ongoing Natural Course of the Primary Disease

The Posterior Vitreous Detachment (PVD)

Transformation of flap tears to retinal round holes with free opercula, bleeding of bridging vessels and detachment of treated retinal tears all suggest that peripheral vitreous is not detached completely and persistent traction occurs beyond the acute PVD. One-third of patients with rhegmatogenous retinal detachment had ultrasonographic evidence of incomplete posterior vitreous detachment.[78] Both dynamic vitreous biomicroscopy and B-scan ultrasounds provide evidence that incomplete or partial PVD is more prevalent than previously estimated by standard biomicroscopy. These studies find that the prevalence of incomplete PVD is 17% to 44% in the seventh decade of life, slowly decreasing afterward.[79,80] Up to one-fourth of symptomatic, acute, and uncomplicated PVDs show incomplete posterior vitreous separation. Delayed complications related to PVD, such as retinal tears and epimacular membranes, develop more frequently in patients showing incomplete PVD.[81] The common pathway to incomplete PVD and delayed complications is to have an abnormal vitreoretinal adherence. This abnormality often extends diffusely throughout the vitreoretinal interface rather than being limited to a focal area. It helps to explain common surgical and clinical findings such as that eyes with retinal detachment often show persistent posterior vitreous attachments or why they frequently develop macular pucker. In the same way, eyes with macular holes usually show enhanced vitreoretinal attachment and peripheral retinal tears frequently are created when posterior vitreous is separated mechanically from the retina.[82] So, incomplete PVD is found frequently in eyes with abnormal vitreoretinal adherence, which predisposes them to develop late new retinal breaks (Table 25B-1). Provided that adequate treatment is done, the development of such tears is associated unlikely to prophylactic treatment inasmuch as some studies reveal similar rates in untreated eyes.[4,5,9]

Iatrogenia of the Surgical Procedure

Induced posterior vitreous detachment. Though most of the new retinal tears actually are intraoperative, induction of PVD during vitrectomy results in a significant higher incidence of both intraoperative and postoperative retinal breaks.[82] There is approximately a 4% attributable risk of retinal detachment secondary to the peeling of posterior cortical vitreous. Frequently, retinal tears are located in the inferior quadrants because forceful separation of the posterior vitreous is more intense and perpendicular inferiorly than superiorly.

Losing the tamponade effect of the vitreous. Peripheral vitreous gel is necessary to tamponade developmental breaks that frequently appear on the peripheral retina. Postmortem studies show that small peripheral retinal breaks occur in up to 10% of otherwise normal eyes. Lesser lesions of the peripheral retina-like retinal tufts are far more common, affecting up to half of the population.[83] The underlying common factor in these lesions is abnormal vitreoretinal attachments, which are considered developmental in origin. In autopsy series, retinal tears are found in 7% of nonpathologic eyes. Approximately, one-third of these small retinal tears are located within the posterior portion of the vitreous base, between the ora serrata and the posterior border of the vitreous base. Anatomically, this area is characterized by an intimate attachment between the internal retina and the cortical vitreous.[84] The fact that small retinal tags and full thickness retinal tears with flaps or opercula can develop suggest the existence of pure tractional forces within the vitreous base other than the influence of posterior vitreous detachment. Interestingly, these small retinal tears do not develop retinal detachments. Probably, it is due to the tamponade effect of the non detached anterior vitreous. However, small retinal tears that are located between the posterior border of the vitreous base and

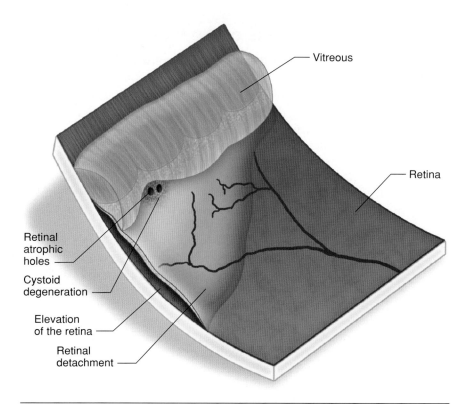

Vitreous

Retina

Retinal atrophic holes

Cystoid degeneration

Elevation of the retina

Retinal detachment

Figure 35B-3 Small retinal holes may originate recurrent retinal detachments due to the fact that properties of vitreous tamponade are lost after vitrectomy.

the equator often are accompanied by limited retinal detachments that do not tend to progress even in the presence of posterior vitreous detachment.[83] Inertial movements of detached vitreous body yield to temporary apposition of the anterior vitreous to the peripheral retina. Thus, allowing for a temporary tamponade effect over any existing peripheral retinal break. Unfortunately, these properties of vitreous tamponade are lost after vitrectomy and retinal detachment may ensue in presence of these developmental small retinal tears **(Fig. 35B-3)**. In addition, forceful hydration of the anterior vitreous during the procedure facilitates anterior vitreous liquefaction. This leads to shrinkage of the anterior vitreous with retraction of the collagenous framework which diminishes the tamponade effect of the anterior vitreous, enhances intraocular currents close to the retina after saccadic eye movements and causes retraction of the anterior vitreous. All these circumstances facilitate not only the development of small flap tears at the level of the posterior vitreous base but also the ensuing retinal detachment. Similar pathogenic mechanisms are involved in aphakic eyes.[85] The clinically visible result is the vitreous retraction appearing in aphakic eyes creating a peripheral traction ridge.

Intraocular expansible gases. Two different mechanisms may participate in developing new retinal tears in eyes treated with gas tamponade. New retinal tears that develop within the first 30 postoperative days are due apparently to unrelieved tractional forces exacerbated by the gas bubble. Usually, these new breaks develop in the superior two-thirds of the fundus, within 3 clock hours of the original break.[29,54] Secondary vitreous base contraction due to gas bubble might explain retinal detachment occurring more than 1 month after vitrectomy **(Fig. 35B-4)**. Secondary breaks due traction on the vitreous base are mostly inferior.[60,65,72] Intravitreal gas may push the cortical vitreous against the retina where it tends to adhere and proliferate, and in some eyes, provoke preretinal traction and new retinal

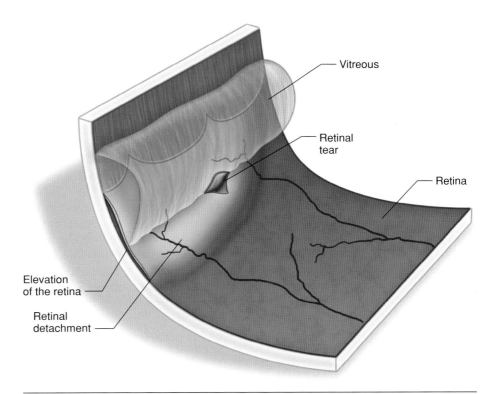

Figure 35B-4 Secondary vitreous base contraction either due to the ongoing process of PVD or to the gas bubble, in cases which had gas tamponade, might explain retinal detachment occurring after vitrectomy.

tears.[28] Preretinal membrane formation stimulated by perfluorocarbon gases has been reported in the intact vitreous of rabbits and cynomolgus monkeys.[86]

Retinopexy: New retinal breaks can develop after prophylactic treatment of retinal breaks or retinal predisposing degenerations in otherwise attached retinas. Newly formed retinal tears often are found close to thermally treated areas **(Fig. 35B-1)**.[5,25] It is almost impossible to prove that they are not precipitated by the treatment itself. When these breaks take place close to the previously treated areas, it seems that thermal coagulation provokes retinal and vitreous changes leading to the formation of secondary retinal breaks closely related to the original chorioretinal scar.[2,5,87] Besides local vitreous traction, likely, chorioretinal vascular insufficiency is involved in new tear developing. The chorioretinal vascular insufficiency may have been produced by the scarring of previous retinopexy in areas adjacent to the recurrent tears or may have developed spontaneously in the areas of retina adjacent to recurrent tears that developed away from the original tear.[26] However, new breaks occurring after photocoagulation in areas of the retina apart from the treated areas probably are not related to the thermal injury of the retina.[4] Interestingly, new retinal tears can also develop in the absence of any thermal treatment of the retina, even when buckling surgery is employed without associated thermal therapy.[9,88] However, new retinal tears tend to cause retinal detachment more frequently when they are located at or close to a previously treated area than when they are apart.[5] This finding suggests that tractional forces are created at or next to treated areas. The scar area serves as anchorage opposing to the pulling of the retina by the tractional forces. Finally, the retina, yielding to traction, tears at the junction of the extensible and immobile retinal areas.[89]

Healing process. Any surgical procedure carried out in the eye will be followed by an inflammatory response resulting from the traumatic disruption of the blood–ocular barrier. Both inflammation and the release of extracellular factors lead to migration and proliferation of cells to form contractile membranes. This process, termed hypocellular gel contraction, would involve the vitreous gel leading to the development of vitreoretinal traction. This type of cell-mediated traction of the cortical vitreous gel may occur via mechanisms other than syncytial hypercellular membranes, which likely occur in cases of well-established PVR.[90] Late retinal redetachment usually are attributed to progressive vitreoretinal traction that either reopens the original retinal breaks, or causes new retinal breaks, or both. Vitreous base traction seems to be an important factor in recurrent retinal detachments occurring later than 6 months after complete retinal reattachment. Frequently, PVR is found associated to new retinal tears but this is likely a secondary phenomenon and not a causative factor in most cases.[21,22,23] Any intraocular entry invariably will be followed by a healing process. Intraocular injections, sclerotomies, accidental punctures, or transcleral injuries generate a fibroproliferative scar in the uvea of the ciliary body that extends into the vitreous body. This fibrous tissue often has vitreous strands adhering to it. Later involution and contraction of the fibrous tissue may originate traction on the retina close to the vitreous and retinal breaks.[63] Many iatrogenic retinal tears are associated with traction at the sclerotomy entry sites occurring postoperatively as the result of fibrovascular healing or contraction of incarcerated vitreous **(Fig. 35B-2)**.[19,91]

⬥ Pearls on How to Prevent It

◆ Think efficiently when indicating the surgical intervention for retinal detachment. Keep in mind that the most important predictor of primary anatomic success and final visual outcome is the choice of initial surgical intervention.[92] In selected cases, scleral buckling surgery still offers better results than vitrectomy.[47,30]

◆ Examine the retinal periphery and treat any retinal break before planned vitrectomy for vitreoretinal diseases other than retinal detachment. It reduces the risk for late retinal detachment.[93]

◆ Reset vitrectomy parameters favoring low aspiration, low flow, and high cutting-rate. Increase the duty-cycle, especially when performing peripheral vitrectomy.[72]

◆ Consider intraoperative use of triamcinolone acetonide, it helps to visualize the vitreous thus reducing the incidence of retinal breaks and retinal detachments in eyes undergoing PPV.[94]

◆ Perform a thorough vitrectomy around breaks, visible degenerations or sclerotomies. If you plan to leave a gas tamponade then trim off the vitreous as complete as possible in order to avoid traction on the peripheral retina by the gas tamponade.[42,95]

◆ Minimize instrumentation and number of instrument changes and ensure good vitreous clearance at sclerotomy sites in 20G PPV. In small gauge PPV, the major amount of vitreous incarceration occurs during the implantation of cannulas. Clean the cannula immediately before removing the cutter from the eye. Use the cutter with high speed and low vacuum inside the cannula in order to get a free egress of the fluid through the cannula. This reassures you that no vitreous is incarcerated inside the cannulas. Repeat this maneuver before removing them at the end of the case. Intraocular cleaning of the port with the cutter releases the anterior–posterior traction without increasing the postoperative rate and degree of hypotony.[70]

◆ Avoid excess vitreous base traction when inducing and extending a PVD to the periphery.[70]

◆ Treatment of retinal degenerations in attached retinas must be done cautiously. Prophylactic photocoagulation of lattice degeneration is associated with 10% incidental new retinal breaks developing adjacent to the treated area. Avoid over-treatment. A healthy rim of retina should be left between the scar and the lattice. Choose cryotherapy if poor pigmented fundi (elderly, myopics, etc.) or in previously failed laser-treated areas.[15]

◆ When performing pneumatic retinopexy, the volume of gas should be kept small. A volume injection of 0.3 to 0.4 cc of SF_6 is preferred to C_3F_8 because it does not expand as much and it disappears much more rapidly.[96]

◆ Examination of the retinal periphery with scleral indentation at the conclusion of the case is mandatory. Treating peripheral retinal breaks reduces successfully the postoperative RD rate to that of an eye without breaks.[76] To distinguish suspicious from true breaks, the use of cryotherapy may help.[74] Remember that two-thirds of retinal tears causing retinal detachment after PPV occur in the superior retina.

◆ Pars plana vitrectomy performed immediately after cataract surgery for retained lens fragments is a viable option and may achieve a better visual outcome, with reduced risk of secondary glaucoma, retinal detachment, or cystoid macular edema.[97,98] Delayed vitrectomy beyond 30 days is associated with poorer outcomes.[77]

◆ Given the favorable outcomes reported with planned PPV, anterior segment surgeons, when facing a ruptured posterior capsule during a cataract procedure, are to be encouraged for removing lens material and vitreous that are accessible from the anterior approach.[99]

◆ Examine retinal periphery of patients who required cataract surgery after retinal procedures and treat risk lesions.[27]

◆ Small gauge cannulated vitrectomy is associated with lower incidence of sclerotomy-related retinal tears.[64,74,100,101] It might decrease trauma to the vitreous and the peripheral retina avoiding excessive tangential vitreous traction toward the sclerotomy. However, adequate instrument stiffness is a requisite for proper peripheral vitrectomy. Otherwise residual peripheral vitreous may contract and create retinal breaks postoperatively.[102,103]

◆ Educate operated patients to asses themselves for retinal detachment symptoms. Perform detailed examination of the peripheral retina at 4 weeks postoperative with either indirect ophthalmoscopy or 3-mirror lens. One-half of concerned patients have asymptomatic retinal detachment and their retinal detachment is discovered on routine postoperative examination.[63,66,72]

◆ In retinal attachment surgery, the use of encircling scleral buckle may decrease the incidence of new retinal breaks through relieving vitreoretinal traction. It also may close undetected small breaks not seen preoperatively, especially in pseudophakic patients.[13,42,50,104,105] However, this hypothesis is not supported by some authors who had found that placing an encircling band did not show any benefit in preventing retinal redetachment when compared to PPV alone.[26,29,31,106,107] Prophylactic scleral buckling, 360-degree peripheral laser and cryotherapy/laser circumscribing the sclerotomies were showed to minimize the incidence of new retinal breaks leading to postoperative RD in PPV for macular disease.[104,108,109] However, they are in fact quite invasive and impose risks of their own. Its use is not generally recommended.

◆ Whenever possible, avoid primary vitrectomy in patients with rhegmatogenous RD and incomplete posterior vitreous detachment; for example, in cases of retinal detachment of young myopic patients and cases with retinal dialysis at the ora serrata. You will avoid inducing iatrogenic retinal breaks in areas of retinal degeneration.[110]

◆ Pearls on How to Solve It

◆ Laser pneumatic retinopexy may be a very successful procedure for the treatment of recurrent retinal detachments after failed scleral buckle surgery. Provided that PVR is not present, newly developed retinal breaks and reopening of original breaks can be treated successfully by pneumatic retinopexy alone. The overall success rate of 70% to 90% is much higher than generally reported for typical pneumatic retinopexy primary repair of retinal detachment. This may be attributable to the previously placed scleral buckle releasing the vitreoretinal traction. Anatomic success was much more likely if the extent of retinal redetachment is less than 2 clock hours. Inferiorly located retinal breaks can achieve a 90% success with motivated patients with the ability to maintain appropriate positioning.[111] Though the lens status seems not to modify the success rate, identification of all retinal breaks is clearly mandatory. Improvement should occur after 1 or 2 days, otherwise other surgical measures are indicated. Laser retinopexy is probably more adequate than cryotherapy since new retinal tears can develop posterior to or overlying the scleral buckle.[10,112]

◆ In cases of recurrent retinal detachment, a new retinal break cannot be found in between 20% and 30% of cases.[113] Vitrectomy facilitates the location of small retinal breaks in the presence of opaque media, a poorly dilating pupil, and of an intraocular lens partially obscured by lens capsule thickening. However, scleral buckling is as effective in the management of uncomplicated rhegmatogenous RDs with undetected breaks as is surgery combining scleral buckling and PPV.[114]

◆ The most important reasons for late failures in retinal attachment surgery are vitreous base traction and periretinal proliferations that clinically appear as new or reopened tears or as PVR. Recurrences show a more difficult retinal situation and require more extensive surgical interventions. Most eyes need to be treated by vitrectomy. The numbers of reoperations to achieve reattachment increases considerably. Functional prognosis is worse when redetachment occurs. Nonetheless, in 50% of eyes useful vision (≥20/50) is retained by repeat surgery.[19,23,24,115] Depending on the underlying cause, recurrent retinal detachments which were treated initially by scleral buckling procedures respond equally well to additional or replacement buckle.[17,30]

◆ Early failures after vitrectomy for rhegmatogenous retinal detachment usually require internal drainage, extended retinopexy, gas tamponade, and sometimes supplementary buckling. Silicone oil tamponade is useful in cases with accompanying PVR.[38] Selected cases of recurrences after vitrectomy for retinal detachment can be successfully treated with fluid–gas exchange.[38,116]

◆ Patients with successful repeated retinal attachment surgery maintain vision at 6 months if PVR is not present.[38]

◆ After pneumatic retinopexy, there is 23% incidence of new retinal breaks.[29] Appropriate management can resolve most cases attaining postoperative visual acuity of 20/50 or better. One-third of cases are successfully managed with cryo/ laser, 21% can undergo repeated pneumatic retinopexy, and 39% may require a scleral buckling procedure. There is no known method for preventing new retinal breaks, 360-degree scatter photocoagulation between the posterior vitreous base and the equator could be an option for aphakic and pseudophakic patients.[51]

◆ Retinal detachments after macular hole surgery occurs after a mean of 4 to 6 weeks postoperative, macular involvement is common.[63,72] A new vitrectomy and gas tamponade are the preferred approaches. Closure of macular hole is generally achieved but the prognosis for visual restoration is guarded. However, one-fifth of cases need more than one surgery and long-term tamponade with silicone oil tamponade.[1,72] Most patients experiencing retinal detachment after epimacular membrane surgery are amenable to vitrectomy and fluid–gas exchange with visual acuity restoration.[72]

Expected Outcomes: What Is the Worst-case Scenario

This imaginary, but not exceptional, scenario illustrates how a new retinal break can have disastrous consequences after an initially successful and "noncomplicated" retinal attachment.

◆ A moderate myopic 50-year-old phakic man had a "macula on" retinal detachment in his right eye with a superior, equatorial retinal tear of 20-degree size located at the "2 o'clock position." The retinal detachment affected both nasal quadrants. His vision was 25/20.

◆ The patient was treated successfully with a PPV, cryo, and SF_6 20% gas.

◆ One year later, the patient developed cataract in the operated eye and underwent somehow complicated cataract surgery with ruptured posterior capsule and intraocular lens placement in the sulcus.

◆ Four weeks postoperatively, the patient has presented with a macula-off retinal detachment. His vision was perception of hands movements. He showed vitreous haze and less than optimal papillary dilation. The retina was detached completely, except for the area of the original tear which remained attached. No break was found. In addition, 360-degree contraction of the vitreous base was noted.

◆ A new vitrectomy in order to complete peripheral vitrectomy and enhance searching of the suspected retinal break was then undertaken.

◆ After peripheral indentation and internal searching, no break was found. After fluid–air exchange and the use of a posterior retinotomy to drain subretinal fluid, a 360-degree endolaser was carried out. The retina was then flat and an air-15% C_3F_8 exchange was done. The patient was asked to keep face down position.

◆ Unfortunately, 2 weeks later, and when there is still gas in the eye, the inferior retina is noted to be detached and fixed retinal folds are appreciated inferiorly.

Comment

In this imaginary case, though the initial surgical approach is not necessarily wrong, it happened that everything that could go wrong, went wrong. Some aspects deserve some reflection.

1. A 50-year-old phakic man will develop cataract after PPV. A cumulative risk for retinal detachment exists with the passing of time after cataract surgery. A 50-year-old patient will face a nonnegligible risk of retinal detachment throughout his life.[117] This possibility will be increased in patients who have been operated on for retinal detachment.[27]

2. An incomplete PVD likely occurs at this age group. In addition, myopic patients frequently have vitreous synchysis with incomplete forms of posterior vitreous detachment.[110] It would not be unusual in this case that the inferior retina show remnants of posterior vitreous still attached.

3. Incomplete peripheral vitrectomy due to the phakic status of the patient is also to be considered. This exposes the eye to unrelieved tractional forces exacerbated by the gas bubble.[29,54]

4. Zonular weakness, inherent to myopic eyes, could worsen after PPV and gas tamponade. This could predispose the eye to complicated cataract surgery, which in turn enhanced inflammation and peripheral vitreous traction.[85]

5. In cases of recurrent retinal detachment, a new retinal break cannot be found in between 20% and 30% of cases.[113] The possibility of a nonflap retinal break has to be considered. A fingernail-like tear which usually appear close to the chorioretinal scar would be gone unidentified easily even with scleral indentation. Indentation below the superior nasal sclerotomy is more demanding.[25]

6. The most important reasons for late failures in retinal attachment surgery are vitreous base traction and periretinal proliferations that appear clinically as new or reopened tears or as PVR. In this setting a redetachment is more likely than a single redetachment.[24] When planning a new surgery, it would be advisable a more aggressive choice such as supplemental encircling band or silicone oil tamponade.

In this fictitious scenario, a more conservative first approach, such as scleral buckling surgery, would avoid this knock-on effect on complications, but someone would think rightly that other options have also complications on their own.

REFERENCES

1. Rizzo S, Belting C, Genovesi-Ebert F. Retinal detachment after small-incision, sutureless pars plana vitrectomy: Possible causative agents. *Graefes Arch Clin Exp Ophthalmol*. 2010;248(10):1401–1406.

2. Heimann H, Zou X, Jandeck C, , et al. Primary vitrectomy for rhegmatogenous retinal detachment: An analysis of 512 cases. *Graefes Arch Clin Exp Ophthalmol*. 2006;244(1):69–78.

3. Smiddy WE, Flynn HW Jr, Nicholson DH, et al. Results and complications in treated retinal breaks. *Am J Ophthalmol*. 1991;112(6):623–631.

4. Robertson DM, Norton EW. Long-term follow-up of treated retinal breaks. *Am J Ophthalmol*. 1973;75(3):395–404.

5. Kanski JJ, Daniel R. Prophylaxis of retinal detachment. *Am J Ophthalmol*. 1975; 79(2):197–205.

6. Combs JL, Welch RB. Retinal breaks without detachment: Natural history, management and long term follow-up. *Trans Am Ophthalmol Soc*. 1982;80:64–97.

7. Boniuk I, Okun E, Johnston GP, et al. Xenon photocoagulation vs. cryotherapy in the prevention of retinal detachment. *Mod Probl Ophthalmol*. 1974;12(0):81–92.

8. Goldberg RE, Boyer DS. Sequential retinal breaks following a spontaneous initial retinal break. *Ophthalmology*. 1981;88(1):10–12.

9. Davis MD. Natural history of retinal breaks without detachment. *Arch Ophthalmol*. 1974;92(3):183–194.

10. Sharma MC, Regillo CD, Shuler MF, et al. Determination of the incidence and clinical characteristics of subsequent retinal tears following treatment of the acute posterior vitreous detachment-related initial retinal tears. *Am J Ophthalmol*. 2004; 138(2):280–284.

11. Mastropasqua L, Carpineto P, Ciancaglini M, et al. Treatment of retinal tears and lattice degenerations in fellow eyes in high risk patients suffering retinal detachment: A prospective study. *Br J Ophthalmol*. 1999;83(9):1046–1049.

12. Schwartz SG, Kuhl DP, McPherson AR, et al. Twenty-year follow-up for scleral buckling. *Arch Ophthalmol*. 2002;120(3):325–329.

13. Rachal WF, Burton TC. Changing concepts of failures after retinal detachment surgery. *Arch Ophthalmol*. 1979;97(3):480–483.

14. Gerhard JP, Flament J. Advantages and complications of non-drainage of subretinal fluid in detached retinal surgery. *Mod Probl Ophthalmol*. 1975;15:185–187.

15. Colyear BH, Pischel DK. Causes of failure in retinal detachment surgery. *Arch Ophthalmol*. 1956;56(2):274–281.

16. Gailloud C, Dufour R, Geinoz J, et al. Failures in retinal surgery. *Mod Probl Ophthalmol*. 1974;12(0):2–14.

17. Lincoff H, Kreissig I, Goldbaum M. Causes of failures in retinal detachment and prophylactic retinal detachment surgery. Reasons for failure in non-drainage. operations. *Mod Probl Ophthalmol*. 1974;12(0):40–48.

18. Zhioua R, Ammous I, Errais K, et al. Frequency, characteristics, and risk factors of late recurrence of retinal detachment. *Eur J Ophthalmol*. 2008 Nov-Dec;18(6): 960–964.

19. Girard P, Mayer F, Karpouzas I. Late recurrence of retinal detachment. *Ophthalmologica*. 1997;211(4):247–250.

20. Fleury J, Bonnet M. Prognostic value of new retinal tears associated with the development of postoperative proliferative vitreoretinopathy. *Graefes Arch Clin Exp Ophthalmol*. 1992;230(5):459–462.

21. Goezinne F, La Heij EC, Berendschot TT, et al. Incidence of redetachment 6 months after scleral buckling surgery. *Acta Ophthalmol*. 2010;88(2):199–206.

22. Kreissig I, Rose D, Jost B. Minimized surgery for retinal detachments with segmental buckling and nondrainage. An 11-year follow-up. *Retina*. 1992;12(3): 224–231.

23. Foster RE, Meyers SM. Recurrent retinal detachment more than 1 year after reattachment. *Ophthalmology*. 2002;109(10):1821–1827.

24. Bopp S, Böhm K. Late recurrences more than 1 year after primary successful surgery for rhegmatogenous retinal detachment. *Klin Monbl Augenheilkd*. 2008; 225(3):227–235.

25. Menezo JL, Suarez R, Francés J. Clinical survey of the forms, number and localization of retinal tears in cases of relapses and recurrences in retinal detachment. *Ophthalmologica*. 1977;174(4):210–216.

26. Seelenfreund MH, Silverstone BZ, Hirsch I, et al. Recurrent tears following successful retinal detachment surgery. *Ann Ophthalmol*. 1986;18(11):319–323.

27. Grand MG. The risk of a new retinal break or detachment following cataract surgery in eyes that had undergone repair of phakic break or detachment: A hypothesis of a causal relationship to cataract surgery. *Trans Am Ophthalmol Soc*. 2003;101: 335–369.

28. Lincoff H, Kreissig I. Extraocular repeat surgery of retinal detachment. A minimal approach. *Ophthalmology*. 1996;103(10):1586–1592.

29. Tornambe PE, Hilton GF. Pneumatic retinopexy. A multicenter randomized controlled clinical trial comparing pneumatic retinopexy with scleral buckling. The Retinal Detachment Study Group. *Ophthalmology*. 1989;96(6):772–783.

30. Haritoglou C, Brandlhuber U, Kampik A, et al. Anatomic success of scleral buckling for rhegmatogenous retinal detachment; a retrospective study of 524 cases. *Ophthalmologica*. 2010;224(5):312–318.

31. Mendrinos E, Dang-Burgener NP, Stangos AN, et al. Primary vitrectomy without scleral buckling for pseudophakic rhegmatogenous retinal detachment. *Am J Ophthalmol*. 2008;145(6):1063–1070.

32. Ahmadieh H, Moradian S, Faghihi H, et al. Pseudophakic and Aphakic Retinal Detachment (PARD) Study Group. Anatomic and visual outcomes of scleral buckling versus primary vitrectomy in pseudophakic and aphakic retinal detachment: Six-month follow-up results of a single operation; report no. 1. *Ophthalmology*. 2005;112(8):1421–1429.

33. Sharma YR, Karunanithi S, Azad RV, et al. Functional and anatomic outcome of scleral buckling versus primary vitrectomy in pseudophakic retinal detachment. *Acta Ophthalmol Scand*. 2005;83(3):293–297.

34. Campo RV, Sipperley JO, Sneed SR, et al. Pars plana vitrectomy without scleral buckle for pseudophakic retinal detachments. *Ophthalmology*. 1999;106(9):1811–1815

35. Lai MM, Ruby AJ, Sarrafizadeh R, et al. Repair of primary rhegmatogenous retinal detachment using 25-gauge transconjunctival sutureless vitrectomy. *Retina*. 2008;28(5):729–734.

36. Johansson K, Malmsjö M, Ghosh F. Tailored vitrectomy and laser photocoagulation without scleral buckling for all primary rhegmatogenous retinal detachments. *Br J Ophthalmol*. 2006;90(10):1286–1291.

37. Mura M, Tan SH, De Smet MD. Use of 25-gauge vitrectomy in the management of primary rhegmatogenous retinal detachment. *Retina*. 2009;29(9):1299–1304.

38. Wickham L, Ho-Yen GO, Bunce C, et al. Surgical failure following primary retinal detachment surgery by vitrectomy: Risk factors and functional outcomes. *Br J Ophthalmol*. 2011;95(9):1234–1238.

39. Hilton GF, Grizzard WS, Avins LR, et al. The drainage of subretinal fluid: A randomized controlled clinical trial. *Retina*. 1981;1(4):271–280.

40. Azad RV, Chanana B, Sharma YR, et al. Primary vitrectomy versus conventional retinal detachment surgery in phakic rhegmatogenous retinal detachment. *Acta Ophthalmol Scand*. 2007;85(5):540–545.

41. Sullivan PM, Luff AJ, Aylward GW. Results of primary retinal reattachment surgery: A prospective audit. *Eye*. 1997;11(6):869–871.

42. Miki D, Hida T, Hotta K, et al. Comparison of scleral buckling and vitrectomy for retinal detachment resulting from flap tears in superior quadrants. *Jpn J Ophthalmol*. 2001;45(2):187–191.

43. Oshima Y, Yamanishi S, Sawa M, et al. Two-year follow-up study comparing primary vitrectomy with scleral buckling for macula-off rhegmatogenous retinal detachment. *Jpn J Ophthalmol*. 2000;44(5):538–549.

44. Gartry DS, Chignell AH, Franks WA, et al. Pars plana vitrectomy for the treatment of rhegmatogenous retinal detachment uncomplicated by advanced proliferative vitreoretinopathy. *Br J Ophthalmol*. 1993;77(4):199–203.

45. Weichel ED, Martidis A, Fineman MS, et al. Pars plana vitrectomy versus combined pars plana vitrectomy-scleral buckle for primary repair of pseudophakic retinal detachment. *Ophthalmology*. 2006;113(11):2033–2040.

46. Kon CH, Asaria RH, Occleston NL, et al. Risk factors for proliferative vitreoretinopathy after primary vitrectomy: A prospective study. *Br J Ophthalmol*. 2000;84(5):506–511.

47. Heimann H, Bartz-Schmidt KU, Bornfeld N, et al., Scleral Buckling versus Primary Vitrectomy in Rhegmatogenous Retinal Detachment Study Group. Scleral buckling versus primary vitrectomy in rhegmatogenous retinal detachment: A prospective randomized multicenter clinical study. *Ophthalmology*. 2007;114(12):2142–2154.

48. Rizzo S, Belting C, Genovesi-Ebert F, et al. Incidence of retinal detachment after small-incision, sutureless pars plana vitrectomy compared with conventional 20-gauge vitrectomy in macular hole and epiretinal membrane surgery. *Retina*. 2010;30(7):1065–1071.

49. Binder S. Repair of retinal detachments with temporary balloon buckling. *Retina*. 1986;6(4):210–214.

50. McAllister IL, Meyers SM, Zegarra H, et al. Comparison of pneumatic retinopexy with alternative surgical techniques. *Ophthalmology*. 1988;95(7):877–883.

51. Hilton GF, Tornambe PE. Pneumatic retinopexy. An analysis of intraoperative and postoperative complications. The Retinal Detachment Study Group. *Retina*. 1991;11(3):285–294.

52. Poliner LS, Grand MG, Schoch LH, et al. New retinal detachment after pneumatic retinopexy. *Ophthalmology*. 1987;94(4):315–318.

53. Grizzard WS, Hilton GF, Hammer ME, et al. Pneumatic retinopexy failures. Cause, prevention, timing, and management. *Ophthalmology*. 1995;102(6):929–936.

54. Tornambe PE, Hilton GF, Brinton DA, et al. Pneumatic retinopexy. A two-year follow-up study of the multicenter clinical trial comparing pneumatic retinopexy with scleral buckling. *Ophthalmology*. 1991;98(7):1115–1123.

55. Dreyer RF. Sequential retinal tears attributed to intraocular gas. *Am J Ophthalmol*. 1986 15;102(2):276–278.

56. Lois N, Wong D. Pseudophakic retinal detachment. *Surv Ophthalmol*. 2003;48(5):467–487.

57. Cole CJ, Charteris DG. Cataract extraction after retinal detachment repair by vitrectomy: Visual outcome and complications. *Eye*. 2009;23(6):1377–1381.

58. Moore JK, Kitchens JW, Smiddy WE, et al. Retinal breaks observed during pars plana vitrectomy. *Am J Ophthalmol*. 2007;144(1):32–36.

59. Kumagai K, Furukawa M, Ogino N, et al. Long-term outcomes of macular hole surgery with triamcinolone acetonide-assisted internal limiting membrane peeling. *Retina*. 2007;27(9):1249–1254.

60. Passemard M, Yakoubi Y, Muselier A, et al. Long-term outcome of idiopathic macular hole surgery. *Am J Ophthalmol*. 2010;149(1):120–126.

61. Park SS, Marcus DM, Duker JS, et al. Posterior segment complications after vitrectomy for macular hole. *Ophthalmology*. 1995;102(5):775–781.

62. Tabandeh H, Chaudhry NA, Smiddy WE. Retinal detachment associated with macular hole surgery: Characteristics, mechanism, and outcomes. *Retina*. 1999;19(4):281–216.

63. Wimpissinger B, Binder S. Entry-site-related retinal detachment after pars plana vitrectomy. *Acta Ophthalmol Scand*. 2007;85(7):782–785.

64. Le Rouic JF, Becquet F, Ducournau D. Does 23-gauge sutureless vitrectomy modify the risk of postoperative retinal detachment after macular surgery?: A Comparison with 20-Gauge Vitrectomy. *Retina*. 2011;31(5):902–908.

65. Banker AS, Freeman WR, Kim JW, et al. Vision-threatening complications of surgery for full-thickness macular holes. Vitrectomy for Macular Hole Study Group. *Ophthalmology*. 1997;104(9):1442–1452;

66. Heier JS, Topping TM, Frederick AR Jr, et al. Visual and surgical outcomes of retinal detachment following macular hole repair. *Retina*. 1999;19(2):110–115.

67. Sjaarda RN, Glaser BM, Thompson JT, et al. Distribution of iatrogenic retinal breaks in macular hole surgery. *Ophthalmology*. 1995;102(9):1387–1392.

68. Al-Harthi E, Abboud EB, Al-Dhibi H, et al. Incidence of sclerotomy-related retinal breaks. *Retina*. 2005;25(3):281–284.

69. Rizzo S, Belting C, Genovesi-Ebert F, et al. Incidence of retinal detachment after small-incision, sutureless pars plana vitrectomy compared with conventional 20-gauge vitrectomy in macular hole and epiretinal membrane surgery. *Retina*. 2010;30(7):1065–1071.

70. Ramkissoon YD, Aslam SA, Shah SP, et al. Risk of iatrogenic peripheral retinal breaks in 20-G pars plana vitrectomy. *Ophthalmology*. 2010;117(9):1825–1830.

71. Theocharis IP, Alexandridou A, Gili NJ, et al. Combined phacoemulsification and pars plana vitrectomy for macular hole treatment. *Acta Ophthalmol Scand*. 2005;83(2):172–175.

72. Guillaubey A, Malvitte L, Lafontaine PO, et al. Incidence of retinal detachment after macular surgery: A retrospective study of 634 cases. *Br J Ophthalmol*. 2007;91(10):1327–1330.

73. Scartozzi R, Bessa AS, Gupta OP, et al. Intraoperative sclerotomy-related retinal breaks for macular surgery, 20- vs 25-gauge vitrectomy systems. *Am J Ophthalmol*. 2007;143(1):155–156.

74. Tan HS, Lesnik Oberstein SY, Mura M, et al. Enhanced internal search for iatrogenic retinal breaks in 20-gauge macular surgery. *Br J Ophthalmol*. 2010;94(11):1490–1492.

75. Tan HS, Mura M, de Smet MD. Iatrogenic retinal breaks in 25-gauge macular surgery. *Am J Ophthalmol*. 2009;148(3):427–430.

76. Moore JK, Scott IU, Flynn HW Jr, et al. Retinal detachment in eyes undergoing pars plana vitrectomy for removal of retained lens fragments. *Ophthalmology*. 2003; 110(4):709–713.

77. Merani R, Hunyor AP, Playfair TJ, et al. Pars plana vitrectomy for the management of retained lens material after cataract surgery. *Am J Ophthalmol*. 2007;144(3):364–370.

78. Capeans C, Lorenzo J, Santos L, et al. Comparative study of incomplete posterior vitreous detachment as a risk factor for proliferative vitreoretinopathy. *Graefes Arch Clin Exp Ophthalmol*. 1998;236(7):481–485.

79. Kakehashi A, Kado M, Akiba J, et al. Variations of posterior vitreous detachment. *Br J Ophthalmol*. 1997;81(7):527–532.

80. Weber-Krause B, Eckardt C. Incidence of posterior vitreous detachment in the elderly. *Ophthalmologe*. 1997;94(9):619–623.

81. Lorenzo Carrero J. Incomplete posterior vitreous detachment: Prevalence and clinical relevance. *Am J Ophthalmol*. 2012;153(3):497–503.

82. Chung SE, Kim KH, Kang SW. Retinal breaks associated with the induction of posterior vitreous detachment. *Am J Ophthalmol*. 2009;147(6):1012–1016.

83. Foos RY, Allen RA. Retinal tears and lesser lesions of the peripheral retina in autopsy eyes. *Am J Ophthalmol* 1967;64(3 suppl):643–55.

84. Hogan MJ. The vitreous, its structure, and relation to the ciliary body and retina. Proctor award lecture. *Invest Ophthalmol*. 1963;2:418–445.

85. Osterlin S. Preludes to retinal detachment in the aphakic eye. *Mod Probl Ophthalmol*. 1977;18:464–467.

86. Lincoff H, Horowitz J, Kreissig I, et al. Morphological effects of gas compression on the cortical vitreous. *Arch Ophthalmol*. 1986;104(8):1212–1215.

87. Byer NE, Colyear BH Jr. New retinal tears following photocoagulation. *Trans Pac Coast Otoophthalmol Soc Annu Meet*. 1965;46:237–259.

88. Fetkenhour CL, Hauch TL. Scleral buckling without thermal adhesion. *Am J Ophthalmol*. 1980;89(5):662–666.

89. Moisseiev J, Glaser BM. New and previously unidentified retinal breaks in eyes with recurrent retinal detachment with proliferative vitreoretinopathy. *Arch Ophthalmol*. 1989;107(8):1152–1154.

90. Williams GA, Blumenkranz MG (1992) Vitreous humor. In: Tasman W, Jaeger EA (eds) *Duane's Foundations of Clinical Ophthalmology*. Vol 2. Rev ed. Philadelphia: Lippincott, Chap 11.

91. Krieger AE. The pars plana incision: Experimental studies, pathologic observations, and clinical experience. *Trans Am Ophthalmol Soc*. 1991;89:549–621.

92. Day S, Grossman DS, Mruthyunjaya P, et al. One-year outcomes after retinal detachment surgery among medicare beneficiaries. *Am J Ophthalmol*. 2010;150(3): 338–345.

93. Hwang J, Escariao P, Iranmanesh R, et al. Outcomes of macular hole surgery in patients treated intraoperatively for retinal breaks and/or lattice degeneration. *Retina*. 2007;27(9):1243–1248.

94. Yamakiri K, Sakamoto T, Noda Y, et al. Reduced incidence of intraoperative complications in a multicenter controlled clinical trial of triamcinolone in vitrectomy. *Ophthalmology*. 2007;114(2):289–296.

95. Kunikata H, Nishida K. Visual outcome and complications of 25-gauge vitrectomy for rhegmatogenous retinal detachment; 84 consecutive cases. *Eye*. 2010;24(6): 1071–1077.

96. Friberg TR, Eller AW. Laser pneumatic retinopexy for repair of recurrent retinal detachment after failed scleral buckle: Ten years experience. *Ophthalmic Surg Lasers*. 2001;32(1):13–18.

97. Yeo LM, Charteris DG, Bunce C, et al. Retained intravitreal lens fragments after phacoemulsification: A clinicopathological correlation. *Br J Ophthalmol*. 1999;83(10): 1135–1138.

98. Chen CL, Wang TY, Cheng JH, et al. Immediate pars plana vitrectomy improves outcome in retained intravitreal lens fragments after phacoemulsification. *Ophthalmologica*. 2008;222(4):277–283.

 99. Rofagha S, Bhisitkul RB. Management of retained lens fragments in complicated cataract surgery. *Curr Opin Ophthalmol.* 2011;22(2):137–40.

100. Scartozzi R, Bessa AS, Gupta OP, et al. Intraoperative sclerotomy-related retinal breaks for macular surgery, 20- vs 25-gauge vitrectomy systems. *Am J Ophthalmol.* 2007;143(1):155–6.

101. Territo C, Gieser JP, Wilson CA, et al. Influence of the cannulated vitrectomy system on the occurrence of iatrogenic sclerotomy retinal tears. *Retina.* 1997;17(5):430–433.

102. Ibarra MS, Hermel M, Prenner JL, et al. Longer-term outcomes of transconjunctival sutureless 25-gauge vitrectomy. *Am J Ophthalmol.* 2005;139(5):831–836.

103. Gupta OP, Ho AC, Kaiser PK, et al. Short-term outcomes of 23-gauge pars plana vitrectomy. *Am J Ophthalmol.* 2008;146(2):193–197.

104. Chang TS, McGill E, Hay DA, et al. Prophylactic scleral buckle for prevention of retinal detachment following vitrectomy for macular hole. *Br J Ophthalmol.* 1999;83(8):944–948.

105. Richardson EC, Verma S, Green WT, et al. Primary vitrectomy for rhegmatogenous retinal detachment: An analysis of failure. *Eur J Ophthalmol.* 2000;10(2):160–166.

106. Stangos AN, Petropoulos IK, Brozou CG, et al. Pars-plana vitrectomy alone vs vitrectomy with scleral buckling for primary rhegmatogenous pseudophakic retinal detachment. *Am J Ophthalmol.* 2004;138(6):952–958.

107. Wickham L, Connor M, Aylward GW. Vitrectomy and gas for inferior break retinal detachments: Are the results comparable to vitrectomy, gas, and scleral buckle? *Br J Ophthalmol.* 2004;88(11):1376–1379.

108. Hager A, Ehrich S, Wiegand W. [Vitreoretinal secondary procedures following elective macular surgery]. *Ophthalmologe.* 2004;101(1):39–44.

109. Koh HJ, Cheng L, Kosobucki B, et al. Prophylactic intraoperative 360 degrees laser retinopexy for prevention of retinal detachment. *Retina.* 2007;27(6):744–749.

110. Stirpe M, Heimann K. Vitreous changes and retinal detachment in highly myopic eyes. *Eur J Ophthalmol.* 1996;6(1):50–58.

111. Mansour AM. Pneumatic retinopexy for inferior retinal breaks. *Ophthalmology.* 2005;112(10):1771–1776.

112. Friberg TR, Eller AW. Laser pneumatic retinopexy for repair of recurrent retinal detachment after failed scleral buckle–ten years experience. *Ophthalmic Surg Lasers.* 2001;32(1):13–18.

113. Moisseiev J, Glaser BM. New and previously unidentified retinal breaks in eyes with recurrent retinal detachment with proliferative vitreoretinopathy. *Arch Ophthalmol.* 1989;107(8):1152–1154.

114. Salicone A, Smiddy WE, Venkatraman A, et al. Management of retinal detachment when no break is found. *Ophthalmology.* 2006;113(3):398–403.

115. El Matri L, Mghaieth F, Baccouri R, et al. Late recurrent retinal detachment after scleral buckling. *J Fr Ophtalmol.* 2006;29(9):991–993.

116. Kulkarni KM, Roth DB, Prenner JL. Current visual and anatomic outcomes of pneumatic retinopexy. *Retina.* 2007;27(8):1065–1070.

117. Russell M, Gaskin B, Russell D, et al. Pseudophakic retinal detachment after phacoemulsification cataract surgery: Ten-year retrospective review. *J Cataract Refract Surg.* 2006;32(3):442–445.

118. Ramkissoon YD, Aslam SA, Shah SP, et al. Risk of iatrogenic peripheral retinal breaks in 20-G pars plana vitrectomy. *Ophthalmology.* 2010;117(9):1825–1830.

119. Romero-Aroca P, Almena-Garcia M, Baget-Bernaldiz M, et al. Differences between the combination of the 25-gauge vitrectomy with phacoemulsification versus 20-gauge vitrectomy and phacofragmentation. *Clin Ophthalmol.* 2009;3:671–679.

120. Ho LY, Doft BH, Wang L, et al. Clinical predictors and outcomes of pars plana vitrectomy for retained lens material after cataract extraction. *Am J Ophthalmol.* 2009;147(4):587–594.

Due to Proliferative Vitreoretinopathy

PHILIP J. BANERJEE AND DAVID G. CHARTERIS

✦ The Complication: Definition

Proliferative vitreoretinopathy (PVR) is the most common cause of anatomic failure in retinal detachment surgery and is generally regarded as having an incidence of 5% to 11% of all rhegmatogenous retinal detachments.[1] PVR can be considered a wound healing response in specialized tissue, which results in the formation of fibrocellular membranes on both surfaces of the retina and the posterior hyaloid face. Contraction of these membranes can result in distortion of the normal retinal topography with visually detrimental sequelae, and/or tractional retinal detachment, with the reopening of pre-existing breaks or the formation of new ones.

Initially, the condition was referred to as massive vitreous retraction (MVR) syndrome or massive preretinal retraction (MPR) syndrome on the premise that the primary pathology was centered in the vitreous.[2] Later, to acknowledge the role of preretinal membrane formation, this was modified to massive preretinal proliferation (MPP).[3]

A unifying classification system was published in 1983 by the Retina Society Terminology Committee, coining the term "proliferative vitreoretinopathy (PVR),"[1] which was later updated in 1991 to the classification system commonly used in daily practice (see Tables 35C-1 and 35C-2).[4]

Although the current classification system has served to standardize terminology and clinical descriptions when dealing with PVR, it is limited with respect to a lack of inclusion of clinically important information such as number, size, and location of retinal breaks, factors known to be significant in the risk of development and progression of PVR.[3] **Figures 35C-1** through **35C-3** provide examples of PVR, and their corresponding grading.

Table 35C-1 • Updated Proliferative Vitreoretinopathy Grade Classification[4]	
Grade	**Features**
A	Vitreous haze, vitreous pigment clumps, pigment clusters on inferior retina
B	Wrinkling of inner retinal surface, retinal stiffness, vessel tortuosity, rolled and irregular edge of retinal break, decreased mobility of vitreous
CP 1-12	Posterior to equator; focal, diffuse, or circumferential full-thickness folds,[a] subretinal strands[a]
CA 1-12	Anterior to equator; focal, diffuse or circumferential full-thickness folds,[a] subretinal strands,[a] anterior displacement,[a] condensed vitreous strands

[a]Expressed in terms of the total number of clock hours involved.

Table 35C-2 • Updated Proliferative Vitreoretinopathy Contraction Type Classification[4]		
Type	**Location (In Relation to Equator)**	**Features**
Focal	Posterior	Starfold posterior to vitreous base
Diffuse	Posterior	Confluent starfolds posterior to vitreous base; optic disc may not be visible
Subretinal	Posterior/anterior	Proliferation under the retina; annular strand near disc; linear strands; moth eaten-appearing sheets
Circumferential	Anterior	Contraction along posterior edge of vitreous base with central displacement of retina; peripheral retina stretched; posterior retina in radial folds
Anterior	Anterior	Vitreous base pulled anteriorly by proliferative tissue; peripheral retinal trough; displacement ciliary processes may be stretched, may be covered by membrane; iris may be retracted

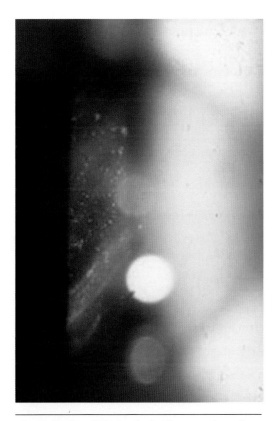

Figure 35C-1 PVR Grade A. Pigment clumping in the vitreous.

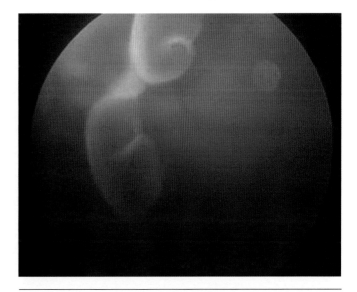

Figure 35C-2 PVR Grade B. A rolled edge to a giant retinal tear.

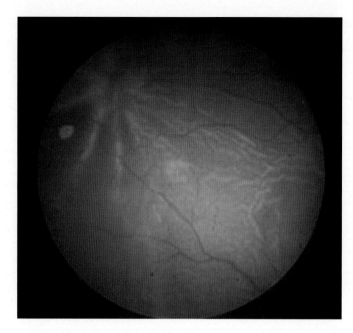

Figure 35C-3 PVR Grade C. P2– a focal starfold of approximately 2 clock hours, posterior to the equator.

 Risk Factors

There are a number of risk factors which have been implicated in the occurrence of PVR, but primarily the following two situations are universally agreed upon[5,6]:

◆ Preoperative PVR (the pathophysiologic process has already begun and may be exacerbated by surgery)

◆ Preoperative choroidal detachment (associated with marked breakdown of the blood retinal barrier and/or inflammation)

In addition, the following situations have also been found to be risk factors which predispose eyes to develop PVR:

◆ Giant retinal tear[6,7]

◆ Large/multiple retinal breaks (cumulative break area greater than 3 disc areas)[6,7]

◆ Retinal detachment greater than 2 quadrants[6]

◆ Retinal tears associated with vitreous hemorrhage[6,8]

◆ Long duration of retinal detachment[9]

◆ Signs of uveitis[6] or increased inflammation after trauma

◆ Previous retinal detachment surgery (particularly vitrectomy)[5]

◆ Intraoperative or postoperative vitreous hemorrhage[6]

◆ Large retinal areas treated with cryopexy[5]

◆ Postoperative choroidal detachment[6]

Eyes with any of these risk factors should be monitored more closely postoperatively.

Pathogenesis: Why Does It Occur

The pathophysiology of PVR is a complex and, as yet, incompletely understood process. As a simplified overview, it is helpful to consider it to be the result of the following components:

◆ Cellular accumulation and proliferation

◆ Extracellular matrix production

◆ Fibrin deposition

◆ Contraction of formed membranes

Cellular Accumulation and Proliferation

Four categories of cells have been identified in PVR membranes; (1) retinal pigment epithelial cells (RPE), (2) glial cells, (3) fibroblasts, and (4) inflammatory cells (macrophages and lymphocytes). Experimental and clinical studies have emphasized the importance of RPE cell chemotaxis, proliferation, and metaplastic differentiation into a fibroblast morphology under the effect of local growth factors/cytokines. More recent studies have demonstrated a central role of retinal glial cell activation and extension into periretinal membranes.[10,11] Infiltrating inflammatory cells are also thought to play a role in the pathogenesis of PVR.

Extracellular Matrix Production and Fibrin Deposition

Collagen (predominantly types I and III) and fibronectin, derived from RPE and glial cells, are key components in PVR membrane formation. Fibrin may also provide a growth surface for the formation of complex vitreal and epiretinal PVR membranes.

Contraction of Formed Membranes

Contraction of tissue across a wound on a planar surface serves to appose the wound edges and close the wound, as occurs on the skin. However, on the inner spherical surface of the eye, the vector of pull is centripetally, thereby dragging tissue toward its center.[12] The contraction of the complex periretinal and vitreous membranes mentioned above is responsible for the clinical picture of PVR and the potential failure of retinal reattachment surgery.

Figure 35C-4 illustrates the sequence of events which occur when a retinal detachment is complicated by PVR and allowed to follow its natural history.

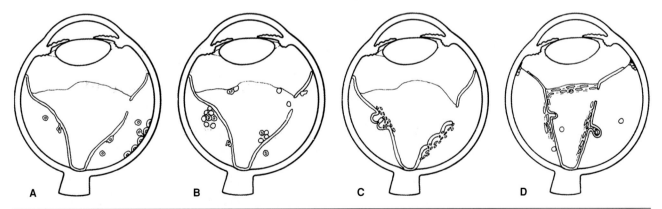

Figure 35C-4 A: Cellular activation, proliferation, and migration following a rhegmatogenous RD. **B:** Formation of fibrocellular membranes. (Note also glial extension from retina at this stage.) **C:** Contraction of epi and subretinal membranes. **D:** Fixed fold formation leading to funnel RD. (Courtesy of P. Leaver and T. Tarrant.)

Table 35C-3 • Perioperative Management Tips

Risk Factor/Clinical Scenario	Management Tips
Pre-existing inflammation	1. Intensive topical steroids 2. Consider systemic steroids 3. Consider deferring surgery
Choroidal detachment/evidence of blood retinal barrier breakdown	1. Intensive topical steroids 2. Topical nonsteroidal anti-inflammatory drugs
High risk detachment, e.g., GRT, pre-existing PVR, and trauma	1. Avoid cryotherapy (as disperses viable RPE cells) 2. Consider adjunctive agent (see below[a])
Pre-existing vitreous hemorrhage	1. Meticulous vitrectomy to clear blood (and therefore fibrin) and RPE cells

[a]Risk factors for the development of proliferative vitreoretinopathy (PVR) and perioperative manoeuvres to avoid them/treat them

As yet, there is no definitive treatment to prevent the formation of PVR. Nevertheless it is of value to identify patients who are at high risk and treat any modifiable risk factors accordingly. Table 35C-3 illustrates examples of such cases and suggested measures to take either preoperatively, intraoperatively, or both if appropriate.

A number of the aforementioned clinical scenarios/risk factors may coexist, and it may be useful to use a combination of the techniques described in the second column of Table 35C-3.

Table 35C-4 • Previously Investigated Adjunctive Agents

Adjunct	Target	Therapeutic Benefit	Evidence Strength
Daunorubicin[13]	Cellular proliferation	Reduce reoperations but no effect on outcome	I b
5FU (5-fluorouracil)[14]	Cellular proliferation	Improved surgical outcome	III
Combined 5FU + LMWH (low molecular weight heparin)[15–17]	Cellular proliferation and extracellular matrix	Improved surgical outcome in high risk cases	I b
Retinoids[18]	Cellular proliferation	No benefit	II b
Colchicine[19]	Cellular proliferation	No benefit	II a
Irradiation[20]	Cellular proliferation	No benefit	I b
Corticosteroids[21–26]	Cellular proliferation and blood–ocular barrier breakdown	No benefit with systemic use/reduction of postoperative inflammation, but conflicting evidence for surgical outcome with Intravitreal triamcinolone (IVTA)	Varying levels of evidence

Adjunctive Agents*

An increased understanding of the pathophysiology of PVR has led to strategies, which target specific pathways in its formation, with the aim of developing adjunctive agents to be used as preventative treatment. Table 35C-4 highlights agents that have been trialed clinically, their target, their proposed therapeutic benefit, and the strength of evidence which supports their use.

Pearls on How to Solve It/Pearls on How to Prevent It

Surgery for PVR-related detachments follows the same basic principles of any rhegmatogenous retinal detachment surgery namely:

◆ Closure/sealing of retinal breaks

◆ Complete release of preretinal traction

   The addition of a third factor can be added for PVR cases:

◆ Prevention of reproliferation

Deciding When to Proceed with Surgery

The decision to operate on a retinal detachment must always be weighed up against the likely visual outcome that has been demonstrated to be limited in many cases.[27] Very advanced PVR pathology where the fellow eye is healthy may not justify surgical intervention.

Surgical Tips

1. *Timing of surgery:* Better surgical results are likely in an uninflamed eye with only limited blood–ocular barrier breakdown. It may therefore be beneficial to delay surgery to allow anti-inflammatory treatment to take effect. A prolonged delay of several weeks may, however, reduce the potential visual recovery of the retina and is not advised.

2. *Patient expectations:* The patient should be advised/counselled that (a) the problem is not straightforward, (b) there is an uncertain visual outcome, (c) there is a possible series of operations, and (d) the need for postoperative posturing.

3. Vitrectomy techniques form the basis of surgery with scleral buckling having only a limited role.

4. Epi- and subretinal membranes should, where possible, be peeled with a surgical pick and/or forceps. Care should be taken not to use excessive force as the membranes may have glial continuity to the adjacent retina[11] and iatrogenic tractional retinal breaks may result. Posterior membranes should be removed prior to performing a retinectomy.

5. Residual anterior traction can be countered by using a scleral buckle or performing a retinectomy. Scleral buckle, used in combination with vitrectomy, can relieve moderate degrees of anterior vitreoretinal traction but may cause motility problems (exacerbated by poor central VA) and in some cases chronic low- grade inflammation.

6. When a retinectomy is performed to relieve basal traction it is usually at least 180 degrees of the ocular circumference. Occasionally a smaller retinectomy is useful in unusual cases, for example, focal PVR in trauma.

7. The following are important in performing a retinectomy: (a) Removing all posterior membranes prior to retinectomy, (b) applying diathermy to retinectomy edges/retinal vessels, (c) Remove all anterior retina to prevent ischemia/re-proliferation.

---

*See Appendix.

8. Silicone oil and long-acting (C_3F_8) intraocular gas can both provide adequate internal tamponde for PVR cases.[28] Silicone oil is, however, often preferred—It provides a more stable postoperative situation with limited progression of recurrent retinal detachment and less hypotony.

9. Postoperative cystoid macular edema (CMO) is a common complication, which can reduce visual outcomes.[29] Intensive anti-inflammatory treatment can reduce CMO and improve visual results.

✥ Expected Outcomes: What Is the Worse-case Scenario

Development of PVR results in markedly reduced visual outcomes compared to retinal detachment not complicated by PVR with only 11% to 25% of patients achieving a visual acuity of 20/100.[30–32]

In the context of repeat vitreoretinal surgery, the rare occurrence of sympathetic ophthalmia, estimated to be approximately 1 in 800 vitrectomies, should be considered.[33,34]

Managing patients with retinal detachments complicated by PVR remains a challenging yet often rewarding part of vitreoretinal surgery, with the ability to reattach the retina in the majority of cases. Although some patients require multiple procedures, vitreoretinal surgeons feel justified in continuing to operate on these complex cases and patients view their attempts as worthwhile.

REFERENCES

1. The classification of retinal detachment with proliferative vitreoretinopathy. *Ophthalmology.* 1983;90(2):121–125.
2. Machemer R. Proliferative vitreoretinopathy (PVR): A personal account of its pathogenesis and treatment. Proctor lecture. *Invest Ophthalmol Vis Sci.* 1988;29(12): 1771–1783.
3. Machemer R, Laqua H. Pigment epithelium proliferation in retinal detachment (massive periretinal proliferation). *Am J Ophthalmol.* 1975;80(1):1–23.
4. Machemer R, Aaberg TM, Freeman R, et al. An updated classification of retinal detachment with proliferative vitreoretinopathy. *Am J Ophthalmol.* 1991;112(2): 159–165.
5. Cowley M, Conway BP, Campochiaro PA, et al. Clinical risk factors for proliferative vitreoretinopathy. *Arch Ophthalmol.* 1989;107(8):1147–1151.
6. Girard P, Mimoun G, Karpouzas I, et al. Clinical risk factors for proliferative vitreoretinopathy after retinal detachment surgery. *Retina.* 1994;14(5):417–424.
7. Yanyali A, Bonnet M. Risk factors of postoperative proliferative vitreoretinopathy in giant tears. *J Fr Ophtalmol.* 1996;19(3):175–180.
8. Duquesne N. Bonnet M, Adeleine P. Preoperative vitreous hemorrhage associated with rhegmatogenous retinal detachment: A risk factor for postoperative proliferative vitreoretinopathy? *Graefes Arch Clin Exp Ophthalmol.* 1996;234(11): 677–682.
9. Tseng W, Cortez RT, Ramirez I, et al. Prevalence and risk factors for proliferative vitreoretinopathy in eyes with rhegmatogenous retinal detachment but no previous vitreoretinal surgery. *Am J Ophthalmol.* 2004;137(6):1105–1115.
10. Sethi CS, Lewis GP, Fisher SK, et al. Glial remodeling and neural plasticity in human retinal detachment with proliferative vitreoretinopathy. *Invest Ophthalmol Vis Sci.* 2005;46(1):329–342.
11. Charteris DG, Downie J, Aylward GW, et al. Intraretinal and periretinal pathology in anterior proliferative vitreoretinopathy. *Graefes Arch Clin Exp Ophthalmol.* 2007; 245(1):93–100.
12. Williamson TH. Proliferative Vitreoretinopathy. In H Marion Philipp H, ed. *Vitreoretinal Surgery.* Berlin, Heidelberg, Germany: Springer-Verlag; Chap 7, 2008:99.

13. Wiedemann P, Hilgers RD, Bauer P, et al. Adjunctive daunorubicin in the treatment of proliferative vitreoretinopathy: Results of a multicenter clinical trial. Daunomycin Study Group. *Am J Ophthalmol.* 1998;126(4):550–559.

14. Blumenkranz M, Hernandez E, Ophir A, et al. 5-fluorouracil: New applications in complicated retinal detachment for an established antimetabolite. *Ophthalmology.* 1984;91(2):122–130.

15. Asaria RH, Kon CH, Bunce C, et al. Adjuvant 5-fluorouracil and heparin prevents proliferative vitreoretinopathy: Results from a randomized, double-blind, controlled clinical trial. *Ophthalmology.* 2001;108(7):1179–1183.

16. Charteris DG, Aylward GW, Wong D, et al. A randomized controlled trial of combined 5-fluorouracil and low-molecular-weight heparin in management of established proliferative vitreoretinopathy. *Ophthalmology.* 2004;111(12):2240–2245.

17. Wickham L, Bunce C, Wong D, et al. Randomized controlled trial of combined 5-Fluorouracil and low-molecular-weight heparin in the management of unselected rhegmatogenous retinal detachments undergoing primary vitrectomy. *Ophthalmology.* 2007;114(4):698–704.

18. Fekrat S, de Juan E Jr, Campochiaro PA. The effect of oral 13-*cis*-retinoic acid on retinal redetachment after surgical repair in eyes with proliferative vitreoretinopathy. *Ophthalmology.* 1995;102(3):412–418.

19. Berman DH, Gombos GM. Proliferative vitreoretinopathy: Does oral low-dose colchicine have an inhibitory effect? A controlled study in humans. *Ophthalmic Surg.* 1989;20(4):268–272.

20. Binder S, Bonnet M, Velikay M, et al. Radiation therapy in proliferative vitreoretinopathy. A prospective randomized study. *Graefes Arch Clin Exp Ophthalmol.* 1994;232(4):211–214.

21. Jonas JB, Hayler JK, Panda-Jonas S. Intravitreal injection of crystalline cortisone as adjunctive treatment of proliferative vitreoretinopathy. *Br J Ophthalmol.* 2000; 84(9):1064–1067.

22. Koerner F, Merz A, Gloor B, et al. Postoperative retinal fibrosis—A controlled clinical study of systemic steroid therapy. *Graefes Arch Clin Exp Ophthalmol.* 1982;219(6): 268–271.

23. Williams RG, Chang S, Comaratta MR, et al. Does the presence of heparin and dexamethasone in the vitrectomy infusate reduce reproliferation in proliferative vitreoretinopathy?. *Graefes Arch Clin Exp Ophthalmol.* 1996;234(8):496–503.

24. Munir WM, Pulido JS, Sharma MC, et al. Intravitreal triamcinolone for treatment of complicated proliferative diabetic retinopathy and proliferative vitreoretinopathy. *Can J Ophthalmol.* 2005;40(5):598–604.

25. Wickham L. Intensive anti-inflammatory therapy as an adjuvant treatment for established proliferative vitreoretinopathy, *ARVO* 2007 Abstract.

26. Ahmadieh H, Feghhi M, Tabatabaei H, et al. Triamcinolone acetonide in silicone-filled eyes as adjunctive treatment for proliferative vitreoretinopathy: A randomized clinical trial. *Ophthalmology.* 2008;115(11):1938–1943.

27. Andenmatten R, Gonvers M. Sophisticated vitreoretinal surgery in patients with a healthy fellow eye. An 11-year retrospective study. *Graefes Arch Clin Exp Ophthalmol.* 1993;231(9):495–499.

28. Vitrectomy with silicone oil or perfluoropropane gas in eyes with severe proliferative vitreoretinopathy: Results of a randomized clinical trial. Silicone Study Report 2. *Arch Ophthalmol.* 1992;110(6):780–792.

29. Benson SE, Grigoropoulos V, Schlottmann PG, et al. Analysis of the macula with optical coherence tomography after successful surgery for proliferative vitreoretinopathy. *Arch Ophthalmol.* 2005;123(12):1651–1656.

30. Lewis H, Aaberg TM. Causes of failure after repeat vitreoretinal surgery for recurrent proliferative vitreoretinopathy. *Am J Ophthalmol.* 1991;111(1):15–19.

31. Lewis H, Aaberg TM, Abrams GW. Causes of failure after initial vitreoretinal surgery for severe proliferative vitreoretinopathy. *Am J Ophthalmol.* 1991;111(1):8–14.

32. Wickham L, Ho-Yen GO, Bunce C, et al. Surgical failure following primary retinal detachment surgery by vitrectomy: Risk factors and functional outcomes. *Br J Ophthalmol.* 2011;95(9):1234–1238.

33. Kilmartin DJ, Dick AD, Forrester JV. Sympathetic ophthalmia risk following vitrectomy: Should we counsel patients? *Br J Ophthalmol.* 2000;84(5):448–449.

34. Grigoropoulos VG, Benson S, Bunce C, et al. Functional outcome and prognostic factors in 304 eyes managed by retinectomy. *Graefes Arch Clin Exp Ophthalmol.* 2007;245(5):641–649.

APPENDIX

Levels of evidence, Centre for Evidence-Based Medicine, June 2010

◆ Ia: Systematic review or meta-analysis of Randomised Controlled Trial (RCTs).

◆ Ib: At least one RCT.

◆ IIa: At least one well-designed controlled study without randomization.

◆ IIb: At least one well-designed quasiexperimental study, such as a cohort study.

◆ III: Well-designed nonexperimental descriptive studies, such as comparative studies, correlation studies, case–control studies, and case series.

◆ IV: Expert committee reports, opinions, and/or clinical experience of respected authorities.

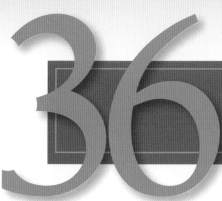

ENDOPHTHALMITIS IN the MICROINCISION VITRECTOMY SURGERY ERA

YUSUKE OSHIMA

 The Complication

Acute-onset postvitrectomy endophthalmitis is uncommon, but remains one of the most serious complications associated with devastating visual loss or blindness despite appropriate treatment.[1-3] The reported incidence rates of infectious endophthalmitis varied from procedure to procedure, for example, 0.082% following cataract extraction, 0.178% following penetrating keratoplasty, 0.124% following glaucoma surgeries, and 0.046% after pars plana vitrectomy (PPV).[4] Similar to the incidence rates following cataract surgery, which dropped to around 0.04% in most recent studies,[5] the incident rates after conventional 20G vitrectomy have decreased from 0.15% to 0.03%–0.05% during the past decades because of improved surgical techniques and recognition of the importance of perioperative antiseptic preparations.[3,6,7] Taking the place of the conventional 20G vitrectomy, transconjunctival microincision vitrectomy surgery (MIVS) with 23G or 25G instrumentation has become commonplace today because of the potential for greater patients comfort, shorter operating time, and less surgically induced inflammation with rapid visual recovery. However, along with the recent trend toward more frequent use of and expanding indications for MIVS, there was a growing concern that MIVS with either 23G or 25G instrumentation may increase the risk of postoperative endophthalmitis compared with conventional 20G vitrectomy because of the transconjunctival approach and sutureless nature of MIVS.[8]

Clinical Characteristics of Postvitrectomy Endophthalmitis

Patients with a clinical diagnosis of infectious endophthalmitis after vitrectomy surgery can be identified based on standard features, including anterior chamber cell and fibrin, vitreous cell and fibrin, hypopyon, blurred/reduced vision, lid swelling, and pain in advanced cases (**Fig. 36-1**). Clinical features and surgical history are clinically important for the diagnosis. However, the diagnosis is often difficult to make because the normal postoperative pain and intraocular inflammation after vitrectomy may mask the symptoms.

Although bacteria, fungi, and viruses are all capable of producing infectious endophthalmitis, the causative organisms of postvitrectomy endophthalmitis are gram-positive in 75% to 95% of the reported cases.[1-7] Although microbiologic data for bacteria isolation from the aqueous humor, vitreous, and/or tap are very helpful for diagnosis and subsequent treatment of endophthalmitis, a significant percentage of cases of apparent infectious endophthalmitis proved to be culture-negative.

 Causative Factors

Several potential predisposing factors contributing to infectious endophthalmitis following MIVS have been proposed including the inoculation of bacteria into the vitreous cavity, vitreous wick in the sclerotomies, the absence of subconjunctival

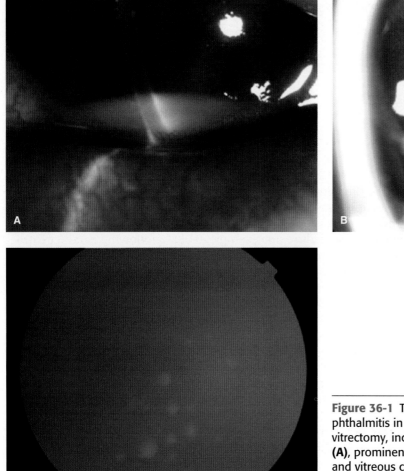
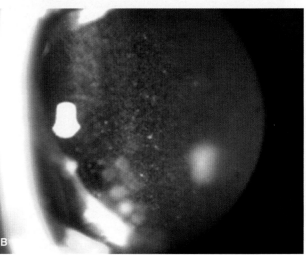

Figure 36-1 Typical findings of acute infectious endo-phthalmitis in a patient who had undergone pars plana vitrectomy, including hypopyon in the anterior chamber **(A)**, prominent inflammatory cells in the anterior chamber and vitreous cavity **(B)**, and fundus obscured with vitreous opacities **(C)**.

antibiotics, less vitreous removal during small gauge vitrectomy, lower infusion rates, and the wound self-sealing related issues. Of these, the most important is incomplete self-sealing of a sutureless sclerotomy, which may cause postoperative hypotony and/or facilitate the presence of a vitreous wick in the sclerotomies, allowing ocular surface bacteria to easily enter the vitreous cavity after surgery. Thanks to better understanding of wound structure reached by recent histologic examinations and optical coherence tomography (OCT)-based imaging studies,[9] a straight incision is revealed to result in wound leakage regardless of the intraocular pressure, while an oblique incision will lead to adequate wound adaptation with self-sealing. Refinements in surgical instruments (e.g., newly designed trocar blades) and techniques (e.g., conjunctival displacement with oblique incision) have improved the rigidity of the sutureless wound structures and minimized wound-sealing-related complications and the risk of bacterial inoculation after surgery.[10,11]

Postoperative infectious endophthalmitis in most intraocular surgeries is generally caused by the introduction of microorganisms at the time of surgery. Recent studies indicate that causative organisms in infection after cataract surgery are usually genetically identical to the patients' own flora.[12,13] Bacteria routinely enter the anterior chamber during surgery and can remain in the anterior chamber at the end of surgery as the potential source of infection.[14] In MIVS, direct inoculation of ocular surface flora into the vitreous cavity through transconjunctival instrument insertion during surgery may account for the increased risk of postoperative endophthalmitis. Bacterial contamination of the anterior chamber during surgery has been proved to be responsible for most postoperative infectious endophthalmitis.[14] Although the mechanism of bacterial inoculation into the vitreous cavity in patients with post-MIVS endophthalmitis remains uncertain, studies on other ophthalmic procedures (e.g., cataract surgery and intravitreal injection) have shown that surgical instruments used for penetrating the ocular surfaces can be highly contaminated with bacteria.[15] These findings led us to assume that infectious endophthalmitis may be caused by direct inoculation of ocular surface flora into the vitreous cavity by penetrating instruments, that is, the trocar-cannula system used during transconjunctival MIVS, repeated insertion of instruments through the cannulas, and intravitreal injection of fluid or gas transconjunctivally.

In a prospective study,[16] transconjunctival MIVS with 25G instrumentations was revealed to have a significantly higher incidence of vitreous contamination at the beginning of surgery compared with conventional 20G pars plana vitrectomy. The multivariate model showed the transconjunctival MIVS has a risk of bacterial contamination in the vitreous cavity 11 times higher than that in the 20G vitrectomy group. Most of the bacterial strains isolated from the vitreous cavity are consistent with strains isolated from the conjunctival specimens, suggesting the possibility of direct inoculation of ocular surface flora into the vitreous cavity through transconjunctival instrument insertion and bacterial contamination of the vitreous cavity is highly prevalent in eyes with transconjunctival MIVS.

Other than the above-described risk factors specifically related to MIVS, conjunctival flora and bacterial contamination in patients with chronic conjunctivitis, blepharitis, or dacryocystitis are the well-known risk factors increasing the chance of postoperative endophthalmitis. Systemic backgrounds such as diabetes and immunodeficiency (compromised host) may also contribute to increasing the risk of infection.

Current Incidence Rates

Acute-onset infectious endophthalmitis after MIVS was first reported in 2005, occurring in a patient treated with a 25G system.[17] To date, several studies have reported the incidence of acute-onset endophthalmitis after transconjunctival MIVS compared with that after conventional 20G PPV.[18–24] However, the reported incidence varies across studies (0% to 1.55%) because most reports are based on the experience of individual institutions or groups of surgeons with cluster biases, because differences in preoperative prophylactic regimens and antiseptic techniques or manipulation exist among facilities, and because statistically valid data often are limited by small sample sizes. To minimize the potential confounding bias when studying a rare event in a retrospective fashion, the Japan MIVS Study Group conducted a multicenter survey and a systematic overview of the recent literature. They combined the results of multiple studies to obtain the best available perspective of the recent trends in acute-onset endophthalmitis after MIVS.[25] The Japan MIVS study group performed a clinical database search at 27 institutions involving 43,868 consecutive patients who underwent vitrectomy between 2003 and 2008 to identify all patients with infectious endophthalmitis after vitrectomy. All surgeries were performed with a standard perioperative antiseptic preparation using povidone-iodine and fluoroquinolone antibiotics. The endophthalmitis rates from the multicenter survey were 0.034% (10/29,030) cases after 20G PPV and 0.054% (8/14,838 cases) after 23G or 25G MIVS, with no significant differences ($P = 0.603$) between groups. Although the incidence in 25G cases (6/8,238 cases; 0.073%) was greater than in 23G cases (2/6,600 cases; 0.030%), the difference was not significant. At almost the same time as our study, the Pan-American Collaborative Retina Study Group also conducted a multicenter study of 12 institutions throughout Latin America. The study involved 35,427 patients who underwent vitrectomy between 2005 and 2009.[26] The postvitrectomy incidence rates were similar to ours: 0.021% (4/19,865 cases) for 20G PPV, 0.028% (3/10,845 cases) for 23G MIVS, and 0.021% (1/4,717 cases) for 25G MIVS, with no significant differences among groups.

A systematic review of studies reported the endophthalmitis rates after MIVS versus 20G PPV to assess the pooled incidence of postvitrectomy endophthalmitis. Meta-analyses from a total of 77,956 cases at the baseline showed that the pooled endophthalmitis rates after MIVS (0.08%; 95% confidence interval [CI], 0.030% to 0.164%) and after 20G PPV (0.030%; 95% CI, 0.012% to 0.048%) did not differ significantly ($P = 0.207$, pooled risk difference; 0.0005 [95% CI, 0.0002 to 0.0012]). Reasonably, the incidence rates of MIVS are slightly greater than that after conventional 20G PPV because of the transconjunctival approach and sutureless nature of MIVS.

Pearls on How to Prevent It

♦ Commensal bacterial contamination of the ocular surface and intraocular inoculation of the flora during transconjunctival procedures may be inevitable even with any prophylactic regimens. However, preoperative preparation with povidone-iodine and perioperative antibiotic administration (e.g., topical administration of 0.5% moxifloxacin 5 times daily for 3 days before surgery and 1.25% povidone-iodine just before starting surgery) can decrease the virulent organisms on the ocular surface (Fig. 36-2); this approach may minimize the chance of serious progression of endophthalmitis due to virulent organisms and achieve better visual recovery, even if infectious endophthalmitis unfortunately occurs.

♦ Creating a rigid self-sealing wound and, consequently, tight wound closure, is an essential cornerstone in reducing the incidence rates of postoperative endophthalmitis. For high-risk patients such as high myopic eyes with thin

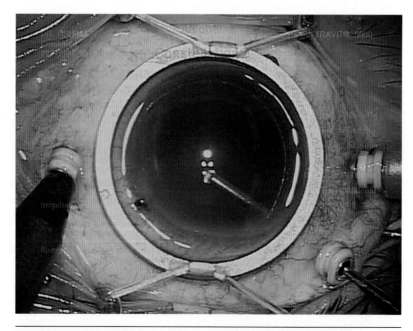

Figure 36-2 Preoperative setting in a case with transconjunctival 25G microincision vitrectomy system. A special surgical drape tinned with povidone-iodine was used to completely cover the lid margin followed by 0.125% topical povidone-iodine drops before starting surgery.

Table 36-1 • Preferable Regimen for Preventing Infectious Endophthalmitis in the MIVS Era

- *Preoperative preparation*
  - Antiseptic preparation with povidone-iodine and topical antibiotics
  - Careful draping to completely cover the lid margin (povidone-iodine-tinned surgical drape would be much preferable)
  - Speculum with drain-aspiration system would be desirable

- *Intraoperative setting and procedures*
  - Displacing the conjunctiva to misaligning the conjunctival and scleral incisions
  - Creating rigid self-sealing wounds (oblique incision)
  - Extensive vitrectomy with sufficient intraocular irrigation
  - Wash out the conjunctival flora with BSS or povidone-iodine during surgery

- *At the end of surgery*
  - Completing wound adaptation
  - Cutting off or removal of the vitreous wick, using a cotton bar or forceps to pick up the vitreous wick and cut it off with a spring scissors
  - Suture placement as appropriate
  - Conjunctival coverage to the sclerotomy
  - Wash out the conjunctival flora once again with povidone-iodine

- *Postoperative attention*
  - Antibiotic administration and patient instruction (no rubbing!)

---

sclera and young patients with soft sclera, addition of sutures should be considered.

◆ Undertaking an extensive vitrectomy with sufficient intraocular irrigation during surgery.

◆ Placing a suture to seal any sclerotomy, if necessary (i.e., if leak is observed at the end of the procedure).

◆ Postoperative topical antibiotics. Moxifloxacin or gatifloxacin, the fourth-generation fluoroquinolones, are equally effective against gram-positive and gram-negative entities. In contrast preventive administration of vancomycin should be handled with utmost delicacy, because vancomycin represents one of the few rescue antibiotics for resistant strains we have available. The recommended perioperative preparation and standardized surgical procedures are listed in Table 36-1.

◆ The author advises irrigating the conjunctiva with povidone-iodine solution at the end of surgery routinely to wash out any flora and pathogen from the ocular surface.

Pearls on How to Solve It

◆ When infectious endophthalmitis after vitrectomy is suspected, sample collection for strain identification immediately followed by urgent treatments should be started as soon as possible. Since there currently are no established therapeutic guidelines specifically for postvitrectomy endophthalmitis, initial treatment with intravitreal antibiotics is a well-known and widely acceptable first line of choice. Even though the Endophthalmitis Vitrectomy Study (EVS) found no significant benefit for systemic antibiotic treatment,[27] this attitude focusing on bacterial endophthalmitis after cataract surgery has been argued over time. Considering that the concentration of intravitreally injected antibiotics can be rapidly decreased in the vitrectomized eye, both routes of administration, intra-vitreal as well as systemic, should be used to obtain a sufficient dose to eradicate the pathogens and prevent the formation of resistant strains. Since infectious endophthalmitis is often accompanied with extensive tissue destruction due to infiltration of leuckocytes and monocytes, additional anti-inflammatory treat-ment with corticosteroids is recommended timely to tackle against the inflam-matory reaction. A sub-Tenon or subconjunctival steroid injection may be a good option to administrate 3 to 5 days following initiation of antibiotics if intraocular inflammation is present.

◆ Pars plana vitrectomy either with 20G or smaller instruments continues to play a role in endophthalmitis therapy. The EVS and subsequent guidelines for the treatment of endophthalmitis recommend PPV only in eyes presenting with initial vision of hand motions or less. This recommendation on acute endophthalmitis after cataract extraction should not be generalized, however, to infection associated with other situations because of the differences in clinical circumstances and pathogenesis. Recent studies reported that com-plete vitrectomy yields far better results after postoperative endophthal-mitis than those published in the EVS in 1995.[27] The availability of better understanding of the pathology, surgical techniques, technical equipment, instruments, illumination, and optic systems, compared to 1990s, may have significantly reduced the risk associated with PPV at that time.[28] Recently, there is a clear trend toward early vitrectomy for extensive vitreous removal and washing out the pathogen with intraocular irrigation of broad-spectrum antibiotics during vitrectomy (balance salt solution (BSS) containing 20 µg/mL of vancomycin and 50 µg/mL of ceftazidime) for the treatment of acute postvitrectomy endophthalmitis.

Since simply washing out bacterial pathogens and inflammatory cytokines from the vitreous cavity are the aim of this procedure, it is unnecessary to aggressively remove the exudates or membranes strongly adherent to the fragile retina. Most of such exudates or membranes will be spontaneously resolved or can be removed subsequently if remained. Removal of the intraocular lens (IOL), if present, is also unnecessary. Instead, posterior capsulotomy with peripheral shaving to remove residual vitreous as much as possible would be advisable. However, care should be taken to avoid iatrogenic retinal breaks and surgically induced retinal detachment, which are the most serious.

✛ Prognosis and Visual Outcomes

Historically, visual outcomes in patients with endophthalmitis after pars plana vitrectomy generally were poor, and vision could decrease to loss of light percep-tion in many cases.[1-7] The clinical condition that was present at the onset and the pathogenicity of the bacteria involved were the primary determinants of the outcome. However, the final visual outcomes in patients with endophthalmitis after MIVS in the recent series were relatively much better compared with those after conventional 20G vitrectomy, despite no significant differences in the base-line characteristics and treatment regimens for postvitrectomy endophthalmitis among the groups.[25]

The visual outcomes of acute-onset postoperative endophthalmitis gen-erally are associated with organism virulence and the spectrum of bacterial sensitivity of the antibiotics used to treat endophthalmitis. All organisms iso-lated in the recent series responded to vancomycin and ceftazidime, which may account for the better visual recovery in our series. Although commensal bacterial contamination of the ocular surface and intraocular inoculation of the flora during surgery may be inevitable with any prophylactic regimens, preoperative preparation with povidone-iodine and perioperative antibiotic administration may decrease the virulent organisms on the ocular surface. Early detection of clinically evident endophthalmitis and timely administration of appropriate antibiotics are important for acute-onset endophthalmitis after surgery and may minimize progression of endophthalmitis and thus achieve better visual recovery.

Retinal detachment complicated with endophthalmitis and retinal detachment after vitrectomy for endophthalmitis are rare but may be the most serious situation that can be encounter. Under these circumstances, the detached retina is often difficult re-attached, especially in those complicated with advanced retinal ischemia. Almost all cases in such challenging situation require long-term tamponade with silicone oil for reattaching the detached retina. In most cases, visual outcomes are generally poor.

REFERENCES

1. May DR, Peyman GA. Endophthalmitis after vitrectomy. *Am J Ophthalmol.* 1976; 81:520–521.
2. Blankenship GW. Endophthalmitis after pars plana vitrectomy. *Am J Ophthalmol.* 1977;84:815–817.
3. Ho PC, Tolentino FI. Bacterial endophthalmitis after closed vitrectomy. *Arch Ophthalmol.* 1984;102:207–210.
4. Aaberg TM Jr, Flynn HW Jr, Schiffman J, et al. Nosocomial acute-onset postoperative endophthalmitis survey. A 10-year review of incidence and outcomes. *Ophthalmology.* 1998;105:1004–1010.
5. Eifrig CWG, Flynn HW Jr, Scott IU, et al. Acute-onset postoperative endophthalmitis: Review of incidence and visual outcome (1995–2001). *Ophthalmic Surg Lasers.* 2002;33:373–378.
6. Cohen SM, Flynn HW Jr, Murray TG, et al. Endophthalmitis after pars plana vitrectomy. The Postvitrectomy Endophthalmitis Study Group. *Ophthalmology.* 1995; 102:705–712.
7. Eifrig CW, Scott IU, Flynn HW Jr, et al. Endophthalmitis after pars plana vitrectomy: Incidence, causative organisms, and visual acuity outcomes. *Am J Ophthalmol.* 2004;138:799–802.
8. Lewis H. Sutureless microincision vitrectomy surgery: Unclear benefit, uncertain safety. *Am J Ophthalmol.* 2007;144:613–615.
9. Taban M, Ventura AA, Sharma S, et al. Dynamic evaluation of sutureless vitrectomy wounds: An optical coherence tomography and histopathology study. *Ophthalmology.* 2008;115:2221–2218.
10. Shimada H, Nakashizuka H, Mori R, et al. 25-Gauge scleral tunnel transconjunctival vitrectomy. *Am J Ophthalmol.* 2006;142:871–873.
11. Shimada H, Nakashizuka H, Hattori T, et al. Conjunctival displacement to the corneal side for oblique-parallel insertion in 25-gauge vitrectomy. *Eur J Ophthalmol.* 2008;18:848–851.
12. Dickey JB, Thompson KD, Jay WM. Anterior chamber aspirate culture after uncomplicated cataract surgery. *Am J Ophthalmol.* 1991;112:278–282.
13. Beigi B, Westlake W, Mangelschots E, et al. Perioperative microbial contamination of anterior chamber aspirates during extracapsular cataract extraction and phacoemulsification. *Br J Ophthalmol.* 1997;81:953–955.
14. Speaker MG, Milch FA, Shah MK, et al. Role of external bacterial flora in the pathogenesis of acute postoperative endophthalmitis. *Ophthalmology.* 1991;98:639–649.
15. De Caro JJ, Ta CN, Ho HK, et al. Bacterial contamination of ocular surface and needles in patients undergoing intravitreal injections. *Retina.* 2008;28:877–883.

16. Tominaga A, Oshima Y, Wakabayashi T, et al. Bacterial contamination of the vitreous cavity associated with transconjunctival 25-gauge microincision vitrectomy surgery. *Ophthalmology.* 2010;117:811–817.

17. Taylor SR, Aylward GW. Endophthalmitis following 25-gauge vitrectomy. *Eye.* 2005; 19:1228–1229.

18. Kunimoto DY, Kaiser RS. Incidence of endophthalmitis after 20- and 25-gauge vitrectomy. *Ophthalmology.* 2007;114:2133–2137.

19. Shaikh S, Ho S, Richmond PP, et al. Untoward outcomes in 25-gauge versus 20-gauge vitreoretinal surgery. *Retina.* 2007;27:1048–1053.

20. Scott IU, Flynn HW Jr, Dev S, et al. Endophthalmitis after 25-gauge and 20-gauge pars plana vitrectomy: Incidence and outcomes. *Retina.* 2008;28:138–142.

21. Shimada H, Nakashizuka H, Hattori T, et al. Incidence of endophthalmitis after 20- and 25-gauge vitrectomy causes and prevention. *Ophthalmology.* 2008;115:2215–2220.

22. Chen JK, Khurana RN, Nguyen QD, et al. The incidence of endophthalmitis following transconjunctival sutureless 25- vs 20-gauge vitrectomy. *Eye (Lond).* 2009;23: 780–784.

23. Hu AY, Bourges JL, Shah SP, et al. Endophthalmitis after pars plana vitrectomy a 20- and 25-gauge comparison. *Ophthalmology.* 2009;116:1360–1365.

24. Parolini B, Romanelli F, Prigione G, et al. Incidence of endophthalmitis in a large series of 23-gauge and 20-gauge transconjunctival pars plana vitrectomy. *Graefes Arch Clin Exp Ophthalmol.* 2009;247:895–898.

25. Oshima Y, Kadonosono K, Yamaji H, et al. (for the Japan Microincision Vitrectomy Surgery Study Group). Multicenter survey with a systematic overview of acute-onset endophthalmitis after transconjunctival microincision vitrectomy surgery. *Am J Ophthalmol.* 2010;150:716–725.

26. Wu L, Berrocal MH, Arévalo JF, et al. Endophthalmitis after pars plana vitrectomy: Results of the Pan American Collaborative Retina Study Group. *Retina.* 2011;31: 673–678.

27. Results of the Endophthalmitis Vitrectomy Study. A randomized trial of immediate vitrectomy and of intravenous antibiotics for the treatment of postoperative bacterial endophthalmitis. Endophthalmitis Vitrectomy Study Group. *Arch Ophthalmol.* 1995;113:1479–1496.

28. Kuhn F, Gini G. Ten years after…are findings of the Endophthalmitis Vitrectomy Study still relevant today? *Graefe's Arch Clin Exp Ophthalmol.* 2005;243:1197–1199.

37

SYMPATHETIC OPHTHALMIA

JOHN V. FORRESTER AND LUCIA KUFFOVÁ

◆ The Complication: Definition

Sympathetic ophthalmia (SO) has been recognized as a specific condition since the time of Hippocrates.[1] SO is defined as a progressive sight-threatening intraocular inflammatory condition (panuveitis), which develops in the second (fellow) eye after penetrating injury. The injured eye is termed the exciting eye, that is, the eye that "excites" inflammation in the second or "sympathizing" eye. Although blunt injury[2] as well as other nonpenetrating injuries such as laser[3] or ruthenium red brachytherapy for ocular melanoma[4] have been linked to SO, the evidence is weak and penetrating injury to the exciting eye is generally regarded as a *sine qua non* for the development of SO. In particular, damage to the uveal tract, especially the ciliary body and the peripheral retina[5] are reckoned to be important clinical correlates of SO risk.

SO was first described in the English language by William MacKenzie[6] **(Fig. 37-1)** who termed the condition sympathetic ophthalmitis. While the etiology of the disease remained obscure, and infectious causes did not seem to explain its restricted presentation to ocular tissue, when the concept of autoimmunity ("horror autoxicus") was formulated, SO was recognized to be a *prima facie* example of an organ-specific autoimmune disease[7] and probably the first autoimmune disease to be described as such.

SO is a rare condition, but its incidence historically has waxed and waned with clusters of cases occurring in association with wars including the recent war in Iraq.[8] Eye injuries from shrapnel were common during the First World War relating to the vast number of casualties.[9] As microsurgical techniques have improved with good

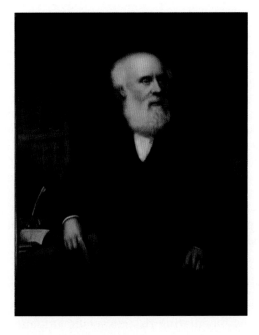

Figure 37-1 Portrait of Sir William Mackenzie, the author of First textbook of Ophthalmology in the English Language who coined the phrase "sympathetic ophthalmia." (With kind permission of Royal College of Physicians and Surgeons of Glasgow.)

wound closure, the incidence of SO due to nonsurgical trauma has decreased. However, with the expansion of vitreoretinal (VR) surgery and the possibility of multiple procedures being performed on one eye in an attempt to achieve anatomical retinal stability in cases of retinal detachment, the risk of SO has emerged as one of the significant complications of VR surgery and the main cause of SO in peacetime.[10]

Risk Factors

The incidence of SO at the present time is around 0.03/100,000 population in developed countries.[11] As indicated above, SO is a consequence of penetrating injury to the exciting eye. Penetration of the globe may be accidental or nonaccidental (surgical). In accidental injuries, the type of injury has a significant bearing on the likelihood of SO. Injuries which involve the uveal tract, particularly the highly vascular ciliary body,[5] have a higher risk of association with SO than, for instance, penetrating injuries which involve only the central cornea. Other wound-related factors include (a) large wounds with prolapse of uveal and retinal tissue, and (b) inadequate surgical closure of the wound with persistent wound leaks and retained uveal tissue in the repaired wound.

Nonaccidental (surgical) penetrating injuries of the eye may also be associated with SO. The commonest association is with VR surgery.[10] In patients where multiple VR procedures were required to achieve retinal stability, the globe may have been penetrated more than 30 times. This, in itself, would constitute an increased risk, but other factors such as postoperative hypotony, leaking sclerotomies, and persistent retinal detachment with proliferative vitreoretinopthy (PVR) all increase the risk of SO.[12] The recent trend to sutureless 23G and 25G vitrectomy with the associated complication of postoperative hypotony[13] has heightened the risk of SO, where it has been reported even after a single vitrectomy procedure.[14]

Interestingly intraocular infection (endophthalmitis) is not considered to be associated with increased risk of SO.[5,15,16] The perceived risk of endophthalmitis in cases of retained intraocular foreign body (IOFB) may be less than previously thought,[15] and delay in surgery under more controlled conditions may reduce the risk of SO.

Systemic factors may rarely increase the risk of SO. The genetic allotypes HLA-DRB1*04 and DQA1*03 are linked to increased risk of SO as are other single nucleotide polymorphisms (SNPs) such as the IL10-1082 SNP and the glucocorticoid (GCC) promoter haplotype GCC IL10-1082G, -819C, -592C.[17] Speculatively this type of genotype analysis may predict responsiveness to therapy.[18] Interestingly, HLA DR 0405 is also a genetic susceptibility factor for Vogt–Koyanagi–Harada (VKH) disease[19,20] in which autoimmunity to melanin or melanin-related proteins such as Trp2 is thought to be causative.[21,22]

SO is considered an autoimmune condition in part because of immunologic ignorance[23] in which "sequestered" ocular auto-antigens escape from immunologic privilege and activate the immune system when the eye is penetrated (see next section). Accordingly a belief has emerged that if the potentially exciting eye has been severely injured, with little prospect of visual recovery, the immune system will not be activated provided that the injured eye is enucleated within 1 week of injury, and the risk of SO can be minimized. A corollary of this is that once SO has developed which usually occurs within 1 to 3 months after injury, there is little value in removing the exciting eye at this stage. The immunologic basis for this viewpoint, however, may not be robust (see next section).

Pathogenesis: How and When Does It Occur

Experimental models of autoimmune disease are extremely valuable and are commonly induced by inoculating tissue-specific autoantigen subcutaneously in

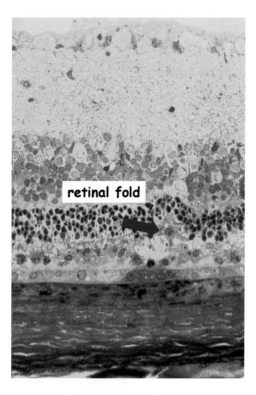

retinal fold

Figure 37-2 Experimental autoimmune uveo-retinitis (EAU) induced in the guinea pig with retinal S antigen in complete Freund's adjuvant.

an oily emulsion, containing an adjuvant with homogenized mycobacterial components (complete Freunds adjuvant, CFA).[24] This directly activates the innate immune system and permits presentation of the autoantigen to antigen-specific T cells. These cells rapidly expand in the draining lymph node and home to the tissues where, on contact with antigen, they are further activated and induce tissue destruction.[25]

As indicated above, because of the failure to identify an infectious etiology, SO is considered the prototypic, quintessential organ-specific autoimmune disease. Early experimental studies sought the source of the autoantigen in uveal tissue but it was not until Wacker and Lipton[26] used retinal tissue instead of uveal tissue to sensitize animals that a reliable model of SO-like disease could be established [experimental autoimmune uveoretinitis, EAU[27]] (Figs. 37-2 and 37-3). Since then the major source of ocular autoantigen has been located to the retina, particularly the photoreceptor cell. However, most of these antigens have been identified as possible inducers of posterior uveitis generally, while SO has more recently been linked to antigens in choroidal melanocytes[28] as has VKH disease (see above).[29]

Whatever the source of the antigen, the clinical manifestations of SO overlap extensively with other forms of posterior uveitis such as multifocal choroiditis. SO is a variant of "granulomatous" uveitis in which the Dalen-Fuchs (DF) nodule is considered a paradigmatic sign (Fig. 37-4), but clinically and pathologically DF nodules resemble many similar lesions in other "white dot" syndromes[30] (Fig. 37-5).

EAU induced by retinal or uveal antigens is mainly a CD4 T-cell-mediated disease, mediated by IFNγ and IL17 (Th1/Th17) in which much of the tissue damage is caused by activated M1 macrophages.[31-33] SO histopathologically has also been shown to be Th1/Th17- and M1 macrophage-mediated[34] (Fig. 37-6). Hypersensitivity to uveoretinal antigens has been shown in some cases of SO, but there is no definitive antigen-specific diagnostic test and diagnosis of the disease remains clinical (see below).

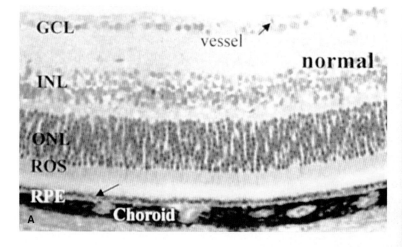

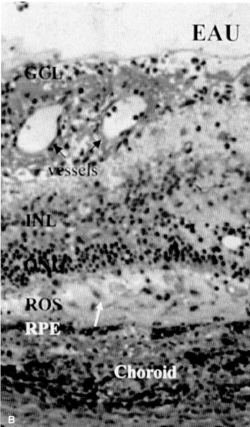

Figure 37-3 Severe EAU in the B10R11 mouse with retina vasculitis and extensive retinal swelling and damage. **A:** Normal retina. **B:** EAU. GCL, ganglion cell layer; INL, inner nuclear layer; ONL, outer nuclear layer; ROS, rod outer segments; RPE, retinal pigment epithelium.

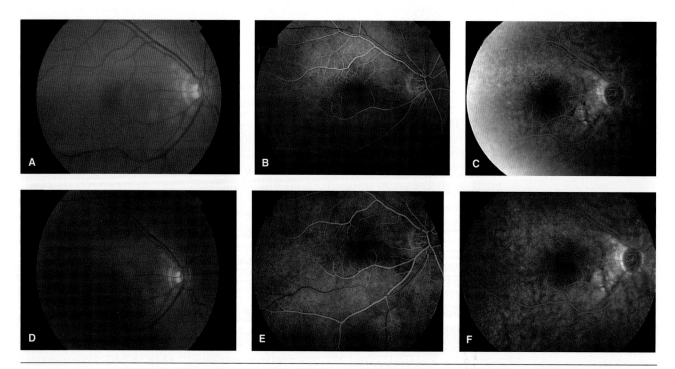

Figure 37-4 Case of SO with early lesions occurring close to the optic nerve in the region of the papillomacular bundle. **A–C:** Before therapy; **D–E:** on immunosuppression. **A, D:** Fundus photographs; **B, E:** early phase fluorescein angiograms. **C, F:** Late phase fluorescein angiograms.

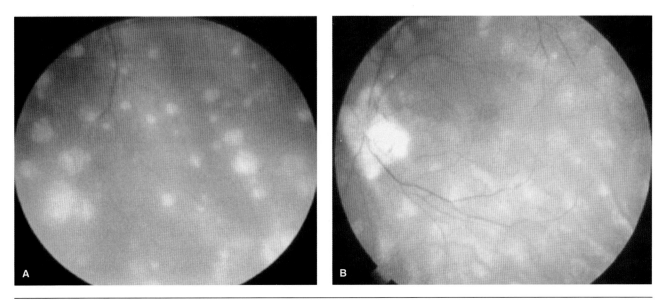

Figure 37-5 Comparison of two "white dot syndromes." **A:** Sympathetic ophthalmia. **B:** Birdshot chorioretinopathy.

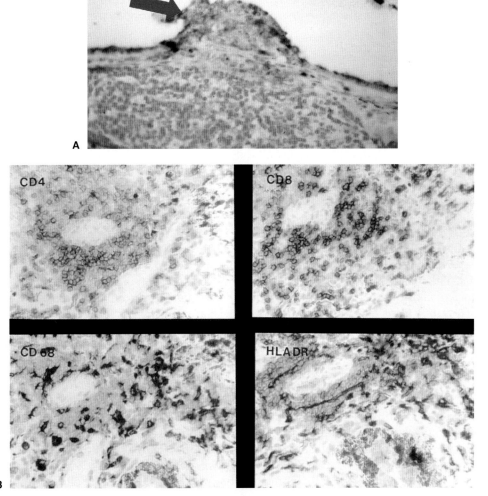

Figure 37-6 A: Histologic section of inciting eye from a case of SO. (Courtesy of Professor WR Lee.) The microgranuloma at the chorioretinal interface is termed a Dalen-Fuchs' nodule (*arrow*). Iron staining macrophages in the granuloma are stained blue. **B:** Montage of immunohistochemistry of choroidal granuloma in the case of SO, stained for CD4+ and CD8+ T cells, CD68+ macrophages, and MHC Class II antigen presenting dendritic cells.

Pearls on How to Prevent It

SO assumes that penetration of the globe has occurred or is planned (surgery). Prevention of SO, or at least minimizing the risk of SO, can be optimized by considering the following.

Accidental Injury

◆ Careful clinical evaluation of the wound (size, site, nature, retained IOFB, etc.).

◆ Timely (high priority) primary surgical closure of the wound without leaks and removal/abscission of wound-retained uveal tissue.

◆ Removal of the eye if severely and irretrievably wounded. Eyes with no perception of light on first or second day examination may still recover some vision.[35,36] Clinical assessment of anatomical integrity by assessing intraocular pressure (IOP), by ultrasound, or other imaging techniques may help to identify vitreous and suprachoroidal hemorrhage, retinal detachment, etc. CT scanning for IOFB is also important.

◆ From an immunologic viewpoint, sensitization of T cells to ocular antigens after release from the injured globe occurs very fast (within hours) and probably reaches its first peak about 3 to 4 days after injury. Further rounds of antigen exposure over weeks and months continue to activate memory T cells to a pathogenic state. Therefore, if there is any question of trying to retain the eye, high doses of systemic steroids to minimize sensitization of T cells would be recommended. Although topical steroids will not prevent SO, they will reduce the level of inflammation in the injured eye and subsequently reduce overall innate immune responses.

Nonaccidental (Surgical) Injury

◆ Minimizing the number of surgical procedures, especially VR procedures.

◆ Ensuring retinal stability (anatomical re-attachment).

◆ Aggressive control of associated intraocular inflammation, using systemic immunosuppression if required (see below).

◆ Careful patient counselling *regarding* risks of SO.

 Pearls on How to Solve It

◆ If detected early, SO can be managed well. The most important factor is awareness of the possibility of SO and recognition of early signs. In particular, photophobia especially in children is an important symptom and so a careful history is essential. The most common presenting symptom is slight blurring in vision. The presence of chorioretinal Dalen-Fuchs nodules is not a prerequisite for the diagnosis of SO. Subtle signs of anterior uveitis (Grade 1 flare, cells)[37] are sufficient to initiate systemic treatment and regular case review with fundoscopy, fluorescein angiography[38] **(Fig. 37-4)**, optical coherence tomography (OCT),[39] and autofluorescence to detect early macular or peripheral changes of posterior uveitis.

◆ Treatment of SO with long-term control of inflammation has greatly improved with the introduction of immunosuppressive drugs. Management is as for any form of sight-threatening posterior intraocular inflammation.[40] Control of the initial stages of inflammation in the sympathizing eye is rapidly achieved with the use of intravenous pulse methylprednisolone (1.0G daily for 3 days) followed by high dose oral steroids (1.0 mg/kg) tapering rapidly. Simultaneous renal, hematologic, and biochemical screening with drug counselling should also be performed and assuming normal health for the patient, introduction of an appropriate second-line immunosuppressant may be required. Such drugs include cyclosporine, tacrolimus, mycophenolate mofetil, and azathioprine.[41]

◆ Occasionally refractory cases occur, which may respond to biologics (anti-TNFα)[42] and even IFNα.[43]

◆ If inflammatory subretinal neovascularization develops, intravitreal anti-VEGF therapy may be considered.[44]

◆ A constant question in managing SO is whether or not to remove the exciting/injured eye if this has been retained beyond 1 week (see above). In particular, if the injured, exciting eye has some degree of visual function that the patient wishes to retain this can present a management dilemma. Immunologically, antigen drains within minutes to hours from an eye in which the blood ocular barrier has been broken and initial activation of T cells takes place within 2 to 3 days.[45,46] This initial response subsides within 3 to 4 weeks with induction of antigen-specific memory cells. Such cells are not activated unless re-exposed to further antigen. Since the peak onset of SO occurs between 2 and 3 months after injury,[8] it can be concluded that reactivation of memory T cells is likely to be derived from persistent systemic leakage of antigen from the injured eye into the reticular-endothelial (lymphovascular) system. Accordingly, when SO develops, there is a strong case for removing the exciting eye even many weeks to months after the original injury since this will remove a source of antigen drainage to the lymph nodes and spleen which continues to activate memory T cells. Enucleation rather than evisceration also reduces the risk of SO.[47]

◆ Expected Outcomes: What Is the Worst-case Scenario

Without active intervention (immunosuppressive treatment) and removal of the source of antigen (the exciting eye), the worst-case scenarios are some of continued sight threatening inflammation and progressive blindness. With carefully controlled but early and robust management, vision can be preserved and in time (months to years) patients with SO can become drug-free.

REFERENCES

1. Albert DM, Diaz-Rohena R. A historical review of sympathetic ophthalmia and its epidemiology. *Surv Ophthalmol.* 1989;34:1–14.
2. Lin X, Zhong X. A clinical analysis of 30 cases of sympathetic ophthalmia. *Yan Ke Xue Bao.* 1996;12:191–192.
3. Su DH, Chee SP. Sympathetic ophthalmia in Singapore: New trends in an old disease. *Graefes Arch Clin Exp Ophthalmol.* 2006;244:243–247.
4. Ahmad N, Soong TK, Salvi S, et al. Sympathetic ophthalmia after ruthenium plaque brachytherapy. *Br J Ophthalmol.* 2007;91:399–401.
5. Punnonen E. Pathological findings in eyes enucleated because of perforating injury. *Acta Ophthalmol (Copenh).* 1990;68:265–269.
6. Mackenzie W. *A Practical Treatise on the Diseases of the Eye.* London: Longman, Rees, Orme, Brown & Green, 1830.
7. Faure JP. Autoimmunity and the retina. *Curr Top Eye Res.* 1980;2:215–302.
8. Galor A, Davis JL, Flynn HW Jr, et al. Sympathetic ophthalmia: incidence of ocular complications and vision loss in the sympathizing eye. *Am J Ophthalmol.* 2009;148: 704–710.e2.
9. Wong TY, Seet MB, Ang CL: Eye injuries in twentieth century warfare: A historical perspective. *Surv Ophthalmol.* 1997;41:433–459.

10. Kilmartin DJ, Dick AD, Forrester JV. Sympathetic ophthalmia risk following vitrectomy: Should we counsel patients? *Br J Ophthalmol.* 2000;84:448–449.

11. Kilmartin DJ, Dick AD, Forrester JV. Prospective surveillance of sympathetic ophthalmia in the UK and Republic of Ireland. *Br J Ophthalmol.* 2000;84:259–263.

12. Grigoropoulos VG, Benson S, Bunce C, et al. Functional outcome and prognostic factors in 304 eyes managed by retinectomy. *Graefes Arch Clin Exp Ophthalmol.* 2007;245:641–649.

13. Spirn MJ. Comparison of 25, 23 and 20-gauge vitrectomy. *Curr Opin Ophthalmol.* 2009;20:195–199.

14. Haruta M, Mukuno H, Nishijima K, et al. Sympathetic ophthalmia after 23-gauge transconjunctival sutureless vitrectomy. *Clin Ophthalmol.* 2010;4:1347–1349.

15. Colyer MH, Weber ED, Weichel ED, et al. Delayed intraocular foreign body removal without endophthalmitis during Operations Iraqi Freedom and Enduring Freedom. *Ophthalmology.* 2007;114:1439–1447.

16. O'Donnell BA, Kersten R, McNab A, et al. Enucleation versus evisceration. *Clin Experiment Ophthalmol.* 2005;33:5–9.

17. Atan D, Turner SJ, Kilmartin DJ, et al. Cytokine gene polymorphism in sympathetic ophthalmia. *Invest Ophthalmol Vis Sci.* 2005;46:4245–4250.

18. Glover N, Ah-Chan JJ, Frith P, et al. Unremitting sympathetic ophthalmia associated with homozygous interleukin-10-1082A single nucleotide polymorphism. *Br J Ophthalmol.* 2008;92:155–156.

19. Davis JL, Mittal KK, Freidlin V, et al. HLA associations and ancestry in Vogt-Koyanagi-Harada disease and sympathetic ophthalmia. *Ophthalmology.* 1990;97:1137–1142.

20. Du L, Kijlstra A, Yang P. Immune response genes in uveitis. *Ocul Immunol Inflamm.* 2009;17:249–256.

21. Damico FM, Cunha-Neto E, Goldberg AC, et al. T-cell recognition and cytokine profile induced by melanocyte epitopes in patients with HLA-DRB1*0405-positive and -negative Vogt-Koyanagi-Harada uveitis. *Invest Ophthalmol Vis Sci.* 2005;46:2465–2471.

22. Yamaki K, Kondo I, Nakamura H, et al. Ocular and extraocular inflammation induced by immunization of tyrosinase related protein 1 and 2 in Lewis rats. *Exp Eye Res.* 2000;71:361–369.

23. Forrester JV, Xu H, Lambe T, et al. Immune privilege or privileged immunity? *Mucosal Immunol.* 2008;1:372–381.

24. Caspi RR. Understanding autoimmune uveitis through animal models. The Friedenwald Lecture. *Invest Ophthalmol Vis Sci.* 2011;52:1872–1879.

25. Forrester JV. Intermediate and posterior uveitis. *Chem Immunol Allergy.* 2007;92:228–243

26. Wacker WB, Lipton MM: Experimental allergic uveitis: Homologous retina as uveitogenic antigen. *Nature.* 1965;206:253–254.

27. Wacker WB, Donoso LA, Kalsow CM, et al. Experimental allergic uveitis. Isolation, characterization, and localization of a soluble uveitopathogenic antigen from bovine retina. *J Immunol.* 1977;119:1949–1958.

28. Damico FM, Kiss S, Young LH: Sympathetic ophthalmia. *Semin Ophthalmol.* 2005;20:191–197.

29. Damico FM, Kiss S, Young LH: Vogt–Koyanagi–Harada disease. *Semin Ophthalmol.* 2005;20:183–190.

30. Ben Ezra D, Forrester JV: Fundal white dots: The spectrum of a similar pathological process. *Br J Ophthalmol.* 1995;79:856–860.

31. Oh HM, Yu CR, Lee Y, et al. Autoreactive memory CD4+ T lymphocytes that mediate chronic uveitis reside in the bone marrow through STAT3-dependent mechanisms. *J Immunol.* 2011;187:3338–3346.

32. Wang L, Yu CR, Kim HP, et al. Key role for IL-21 in experimental autoimmune uveitis. *Proc Natl Acad Sci U S A.* 2011;108:9542–9547.

33. Banerjee S, Savant V, Scott RA, et al. Multiplex bead analysis of vitreous humor of patients with vitreoretinal disorders. *Invest Ophthalmol Vis Sci.* 2007;48:2203–2207.

34. Furusato E, Shen D, Cao X, et al. Inflammatory cytokine and chemokine expression in sympathetic ophthalmia: A pilot study. *Histol Histopathol*. 2011;26:1145–1151.

35. Salehi-Had H, Andreoli CM, Andreoli MT, et al. Visual outcomes of vitreoretinal surgery in eyes with severe open-globe injury presenting with no-light-perception vision. *Graefes Arch Clin Exp Ophthalmol*. 2009;247:477–483.

36. Yeung L, Chen TL, Kuo YH, et al Severe vitreous hemorrhage associated with closed-globe injury. *Graefes Arch Clin Exp Ophthalmol*. 2006;244:52–57.

37. Jabs DA, Nussenblatt RB, Rosenbaum JT. Standardization of uveitis nomenclature for reporting clinical data. Results of the First International Workshop. *Am J Ophthalmol*. 2005;140:509–516.

38. Sharp DC, Bell RA, Patterson E, et al. Sympathetic ophthalmia. Histopathologic and fluorescein angiographic correlation. *Arch Ophthalmol*. 1984;102:232–235.

39. Gupta V, Gupta A, Dogra MR, et al. Reversible retinal changes in the acute stage of sympathetic ophthalmia seen on spectral domain optical coherence tomography. *Int Ophthalmol*. 2011;31:105–110.

40. Dick AD. Immune mechanisms of uveitis: Insights into disease pathogenesis and treatment. *Int Ophthalmol Clin*. 2000;40:1–18.

41. Imrie FR, Dick AD. Nonsteroidal drugs for the treatment of noninfectious posterior and intermediate uveitis. *Curr Opin Ophthalmol*. 2007;18:212–219.

42. Gupta SR, Phan IT, Suhler EB. Successful treatment of refractory sympathetic ophthalmia in a child with infliximab. *Arch Ophthalmol*. 2011;129:250–252.

43. Plskova J, Greiner K, Forrester JV. Interferon-alpha as an effective treatment for noninfectious posterior uveitis and panuveitis. *Am J Ophthalmol*. 2007;144:55–61.

44. Julian K, Terrada C, Fardeau C, et al. Intravitreal bevacizumab as first local treatment for uveitis-related choroidal neovascularization: Long-term results. *Acta Ophthalmol*. 2011;89:179–184.

45. Kuffova L, Netukova M, Duncan L, et al. Cross presentation of antigen on MHC class II via the draining lymph node after corneal transplantation in mice. *J Immunol*. 2008;180:1353–1361.

46. Kuffova L, Lumsden L, Vesela V, et al. Kinetics of leukocyte and myeloid cell traffic in the murine corneal allograft response. *Transplantation*. 2001;72:1292–1298.

47. Birnbaum AD, Tessler HH, Goldstein DA. Sympathetic ophthalmia in Operation Iraqi Freedom. *Am J Ophthalmol*. 2010;150:758–759.

SECTION II

PREVENTING SURGICAL COMPLICATIONS BY THE USE OF NON-TECHNICAL SURGICAL SKILLS

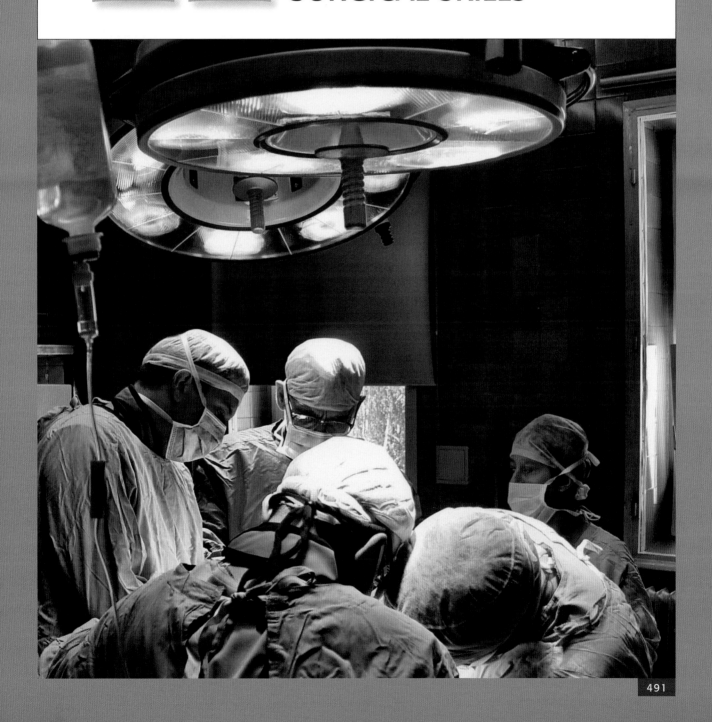

REDUCING COMPLICATIONS THROUGH NONTECHNICAL SURGICAL SKILLS

RHONA FLIN AND AUGUSTO AZUARA-BLANCO

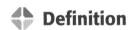 **Definition**

Although vitreoretinal surgery may be the most skilful and sophisticated surgical specialty in ophthalmology, the surgical profession increasingly recognizes that across specialties, there is more to good practice than having extensive clinical knowledge, as well as high level technical and surgical skills. Aspects of performance such as decision making, leadership, and team working are essential for optimal surgical outcomes.

Studies into medical error show that it is frequently these "behavioral" aspects of performance that are pathogenic causal factors rather than individuals not having the necessary technical expertise.[1,2] Communication was found to be a causal factor in 43% of errors made in surgery.[3] In another study, cognitive and diagnostic errors in the operating room contributed to 27% of claims against a health care organization.[4] Among surgical specialties, ophthalmology occupied the first place in surgical errors due to wrong intraocular lens implantation.[5] The second most common error in ophthalmic surgery is administering local anesthetic to the wrong eye. Errors including operating in the wrong site/or wrong patient/procedure are rare but unacceptable for the public.[5,6] Therefore, technical skills are not, of themselves, sufficient to preserve patient safety and, attention is drawn to ophthalmic surgeons' nontechnical skills. This term comes from European aviation where nontechnical skills are defined as "the cognitive and social skills that complement technical skills to achieve safe and efficient operations".[7]

Risk Factors

Eye surgery, and specifically vitreoretinal surgery, has some characteristics that may increase the risk for complications, including:

1. High volume and high turnover ophthalmic surgery increase the potential for errors, such as choosing a wrong IOL, or using a different tamponade or gas in vitreoretinal surgery, or advising an erroneous postoperative head position or postoperative topical medication. Injecting anti-VEGF in a wrong eye in elderly patients with bilateral age-related macular degeneration is likely to happen if there are no solid systems in place (e.g., confirm and mark the eye before treatment).[8,9]

2. Vitreoretinal surgery is now commonly performed under local anesthesia and with the patient awake. Special attention to verbal communication among team members in the operative environment is needed. For example, if a complication occurs, or if a maneuver by a trainee needs to be corrected, interaction between the surgeons and other members of the team need to take into account that the patient is aware of the conversations. This can also present particular challenges for training.

493

3. This type of surgery is heavily reliant on highly specialized equipment (e.g., vitrectomy, phacoemulsification, and laser) and microscopic procedures. The surgical team needs to have a clear understanding of what needs to be calibrated and checked, when, and what to do when the equipment fails.

Nontechnical Skills

If we turn to other complex, risky work settings (e.g., aviation, oil and gas exploration, and nuclear power), analyses of their accidents and complications reveal that the underlying causes often originate from failings that are not due to deficiencies in technical skills but in the "nontechnical" skills, described above. When the aviation industry recognized this as one source of their safety problems, they asked teams of psychologists and experienced pilots to identify the key nontechnical skills to maintain safe operations and to devise methods for training and assessment. The resulting training is known as crew resource management (CRM) and is mandated by the aviation regulators for flight crew, along with regular assessment of their CRM skills.[7]

Traditionally, medical education has focussed on developing clinical expertise and technical skills. Aspects of performance that relate to nontechnical skills, such as decision making, leadership, and team working, which provide a vital underpinning for effective performance, have only recently been addressed explicitly in surgery and anesthesia. Surgeons' nontechnical skills relate to behaviors necessary for safe and effective practice in a clinical context which are not directly related to the use of medical expertise, drugs, or equipment.[10] Evidence from observations of performance in theater clearly indicates that nontechnical skills constitute a critical component of competence and deficiencies can lead to complications and poor outcomes for patients.[11] Conversely, some surgeons can be seen to demonstrate their nontechnical skills as an integral part of their work.[12] Such areas of competence should receive explicit attention during surgical training to ensure individuals are aware of what constitutes good practice and have the requisite skills to deliver this.

In order to develop training and assessment programs related to nontechnical aspects of surgeons' task performance, a basic taxonomy of nontechnical skills for the specified task set was required. The design process was based on the methods used previously to produce the nontechnical skill sets and associated behavioral assessment tools for airline pilots and anesthetists.[13] With sponsorship from National Education for Scotland and the Royal College of Surgeons Edinburgh, a nontechnical skills taxonomy for surgeons (NOTSS) was developed by a team of Scottish surgeons working with industrial psychologists and an anesthetist.[10] The system developers used several methods of task analysis (literature review, observations, questionnaire survey, and interviews) to identify the key nontechnical skills for the intraoperative phase of surgery. This skill set was refined and examples of good and poor behaviors produced for each element by working with panels of with subject matter experts (consultant surgeons) to devise a prototype taxonomy and a behavioral rating scale. This was evaluated in trials with groups of consultant surgeons who rated observed behavior of surgeons portrayed in standardized video scenarios of operations using the NOTSS rating tool.[10] Preliminary usability testing of the NOTSS rating system indicated that consultant surgeons could use this instrument with acceptable accuracy and reliability. It allows consultant (attending) surgeons to give feedback to colleagues and trainees based on structured observations of nontechnical aspects of performance during intraoperative surgery.[14]

The main categories and elements of the NOTSS system[15] are shown in Tables 38-1 through 38-4. Each skill category is now considered in turn with specific reference to the minimization of complications of vitreoretinal surgery.

Table 38-1 • Elements of Situation Awareness in NOTSS	
Category	**Elements**
Situation awareness	Gathering information
	Interpreting information
	Anticipating future states

Situation Awareness

The term situation awareness comes originally from the military in relation to knowing where the enemy was located. Most of the research on situation awareness has been developed in aviation settings, both military and commercial, but the term is now being widely adopted in other occupations, including surgery.[16]

The definition of situation awareness in NOTSS is "developing and maintaining a dynamic awareness of the situation in theatre based on assembling data from the environment (patient, team, time, displays, equipment); understanding what they mean, and thinking ahead about what may happen."[15] Situation awareness is essentially what psychologists call perception or attention. It is a continuous monitoring of the environment, noticing what is going on, and detecting any changes in the environment. The main components of situation awareness in NOTSS are shown in Table 38-1.

Situation awareness is an essential cognitive process used throughout a surgical procedure for building and maintaining awareness of the operative site, patient status, and ongoing events in theater. In vitreoretinal procedures, surgeons need particularly high situation awareness, especially when reviewing preoperative patient notes to ensure the team and equipment are ready for the surgical procedure to be performed (e.g., choosing between extrascleral or vitrectomy for retinal detachment repair, identifying the retinal tear position, preselecting the intraocular lens, and type of tamponade), optimizing operating conditions (microscope and viewing tools), and having contingency plans ("plan B"). During a procedure, skills of anticipation are critical when there are expected or unexpected complications.

The term "situation assessment" describes the first stage of decision making in operational settings when a specific, focussed diagnosis of the current situation is made in order to take action. This is based on the ongoing situation awareness (i.e., monitoring) and the need for a new situation assessment is usually triggered by a significant change in the task environment, for example, loss of fluid and collapse of the eye, puncture of the sclera during a buckle procedure, and appearance of iatrogenic retinal tear.

Decision Making

Decision making is defined in NOTSS as "skills for diagnosing the situation and reaching a judgment in order to choose an appropriate course of action."[15] In most dynamic tasks, there is a continuous cycle of monitoring and re-evaluating the work environment, then taking appropriate action. Decision making does not just involve one method—different decision-making techniques may be used at different times, depending on circumstances. Conditions for decision making can vary in relation to time pressure, task demands, feasibility of options, and what level of constraint, support, and resource exists for the decision maker. Four main components of decision making in NOTSS are shown in Table 38-2.

Table 38-2 • Elements of Decision Making in NOTSS

Category	Elements
Decision making	Situation assessment/defining problem
	Generating and considering one or more response options
	Selecting and implementing an option
	Outcome review

There is surprisingly little research into surgeons' intraoperative decision making[17] but recent studies[18,19] show that general surgeons use a mixture of these techniques.

In vitreoretinal procedures, surgeons require high-level decision skills because of the relatively high variability in surgical techniques and intraoperative outcomes. In particular the vitreoretinal surgeon must be able to consider alternative options during the operation, for example, if the view is getting cloudy because the surgery is taking longer than expected and the lens becomes hazy, should he/she remove the lens or should he/she continue the surgery with no lens removal despite the not so clear view of the retina?; if an inferior retinal tear is found while performing vitrectomy in an eye with a subtotal retinal detachment, should he/she continue with vitrectomy alone or add an inferior buckle? Should he/she use a tamponade that sinks, rather than one that floats? They must also be able to take rapid action and know what to do when the situation demands an immediate response, for example, if the eye collapses during a vitrectomy, the surgeon should quickly make sure that the there is no compression or kinking of the tubing, that the infusion line is inside the vitreous cavity, that there is remaining fluid in the bag, and instruct to raise the bag urgently or increase the infusion pressure if the pressure is being controlled though the vitrectomy machine.

Communication and Teamwork

The definition of communication and teamwork in NOTSS is "skills for working in a team context to ensure that the team has an acceptable shared picture of the situation and can complete tasks effectively" (Table 38-3).[15]

As mentioned above, communication failures are a known cause of adverse events in all teamwork domains and surgery is no exception as recent studies of theater teams demonstrate.[11] Intraoperative communication may be compromised in cases undergoing vitreoretinal surgeries under local anesthetic, especially if there is an unexpected complication or adverse event. Using inappropriate or confusing code words may lead to additional problems using inappropriate code words of poor behavior during vitreoretinal surgery would include starting the operation without ensuring the equipment is ready, or failing to communicate operative plans or concerns to the team.

Table 38-3 • Elements of Communication and Teamwork in NOTSS

Category	Elements
Communication and teamwork	Exchanging information
	Establishing a shared understanding
	Co-ordinating team activities

Table 38-4 • Elements of Leadership in NOTSS	
Category	**Elements**
Leadership	Setting and maintaining standards
	Supporting others
	Coping with pressure

Leadership

Leadership is defined in NOTSS as "leading the team and providing direction, demonstrating high standards of clinical practice and care, and being considerate about the needs of individual team members."[15] There is surprisingly little evidence on the leadership behaviors shown by surgeons while operating or how they influence team and patients outcomes, with the exception of some recent psychological research (Table 38-4).[20]

Good leadership for a vitreoretinal surgeon includes remaining calm (or apparently calm) and making appropriate decisions under pressure, requiring that all team members observe standards (e.g., sterile field), providing constructive criticism to team members, and establishing rapport with team members.

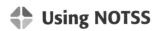 **Using NOTSS**

NOTSS can be used as a syllabus for training, a rating system for observation and feedback, self-assessment, and as a framework for incident analysis at morbidity and mortality meetings or in incident investigation. Some simple tips relating to ophthalmic surgeons' nontechnical skills are given in Table 38-5.

The NOTSS framework is likely to be introduced as part of performance-based assessment for UK surgeons. The Royal Australasian College of Surgeons incorporated NOTSS into their new professional standards in 2009[21] and current projects in Japan, Denmark, and the Netherlands are customizing NOTSS for surgeons in these

Table 38-5 • Pearls for Using Nontechnical Skills in Surgery
• Be considerate to your team (do not shout which distracts and reduces situation awareness)
• Before starting the surgery use a standard safety check list and check the relevant equipment and materials are ready for the case (e.g., type of gas, oil, intraocular lens)
• Communicate your concerns and potential complications, anticipate possible "expected" complications
• Check shared team awareness, e.g., changing circumstances, complication developing, anticipating for a change of plan
• Keep calm (or apparently calm), maintain efficient communication while under pressure
• Provide feedback to the team after the case on what has been done well and not well
• In cases under local anesthetic, have an agreed communication strategy both with the patient and with the team, including how to manage unexpected events

countries, as well as interest noted by the American Board of Surgeons. However, eye surgeons did not participate in the development of NOTSS, nor is there a version of NOTSS which is suited to the particular working conditions of ophthalmic surgery, e.g., conscious patients.[22] The Royal College of Ophthalmologists does not recommend any specific training in nontechnical skills to date, although provides valuable advice on patient safety.[23]

✥ Acknowledgments

Health Services Research Unit is funded by the Chief Scientist Office of the Scottish Government Health Directorates (AAB). The Scottish Patient Safety Research Network is now funding a study of Ophthalmic NOTSS at the University of Aberdeen.

REFERENCES

1. Catchpole K, Panesar SS, Russell J, et al. National Patient Safety Agency 2009, National Reporting and Learning Service, Surgical safety can be improved through better understanding of incidents; Reference 1116. Available online at http://www.nrls.npsa.nhs.uk/resources/type/data-reports/?entryid45=63054. Last accessed on 24th July 2010.
2. de Leval MR, Carthey J, Wright DJ, et al. Human factors and cardiac surgery: A multicenter study. *J Thorac Cardiovasc Surg.* 2000;119:661–672.
3. Gwande AA, Zinner MJ, Studdert DM, et al. Analysis of errors reported by surgeons at three teaching hospitals. *Surgery.* 2003;133:614–621.
4. Wilson J. A practical guide to risk management in surgery: Developing and planning. *Health Care Risk Resources International—Royal College of Surgeons Symposium Edinburgh,* 1999.
5. Simon JW, Ngo Y, Khan S, et al. Surgical confusions in ophthalmology. *Arch Ophthalmol.* 2007;125:1515–1522.
6. White M, Gupta M, Utman S, et al. Importance of site marking in ophthalmic surgery. *The Surgeon.* 2009;7(2):82–85.
7. Flin R, O'Connor P, Crichton M. *Safety at the Sharp End: A Guide to Non-Technical Skills.* Farnham: Ashgate, 2008.
8. Kelly SP, Barua A. A review of safety incidents in England and Wales for vascular endothelial growth factor inhibitor medications. *Eye.* 2011;25:710–716.
9. Kelly SP, Jalil A. Wrong intraocular lens implant; learning from reported patient safety incidents. *Eye.* 2011;25:730–734.
10. Yule S, Flin R, Maran N, et al. Surgeons'non-technical skills in the operating room: Reliability testing of the NOTSS behavior rating system. *World J Surg.* 2008;32:548–556.
11. Mitchell L, Flin R, eds. *Safer Surgery. Analysing Behaviour in the Operating Theatre.* Farnham: Ashgate, 2009.
12. Edmondson A. Speaking up in the operating room: How team leaders promote learning in interdisciplinary action teams. *J. Management Studies.* 2003;40:1419–1452.
13. Flin R, Patey R, Glavin R, et al. Anaesthetists' Non-Technical skills (ANTS). *Br J Anaesth.* 2010;105:38–44.
14. Yule S, Flin R, Rowley D et al. Debriefing Surgeons on Non-technical Skills (NOTSS). *Cognition Technol Work.* 2008;10:265–274.
15. Flin R, Yule S, Paterson-Brown S, et al. *The Non-Technical Skills for Surgeons (NOTSS) System Handbook v 1.2.* University of Aberdeen. Available on www.abdn.ac.uk/iprc/notss, 2006.
16. Way LW, Stewart L, Gantert W, et al. Causes and prevention of laparoscopic bile duct injuries. *Ann Surg.* 2003;237:460–469.

17. Flin R, Youngson G, Yule S. How do surgeons make intraoperative decisions. *Qual Saf Health Care.* 2007;16:235–239.

18. Pauley K, Flin R, Yule S, et al. Surgeons' intra-operative decision making and risk management. *Am J Surg.* 2011;202:375–381.

19. Moulton C, Regehr G, Lingard L, et al. Slowing down when you should: Initiators and influences of the transition from the routine to the effortful. *J Gastrointest Surg.* 2010;14(6):1019–1026.

20. Henrickson Parker SE, Yule S, Flin R, et al. Towards a model of surgeons' leadership in the operating room. *BMJ Qual Saf.* 2011;20:570–579.

21. Dickinson I, Watters D, Graham I, et al. Guide to the assessment of competence and performance in practising surgeons. *ANZ J Surg.* 2009;79:198–204.

22. Azuara-Blanco A, Reddy A, Wilkinson G, et al. Safe eye surgery: Non-technical aspects. *Eye.* 2011;25:1109–1111.

23. Kelly SP. Royal College of Ophthalmologists. Guidance on patient safety in ophthalmology from the Royal College of Ophthalmologists. *Eye.* 2009;23:2143–2151.

Index

Page numbers followed by "f" indicate figure and Page numbers followed by "t" indicate table.